W9-DHW-543

Reviewers

Sandra A. Almeida, M.D., M.P.H., is a board-certified preventive medicine physician with a specialty in exercise medicine and musculoskeletal injury management. She is the assistant coordinator of the Sports & Exercise Medicine Track of the UCSD-SDSU General Preventive Medicine Residency Program. She also works as an expert consultant to the U.S. military and private industry in the areas of exercise research, injury prevention and management, and exercise-program development.

Peter M. Aufsesser, Ph.D., is the director of the Fitness Clinic for Individuals with Disabilities at San Diego State University. In addition, he is the coordinator of the adapted physical education program and the pre-physical therapy advisor.

Brock Beamer, M.D., received his graduate medical and geriatric fellowship training at the Johns Hopkins University School of Medicine, separated by Internal Medicine residency and chief-residency at the UCLA-San Fernando Valley Program. Dr. Beamer currently is an assistant professor of medicine in the Division of Geriatric Medicine and Gerontology at Johns Hopkins University School of Medicine. He is supported in part by The Brookdale Foundation.

Christine "CC" Cunningham, M.S., is an NATABOC-certified athletic trainer with extensive experience as a personal trainer. Formerly the director of programming for First Fitness, Inc., she is now a private consultant specializing in fitness-program development and education. She is a frequent writer and lecturer and an American Council on Exercise Master Practical Trainer.

Scott D. Flinn, M.D., is the director of the Sports Medicine Clinic at Marine Corps Recruit Depot, Parris Island, S.C. He is a board-certified family practice physician, and completed his Primary Care Sports Medicine Fellowship at Sharp/San Diego Family and Sports Medicine affiliated with Stanford University.

Laura A. Gladwin, M.S., is president of LGA Fitness Consulting, Fairport, N.Y., which specializes in senior-fitness program development. She also is a special advisor to the California Governor's Council on Physical Fitness and Sports, serving on the Older Adult Committee. Ms. Gladwin chairs the Board of Certification and Training for AFAA and is a former faculty of the Department of Kinesiology and Health Promotions and Senior Fitness Certificate Program at California State University, Fullerton. She is an author and international presenter with more than 25 years experience.

Carol Mae Gordon, Ph.D., P.T., O.C.S., is a private practice physical therapist with 25 years of experience. She is certified as Orthopedic Clinical Specialist by the A.P.T.A. and earned her doctorate in neurophysiology from Northwestern University.

Angela S. Guarda, M.D., is assistant professor of medicine at Johns Hopkins University in Baltimore, Md., and director of the Eating and Weight Disorders Program at the Johns Hopkins School of Medicine. Dr. Guarda is a board-certified psychiatrist who specializes in the treatment of bulimia nervosa, anorexia nervosa and binge eating.

Mark Jackman, Ph.D., owns LIFE SIGNS[sm] HEALTH FITNESS in Durham, N.C., providing fitness, weight management and lifestyle coaching for individuals, many who possess health challenges. He earned his doctorate from Duke University where he conducted epidemiological research in occupational stress. Dr. Jackman is an ACE-certified Personal Trainer and Lifestyle & Weight Management Consultant, was involved in development of the CES Exam and has written articles for ACE.

Glen Morgan, Ph.D., is a clinical psychologist currently with the National Institutes of Health in Rockville, Md. He has more than 14 years of experience as a professor of family medicine and as a practicing clinician. His research has focused upon preventive behavioral medicine, with special emphasis in primary-care interventions

David C. Nieman, Dr.P.H., is a professor of health and exercise science, and director of the Human Performance Laboratory at Appalachian State University, Boone, N.C. He is the author of seven books on exercise, nutrition and health.

Thomas G. O'Connell, M.S., A.T.C./L., is the head athletic trainer at Glenbrook North High School in Northbrook, Ill. He has served on the High School Athletic Trainers' Association and the National Athletic Trainers' Association.

Naresh M. Punjabi, M.D., is a senior postdoctoral fellow in the Division of Pulmonary and Critical Care Medicine at Johns Hopkins

University. He completed his undergraduate training in biomedical engineering at Northwestern University and attended medical school at the University of Chicago, Pritzker School of Medicine. He is currently enrolled in the Graduate Training Program in Clinical Investigation at the Johns Hopkins University School of Hygiene and Public Health.

J. Mark Roberts, M.D., is associated with the Allan McGauin Sports Medicine Center at the University of British Columbia (UBC) in Vancouver, B.C. Dr. Roberts received his B.S. in zoology from the University of California, Davis, his medical degree and residency in internal medicine from the University of California, San Diego, and a fellowship in sports medicine at UBC. He is a diplomat of the American Board of Internal Medicine and the Canadian Academy of Sports Medicine.

Brad A. Roy, Ph.D., F.A.C.S.M., is the director of The Summit, Kalispell Regional Medical Center's 117,000-square-foot facility for health promotion and fitness in Kalispell, Mont. Dr. Roy has more than 20 years of experience working with clinical patients in the rehabilitation setting and has successfully consulted with numerous world-class athletes. He received a bachelor's degree in physical education from Point Loma Nazarene College, a master's degree in exercise physiology from San Diego State University and his doctorate in exercise physiology from Columbia Pacific University.

Christine Seidl is an adapted physical education teacher at the Summit School for Developmentally Disabled Children in Ville St. Laurent, Quebec. She also is a member of the Leadership Development Initiative for People with a Disability for the Canadian Society for Exercise Physiology.

Janet M. Shaw, Ph.D., is an assistant professor in the Department of Exercise and Sports Science at the University of Utah. She helped develop an instructional exercise video for the Oregon State University Extension Service for a statewide educational program titled "Women and Osteoporosis."

Bradford H. Stiles, M.D., is a primary care and sports medicine physician at the University of California, San Diego, Medical Center, and is a staff physician at Kaiser Permanente Medical Center, Department of Occupational Medicine.

Table of
Contents

Foreword

Millions of Americans suffer from chronic disease. And even more Americans have received some form of medical rehabilitation for an injury or illness. Most of these people have something in common — they can enhance their quality of life with a well-designed program of exercise and physical activity.

Until now, the fitness options available to these people have been largely limited to participation in fitness centers and community recreation programs. And the expertise of the staff at these clubs has varied considerably. If it is a progressive, quality club, you will usually find staff members who have passed some type of national certification program or may even hold a college degree in physical education. But most likely, you will not find individuals who have had specific education and experience in dealing with the special needs of people who are not entirely healthy.

The number of people who can benefit from more highly qualified fitness professionals working with them is staggering. At any given time, some 14 million Americans are living with heart disease, another 40 million are struggling to overcome the debilitating effects of arthritis, while obesity plagues approximately 58 million, possibly more depending on the standard of obesity used. And there are other conditions,

such as hypertension, osteoporosis, diabetes and back pain, that affect millions more.

To give these fitness consumers the confidence they need to engage in physical activity, they need someone with in-depth knowledge of their limitations and the appropriate types of activity that will most benefit them. They need a Clinical Exercise Specialist.

Not only should the ACE-certified Clinical Exercise Specialist provide the individual with more confidence, ACE hopes to provide the medical community with more confidence in making referrals to fitness professionals. We believe the ACE-certified Clinical Exercise Specialist can do just that.

This is an incredible opportunity to not only reap the rewards of helping people improve their health, perhaps even establish a level of wellbeing higher than what they had previously experienced, but to advance your own career as well. You will, after all, be tapping into a market that, as previously mentioned, has been largely ignored. The possibilities for growth and professional recognition are tremendous.

Sheryl Marks Brown
Executive Director

Introduction

The development of the *Clinical Exercise Specialist Manual* naturally followed the development of the job analysis for the Clinical Exercise Specialist certification examination. A job analysis process is the proper first step in creating a valid and reliable certification examination. Creating this analysis involved gathering more than 20 specialists from a variety of fields, each of which were related to the job of the ACE-certified Clinical Exercise Specialist. Their task was to identify the knowledge and skills required by an individual working as an ACE-certified Clinical Exercise Specialist. After the job analysis was completed, it was sent out for validation to 2,000 currently practicing professionals. This validated document, which also is referred to as the Exam Content Outline, appears in Appendix C.

In the development of the certification and this manual we were very careful to avoid scope-of-practice conflicts with other healthcare professionals. The ability to obtain exercise and activity guidelines from a client's physician or other appropriate healthcare professional is fundamental to the role of the ACE-certified Clinical Exercise Specialist. Furthermore, the ACE-certified Clinical Exercise Specialist must recognize their limitations and know how they fit into today's complex healthcare system. All authors followed these guidelines while writing their individual chapters.

The ACE-certified Clinical Exercise Specialist has demonstrated they have met the requirements to safely and effectively assist a client who has been cleared by their physician following treatment or rehabilitation to take part in independent physical activity. It is important that the reader understand we are not educating and certifying trainers to continue treatment or rehabilitation but, rather, to take over once an individual has received adequate care from the healthcare system. The ACE-certified Clinical Exercise Specialist forms an important bridge between rehabilitation and a health club or home-based exercise program.

We have recruited some of the most respected members of the exercise science and healthcare communities to contribute chapters to this book. The text is divided into eight sections. The first section, chapters one through four, provides a thorough introduction to the role of the ACE-certified Clinical Exercise Specialist. Chapter One covers the actual work of the ACE-certified Clinical Exercise Specialist, from the evolution of the job and its scope of practice, through the professional and legal issues pertinent to trainers working with clients with health challenges. Chapter Two, "Screening and Assessment for Exercise Programming," gives you an overview of this process with an emphasis on the additional responsibilities of ACE-certified Clinical Exercise Specialists. Chapter Three, "Working with Clients with Health Challenges," delves into the additional challenges both ACE-certified Clinical Exercise Specialists and clients face when working together following a chronic disease diagnosis and/or treatment. Chapter Four addresses how the ACE-certified Clinical Exercise Specialist can effectively communicate with healthcare professionals.

The remaining seven sections of the text feature chapters that cover the process of working with a client with a given disorder or health challenge. Each chapter begins with an overview of the basics of the disorder, which is followed by client assessment, exercise programming and case studies. Each of the chapters also include tables listing the recommended assessment questions a ACE-certified Clinical Exercise Specialist should ask a referring healthcare professional, and the activity guidelines typically given to a client who is released to take part in independent physical activity. If these tables are not present in a given chapter it is because their content was too lengthy to put in table form, so the information is available in the text of the chapter. Each chapter also includes a current reference list.

This text provides the foundation for assisting health-challenged clients to adopt more active lifestyles, but it is just that — a foundation. Experience as a personal trainer is paramount, but it also requires an ability to take information and make decisions as a result of that experience.

It is our hope that you will use this text as the cornerstone of your library, in preparation for the ACE Clinical Exercise Specialist certification exam and also as a comprehensive reference text for working with clients in the future. Finally, we are very excited about this manual and the potential role that the ACE-certified Clinical Exercise Specialist can play in helping more people enjoy active, healthier lifestyles.

Richard T. Cotton
American Council on Exercise

Ross E. Andersen
Johns Hopkins School of Medicine

Section One

Introduction

CHAPTER 1

The ACE-certified Clinical Exercise Specialist

DAVID E. UPTON

David E. Upton, Ph.D., has a doctorate in exercise physiology and doctoral and postdoctoral education in nutrition and psychology. His consulting firm, The David Upton Company, Inc., of Fort Worth, Texas, provides lectures, seminars and consulting services on the attainment of wellness to individuals and corporations. His firm also provides consulting to businesses in the design, development and operation of fitness facilities. Dr. Upton is a member of the ACE Board of Directors, chairman of the ACE Personal Trainer Certification committee, and has been actively involved in the development of the ACE Clinical Exercise Specialist Certification.

Overview

Scope
of Practice

Professionalism

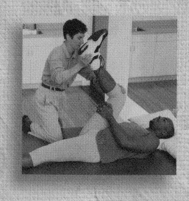

he ACE Clinical Exercise Specialist Certification was created to fill the need of individuals who are given clearance to exercise following treatment for a disease, injury or other health challenge, but lack the necessary skills and knowledge to carry out this directive on their own.

Though the tide is turning toward lifestyle modification as a means for improving quality of life in the presence or absence of disease, many physicians lack formal education and practical experience in such related areas as exercise physiology, motivation, goal setting, biomechanics, and exercise technique. As

such, patients are left on their own to fulfill this aspect of their discharge instructions — to begin or return to physical activity and exercise.

As an ACE-certified Clinical Exercise Specialist (CES), you can help fill this void by providing a comprehensive understanding of the academic and practical aspects of the clinical exercise sciences. The remainder of this chapter focuses on the prerequisites for certification (see Table 1.1), scope of practice, and the professional, legal and ethical implications of the CES.

Scope of Practice

In conjunction with other healthcare professionals, as an ACE-certified Clinical Exercise Specialist you will design, implement and manage exercise, physical activity and appropriate lifestyle programs for individuals following treatment or rehabilitation for clinically documented chronic disease, musculoskeletal injury and/or disability. The CES is NOT in the practice of providing the services of their profession to the immediate, primary, post-surgical or post-trauma rehabilitation patient. Rather, the CES provides a safe and effective bridge for the patient to cross from the structured clinical treatment and/or rehabilitation environment to mainstream community or home-based exercise.

Bridging the Gap

The role of the CES may be likened to a bridge that extends between the healthcare community and the patients it treats and releases. Though medically cleared to exercise, these individuals may lack the necessary knowledge and resources to continue progressing toward an optimal quality of life. The CES, however, does possess the requisite knowledge and resources, and can assist in carrying out the instructions of the healthcare professional while providing support and guidance to the individual.

The CES and the Healthcare Community

As an ACE-certified Clinical Exercise Specialist you will work closely with members of the healthcare community, including physicians (both allopathic and osteopathic), chiropractors, physical therapists, nutritionists, psychologists, nurse practitioners and physicians' assistants. It is imperative that you explicitly state your bounds of competence and areas of academic and experiential exper-

tise to any healthcare professional prior to accepting referrals. Furthermore, differentiation between a CES and other fitness practitioners, certified or uncertified, such as personal trainers or exercise technologists, must be clearly yet concisely represented. In the mind of many healthcare professionals, personal trainers are closely likened to those who appear on infomercials promoting some sort of quick-fix program or equipment. The American Council on Exercise works hard to change this image for both ACE-certified Personal Trainers and ACE-certified Clinical Exercise Specialists.

Both you and the associated healthcare professional must understand and accept the following operational premise:

The ACE-certified Clinical Exercise Specialist is NOT in the practice of providing the services of their profession to the immediate, primary, post-surgical or post-trauma rehabilitation patient. Rather, the ACE-certified Clinical Exercise Specialist provides a safe and effective bridge for this patient to cross from the structured rehabilitation environment to mainstream community or home-based exercise.

It is unfortunate, but all too common, for many patients to be released from the structured treatment or rehabilitation environment to find their own way. As a result, many patients do not follow through with the recommendation to participate in an exercise program and, consequently, their condition does not improve or, in some cases, worsens. As a CES you can alter this negative outcome for individuals following disease challenges or injuries by designing and implementing exercise and lifestyle programs that are based on their healthcare professionals' instructions.

Optimally, your expertise will be recognized by the healthcare professional and you will play an active role on the treatment team. This cooperative effort typically results in a more comprehensive program for the client. In other cases, you may serve only as a technician whose role is to implement the directives set forth by the healthcare professional.

Your position as a CES on this interaction continuum is directly related to your ability to demonstrate your competence and responsibility. Remember, the healthcare professional is being asked to place not only their confidence in you, but a portion of their professional liability and the safety of their patients as well. The burden of proof is your responsibility.

An excellent way to represent yourself to the healthcare community is to prepare a concise brochure that includes: college attended, major and minor areas of study, certifications, areas of expertise, your philosophy and a statement of purpose. In addition, you should provide information regarding your policy for handling cases or situations that fall outside your realm of expertise (referral structure), your length of time in practice, your method of follow-up with referring healthcare professionals and a few examples of the work you've done. Lastly, include brief statements as to how your services carry out the objectives of the healthcare professional and benefit their patients. You might also consider providing the healthcare professional with current articles from peer-reviewed journals regarding the effectiveness of exercise programs for specific diseases and/or disabilities.

Effective communication is essential to the development of a productive working relationship between you and healthcare professionals. Be respectful of their time and concentrate on making a positive impression from the outset whether that be via phone, written communication or in person.

The CES and the Consumer

As an ACE-certified Clinical Exercise Specialist, you may provide services to individuals whose healthcare profession-al has determined that the addition of an exercise program and/or a lifestyle modification plan will benefit the treatment of their disease or disability. Given a formal relationship between you and the referring healthcare professional, this individual will likely come to you with program directives and medical clearance protocols, which will be based upon the previously established working standard.

In other cases, the individual with a given disease or disability may come to you first without the referral from their healthcare professional. For example, a 46-year-old diabetic, post-bypass surgery, the friend of one of your clients, may come to you for help with the design and implementation of an exercise program. In this case, it is imperative that you open a line of communication with that client's healthcare provider. Upon initial contact, it is advisable to present the healthcare professional with your brochure, as well as an overview of the scope of the program you plan for this particular client. Medical clearances must be obtained and the healthcare professional must establish program guidelines and limitations. You should prepare a package of simple, concise forms through which this information may be obtained (sample forms are provided in Chapters 2 and 4 of this manual).

You may not move forward with this client until this information has been returned. Failure to obtain the appropriate physician clearance and physical activity guidelines creates a physical risk to the client and a significant liability risk to you and your company. This latter exam-

---

Table 1.1
Clinical Exercise Specialist Eligibility Requirements

1. Current CPR (through the date of the exam)	OR
2. 300 hours of work experience designing and implementing exercise programs for apparently healthy and/or high risk individuals, to be documented by a qualified professional (e.g., allied health professional, fitness director, club manager, professor, teacher, etc.)	3b. Current ACE, ACSM or NSCA certification ACE-certified Personal Trainer ACSM-Certified Exercise Technologist ACSM-Certified Exercise Specialist ACSM-Certified Health Fitness Director ACSM-Certified Program Director NSCA-Certified Strength & Conditioning Specialist Petition for Application
3a. Bachelor of Science/Bachelor of Arts in one of the following fields: Physical Education (courses in: Exercise Physiology, Programming and Leadership) Exercise science Kinesiology Exercise physiology Adapted physical education Athletic training Physical therapy	An applicant who does not meet requirement 3a or 3b above may petition to take the exam with one of the following qualifications: a. Bachelor of Science/Bachelor of Arts in other related fields (e.g., nursing, occupational therapy, etc.) b. Other nationally recognized fitness certifications

ple will likely represent the primary scenario for the acquisition of clients.

Close, cooperative, ongoing interaction between you and the healthcare professional should be standard operating procedure. This is best accomplished by the use of standardized progress reports sent to the healthcare professional at predetermined intervals. These reports, which should be kept simple and concise, should include requests for program modification guidelines as needed. It is best to establish an arrangement whereby the healthcare professional need respond only if modifications to their most recent recommendations and/or limitations are needed.

Unlike the ACE-certified Personal Trainer, who by definition is certified to work with "asymptomatic, apparently healthy individuals," ACE-certified Clinical Exercise Specialists are certified to work with "individuals following treatment and/or rehabilitation for clinically documented chronic disease, musculoskeletal injury and/or disabilities." As such, an overwhelming majority of your clients will require, at the very least, a medical clearance. Failure to accept and adhere to this definition will place you outside your scope of practice, which not only jeopardizes the safety of your client but compromises the integrity of the profession and puts you at a significant liability risk.

Traits of a Successful Clinical Exercise Specialist

Success, as it applies to the ACE-certified Clinical Exercise Specialist, is the ability to derive acceptable compensation, financial or otherwise, for consistently providing safe, effective and beneficial services to the client within the stated scope of practice. Knowing one's limitations is critical to success in any profession.

The depth of knowledge in the performance domains of the ACE-certified Clinical Exercise Specialist is far too vast to master in its entirely. Obviously, there are some basic and advanced concepts and skills that should be readily available for immediate recall. However, there is a far greater pool of ever-changing knowledge that is not committed to memory. One of the most important characteristics of the successful ACE-certified Clinical Exercise Specialist is the ability to

acquire additional knowledge and apply it to new situations. In addition to acquiring a substantial clinical and general knowledge base that is utilized on a daily basis, The ACE-certified Clinical Exercise Specialists have learned how to learn. They know how and where to acquire needed new knowledge to supplement their existing expertise in order to continue providing safe and effective programs for their clients. This may be accomplished through the development of a network of recognized experts and applicable primary and secondary resources, such as textbooks and journals.

Professionalism

Professionalism or professional conduct can be divided into two primary categories: ethical and legal. Ethics implies a moral standard or a code that inherently differentiates right from wrong. Professional associations often monitor the ethical conduct of their members. With regard to the CES, the American Council on Exercise has created a code of ethics that governs the professional conduct of its certified professionals (see Table 1.2).

Ethics

The ethical aspects of professionalism include knowing your limitations, that is, your bounds of competence. Based on this knowledge, you should develop your individual scope of practice that is safely located within the CES scope of practice. Therefore, based on your individual areas of competence, it is acceptable to exclude certain diseases, injuries and/or disabilities from your practice. It is not acceptable, however, for your practice as a CES to venture outside the boundaries of the overall scope of practice for this profession.

Legal

Legal conduct violations are, as the term suggests, violation of a given law. The laws in question could be in the areas of contract law, tort law or criminal law. Activities outside of the boundaries established by the scope of practice of the ACE-certified Clinical Exercise Specialist are a violation not only of the ethical standards of the profession, but of the legal standards of society as well. You have a responsibility to deliver services to the public in accordance with an acceptable "standard of care." Providing substandard services also may be a violation of legal standards.

In the event that legal standards are violated, the judicial system will impose a penalty commensurate with the nature and severity of the violation and resulting damages. The penalty imposed upon ACE-certified Clinical Exercise Specialists can range in severity from sanctions and/or limitations placed on their practice, to financial consequences and even incarceration. It is beyond the scope of this chapter to cover the specifics of all the legal aspects of this profession. For more information, refer to the suggested reading list at the end of this chapter.

Risk Management

There are risks associated with every profession and you would be well advised to do everything in your power to minimize these risks. Risk management begins with your choice of business structure: sole proprietorship, partnership or corporation. Each of these structures has inherent advantages and disadvantages, and the advice of both an attorney and an accountant can help you to determine which structure is best suited to your needs. Once you have established your business structure, you can begin to develop your operational systems.

The first level of operational systems relates to the mode by which you and/or your company conducts your business dealings. This includes, but is not limited to:

- written scope of practice
- statement of purpose or mission statement
- policies and procedures that govern interactions with clients and employees
- employee contracts
- employee manual
- independent contractor agreements
- fees for service provided
- billing and accounting practices
- facility and equipment inspection protocols
- contracts for services

The next level of operational systems involves your methods and techniques for collecting, recording and storing client data. Data collection forms include, but are not limited to:

- Waiver of Liability
- Informed Consent
- Health History
- Medical History
- Medical Clearance
- Coronary Risk Analysis
- Release of Information
- Progress Report
- Request for Update of Medical Clearance
- Lifestyle Information
- Fitness Testing and Screening
- Workout Records
- Daily Client Correspondence/Notes

Once you have completed and/or executed any data-collection form, it immediately becomes part of that client's confidential record, which should be maintained in individual client files located in a secure storage environment. Adherence to policies regarding client confidentiality is an ethical issue and, depending on the nature of the record and your geographical location, may be a legal obligation as well. Therefore, it is imperative that these records remain secure and available for review by, and/or discussion with, only those whom the client has designated as appropriate in an executed release-of-information document.

**Table 1.2
ACE Code of Ethics**

ACE-certified Professional Code Of Ethics

As an ACE-certified Professional, I am guided by the American Council on Exercise's principles of professional conduct whether I am working with clients, the public or other health and fitness professionals. I promise to:
- Provide safe and effective instruction.
- Provide equal and fair treatment to all clients.
- Stay up-to-date on the latest health and physical activity research and understand its practical application.
- Maintain current CPR certification and knowledge of first-aid services.
- Comply with all applicable business, employment and copyright laws.
- Protect and enhance the public's image of the health and fitness industry.
- Maintain the confidentiality of all client information.
- Refer clients to more qualified fitness, medical or health professionals when appropriate.

ACE-certified Clinical Exercise Specialists in private practice must secure and maintain sufficient and comprehensive professional and general liability insurance policies. These policies must be active prior to the delivery of any services, and may be obtained through professional associations. Shop several carriers and critically review the policy language, paying special attention to the exclusions section. Any questions about what is covered and excluded from the proposed policy, and how this corresponds to the services that you provide, must be addressed with the agent prior to activating the policy.

ACE-certified Clinical Exercise Specialists under the employ of a rehabilitation clinic, fitness center, physician or other entity may not need to obtain an individual general liability policy. However, it is advisable to explore the feasibility of obtaining an individual professional liability policy. Request written confirmation from your employer as to the nature and extent of your coverage under their policy and consult with an insurance professional and/or qualified attorney.

Lastly, you can decrease your risk exposure by staying current with the constantly updating knowledge base within the profession. This may be accomplished by reviewing research and professional publications within your scope of practice and by participating in continuing education programs and workshops. These workshops afford you the opportunity to expand your base of knowledge and to network with other ACE-certified Clinical Exercise Specialists. Incorporating this added knowledge into your daily practice will improve the quality of service you offer and ensure that you are adhering to the "standard of care" for your profession. In addition, participation in continuing education programs is a requirement for maintaining your certification.

Conclusion

Ideally, as an ACE-certified Clinical Exercise Specialist, you will function as a contributing member of a treatment team whose mission is to improve the quality of life for an individual returning to physical activity following treatment or rehabilitation for a disease, injury and/or disability. Your input regarding the need, design and implementation of the exercise and physical activity components of the client's treatment pro-

gram will be as valued by the team as that provided by the internist, orthopedist, physical therapist or diabetes educator. Furthermore, the value of your service will be recognized by insurance companies as a means of reducing expenditures and thereby qualify for reimbursement. Today's environment, however, has not reached this ideal.

The present healthcare system often falls short in the support provided to patients following their discharge, leaving them on their own to follow the ambiguous directive to begin an exercise program. As an ACE-certified Clinical Exercise Specialist, you can assist many of these patients by providing the needed bridge between medical clearance and independent exercise and improved well-being. It is up to you, however, to demonstrate your ability and willingness to fill this need by remaining within your scope of practice, knowing and respecting your limitations, educating both the healthcare community and the public and upholding high standards of professionalism. Adhering to these standards will go a long way toward creating that ideal environment in which the ACE-certified Clinical Exercise Specialist is considered a valued member of the treatment team.

Suggested Readings

American Council on Exercise. (1996). Cotton, R.T. (Ed.) *ACE Lifestyle & Weight Management Consultant Manual.* San Diego, Calif.: American Council on Exercise

American Council on Exercise. (1996). Cotton, R.T. (Ed.) *ACE Personal Trainer Manual* (2nd ed.). San Diego Calif.: American Council on Exercise

Koeberle, B. (1990). *Legal Aspects of Personal Fitness Training.* Canton, Ohio.: Professional Reports Corporation

Riegelman, R.K. & Hirsch, R.P. (1996). *Studying a Study and Testing a Test: How to Read the Health Science Literature.* Lippincott-Raven.

CHAPTER 2

Screening and Assessment for Exercise Programming

LARRY S. VERITY
KAREN M. WILLIAMS

Larry S. Verity, Ph.D., F.A.C.S.M., is a professor of exercise physiology in the Department of Exercise and Nutritional Sciences at San Diego State University. He is a Fellow of the American College of Sports Medicine and is certified as an Exercise Specialist. He has served as a writing consultant with the American Council on Exercise, and has published reviews and original manuscripts on diabetes and exercise in referred publications. He has had type 1 diabetes for 22 years and is without complications.

Karen M. Williams, M.S., holds a master's degree in exercise science from Brigham Young University. She is an independent fitness consultant specializing in sports medicine research and exercise program development. She has developed training programs for the military as well as the individual and has contributed to several research publications.

Health History
Informed Consent
Client Education

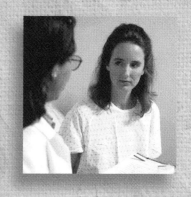

Physical activity plays an important role in improving the health of individuals who face health challenges such as type 2 diabetes, obesity, hypertension, cancer, AIDS, neurological disorders, low-back pain and selected psychological disorders (USDHHS, 1996). Similarly, individuals engage in physical activity as a part of rehabilitation for orthopedic problems, cardiovascular diseases, pulmonary disorders, neurological conditions and immune dysfunction.

You have the opportunity to establish a needed link between the health-challenged client who wants to participate in physical activity and their healthcare professional. The value you offer is the ability to provide safe and effective exercise programming for your client, and skill in motivating and supporting him as he strives to reach his goals. This chapter will provide you with the tools necessary for conducting proper screening and assessment, as well as designing effective programs, for clients with metabolic, cardiovascular, neurological and psychological disorders.

The first step for ensuring your clients perform safe and effective physical activity is to thoroughly screen and assess them. Screening is the initial process by which you separate individuals who may be appropriate for your services from those who clearly are not. Assessment is the process of determining the significance or importance of various factors that contribute to, or complicate, your client's exercise programming. A thorough screening and assessment process protects both you and your client by ensuring that the needs of a potential client can be met by the services you can legitimately and ethically provide. To do this, you must understand your client's health disorder and its impact on the ability to perform physical activity. Moreover, a comprehensive screening and assessment process helps instill client confidence in your abilities as a competent trainer who offers quality services.

The knowledge you use in screening and assessment will come, in part, from your training, experience and knowledge of the current scientific literature. It may also be necessary to consult established exercise guidelines from professional groups such as the American College of Obstetricians and Gynecologists (ACOG), the American College of Sports Medicine (ACSM) or the American Heart Association (AHA).

It is also crucial that you be effective in communicating with your client's healthcare providers. This communication is a two-way street where you obtain guidance from your client's healthcare provider and, in return, report to the provider on your client's progress. Chapter 3 provides guidelines for communicating effectively with healthcare professionals.

Tools for Screening, Evaluation and Assessment

Screening and assessment require that you collect both subjective and objective data from your client that will allow you to build an individualized training program. Proper tools and the information they generate will allow you to:

➤ Determine how the client's perceived problem relates to all levels of physical activity.

➤ Ask about old and new musculoskeletal injuries and use the information obtained to accurately develop a plan for testing and programming.

➤ Choose exercise tests that relate to functional outcomes and meet the special needs of the disorder or condition.

➤ Select exercise tests that can be modified to fit each client's needs.

➤ Identify and learn about any other conditions (e.g., hypertension may coexist with rheumatoid arthritis) that may influence exercise performance.

➤ Obtain a list of any medications the client is currently taking and know how each drug may affect exercise performance results, particularly the cardiovascular response to physical exertion.

The identification of goals is an important part of the health screening process. Interviews and surveys are useful tools in determining the goals of your client. You must also determine the goals of your client's healthcare team. Obtain this information by adding a "goals" section to the physician release form. These tools will offer you invaluable information about the needs of your client and will assist the client in setting realistic goals.

The Health History

The pre-activity health history not only allows you to gain valuable insight into your client's condition and history, but also provides you with the opportunity to educate your client on the benefits of physical activity and therefore motivate them to participate.

The screening assists you in identifying clients with:

• medical contraindications to exercise
• risk factors for coronary heart disease (CHD) that require medical clearance prior to participation in physical activity
• clinically significant disease that requires a medically supervised activity program (e.g., CHD, pulmonary disease, orthopedic concerns, neurological issues, metabolic disease, immune disorders)

- multiple, coexisting health conditions that require increased and/or special attention

In addition, administering a health screening allows you to:

- become more familiar with the client's health condition and abilities
- gain your client's confidence in you as a thorough, concerned fitness professional
- reduce the likelihood of legal problems by acknowledging the client's health condition and adhering to recommended activity guidelines specific to the health challenge
- increase communication between you, the client and their healthcare professionals

Because CHD may either be present as a single condition or may coexist with other health disorders (e.g., physical, neuromuscular and psychological conditions), it is essential that you screen all clients for cardiovascular risk factors before initiating an exercise program (ACSM, 1997; CSEP, 1998). Research has shown that physical activity precipitates an increased risk for cardiovascular incidents, especially in clients with medically significant risk factors. It also is recommended that you screen your clients for risk factors related to their specific disorder, as each health condition produces unique responses.

Currently, both the American Heart Association and American College of Sports Medicine have identified several positive CHD risk factors that directly contribute to the progression and/or presence of the disease. A single negative CHD risk factor also has been identified and actually lessens the progression and/ or aids in the regression of the disease. Table 2.1 presents a list of those CHD risk factors that you should screen for in all prospective clients.

Use these objective CHD risk factors (ACSM, 1995; Howley & Franks, 1997) to determine the cardiovascular health status (i.e., apparently healthy, increased risk, known disease) of clients with specific disorders. Once you determine your client's cardiovascular health status, follow the recommended guidelines (ACSM, 1995) regarding the necessity of an exercise stress test, and referral for physician-supervised submaximal or maximal exercise testing (see Table 2.2).

The PAR-Q, PARmed-X and HHQ

A number of screening tools may be used to gather information about your client. Though the PAR-Q (Figure 2.1) is a particularly useful questionnaire that is easy to administer, it may be inadequate as a sole means of assessing relative cardiovascular health and other physical, neuromuscular and psychological conditions. Use of additional questionnaires, such as the PARmed-X (Figure 2.2) or a comprehensive health history questionnaire (HHQ) (Figure 2.3), may assist in gathering information.

The PARmed-X identifies any existing contraindications to exercise (CSEP, 1998). Administer this questionnaire by having the client complete the PAR-Q, as well as sections A through D on the PARmed-X questionnaire. The client then should take the form to their physician to gain medical approval. The PARmed-X also allows the physician to offer specific recommendations for programming and progression.

Psychological Factors

Although the health screening process typically covers a client's physiological condition, you should also address the psychological health of

---

Table 2.1
Coronary Heart Disease Risk Factors

Positive Risk Factors	
• **Age** (men > 45 yrs; women > 55 yrs) When age exceeds these ranges, the client should undergo a stress test	• **Diabetes mellitus** (IF type 2, > 40 yrs of age; IF type 1, 15 yrs duration and/or > 30 yrs of age))
• **Family history** (premature disease or heart attack in an immediate relative: male < 55 yrs; female < 65 yrs.)	• **Current smoker**
• **Hypertension** (SBP >140 mmHg and/or DBP>90 mmHg)	• **Obesity**+ (BMI > 30, or Body weight > 120 percent of ideal body weight) +Note: Obesity is currently being considered as an independent major risk factor by AHA & ACSM
• **High cholesterol** (Chol > 200 mg/dl; HDL < 35 mg/dl)	**Negative Risk Factor**
• **Physical inactivity**	• HDL > 60 mg/dl.

From: *ACSM's Guidelines for Exercise Testing and Prescription,* 5th ed., (1995), pp. 18

your client. While most trainers are not qualified to evaluate a client's psychological status, you can use your professional experience, observations and intuition to determine your client's stage of readiness for adopting and maintaining an active lifestyle. These same skills can help you identify the most appropriate strategy for handling a specific client. If the client is currently under a mental health professional's or physician's care for a psychological disorder, it may be advisable to contact the professional for any guidance they may wish to provide.

Know a Client's Medications

In the health history, obtain a list of all medications that the client is taking, and understand their effects on all of the major organ systems of the body (ACSM, 1997). Determine if prescribed medications adversely affect the body's response to physical exertion. Clients who take heart-rate-altering medications (HRAM) are not candidates for a submaximal assessment to determine aerobic capacity; however, you may need to assess the amount of work that a client can perform at a specific heart rate without estimating aerobic capacity. This will determine the client's ability to perform work at a predetermined heart rate identified by their physician. Lists of questions you may want to ask physicians regarding medications for specific conditions are provided in each chapter of this manual.

Once your client has obtained physician approval to exercise, and you feel you have a solid understanding of the effects of your client's health condition and the medications they are taking on their physical activity performance, you must prepare for emergency sit-

uations. Research potential emergencies associated with your client's condition/s and be prepared to handle any adverse events associated with increasing physical effort. Each chapter will identify risks associated with a specific disorder and recommend emergency procedures.

Informed Consent and Liability Waivers

It is recommended that you review an informed consent form with your client and have them sign it. Though a signed informed consent form does not prevent litigation, it does improve the client's understanding of the nature of assessment tests by ensuring they are given both verbal and written instructions. Most informed consent forms include the following information in an effort to prepare the client for the exercise evaluation:

- objectives of the intended test battery or assessments
- explanation of all tests to be administered
- description of all risks related to each assessment
- instruction that the client is free to withdraw from the tests at any time
- explanation that the client may abstain from completing a questionnaire
- indication that all client information is confidential
- encouragement to ask questions about any of the tests at any time

The laws pertaining to consents and waivers vary from state to state and country to country, so it is inappropriate and in fact exposes you to legal risk if you copy samples printed in various

Table 2.2
Recommended Clinical Exercise Test and Physician Supervision Prior to Participating in Physical Activity

	Medical Exam and Clinical Stress Test Recommendations for:				
	Apparently Healthy		Increased Risk		Known Disease
	Younger	Older	No Symptoms	Symptoms	
Moderate activity	No	No	No	Yes	Yes
Vigorous exercise	No	Yes	Yes	Yes	Yes
	Physician Supervision Recommended During Exercise Testing:				
	Apparently Healthy		Increased Risk		Known Disease
	Younger	Older	No Symptoms	Symptoms	
Submaximal testing	No	No	No	Yes	Yes
Maximal testing	No	Yes	Yes	Yes	Yes

From: *ACSM's Guidelines for Exercise Testing and Prescription*, 5th ed., (1995) pp. 25

texts. A more in-depth discussion of these forms (and examples) can be found in the *ACE Personal Trainer Manual* and the *ACE Lifestyle and Weight Management Consultant Manual* and in publications by the Professional Reports Corporation. You should develop your consent and waiver forms with the assistance of an attorney with a specialty in such a process and licensed to practice in your state.

In rare instances, you may work with a client who does not want to obtain physician approval for participation in physical activity. It is important that you have the client sign a legally prepared document that releases you, and the facility in which you work, from any liability related to injury that results from exercise testing and/or programming. From both a medical and legal perspective, it is probably best to obtain physician clearance for all clients with an identified health condition even if a clearance is not explicitly recommended in any of the established guidelines.

You must protect yourself and your client from any untoward outcomes of physical activity. Limit the likelihood of litigation by using informed consent and liability waiver forms when working with clients with health challenges, particularly those with cardiovascular, neuromuscular, metabolic and hematological disorders.

Choosing Assessment Tests

Take care when selecting tests for client evaluation. Assessments must be known to be accurate, reliable and easy to administer (consider equipment cost, difficulty of assessment and adaptability to special needs). In general, test types include resting cardiovascular function, anthropometry, submaximal aerobic fitness capacity, muscular fitness measures, joint range of motion (flexibility) measures for both upper- and lower-body extremities, and neuromuscular assessments (Table 2.3).

The client's health condition dictates the type of fitness tests needed and the order in which these tests are administered. For example, a cardiac client may undergo an entirely different battery of tests than those administered to a client with a neurological disorder. Some disorders require that clients improve their functional fitness. Therefore, when work-

ing with clients with disorders ranging from cardiovascular, metabolic and pulmonary disease, to orthopedic, immune and neurological disorders, you may need to administer assessments that focus on functional performance (CSEP, 1998; USDHHS, 1996) to measure improvements related to performing activities of daily living.

Once the battery of assessment tests is complete, interpret the results for your client in an accurate and positive manner. Any comparisons that you offer should be made to relative age- and gender-matched persons, particularly for cardiorespiratory and musculoskeletal fitness, and anthropometric assessments.

Client Education

You should include fitness counseling as a routine part of client education. The majority of fitness counseling overviews results from the screening and assessments, and identifies realistic goals for the client to achieve. Additionally, you can use fitness counseling as an educational opportunity to address health and behavioral issues, as well as reiterate the benefits of physical activity specific to a client's illness. Along these lines, you need to be an effective educator who knows the barriers to client education include lack of priority setting, lack of time and insufficient knowledge or skill (Hansen & Streff, 1995). To address these barriers and move your client toward a successful physical activity program, you must understand the adult learner. A successful fitness counseling session moulds at least these four phases of adult learning:

➤ Adult learners need an active and controlling role in deciding what will be learned.
➤ Learning improves when the material is relevant to a learner's experience.
➤ Like children, adults usually have phases of growth with corresponding developmental tasks.
➤ Adults are most motivated to learn what is immediately applicable in their life setting (Padberg & Padberg, 1990).

As the fitness counselor, you must individualize the counseling session to your client and offer an opportunity to establish realistic personal goals. Many people with health challenges who are motivated enough to start a physical activity program have some goal(s) in mind. Thus, an effective fitness counselor listens carefully to their client's needs and reasons for beginning an activity program. Unfortunately, the client who starts out motivated does not always remain motivated. Trainers play a pivotal role in assisting the client with an illness or disorder to understand their current health and fitness status, develop a structured plan of achievable goals at the outset of the program, and help the client to sustain a motivation level whenever it begins to fade. Knowing about the client's past is crucial to understanding the client's present needs and prospective goals. Therefore, you may want to ask such questions as:

Table 2.3
Assessment of Clients with a Health Challenge

PARAMETER	ASSESSMENT	SPECIAL CONSIDERATIONS
RESTING CARDIOVASCULAR FUNCTION		
• Heart rate	30-60 secs measure	Abnormal: HR > 100 bpm
• Systolic/diastolic blood pressure	two measures 3-5 min apart	Abnormal: SBP > 140 mmHg
		and/or DBP > 90 mmHg
ANTHROPOMETRY		
• Height and weight	record: in/lbs or cm/kg	
• Body Mass Index (BMI)	determined via: weight (kg) ∏ height (m2)	When BMI > 29, initiate weight mgmt. strategies: indicates obesity
• Circumference measures	waist, hip, upper arm, upper thigh	Good measures to confirm loss of inches
	Waist-to-hip ratio (WHR)	Abnormal: men > 0.9; women > 0.8
• Skinfold measures	Recommended: waist, iliac, thigh, subscapular, chest, mid-calf, midaxillary	Requires accurate anatomic location of skinfold sites to determine body fat
SUBMAXIMAL AEROBIC FITNESS ASSESSMENT		
• Aerobic capacity	In lab setting, use various ergometers: upright bicycle, recumbent bicycle, treadmill, and arm. In field, use walking test.	Use of standard protocol may require modification for some health challenges
	DATA: HR and RPE	Both are good indicators of effort
• Endurance performance	Functional assessment must focus on mode of activity usually performed DATA: TIME to complete known distance	Good means to assess progress for clients who are limited (e.g., cardiac, pulmonary, arthritic, disabled, etc.)
MUSCULAR FITNESS MEASURES		
• Muscle strength	1-RM of any muscle group	Not appropriate for all persons: Handgrip dynamometer Caution in using these tests Prior strength training and cuing important for performing correctly
•Muscle endurance	Number of repetitions before fatigue using: curl-ups, pull-ups, YMCA bench press, or any muscle group	Tests are available with norms; but not all persons can perform such tests. Address specific ability of client to perform repeated movements of any muscle group. Use RPE as a guide to fatigue.
• Joint range of motion (Flexibility)	Upper extremities with goniometer or standardized instrument and lower extremities with goniometer or standardized instrument	Shoulder flexion/extension/ab- and adduction/ internal/external rotation. Focus on functional ADL outcomes Sit-n-Reach (low back); hip flexor/ extensor; hip ad- and abduction; hamstrings & quadriceps; gastoc-soleus complex; ankle flexibility Focus on functional ADL outcomes — related to balance, coordination imbalance
NEUROMUSCULAR ASSESSMENTS		
	Eye-hand coordination, Reaction time Gait analysis	Usually performed in lab setting on persons with neuromuscular deficits

- *What do you want from the program?*
- *What has prevented you from doing this before?*
- *What is your plan of action?*

By engaging in this conversation, you will identify areas of unrealistic expectations, improve your client's sense of self-direction, and gain important information about the focus of education, knowledge and/or skills for your client. Most importantly, fitness counseling can help to establish, focus on, and achieve realistic goals for clients with specific illnesses or challenges.

Pre-exercise Session Assessment

To ensure safe conduct of each exercise session, it is imperative that you administer a brief pre-exercise session assessment. Take appropriate vital signs and obtain information on symptoms. Additionally, ask your client if there have been any changes in their symptoms or medications since their last exercise session. Review your client's exercise program and be aware of any signs indicating that your client may be having problems with the exercise program. After you have obtained the necessary information, modify the exercise session to meet your client's present status (ACSM, 1993).

Physical Activity Programming

Exercise programming for clients with health conditions is similar to that for apparently healthy individuals, and program design should be based on client needs and goals. A thorough understanding of the risks and benefits of exercise associated with your client's condition will guide you in developing a safe and effective program. Each session should include a warm-up, activity and cool-down phase. It is imperative that aerobic activity is preceded by a warm-up and followed by a recovery period. In general, most clients with health conditions will require an extended warm-up and cool-down period. Exercise progression should be gradual with an emphasis on increasing duration rather than intensity.

Each client's program should be based on their needs and condition. In general, however, the framework for the program should be based on the FITT acronym. F= frequency (e.g., 3 to 5 times per week); I= intensity (e.g., 60 percent to 90 percent of heart-rate maximum); T= time of activity (e.g., 20 to 60 minutes of continuous or intermittent activity); T= type or mode of activity (e.g., use of large muscle groups via walking, running, cycling, swimming, aerobic/step training, etc.). Modifications to the FITT principle may be necessary for clients with health challenges. It is important to note that many clients with health challenges are sedentary. Therefore, be conservative in the initial stages of exercise programming and make gradual increases in frequency, intensity and time as appropriate. Once you have developed the exercise program, make sure that all of your recommendations are in accordance with established guidelines and recommendations.

The U.S. Surgeon General's Report on Physical Activity and Health recommends that all Americans participate in 30 minutes of moderate physical activity at least five, preferably seven, days per week to obtain the health benefits of physical activity (USDHHS, 1996). Address these benefits with your client to encourage compliance.

Pay close attention to your client's exercise response. The objective data (heart rate, blood pressure, distance completed, time spent exercising) are important; however, the subjective data (RPE, leg pain, work intensity tolerance, shortness of breath, etc.) may be more helpful in appropriately modifying the physical activity to meet your client's needs.

At the present time, specific exercise guidelines for clients with health challenges are lacking. A "10-Step Decision-Making Approach" (Appendix A) can provide you with a model for reasoning through the critical steps of exercise programming for clients with health challenges. Remember that it is your responsibility to stay current in the field of exercise science by conducting a regular review of professional scientific literature and applying the knowledge gained to your exercise programming methods.

References

American College of Sports Medicine. (1993). *ACSM's Resource Manual for Guidelines for Exercise Testing and Prescription.* (3rd ed.) Baltimore: Williams & Wilkins.

Screening and Assessment for Exercise Programming

American College of Sports Medicine. (1995). *ACSM's Guidelines to Exercise Testing and Prescription.* (5th ed.) Baltimore: Williams & Wilkins.

American College of Sports Medicine. (1997). *ACSM's Exercise Management for Persons with Chronic Diseases and Disabilities.* Champaign, Ill.: Human Kinetics.

American College of Sports Medicine. (1998). The recommended quantity and quality of exercise for developing and maintaining cardiorespiratory and musculoskeletal fitness, and flexibility in healthy adults. *Medicine and Science in Sports and Exercise,* 30, 6, 975-991.

Canadian Society for Exercise Physiology (CSEP). (1998). Recommendations for the fitness assessment, programming and counseling of persons with a disability. *Canadian Journal of Applied Physiology,* 23, 2, 119-130.

Hansen, M. & Streff, M.M. (1995). Patient education: Practical guidelines (pp.277-285). In: *Heart Disease and Rehabilitation,* 3rd ed. (M.L. Pollock & D.H. Schmidt, eds.)

Howley, E. & Franks, D.B. (1997). *Health Fitness Instructor's Handbook.* (3rd ed.) Champaign, Ill.: Human Kinetics.

Koeberle, B. (1998). *Legal Aspects of Personal Training.* (2nd ed.) Canton, Ohio: Professional Reports Corporation.

Nieman, D. (1995). *Fitness and Sports Medicine.* (3rd ed.) Palo Alto, Calif.: Bull Publishing.

Padberg, R.M. & Padberg, L.F. (1990). Strengthening the effectiveness of patient education: Applying principles of adult education. *Oncology Nursing Forum,* 17:65-69.

Shephard, R.J. (1990). Fitness in Special Populations. Champaign, Ill.: *Human Kinetics.*

Skinner, J., (Ed.) (1993). *Exercise in Special Populations: Theoretical Basis and Clinical Applications.* (2nd ed.) Philadelphia: Lea & Febiger.

U.S. Department of Health and Human Services (USDHHS). (1996). *Physical activity and health: A report of the Surgeon General.* Atlanta, Ga.: US Department of Health and Human Services, Centers for Disease Control and Prevention.

Weinberg, R.S. & Gould, D. (1995). *Foundations of Sports and Exercise Psychology.* Champaign, Ill.: Human Kinetics.

PAR-Q & YOU (A Questionnaire for People Aged 15 to 69)

Regular physical activity is fun and healthy, and increasingly more people are starting to become more active every day. Being more active is very safe for most people. However, some people should check with their doctor before they start becoming much more physically active. If you are planning to become much more physically active than you are now, start by answering the seven questions in the box below. If you are between the ages of 15 and 69, the PAR-Q will tell you if you should check with your doctor before you start. If you are over 69 years of age, and you are not used to being very active, check with your doctor. Common sense is your best guide when you answer these questions. Please read the questions carefully and answer each one honestly: check YES or NO.

Figure 2.1

The Physical Activity Readiness Questionnaire — PAR-Q (revised 1994)

YES	NO		YES	NO	
☐	☐	1. Has your doctor ever said that you have a heart condition and that you should only do physical activity recommended by a doctor?	☐	☐	5. Do you have a bone or joint problem that could be made worse by a change in your physical activity?
☐	☐	2. Do you feel pain in your chest when you do physical activity?	☐	☐	6. Is your doctor currently prescribing drugs (for example, water pills) for your blood pressure or heart condition?
☐	☐	3. In the past month, have you had chest pain when you were not doing physical activity?	☐	☐	7. Do you know of any other reason why you should not do physical activity?
☐	☐	4. Do you lose your balance because of dizziness or do you ever lose consciousness?			

If you answered Yes to one or more questions:

✔ Talk with your doctor by phone or in person BEFORE you start becoming much more physically active or BEFORE you have a fitness appraisal. Tell your doctor about the PAR-Q and which questions you answered with YES.

✔ You may be able to do any activity you want — as long as you start slowly and build up gradually. Or you may need to restrict your activities to those that are safe for you. Talk with your doctor about the kinds of activities you wish to participate in and follow his/her advice.

✔ Find out which community programs are safe and helpful for you.

If you answered NO honestly to all PAR-Q questions, you can be reasonably sure that you can:

✔ Start becoming much more physically active — begin slowly and build up gradually. This is the safest and easiest way to go.

✔ Take part in a fitness appraisal — this is an excellent way to determine your basic fitness so that you can plan the best way for you to live actively.

DELAY BECOMING MUCH MORE ACTIVE:

✔ If you are not feeling well because of a temporary illness such as a cold or a fever — wait until you feel better; or

✔ If you are or may be pregnant — talk to your doctor before you start becoming more active.

Please note: If your health changes so that you then answer YES to any of the above questions, tell your fitness or health professional. Ask whether you should change your physical activity plan.

Informed Use of the PAR-Q: The Canadian Society for Exercise Physiology, Health Canada, and their agents assume no liability for persons who undertake physical activity, and if in doubt after completing this questionnaire, consult your doctor prior to physical activity.

You are encouraged to copy the PAR-Q but only if you use the entire form.

Note: If the Par-Q is being given to a person before he or she participates in a physical activity program or a fitness appraisal, this section may be used for legal or administrative purposes.

I have read, understood and completed this questionnaire. Any questions I had were answered to my full satisfaction.

_____
Name

_____
Signature   Date

_____
Signature of Parent, Witness or Guardian (for participants under the age of majority)

© Canadian Society for Exercise Physiology. Supported by: Health Santé, Societe canadienne de physiologie de l'exercice, Canada, Canada

Figure 2.2

PARmed-X

Physical Activity Readiness Medical Exam Form (PARmed-X)

The PARmed-X is a physical activity-specific checklist to be used by a physician with patients who have had a positive response to the Physical Activity Readiness Questionnaire (PAR-Q). In addition, the Conveyance/Referral Form in the PARmed-X can be used to convey clearance for physical activity participation, or to make a referral to a medically supervised exercise program.

Regular physical activity is fun and healthy, and increasingly more people are starting to become more active every day. Being more active is very safe for most people. The PAR-Q by itself provides adequate screening for the majority of people. However, some individuals may require a medical evaluation and specific advice (exercise prescription) due to one or more positive responses to the PAR-Q.

Following the participant's evaluation by a physician, a physical activity plan should be devised in consultation with a physical activity professional (CSEP-Certified Fitness Appraiser). To assist in this, the following instructions are provided:

Page 1: Sections A, B, C and D should be completed by the participant BEFORE the examination by the physician. The bottom section is to be completed by the examining physician.

Pages 2 & 3: A checklist of medical conditions requiring special consideration and management.

This section to be completed by participant

A Personal Information:

Name _____

Address _____

Telephone _____

Birthdate _____ Gender _____

Medical No. _____

B PAR-Q: *Please indicate the PAR-Q questions to which you answered YES*

☐ Q1. Heart condition   ☐ Q4. Loss of balance, dizziness   ☐ Q7. Other reason: _____
☐ Q2. Chest pain during activity ☐ Q5. Bone or joint problem   _____
☐ Q3. Chest pain at rest   ☐ Q6. Blood pressure or heart drugs   _____

C Risk Factors For Cardiovascular Disease: *Check all that apply*

☐ Less than 30 minutes of moderate physical activity   ☐ Family history of heart disease
   most days of the week   ☐ High blood pressure reported by physician after
☐ Excessive accumulation of fat around waist   repeated measurements
☐ Currently smoker (tobacco smoking one or more   ☐ High cholesterol level reported by physician
   times per week

Please note: Many of these risk factors are modifiable. Please discuss with your physician.

D Physical Activity Intentions: What physical activity do you intend to do?
_____
_____

This section to be completed by the examining physician

Physical Exam:

| Ht _____ | Wt _____ | BP i)   / |
| | | BP ii)   / |

Conditions limiting physical activity:
☐ Cardiovascular   ☐ Musculoskeletal   ☐ Respiratory   ☐ Abdominal   ☐ Other _____

Tests required:
☐ ECG   ☐ Exercise test   ☐ X-Ray   ☐ Blood   ☐ Urinalysis   ☐ Other _____

Physical Activity Readiness Conveyance /Referral:
Based upon current review of health status, I recommend:
☐ No physical activity   ☐ Only a medically supervised exercise program until further medical clearance

☐ Progressive physical activity
   ☐ with avoidance of: _____   ☐ with inclusion of:_____

   ☐ with physical therapy: _____   ☐ Unrestricted physical activity — start slowly and build up gradually.
Further Information:
        ☐ Attached   ☐ To be forwarded   ☐ Available upon request

*refer to special publications for elaboration as required. Reprinted from the Canadian Society for Exercise Physiology, Inc. 1995.

	Special Prescriptive Conditions	ADVICE
Lung	☐ chronic pulmonary disorders	special relaxation and breathing exercises
	☐ obstructive lung disease	breath control during endurance exercise to tolerance; avoid polluted air
	☐ asthma	avoid hyperventilation during exercise; avoid extremely cold conditions
	☐ exercise-induced bronchospasm	warm up adequately; utilize appropriate medication
Musculoskeletal	☐ low back conditions (pathological, functional)	avoid or minimize exercise that precipitates or exacerbates (e.g., forced extreme flexion, extension and violent twisting); correct posture, proper back exercises
	☐ arthritis — acute (infective, rheumatoid; gout)	treatment, plus judicious blend of rest, splinting, and gentle movement
	☐ arthritis — subacute	progressive increase of active exercise therapy
	☐ arthritis — chronic (osteoarthritis and above conditions)	maintenance of mobility and strength: non-weightbearing exercises to minimize joint trauma (e.g., cycling, aquatic activity, etc.)
	☐ orthopedic	highly variable and individualized
	☐ hernia	minimize straining and isometrics; strengthen abdominal muscles
CNS	☐ convulsive disorder not completely controlled by medication	minimize or avoid exercise in hazardous environ-ments and/or exercising alone (e.g. swimming, mountain climbing, etc.)
	☐ recent concussion	thorough examination if history of two concussions; review for discontinuation of contact sport if three concussions, depending on duration of unconsciousness, retrograde amnesia, persistent headaches, and other objective evidence of cerebral damage
Blood	☐ anemia (<10 gm/dl) ☐ electrolyte disturbances	control preferred; exercise as tolerated
Medications	☐ antianginal ☐ antiarrhythmic ☐ antihypertensive ☐ anticonvulsant ☐ beta-blockers ☐ digitalis preparations ☐ diuretics ☐ ganglionic blockers ☐ others	NOTE: consider underlying condition. Potential for: exertional syncope, electrolyte imbalance, bradycardia, dysrhythmias, impaired coordinations and reaction time, heat intolerance. May alter resting and exercise ECGs and exercise test performance
Other	☐ post-exercise cyncope	moderate program
	☐ heat intolerance	prolong cool-down with light activities; avoid exercise in extreme heat
	☐ temporary minor illness	postpone until recovered
	☐ cancer	if potential metastases, test by cycle ergometry, consider non-weight bearing exercises; exercise at lower end of perspective range (40-56% of heart rate reserve), depending on condition and recent treatment (radiation, chemotherapy; monitor hemoglobin and lymphocyte counts; add dynamic lifting exercises to strengthen muscles, using machines rather than weights

Figure 2.2

PARmed-X
(continued)

Following is a checklist of medical conditions for which a degree of precaution and/or special advice should be considered for those who answered "YES" to one or more questions on the PAR-Q and people over the age of 69. Conditions are grouped by system. Three categories of precautions are provided. Comments under Advice are general, since details and alternatives require clinical judgement in each individual instance.

	Absolute Contraindications	Relative Contraindications	Special Prescriptive Contraindications	ADVICE
	Permanent restriction or temporary restriction until condition is treated, stable, and/or past acute phase.	Highly variable. Value of exercise testing and/or program may exceed risk. Activity may be restricted. Desirable to maximize control of condition. Direct or indirect medical supervision or exercise program may be desirable.	Individualized prescriptive advice generally appropriate. • limitations imposed; and/or • special exercises prescribed May require medical monitoring and/or initial supervision in exercise program	

Cardiovascular	☐ aortic aneurysm (dissecting)
	☐ aortic stenosis (severe)
	☐ congestive heart failure
	☐ crescendo angina
	☐ myocardial infarction (acute)
	☐ myocarditis (active or recent)
	☐ pulmonary or systemic embolism — acute
	☐ thrombophlebitis
	☐ ventricular tachycardia and other dangerous dysrhythmias (e.g., multi-focal ventricular activity)
		☐ aortic stenosis (moderate)
		☐ subaortic stenosis (severe)
		☐ marked cardiac enlargement
		☐ supraventricular dysrhythmias (uncontrolled or high rate)
		☐ ventricular ectopic activity (repetitive or frequent)
		☐ ventricular aneurysm
		☐ hypertension — untreated or uncontrolled severe (systemic or pulmonary)
		☐ hypertrophic cardiomyopathy
		☐ compensated congestive heart failure
			☐ aortic (or pulmonary) stenosis — mild angina pectoris and other manifestations of coronary insufficiency (e.g., post acute infarct)
			☐ cyanotic heart disease
			☐ shunts (intermittent or fixed)
			☐ conduction disturbances
			  • complete AV block
			  • left BBB
			☐ Wolff-Parkinson-White syndrome
			☐ dysrhythmias — controlled
				• clinical exercise test may be warranted in selected cases, for specific determination of functional capacity and limitations and precautions (if any)
				• slow progression of exercise to levels based on test performance and individual tolerance
				• consider individual need for initial conditioning program under medical supervision (indirect or direct)

			☐ intermittent claudication	progressive exercise to tolerance
			☐ hypertension: systolic 160-180, diastolic 105+	progressive exercise; care with medications (serum electrolytes; postexercise syncope, etc.)
Infections	☐ acute infectious disease (regardless of etiology)	☐ subacute/chronic/recurrent infectious diseases (e.g., malaria, others).	☐ chronic infections	variable as to condition
Metabolic		☐ uncontrolled metabolic disorders (diabetes mellitus, hyrotoxicosis, myxedema)	☐ renal, hepatic & other metabolic insufficiency	variable as to status
			☐ obesity ☐ single kidney	dietary moderation and initial light exercises with slow progression (walking, swimming, cycling)
Pregnancy		☐ complicated pregnancy (e.g., toxemia, hemorrhage, incompetent cervix, etc.)	☐ advanced pregnancy (late 3rd trimester)	refer to the "PARmed-X for PREGNANCY"

References: Arraix, G.A., Wigle, O.T., Mao. Y. (1992). Risk Assessment of Physical Activity and Physical Fitness in the Canada Health Survey Follow-Up Study. *I Clin. Epidemiol.* 45, 4 419-428. Mottola, M., Wolfe, LA. (1994). Active Living and Pregnancy, In: A. Quinney. L Gauvin, T. Wall (eds). *Toward Active Living: Proceedings of the International Conference on Physical Activity, Fitness and Health.* Champaign, Ill. Human Kinetics. *PAR-Q Validation Report,* British Columbia Ministry of Health, 1978. Thomas C. Reading, J., Shepard, R.J. (1992). Revision of the Physical Activity Readiness Questionnaire (PAR-Q). *Can. J. Spt. Sci.* 17, 4 338-345.

Physical Activity Readiness Medical Exam Form

Figure 2.3

Health History Questionnaire

Name:____

Home Address:____

Telephone (h): (______) __________________________(w): (______) ______________________

Occupation: ____

Gender: M ________ F ________ Age (yrs): ________ Weight (lbs.): ________ Height (in.):__________

Resting Heart Rate (average of > 2 measures): ________bpm

Resting Blood Pressure (average of > 2 measures): ________/ ________mmHg

Yes	No		
☐	☐	1.	Have you ever been told that you have a heart condition?
☐	☐	2.	Have you ever had a heart attack?
☐	☐	3.	Have you ever been told that you have high blood pressure?
☐	☐	4.	Have you ever had a stroke?
☐	☐	5.	Do you have emphysema?
☐	☐	6.	Do you have chronic bronchitis?
☐	☐	7.	Have you ever felt pain in your chest during physical activity?
☐	☐	8.	Have you ever felt pain in your chest when at rest?
☐	☐	9.	Have you ever been told that you have high cholesterol?
☐	☐	10.	Do you currently smoke?
☐	☐	11.	Do you have diabetes?
☐	☐	12.	Are you a male > 45 years of age?
☐	☐	13.	Are you a female > 55 years of age?
☐	☐	14.	Has an immediate family member (parent or sibling) had a heart attack, stroke or cardiovascular disease before 55 years of age?
☐	☐	15.	Have you ever lost consciousness or lost your balance due to dizziness?
☐	☐	16.	Are you currently being treated for any bone, orthopedic or joint problems that limit your activity level?
☐	☐	17.	Are you currently taking a medication that your doctor prescribed? If YES, please list each medication and why you are taking it.

CHAPTER 3

Working with Clients with Health Challenges

SUSAN BARTLETT

Susan J. Bartlett, Ph.D., is a clinical
psychologist and instructor of medicine at the
Johns Hopkins School of Medicine in
Baltimore, Md. Dr. Bartlett's research and
clinical interests focus on weight and eating
disorders as well as the development of effective
strategies healthcare providers can use to
motivate lifestyle changes
in their patients.

Psychosocial Impact
Process of Change
Building Rapport

When working with clients with health challenges, the psychological needs of clients are equally as important as the clients' physiological needs. Without adequate psychosocial support, individuals will likely fail to reach the goals of a physical activity program. An overview of psychosocial needs and how to address them is outlined in this chapter. Also addressed are methods for communicating with clients to ensure the development of a good working relationship. The chapter concludes with motivational principles and strategies to help inspire clients to adopt new behaviors and maintain them over time.

The Psychosocial Impact of Health Challenges

Newly developed health challenges, including illness or disability, bring new meaning to elements of life that formerly were taken for granted. There may be a new-found appreciation for things such as a loving family or a concerned and flexible employer. For others, the challenge may magnify a loss of ability, such as the ability to climb stairs or walk at a brisk pace.

Events that mark the onset of a health challenge often become a central focus in an individual's life. Examples include having a heart attack or bypass surgery, receiving the diagnosis of cancer or HIV, or having a stroke. Clients who have experienced these events often think of themselves in dichotomous terms. For example, they classify themselves in terms of how they were before the event and how they are after the event. In addition to the physiological consequences of a health challenge, there is usually psychological trauma involved. Signs and symptoms of psychological trauma include, but are not limited to, feelings of fear and helplessness, increased worry and anxiety, and having recurring dreams about the event (American Psychiatric Association, 1994).

People cope with psychological trauma in different ways. Many attempt to avoid any situation that arouses recollection of the event. Thus, someone who has experienced cardiac trouble may be highly fearful of (and wish to actively avoid) the physiological arousal that normally accompanies increased exertion. Thus, sensations such as increased heart rate, shortness of breath and sweating may be perceived as dangerous and distressing to the client. Clients also may be reluctant to change their exercise routine or increase the frequency, intensity or duration of exercise. They may appear anxious about physical activity and have negative feelings about its value. After a health change occurs, many clients focus on the physical limitations of their condition, failing to realize their capabilities. As a result, they perceive themselves as more fragile and weak than they really are. (Note: If the client seems highly traumatized by the event for more than one month, consider contacting other members of their healthcare team. A referral to a mental health specialist to rule out post-traumatic stress disorder may be necessary.)

Reassurance, close monitoring and safety are central themes to integrate when interacting with your clients. Their ability to feel comfortable when exercising often is directly related to their perception of safety, and you can help clients to feel safe in several ways. Active monitoring of the client (during and between exercise) goes a long way to foster comfort. Give clients your full attention when working with them, especially near the beginning of the program when feelings of vulnerability are often high. Heart-rate monitors and/or regular pulse checks can ease a client's fear about exercising too hard. Openly discussing the signs and symptoms that are both normal and problematic before and after exercise conveys knowledge and professionalism, and helps to reduce anxiety. Be careful not to dismiss or minimize any concern the client voices about their health or well-being. Listen for comments that sound like jokes or are mildly sarcastic, as they may ex-

Table 3.1

Client Information to Obtain from Medical Professionals

1) Are there any chronic medical conditions present? If so, how will they affect an exercise program?

2) What precautions should I take when working with this client?

3) Are there any limitations that I should be aware of when developing an exercise program?

4) What medication(s) is this client taking? Will any of them affect an exercise program?

5) Are there any symptoms/signs I should be aware of during exercise? (shortness of breath, chest pains, etc.)

6) How would you like me to keep you informed of this client's progress? (phone call, letter, etc.)

press true fears. An example would be the client who laughs while saying, "I hope this doesn't cause another stroke."

Facing a health challenge also can intensify emotional struggles. To adapt psychologically, clients often must develop patience, tolerance and a willingness to accept help. Progressive illnesses, such as cardiovascular disease, carry an additional burden, as the need to monitor signs and symptoms of disease progression can make the health challenge seem all-consuming to clients. Your knowledge and experience can help the client develop the appropriate level of self-monitoring and provide perspective to the role of exercise. Many times, physical activity is the optimal pathway to increasing functional capacity and helping clients feel better both physically and mentally.

Health challenges bring the need for ongoing adaptation. Sometimes these adaptations are outwardly noticeable and, therefore, make it harder for the client to "blend into the background." Even when the challenge is not visible, it serves as a reminder to the client that they are different. This difference may become a source of shame or can be perceived as evidence that the person has now become a burden to family and friends. An example may be an older woman with chronic obstructive pulmonary disease who requires oxygen with any activity. Carting the oxygen canister wherever she goes is a necessary but cumbersome and sometimes humiliating task. In the same way, individuals who are wheelchair bound may feel self-conscious about having to use a different entrance or route into a building. These individuals also may be concerned that they are taking too long or not moving quickly enough for you, their trainer. Be sensitive to the ways in which health challenges can significantly raise self-consciousness and respond promptly when clients voice concerns about inconveniencing you.

Both you and the client can uncover the best approach to physical activity largely through trial and error. To help this process along, it is crucial to have sensitivity, tolerance and empathy for where the client is at the moment. Understanding the impact that health challenges have on one's body, mind and spirit is critical when designing the optimal exercise program. The next section provides an overview of how to communicate this understanding effectively to clients and, in return, ways to hear what they are really saying.

Elements of Effective Communication

Communication is how we convey and receive information to and from others. The ability to communicate is the primary factor in working effectively with clients, and involves creating the optimal atmosphere, listening closely to what is said and what remains unsaid, and building rapport.

Select the Right Environment

Take care when selecting the environment in which your meeting is held. Be sure clients will have the privacy and time necessary to convey their concerns and wishes to you. Interviews that are rushed, interrupted or held in areas where others can overhear may imply a lack of sensitivity and respect.

Listen Carefully

Clients need to know two things: 1) that you hear what they are telling you, and 2) that you understand what they are saying. Both verbal and nonverbal cues demonstrate to the client that they are being heard and understood.

Active listening techniques use verbal cues that have been shown to enhance communication. By including brief prompts such as "um hmm" and "go on," you signal that you are following the client and encouraging them to continue. Brevity in the prompt is important in acknowledging that you are listening without interrupting the person's thoughts.

There are times, however, when it is beneficial to interrupt the conversation to probe for more specific information. You may need to clarify the sequence of events, for example, related to the treatment of a condition. Obtaining an accurate timeline of events and recording this in your notes likely will prove helpful several months later. Often, it is helpful to slow a client's recount of details, summarize briefly from time to time, and ask for specific information. For example:

Joe, you injured your knee 15 years ago during high school football and stayed out the rest of the season, but received no other treatment. You continued to remain physically active playing basketball several times a week through your early 20s, until you felt pain in your knee when you were skiing four years ago. When you knew there was a problem, who did you see first and what was done?

Obtain more than the basic physical or medical details of your client's condition, and try to understand any emotional reactions to the injury or illness. Open-ended questions such as "Tell me more about…" and "How did you feel about…" encourage the discussion to continue. Monitor your responses to client statements to ensure that they are nonjudgmental in tone and that they help clients feel comfortable about disclosing personal information.

Nonverbal techniques are equally important. Maintaining eye contact demonstrates your interest. Therefore, it is important to avoid taking detailed notes during your discussions. Body posture also conveys your comfort level with the client and the information being disclosed. Lean slightly forward and maintain an open posture to decrease any apprehension the client may have about initially meeting with you. Avoid sitting back in the chair and/or crossing your arms. During an initial interview with a new client that is scheduled for 7 p.m., make sure your body language does not convey that you are tired and anxious to go home.

Watch your client's body language, as well, to look for cues that suggest the client may be anxious or reticent to disclose information. Frequent shifting in the chair, looking away from you, fidgeting or frequently looking at one's watch all are signals that the client may feel uncomfortable. When you notice these signs, it often is helpful to acknowledge the discomfort and let the client know you understand it is difficult to talk openly about personal issues. For example, Hector is a 53-year-old business executive who completed cardiac rehab, and wants you to develop and supervise a comprehensive wellness program for him. Hector's life has changed in many ways since his heart attack. He is a proud man who is used to being in charge, and traditionally others have come to him for help. To optimize your ability to work with Hector, you must understand the psychosocial impact the heart attack has had, as well as the physical limitation that has been imposed by the heart attack. The following represents an attempt to acknowledge Hector's visible discomfort in talking about his current circumstances, while setting the stage for further discussion:

It can be difficult for many people to talk about their heart attack and its effects. It's helpful for me to understand what your rehab experience has been like, trying several new medications and dealing with their side effects. I also appreciate the fact that you're willing to share with me that your heart attack has affected your relationship with your wife and your colleagues at work.

If there are things you don't want to discuss today, that's fine too. We can always talk about some of these issues, or any others, in more detail as we get to know each other.

Building Rapport

Your effectiveness in working with a client often is directly related to the strength of your relationship with that person. Trust is the foundation of a strong alliance. Carl Rogers, a noted psychologist, identified three conditions that must be present in the development of trust: empathy, unconditional positive regard and genuineness (Rogers, 1957). Empathy refers to the ability to "walk in the client's shoes." You convey empathy when you listen actively and work to understand what is being said without making judgments. Unconditional positive regard, or respect, conveys a sincere acceptance of the client as a person, regardless of their status, symptoms or ability to make changes. Positive regard is conveyed with an attitude that says, "I know you can make these changes. We just need to provide you with the right road map." Genuineness reflects your ability to be a real person and to relate to your client as a person. Too often, it is easy to fall into a reserved, professional role and forget to see clients as people first.

When working with clients with special needs, an open line of communication is essential to long-term success. In most cases, the illness or disability your client lives with has had an enormous impact on their lives — physically, emotionally and perhaps even spiritually. The medical treatment they have received has been focused largely on alleviating symptoms and reversing or stalling the disease process. However, dignity, self-esteem and quality of life, which are so insidiously eroded by disease, receive little or no attention. Empathy, respect and genuineness can nurture a relationship and touch the client's spirit, and offer assistance beyond mere physical rehabilitation of the body.

Motivating Clients

Motivation is a central issue that arises again and again when working with any client. In fact, people often may choose a clinical exercise specialist because they hope you are skilled in helping to rekindle motivation when inevitable slumps occur. In the past 15 years, behavioral researchers have focused a great deal of attention on understanding the factors that facilitate adherence to any type of behavior-change program. This section offers a review of current motivational theories, as well as practical tips on how to implement these theories into your day-to-day work.

The Process of Change

In the early 1980s, two psychologists carefully began to study how people changed lifestyle behaviors by observing the process as it occurred. The model became known as the Transtheoretical Model of Stages of Change. Four stages were initially identified. Since then, the model has been expanded to incorporate two additional stages. The Stages of Change are presented in Figure 3.1.

The Stages of Change theory was originally developed after observing the process that smokers and others with addictive behaviors (i.e., substance abusers) undergo. In the last decade, this model has been applied to a number of health-promoting behaviors, most notably exercise adoption and nutritional changes (Prochaska et al., 1995; Prochaska et al., 1992). Results from several studies have shown that when interventions are matched to individual levels of readiness, people can move through the process of change to obtain desired results. For instance, several studies have designed materials promoting physical activity for those in the precontemplation, contemplation and preparation stages. When these materials are matched to the individual's motivational readiness, results show that significantly more people increased the adoption of physical activity (Marcus et al., 1994; Marcus et al., 1992a; Marcus et al., 1992b).

Table 3.2 describes each of the stages, along with stage-specific interventions. One of the principle findings that emerged from this work

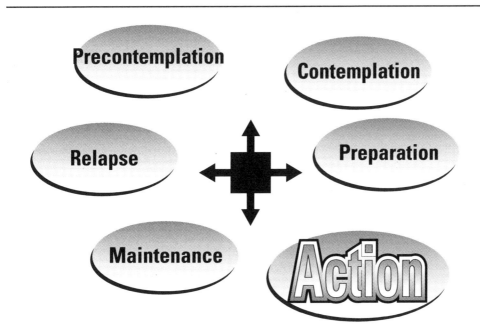

Adapted from Prochaska, Norcross and DiClemente (1995).

Figure 3.1

The Stages of Change

Signs of Readiness to Move into Action

1. **Decreased resistance.** The client stops arguing, interrupting, denying or objecting.
2. **Decreased questions about the problem.** The client seems to have enough information about their problem and stops asking questions. There is a sense of being finished.

   Resolve. The client appears to have reached a resolution, and may seem more peaceful relaxed, calm, unburdened or settled.

   Self-motivational statements. The client makes direct self-motivational statements reflecting problem recognition, concern, openness to change or optimism.

   Increased questions about change. The client asks what they can do about the problem, how people change if they decide to, etc.

   Envisioning. The client begins to talk about what life might be like after a change is made, or begins discussing the advantages of change. Experimenting. Between meetings, the clients may begin making some changes.

Adapted from Miller and Rollnick (1991).

People may remain in the initial stages — precontemplation and contemplation — for months or even years. It is important to be patient and recognize these stages as critical elements in behavior change. Most of the time, to outside observers and even the clients themselves, it appears that nothing is happening. Clearly this is not the case, and the theory suggests that very important cognitive work occurs and moves the person into preparation and action stages. While movement through the stages is linear, it is not always forward; sometimes individuals regress to an earlier stage. In fact, people in the early stages often appear to be stuck and have difficulty moving into preparation and action stages.

A second important discovery related to the stages of change is the observation that different stages rely on different mechanisms of action. For example, people move from precontemplation to contemplation and then preparation through a process known as decisional balance. During this process, clients make subjective evaluations about what will be gained and lost by changing. In the preparation stage, individuals plan, or even perform, some of the behaviors some of the time. They may develop an exercise schedule, plan a start date, buy walking shoes, find an exercise buddy, etc. In other cases of preparation, they may begin to exercise sporadically (but not at an intensity or frequency sufficient to obtain the desired results). An example of a client in the preparation stage would be the person who exercises

is the recognition of the idea that long before people are moved to act (i.e., the stage in which they are making the lifestyle changes to meet their target goals), they experience a series of stages that involve considering the pros and cons and committing to action.

**Table 3.2
Transtheoretical Stages of Change and Recommended Strategies to Facilitate Movement**

Precontemplation - Clients may not perceive their lifestyle as problematic. Acceptance of the client's perspective and less (rather than more) intensive discussions may help motivate precontemplators to move to the next stage.

Contemplation - Clients are willing to consider the problems associated with their current lifestyle and the possibilities offered by changing these behaviors. This stage is characterized by ambivalence and information gathering, processes that may sometimes thwart movement to the next stage. Motivational interviewing may be especially helpful during this stage.

Preparation - Deciding to change behavior and firmly committing to make the change are the hallmarks of this stage. Exploration of potential barriers and requisite coping skills needed to initiate change are helpful during this stage.

Action - Action refers to building a new pattern of behavior over time and typically is thought to take a minimum of three months. Increasing self-efficacy and teaching a problem-solving approach help foster persistence, optimism and a sense of success.

Maintenance/Relapse/Recycling - Maintenance is the process of sustaining behavior change over long periods of time (e.g., several years). As the behaviors become more of a lifestyle, the threat of relapse, or the return to the old patterns, lessens. Relapse prevention techniques help clients avoid or successfully cope with inevitable slips. Recycling through the stages may allow a more rapid transition back into action.

---

one or two times per week, but is unable to consistently exercise more than that. Consider the case of Betty:

Betty is a 60-year-old nurse who has advanced osteoarthritis of the knees. Her orthopedic surgeon does not consider joint replacement surgery to be an option for several years. Instead, he has strongly encouraged her to lose weight and exercise regularly to reduce pain and slow disease progression. Betty has never exercised regularly in her adulthood.

When you begin working together, Betty agrees to walk regularly but admits that, on average, she takes only a 15-minute walk once or twice a week. However, she does do five leg lifts bilaterally each day, and considers this to be partial adherence to her exercise prescription. Betty would be classified as being in the preparation stage. With your support and encouragement (and some good old-fashioned monitoring and accountability), you can hope to nudge her into the action stage (i.e., exercising regularly above the minimum threshold that provides weight loss and desired aerobic and fitness benefits). However, Betty also is at high risk of discontinuing her walking program altogether, as she considers how to fit it in to a busy schedule (i.e., regression back to contemplation).

Betty has become skilled in "thinking" about why it is important to make behavioral changes, but needs to develop skills to actually behave differently. To do this, a strategy is required to move her from the preparation stage to the action stage.

Most exercise programs are devised during the action stage, in which it often is assumed that the person is motivated, committed and willing to follow through with prescribed changes. (Note: These are huge assumptions that are not necessarily true. The person's ability to follow through is due to a host of factors, including the difficulty of the task, history with successful behavior change, etc.) As the "coach," you can shift from enhancing motivation to focusing on providing specific skills to help your client successfully negotiate short-term behavior change.

The fifth stage, maintenance, emphasizes sustaining behaviors over the long term. The reality that nearly 50 percent of all those who begin an exercise program abandon it within six months is a clear indication that much work needs to be done to uncover how we can best support the persistence of behavior change over time. By following the patient over time, you can support change, problem solve around emerging difficulties, keep the program fresh and identify potential relapses. Meeting frequency often varies over time; for example, a client may be comfortable going months between visits, yet at other times, when they are struggling, it may be helpful to meet several times a week.

During the last 10 years, the Stages of Change theory has had a significant impact on how most medical and lifestyle-change programs are delivered. The emphasis has moved from one intervention that is uniformly provided to everyone (e.g., encouragement by the physician to be more physically active) to interventions matched to an individual's stage of readiness. Specific strategies have been developed to move people through the process of change.

Moving Precontemplators and Contemplators to Action

For patients in precontemplation and contemplation, the following strategies have been shown to be helpful:

1. Providing a clear message of importance
2. Motivational interviewing
- *The importance of your message.*

Research has shown that messages provided by healthcare providers do have an impact on clients. With this in mind, if only half of all clinicians provided brief advice to their patients to stop smoking, and only 10 percent of the patients successfully quit, there would be 2 million new nonsmokers in the United States each year and 20 million non smokers within a decade. Do not underestimate the importance your words carry with clients, particularly when they echo those provided by other members of the healthcare team (e.g., physicians, physical therapists, etc.).

Begin by providing a clear, strong and personalized message of the importance of changing behavior. Now is not the time to soft-pedal or convey any sense of ambiguity. Effective messages include statements such as: "Betty, I'm concerned that your weight and sedentary lifestyle are affecting the arthritis in your knees. You can make lifestyle changes that will really make a difference in the way you feel, the amount of pain you have every day, and your overall energy. I want to help you create a lifestyle that is safe and comfortable for you — one that allows you to lose weight and be more physically active." Review basic information linking current diseases or illnesses to the desired changes, and provide any available handouts that reinforce your message.

- *Using motivational interviewing principles.* Motivational interviewing, developed by psychologists William Miller and Stephen Rollnick, is designed to assist people in moving through the Stages of Change (Miller et al., 1992). It is especially helpful in targeting the ambivalence clients often feel about making lifestyle changes. Motivational interviewing relies heavily on the principles of effective communication outlined earlier, including empathy, genuineness and positive regard. (In contrast with Carl Roger's approach, however, motivational interviewing is directive in nature.)

Motivational interviewing is not cheerleading, cajoling or even trying to gently persuade patients to change. It's not about your being a good salesperson for the benefits of healthier living. Rather, motivational counseling has been compared to creating a road map in which you (the coach) actively guide your client through a series of decision points by creating an atmosphere in which they generate their own arguments for change.

Motivational interviewing is a two-step process, and the first is to create a dialogue about the behaviors in question. Your goal is to actively elicit and then reinforce self-motivating statements that the client makes. This is based on the notion that when arguments for change are self-generated, they tend to be much more effective than anything we can say to our clients.

The following are examples of self-motivating statements frequently made by clients:

I suppose this is more of a problem than I thought...
I'm worried about how sedentary I am...
I think it's time for me to make some changes...
I'm going to make these changes...

Whenever you hear these types of statements, reinforce them by looking directly at the client, putting your pen down (if applicable) and acknowledging what the client has just said. A helpful response might be, "I'm really glad to hear you say that." Be enthusiastic when reinforcing these statements, as your clients may make critical evaluations about how important change really is based on your reaction. The enthusiasm, interest and importance you place on this part of the process are thought to have a direct impact on influencing your client's motivational state.

The second step is to create a level of discomfort by looking for and amplifying discrepancies in what each client says. For example, when clients tell you that they really enjoy smoking, ask them how they feel about having to go outside in the cold for a cigarette at work, how they feel about the price of cigarettes, etc. Be respectful when raising these issues and avoid sounding argumentative or judgmental.

For individuals in the early stages of change, your goal is to provide a clear message of importance and discuss problematic behaviors in a nonjudgmental manner. Keep in mind, though, that while most of your clients will fall into this stage of readiness, very few will respond to your advice the first time these issues are raised. Think of your role as the gardener who plants seeds now to harvest benefits later.

Working with Clients in
Preparation and Action Stages

Clients in the preparation and action stages benefit from a different approach. The goal is to increase the frequency of behavior to desired levels and promote long-term adherence. Behavioral skills are important. Your role as a clinical exercise specialist is to identify whether clients have the requisite skills, teach or enhance skills as needed, and provide opportunities to rehearse new behaviors under controlled conditions.

Successful movement into the action stage requires a solid commitment to make and implement behavior changes. Help your client spell out exactly what they are willing to commit to. To be most effective, clients should clearly commit to implementing the targeted behavioral changes by a specified date and time. It is often helpful to record this information directly in the client's file (while the client is still in your office). Encourage the client to write down their commitments as well, either in a daily planner or even on a sticky note that can be placed in a conspicuous location.

Help clients identify barriers to behavior change, including time constraints (real or perceived), and negative moods or thoughts. Help them see the critical relationship between saying, "I just don't feel like exercising today; I'll do it tomorrow," and ultimately giving up their behavior-change goals altogether.

Teach and refine problem-solving skills to help clients effectively anticipate and negotiate these barriers. By defining the problem, generating potential solutions and evaluating the effectiveness of each solution during your time together, you can model the usefulness of this approach. Demonstrate your belief in the process by spending a reasonable percentage of time in each session systematically working through problems. Problem solving also effectively reduces the emotional shame clients experience when they fail to follow through with set goals.

Create a hierarchy of experiences to enhance your client's sense of self-efficacy — an individual's belief or expectation that they are able to behave in a certain manner in a specific situation. Self-efficacy is a consistent predictor of exercise behavior and, in research trials, it has been influenced in the short term to alter activity levels. Sense of self-efficacy is thought to influence both one's choice of activities and selection of environments. For example, most persons avoid activities and situations they believe exceed their coping capabilities, but readily engage in activities and environments that they believe they are capable of handling. Thus, to bolster their confidence, help clients identify activities they have previously enjoyed or are likely to master in the beginning (e.g., a walking program). The overall approach is to first help clients feel competent as an exerciser, then assist them in expanding their choice of activities.

The best way to enhance self-efficacy is through mastery experiences. Short-term success enhances a person's belief in their ability to handle situations. Thus, early in your work together, ensure the goals you have developed with your client maximize the likelihood for short-term success. Structure experiences each week that build upon previous gains to further bolster confidence.

Self-efficacy also is enhanced when an individual experiences a setback, then recovers. Recovery from a setback provides evidence that the person has the skills needed to cope, further reinforcing self-efficacy.

Keep in close contact with clients, especially when they are struggling. When motivation is waning, it often is helpful to touch base, either directly or indirectly, between sessions. Does follow-up really make a difference? Consider that counselors who follow up with clients who are trying to quit smoking in the first few weeks report nearly triple the success rate compared to those who do not. While face-to-face follow-up is always best, a phone call only takes a few minutes and also can make an impact by conveying your interest. Other ways to follow up include having the client call you to leave a message on your voice mail or send an e-mail.

Promoting Maintenance — Keeping it Going

Two psychologists at the University of Washington, Drs. Marlatt and Gordon, carefully studied their patients with addictive disorders (e.g., smoking and substance abuse) to determine why some were successful in sustaining behavior change while others relapsed (Marlatt et al., 1985). They noticed that while most people experienced some slips or even returned briefly to previous behaviors (e.g., smoking a cigarette after quitting), those who were successful long-term thought very differently about a "slip" and behaved differently afterward. It appeared that the marker of who was going to ultimately succeed had little to do with whether they experienced a behavioral lapse and much more to do with how they responded to their slips.

Those who successfully stopped smoking were much more likely to view one cigarette as a slip. In contrast, those who relapsed back to smoking were much more likely to view their regression as evidence that they could not possibly stay off cigarettes long-term.

Relapse Prevention (RP) facilitates the maintenance of behavior change. A key component of RP is the identification of high-risk situations in which a lapse, or return to former behaviors, is likely to occur. Once these situations are identified, you can help the client plan accordingly to bolster coping skills. Consider the example of a client who tells you that in the past taking a vacation resulted in a backlog of work, which in turn prevented her from immediately resuming her training sessions with you. Several weeks later when the client still had not rescheduled an appointment, it became apparent that factors other than the initial backlog were keeping her from being physically active.

By definition, vacations for this client present a high-risk situation that may trigger a relapse. As a result, it is essential that a clear plan be developed before the client's next vacation. For instance, she might be able to anticipate her workload and address it before she leaves. Alternatively, she might not take on additional projects at work shortly before her vacation is scheduled. Finally, she may allocate an additional hour each day to "catch up" in the week after she returns. Other risks for abandoning exercise programs include a period or illness or injury, or any disruption to the person's routine (including you taking a vacation).

Another important component of RP is relabeling, or reinterpreting the meaning of lapses. Too often, our clients see any slip backward as a sign of an inevitable return to baseline. This is rooted in the pervasive wish that we can and will change once and for all, and that there will be no slips with which to cope. In the 1980s, psychologist Stanley Schachter interviewed individuals in the community (not just those who come to behavior-change programs) about their lifetime attempts to quit smoking and lose weight. He reported findings that were considerably different from those reported in research settings (Schachter, 1982). Schachter noted that the average ex-smoker successfully quits on their fifth attempt. Clearly, it appeared that preliminary attempts to quit (i.e., attempts one through four), were a warm-up for lasting success brought about by the fifth try. Thus, a person who tried four times previously but relapsed each time might have considered themselves completely unable to quit when, in reality, they may well have been on the brink of success. Helping clients relabel previous and current experiences with exercise and lifestyle change is essential to keeping

them motivated to persist with their new active lifestyle.

Another factor that offers added insurance during lapses is the client's level of social support. While patients can make changes on their own, research has shown that level of support is a potent predictor of long-term outcome. Help your clients engineer their environment to maximize support systems; friends, family, colleagues, employers and others can be helpful in many ways. A spouse may ensure that your client has the necessary time after work or in the mornings to attend appointments with you, or they may help monitor and prompt exercise between training sessions. It also is important that clients identify who is unlikely to be helpful, as social contacts can be harmful when others sabotage efforts to change. In this situation, the client needs the skills to (gently) confront the saboteur and negotiate more helpful interactions.

Apart from consistent praise, there is no universal method of support that works for everyone. Clients are most likely to receive the help that is most beneficial to them when they directly ask for a specific type of support, such as asking others if they are willing to make dietary and exercise changes with them, providing positive support and encouragement as goals are met, being tolerant of efforts to change (and the inevitable slips) and being available to talk about efforts to change. Each client has their own unique version of what constitutes positive social support. For instance, while some clients may appreciate a spouse or friend who assumes responsibility for prompting physical activity, others may find this an annoyance or even a reason not to exercise. Work with your client to help uncover the strategies that are helpful to them, and teach them how to ask others for help by being very specific in their requests.

One Size Does Not Fit All

Certification as a clinical exercise specialist implies that one has the requisite training in exercise science and a basic level of knowledge and skill in allied sciences such as psychology, counseling and nutrition. Implicit in this breadth of knowledge is the understanding that working with a more complex client base requires the enhanced ability to assess the unique needs of a wide variety of clients and to design programs that are safe and effective. Flexibility is a hallmark of creating and implementing such programs. Thus, experience and education allow you to understand the framework upon which safe and effective programs are constructed, while communication allows you to customize the design to maximize effectiveness.

Your ability to incorporate effective communication and motivational strategies into your day-to-day work with clients will be refined over time. As your experience with counseling grows, so does the sensitivity and intuition that's needed when providing a gentle nudge or more energetic push. Over time, you will develop a style as unique and tailored as the exercise and lifestyle programs you create. Ongoing nurturing of the relationship with clients with special needs can infuse inspiration and confidence into your clients. In return, it engenders a richer and more rewarding experience for you as a clinical exercise specialist.

References and Suggested Reading

American Psychiatric Association. (1994). *Diagnostic and Statistical Manual of Mental Disorders.* (4th ed.) Washington, DC.

Marcus, B.H., Rakowski, W. & Rossi, J.R. (1992a). Assessing motivational readiness and decision making for exercise. *Health Psychology,* 11, 257-261.

Marcus, B.H., Selby, V.C., Niaura, R.S. & Rossi, J.S. (1992b). Self-efficacy and the stages of exercise behavior change. *Research Quarterly for Exercise & Sport,* 63,1, 60-66.

Marcus, B.H. & Simkin, L.R. (1994). The transtheoretical model: Applications to exercise behavior. *Medicine & Science in Sports & Exercise,* 26, 11, 1400-1404.

Marlatt, G. & Gordon, J. (1985). *Relapse Prevention: Maintenance Strategies in Addictive Behavior Change.* New York: Guilford.

Miller, W.R. & Rolnick, S. (1992). *Motivational Interviewing: Preparing People to Change Addictive Behaviors.* New York: Guilford.

Prochaska, J.O., DiClemente, C.C. & Norcross, J.C. (1992). In search of how people change: Applications to addictive behaviors. *American Psychologist,* 47, 1102-1111.

Prochaska, J.O., Norcross, J.C. & DiClemente, C. (1995). *Changing for Good.* New York: Avon.

Rogers, C. (1957). The necessary and sufficient conditions of therapeutic personality change. *Journal of Consulting Psychology,* 21, 95-103.

Schachter, S. (1982). Recidivism and self-cure of smoking and obesity. *American Psychologist,* 37, 436-444.

CHAPTER 4

Communicating Effectively with Healthcare Professionals

JACK L. COX

Jack Cox, M.D., is a family physician who has spent the last 12 years providing medical education and conducting research that emphasizes preventive healthcare. He currently is an associate clinical professor of family and preventive medicine at the University of Utah School of Medicine, and regional medical director for Intermountain Healthcare in Provo, Utah.

Effective Communication
Medical Documentation
Confidentiality Issues

Today's healthcare system increasingly emphasizes team management of clients' health. The healthcare team includes the physician or other primary healthcare provider, and allied healthcare professionals such as clinical exercise specialists, dietitians, and physical and occupational therapists. Consequently, communication within the healthcare community becomes critical as all seek to influence the health and well-being of their clients. Effective communication is one of the most important life skills, and also is the hardest to learn (Covey, 1989). This chapter explains the communication skills necessary to actively participate as a member of the healthcare team. Team communication is greatly enhanced if you know 1) the expertise you bring to the team; 2) the expectations other team members have of you (do they understand your expertise?); 3) your clients' expectations; 4) how to effectively communicate feedback to other team members; and 5) the other team members' expertise.

Types of Healthcare Professionals

Physicians generate the majority of consultations or client referrals for exercise programs. Most health insurance plans require individuals to have a primary care physician who directs referrals to the healthcare team. Primary care physicians usually are family physicians, internists or pediatricians — all specialties that require a three-year, post-medical school residency and board certification. Family physicians take care of both children's and adults' medical care. Internists primarily treat adults. Pediatricians care for children, usually under the age of 18. The Accrediting Council of Graduate Medical Education (ACGME) (www.acgme.com) and the American Medical Association (AMA) (www.ama.org) recognize numerous other specialties, including cardiology, orthopedics, general surgery, sports medicine, etc. You may receive referrals or consults from any of these medical specialists, and knowing something about their specialty will aid you in understanding their expectations and in communicating effectively with them. Additionally, physician assistants (PA) and certified registered nurse practitioners (CRNP) are licensed providers that may send you referrals. They practice with physicians either in primary care or other specialty areas.

Effective Communication

Effective communication with your client's primary care provider should be based on the following objectives:

➤ determining physical limitations to an exercise program
➤ obtaining medical clearance for a specific exercise program
➤ obtaining recommendations regarding an exercise program
➤ introducing yourself and your services
➤ clarifying questions on the client's health
➤ obtaining special considerations related to the client's health (i.e., a chronic disease such as diabetes or hypertension)
➤ providing progress reports on the exercise program, or receiving health status updates

➤ establishing rapport with a potential referral source

Clients may be self-referred or may contact you via a referral from a physician or other healthcare provider. The primary method of referral is either a phone call or a consult. Consults are formal requests for your evaluation of a client that produce recommendations for an exercise program. Physicians also may request that you design and implement the program, giving them regular progress reports. In the case of self-directed referrals, obtain written permission from the client to forward any information about their program and progress to their physician.

If the client has any one of the conditions covered in this text, obtaining their physician's clearance to exercise is necessary before the client begins a program. A phone call or letter to the physician's office requesting client evaluation and suggesting limitations for an exercise program will go a long way in establishing rapport. Your request should include a brief statement of your area of expertise and what modalities you use. Ask for specific recommendations on client limitations, which may include a specific target heart rate, restrictions on using certain muscle groups or joints, or specific complaints to be aware of (chest pain or lightheadedness). Let the physician know what form of communication you will use to keep them updated on the client's progress, (i.e. letter or phone call). You should ask your client to sign a release that allows you to send reports to their physician. Likewise, physicians will require a signed release from clients before sharing medical information with you. See the Confidentiality Issues section.

Feedback to the physician does not occur in a vacuum, but within a system that includes the message sender (you), the receiver of the message (the physician), the actual message, the medium used to send the message (phone call, mail, e-mail) and any distractions that impede reception of the message. Written communications to physicians should be brief, cover the salient points and close with an acknowledgement of appreciation for the referral. An example of a commonly used format includes:

• Client identification (Mrs. Jones is a 53-year-old woman referred for conditioning and strength training).

- Identification of medical conditions of concern and limits that the physician has suggested (She has diabetes mellitus and hypertension, both well controlled by medication. She has been directed to eat a snack prior to aerobic exercise, to carry a snack during exercise to manage hypoglycemia and to maintain hydration).
- A list of prescription and over-the-counter medications that the client has told you they are taking.
- List significant exercise history, sports-participation history, and injuries or surgery that may limit exercise participation.

In your initial letter, cover your evaluation and recommendations for a plan. Include your time frame (how many times per week you will meet with the client, how long sessions will last, the length of time for the program). List any specific target expectations that the client has, and be sure you state that this plan was covered with the client and that they are in agreement. You also may want to list any educational material given to the client.

Follow-up Communication

Follow-up letters simply should list how the client performed with regard to your original plan, and any changes in the program. Mention unexpected occurrences, e.g., low-pulse episodes, feelings of dyspnea (shortness of breath) or light-headedness that caused exercise to cease. You may want to include details about the client's level of satisfaction with their progress, and any other information that will help the physician understand your role in providing care for this client.

Keep a copy of any letters you send in an individual client file and give a copy to the client. As you can see from Figure 4.1, a physician quickly can determine what you have recommended and can tailor future medical therapy to the client's activity. This may become important in adjusting medication. For example, diabetics participating in regular exercise frequently need a lower dose of their diabetic medication.

Barriers to Effective Communication

Awareness of communication barriers can greatly facilitate your working relationship with healthcare providers and can lead to improved coordinated client care. Use common courtesy, clarify expectations and communicate clearly to avoid these frequent barriers to effective communication:

Timeliness of the communication. Does the physician receive your referral letter within days, or within six weeks, of your initial session? Were you able to call or send a letter before the physician had a follow-up visit with the client? Does the physician prefer calls or letters? Tardy communication places the physician in a position in which he is uninformed of what other team members are doing. This decreases the chance that he will send you another referral. If you know your client has scheduled an appointment with their physician that will take place before you can send a letter, consider calling the physician's office to give a brief report on your findings and recommendations. Keep written notes in the client's file that detail any phone conversations you have with them or their physician. Always be prompt in your replies and type them in a professional manner.

Not understanding the findings or recommendations. Physicians generally are unfamiliar with the role that clinical exercise specialists can play in the healthcare team. Therefore, you are in a position to educate physicians on what you have to offer. Your method of doing so may include a phone call to let the physician know that if they have questions, they may use you as a resource. You also might try including some explanation in your referral letters, personally visiting the physician's office or sending them pertinent articles on different aspects of physical training and exercise. As you develop rapport with physicians, you will better understand their information needs. Use clear, concise statements in your letters. Follow the KISS rule (Keep It Short and Simple).

Unclear expectations. The root of most interpersonal, as well as professional, relationships is ambiguous or conflicting expectations (Covey, 1989). Indeed the inability of individuals to convey their intentions and meaning has been one of the prime causes of confusion and violence over the ages, and healthcare is no exception (Cousins, 1983). Make sure you understand what the physician expects of you and strive to deliver it. Be clear about what you have to offer the healthcare team, how to utilize your exper-

Figure 4.1

*Sample Follow-up
Letter*

Dear Dr. Cox:

Grace Jones is a 53-year-old woman whom you referred to me for aerobic conditioning and strength training. She has a 10-year history of adult-onset diabetes and hypertension, which you have indicated are under good control. She currently is taking glyburide (diabetes), prinavil (hypertension) and vitamin C. Her last exercise program, in which she walked two miles each day, ended at least eight years ago. She ran track in college, has no history of significant injuries or surgery, and indicates no other physical limitations. You indicated that Mrs. Jones should be monitored for hypoglycemia symptoms, including excessive sweating, lightheadedness and rapid pulse.

Findings:

Weight: 154 pounds; resting pulse: 80; height: 63 inches; BMI: 27. Her two-minute, post-exercise pulse is 96, at an exercise level of 6 METs. Her flexibility in all extremities and back, as well as her strength in major muscle groups, is moderate for her age. Fat composition using impedance is 28 percent. She demonstrated full range of motion in all major joints without pain.

Recommendation:

Mrs. Jones stated that she liked the stationary bike and the treadmill. I recommended that she start a program of 30 minutes each on alternating days for five days per week with light resistance for the first two weeks. She also should begin resistance training three days per week using moderate weight—one set of 10 reps for each of her major muscle groups in the upper and lower extremities. I demonstrated stretching exercises to be done for 10 minutes prior to exercise and 10 minutes post exercise. I also gave her a handout explaining the stretching exercises and a log for her aerobic and resistance training exercises. I will follow her for the first week daily and then weekly for the first month. She agrees that this is a program she can follow and stated that she understands the program and the risks involved.

Please contact me if there are any questions. I will send you an update letter after Mrs. Jones' first week of participation.

Sincerely,

your name

tise and when it is appropriate to refer an individual to you. Let the physician know what kind of results your clients can expect so that they may provide reinforcement when they see the client.

Reaching beyond your scope. If you do not know an answer or cannot help an individual, admit it. Do not offer medical advice to your clients, no matter if you "know someone with the same condition" or not. You do not want the liability that accompanies these types of decisions. Each member of the healthcare team has a different perspective of the client, but the physician ultimately is accountable in most cases. Physicians communicate quite closely with one another and you quickly can find yourself with no referrals if you are known in the medical community as an "armchair doctor."

The Do's and Don'ts:

Some of the do's and don'ts of good referral communication:

Do's

- Do spend time building credibility with the physician population of your community by sending introductory letters to physicians (Figure 4.2), personally visiting their offices, sending educational materials, making phone calls, advertising in the newspaper and, above all, making sure you provide a valuable service.
- Do send timely, clear, concise referral letters.
- Do set clear goals with the physician as well as the client, and follow through.

- Do establish your practice with a credible facility.
- Do keep clear records, including your referral letters and notes from phone calls, in individual client files. You never know when you will need to refer back to them.
- Do ask questions. The word "doctor" comes from the Latin root meaning "teacher." Most physicians love to share knowledge.
- Do utilize resources to learn about diseases, medications or other health conditions. These resources include professional journals, medical dictionaries, a medical terminology class (check with your local hospital or community college), the Internet, local physicians, local pharmacists and this book.
- Do "seek first to understand and then to be understood" (Covey, 1989) in your communications. In other words, what does the physician want?
- Do look for win-win solutions to communication problems.

Don'ts

- Don't "play doctor." Value your expert position within the healthcare team.
- Don't offer advice, either to clients or physicians, that is not within your scope as a clinical exercise specialist.
- Don't address clients or physicians by their first names until given permission to do so. Both will respect this professional courtesy.
- Don't procrastinate. Make timely appointments with clients, complete and send referral letters soon after the evaluation, and promptly return phone calls.

Medical Documentation

Documentation is a cornerstone in healthcare. "If you did not document it, you did not do it" is the mantra hammered into physicians' heads from the first day of medical school. What documentation is needed for allied health professionals, including clinical exercise specialists, varies by location. Check with local clinical exercise specialists, your state

---

Figure 4.2

*Sample
Introductory Letter
to a Physician*

Dear Dr. Cox:

Diet and lack of exercise account for more than 400,000 deaths annually. Recent studies have shown that only 30 percent of the population exercise regularly; however, another 30 percent state they would like to. Exercise has been shown to improve medical outcomes in chronic diseases such as diabetes, hypertension and coronary artery disease. However, few individuals know how to begin a safe, effective exercise program. I can help.

My name is John Smith and I am a certified clinical exercise specialist at The Health and Fitness Institute in Baltimore. My certification is from The American Council on Exercise (ACE). As an ACE-certified Clinical Exercise Specialist, I have a background in evaluating individuals referred to me by their physicians for design and supervision of the ideal exercise program. My evaluation includes:

Exercise history

Exercise likes and dislikes

Aerobic capacity (METS)

Weight analysis with impedance and BMI calculations

Range-of-motion evaluation

Once I have evaluated the client, with your specific instructions, I tailor an exercise program that usually includes both aerobic and resistance training. I monitor the client's progress and frequently provide you with progress reports and follow-up information.

Our facility provides a wide range of aerobic and resistance-training equipment, a pool for water aerobics and professionally taught aerobic classes.

I would like to offer my services to you and your patients. Enclosed is some material explaining the role of certified clinical exercise specialists, as well as an article on the evaluation of abdominal exercise machines. Please feel free to use me as a resource for this type of information, as well as a referral source for your patients.

I would be happy to further discuss referrals at your convenience. My telephone number is 999-999-9999.

I look forward to working with you to improve your patients' health.

Sincerely,

John Smith

Figure 4.3

*Sample Progress
Note (follow-up
visit)*

12/1/98

S: Mrs. Smith is back today for evaluation of her exercise program. She states she has followed the plan of 20 minutes of stationary cycling at a moderately hard level (pulse max 145) for four days per week, as well as 15 minutes of resistance training three days per week. She states she experienced some soreness for five days, resolved with ibuprofen.

O: Weight: 155   Height: 5'4"   Resting Pulse: 72   BP: 130/80

I observed Mrs. Smith on the bike. Her maximum pulse was 150, exertion moderate. Length of time 20 minutes. She also performed 8 reps with 80 percent of her repetition maximum weight in bicep curls, military press, bench press and leg raises.

A: Mrs. Smith is progressing well and tolerating her exercise program.

P: 1. Increase time on the stationary cycle from 20 minutes to 30 minutes four times per week.

    2. Increase resistance training to 10 reps per station.

    3. Discussed pre- and post-exercise stretching (handout given to Mrs. Smith).

    4. Follow-up appointment in one week.

    5. Letter to Dr. Cox discussing her progress.

Signature

---

laws, your local hospital risk manager or quality-improvement nurse, or a local healthcare attorney. It usually is better to document too much than too little. Remember that all you write can find its way into a court of law, so be professional at all times. Derogatory adjectives have little use in your documentation (e.g., a statement such as, "Mrs. Jones, a 53-year-old demented and belligerent lady" can be used in a harmful manner). Good documentation should help the physician understand what is happening with their client, and can help you plot client progress.

A minimum standard of good documentation should include the client's name, sex, age, phone number, address, emergency contacts, insurance information, medications, medication allergies, and their physician's name, address and phone number. Also include chronic medical conditions (e.g., hypertension, degenerative arthritis of the hips, diabetes, asthma, etc.). A running log of visit dates and times, along with pertinent vital-sign data (i.e., weight, blood pressure, and pre- and post-exercise pulse) should be kept in the front of the file. Copies of referral letters to physicians, notes of phone conversations with physicians or clients, client medical-data release statements and signed consent statements should be kept in the client file. Phone notes can be brief, but should include the date and time, whom you spoke to, and a brief synopsis of the conversation that includes pertinent information.

Progress notes, that is notes of subsequent client visits in which you are involved, are included in the client file with date, time and a brief synopsis of the visit. Progress notes are written accounts of your visits with clients, and should be kept in the client's file by date (be sure to date all entries). Most physicians use a "SOAP" note format to document visits. "SOAP" is an acronym describing the organized structure of the progress note. "S" is for subjective findings (what the patient tells you). "O" is for objective findings (what you observe directly). "A" is for assessment (your conclusions and analysis). "P" is for plan (your plan for exercise, further evaluation, etc.) (Figure 4.3). Sign all notes you put in a client's file.

If another clinical exercise specialist sees your client, their note goes in the same client file. You also may want to keep a log of the client's progress (amount of time on specific aerobic exercises, resistance training, etc.), as well as a list of the educational material you give them. Good documentation is a valuable resource in the longitudinal care of your client. It is difficult to go back and try to reconstruct events or conversations after the fact, so make sure your documentation practices are in place and consistent.

Confidentiality Issues

Few issues in medicine get a quicker response from risk managers or healthcare attorneys than confidentiality. It is one of the greatest liability issues for physicians' offices, which are required to keep client charts in a limited-access area where only personnel with a need to know may access the charts and the information they contain. It is easy to imagine how destructive sensitive medical information could be to an individual if it got out. For example, information on mental conditions, such as depression, or sexually transmitted diseases could wreak havoc with a client. Clients and physicians have an expectation that information shared or collected by you will be handled in a confidential manner. Some general tips on confidentiality include:

- Keep all client files in an area not accessible to the general public (e.g., a locked file cabinet or shelves in a closet).
- Develop a confidentiality policy for your office. It should include the understanding that only personnel working with the client have access to their files. In many offices, unauthorized accessing of client files or charts is grounds for immediate termination from the job. As offices begin to use electronic client files, it also is becoming important to safeguard them against unauthorized access.
- Do not discuss client medical information in areas where others may overhear it. Hold conversations with clients, as well as phone calls with physicians, in a private place.
- If you do not type your letters, know who does. Make sure that they understand your confidentiality policy.
- Obtain written permission from the client to share information with their physician and keep this document in the client's file. The physician must obtain the same type of release before sharing information with you. Do not assume that it is okay to share client information with a client's family members or friends. This can be difficult, especially when friends or relatives ask, "How is Jack doing?" Also use caution when giving information over the phone; know the caller.
- Do not talk to your family and friends about clients.
- Destroy old or unneeded client information appropriately. Many offices have a paper shredder for this purpose.

Confidentiality is a serious issue and should be treated as such. Most hospital risk managers have educational material, instructional videos and other resources on the issue of confidentiality. Contact your local hospital risk manager, and check state and local laws on this subject. A breach in a client's confidentiality is one of the quickest ways to lose your professional credibility. Don't take it for granted.

Summary

This chapter has touched on the highlights of professional communication for the clinical exercise specialist as a member of the healthcare team. Good communication, both with other team members and clients, is critical for your training success as well as theirs. Effective communication takes time. Frequently solicit feedback from clients and other team members.

References

Covey, S. R. (1989). *The 7 Habits of Highly Effective People.* New York: Simon & Schuster, Inc.

Cousins, N. (1983). *The Healing Heart.* New York: W.W. Norton & Company.

Suggested Reading

Covey, S .R. (1989). *The 7 Habits of Highly Effective People.* New York: Simon & Schuster, Inc.

Fisher, R. & Ury, W. (1981). *Getting to Yes.* Boston: Houghton Mifflin.

Ury, W. (1991). *Getting Past No.* New York: Bantam Books.

Section Two

Cardiovascular Disease

CHAPTER 5

Hypertension

SCOTT O. ROBERTS

Scott Owen Roberts, Ph.D., F.A.A.C.V.P.R., is an assistant professor at Texas Tech University in Lubbock. He has more than 15 years experience as a clinical exercise physiologist, and is a fellow of the American Association of Cardiovascular and Pulmonary Rehabilitation and an ACSM Certified Exercise Program Director. Dr. Roberts has published numerous original scientific articles, trade articles, chapters and books, including Exercise Physiology: Exercise Performance, and Clinical Applications and Clinical Exercise Testing and Prescription: Theory and Application. He also served as a section editor for ACSM's Exercise Management for Persons with Chronic Diseases and Disabilities. Dr. Roberts has served as a member of ACE's Aerobics Instructor Examination and Personal Trainer Committees.

Client Assessment

Rate of Progression

Suggestions for Health Enhancement

Blood pressure, or more accurately, mean arterial blood pressure, is the primary driving force propelling blood to the tissues. Resting blood pressure in healthy individuals averages 120/80 mmHg. The first number, 120, is defined as systolic blood pressure, and represents the pressure of the blood against the artery walls during the contraction phase of the heart. The second number, 80, is defined as diastolic blood pressure, and represents the pressure against the artery walls when the heart is resting between beats. Mean arterial blood pressure is the average (difference between systolic and diastolic) blood pressure throughout the arterial system, and can be estimated with the following formula: Mean Arterial Blood Pressure = 1/3 (systolic-diastolic) + diastolic. The calculation is based on a diastole duration that is approximately three times greater than systole at rest. This relationship changes with an increase in heart rate. During exercise, systolic and mean arterial blood pressure increase and diastolic blood pressure remains close to, or slightly less than, resting values (<80 mmHg). Mean resting means arterial blood pressure averages just under 100 mmHg at rest. Blood pressure is a product of cardiac output (the sum of all the blood ejected from the heart per minute) multiplied by total peripheral resistance. Thus, if either side, or both, of the equation increases or decreases, blood pressure rises or falls.

Mean Arterial Blood Pressure =
Cardiac Output x *Total Peripheral Resistance*

Blood pressure is very closely regulated by specialized pressure sensors throughout our body that ensure it 1) does not fall too low and compromise adequate flow to tissues, or 2) rise too high and increase the work of the heart and blood vessels. Under normal conditions, the body is able to regulate mean arterial blood pressure so that it rises and falls according to the demands being placed on the body. For example, during continuous graded exercise, cardiac output increases and total peripheral resistance decreases slightly, leading to an increase in systolic blood pressure, and little or no increase in diastolic blood pressure (Figure 5.1). Occasionally, blood-pressure-control mechanisms do not function properly or adequately, and are unable to compensate for demands placed on the body. One of the resulting conditions is hypertension.

Figure 5.1

Normal Responses To Blood Pressure During Exercise

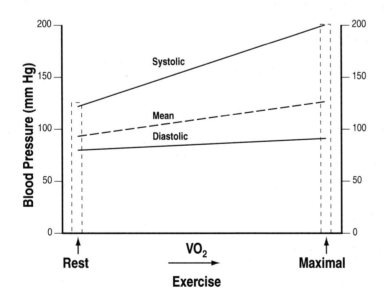

Overview of Hypertension

Hypertension is defined as a chronically elevated blood pressure greater than 140/90 mmHg measured on two or more separate occasions. A person currently taking antihypertensive medication also may be classified as hypertensive.

As many as 50 million Americans have chronically elevated blood pressure, or are taking antihypertensive medication (NHANES III, The fifth report of the Joint National Committee on Detection, Evaluation and Treatment of High Blood Pressure). Hypertension is related to the development of heart disease, increased severity of atherosclerosis, stroke, congestive heart failure, left-ventricular hypertrophy, aortic aneurysm and peripheral disease. In addition, hypertension:

➤ causes the heart to work harder, resulting in enlargement of the heart (cardiac or left-ventricular hypertrophy)
➤ reduces the elasticity of the arteries (resulting in arteriosclerosis)
➤ causes narrowing of the arteries (resulting in atherosclerosis)
➤ increases the risk of blood clot formation (resulting in myocardial infarction or stroke)

The majority of individuals with high blood pressure are not undergoing therapy to control their blood pressure. In fact, many do not even know they have a problem. The cause of high blood pressure in 90 percent to 95 percent of cases is unknown; however, once detected, these cases can be controlled. If left untreated, hypertensive individuals have a three-to-four-times higher risk of developing coronary artery disease, and up to a seven-times higher risk of having a stroke.

Exercise and Hypertension

Exercise training is an important part of controlling hypertension. Regular aerobic exercise appears to reduce both systolic and diastolic blood pressure by an average of about 10 mmHg. Although the exact mechanisms responsible for the reduction in blood pressure following exercise training are not completely understood, it appears that exercise causes a reduction in cardiac output and total peripheral resistance at rest, and/or reduced sympathetic activity. Based on the available literature, the American College of Sports Medicine recently released a position statement on exercise and hypertension that recommends endurance exercise training as a nonpharmacological strategy to reduce the incidence of hypertension in susceptible individuals.

The available evidence indicates that endurance exercise training by individuals at high risk for developing hypertension will reduce the rise in blood pressure that occurs with time. Thus, it is the position of the American College of Sports Medicine that endurance exercise training is recommended as a nonpharmacological strategy to reduce the incidence of hypertension in susceptible individuals. The exercise recommendations to achieve this effect are generally the same as those prescribed for developing and maintaining cardiovascular fitness in healthy adults. However, exercise training at somewhat lower intensities appears to lower blood pressure as much as, or more than, exercise at higher intensities, which may be more important in specific hypertensive populations.

Portions adapted from American College of Sports Medicine Position Stand on Physical Activity, Physical Fitness and Hypertension.

In addition to exercise, individuals should follow the lifestyle-modification guidelines listed below. If lifestyle modification does not work, or if blood pressure is severely high, the client's physician may prescribe medication to lower and control blood pressure. In addition to regular aerobic exercise, the Joint National Committee on Detection, Evaluation and Treatment of High Blood Pressure makes the following recommendations to lower and control blood pressure:

- If overweight, lose weight.
- Limit alcohol intake to less than 1 ounce per day.
- Reduce sodium intake to less than 2.3 grams per day.
- Stop smoking.
- Reduce dietary fat, saturated fat and cholesterol.
- Maintain adequate dietary potassium, calcium and magnesium intake.

Client Assessment

The majority of individuals with diagnosed hypertension can safely enjoy exercise. However,

---

Table 5.1
Facts about Hypertension

- Hypertension is one of the most prevalent chronic diseases in the United States.
- As many as 50 million Americans have chronically elevated blood pressure, or are taking antihypertensive medication.
- Hypertension is a primary risk factor for heart disease, increased severity of atherosclerosis, stroke, congestive heart failure, left-ventricular hypertrophy, aortic aneurysm and peripheral vascular disease.
- African Americans are at higher risk for hypertension than Caucasians.
- Risk for hypertension is increased in individuals with high total cholesterol levels and impaired glucose tolerance, cigarette smokers, and those with abnormal electrocardiograms.
- The majority of individuals with high blood pressure are not undergoing any therapy to control their blood pressure; many do not even know they have a problem.
- The cause of 90 percent to 95 percent of high-blood-pressure cases is unknown, however, once detected, the disease can be controlled.

- Hypertensive individuals have a three-to-four-times greater risk of developing coronary artery disease, and up to seven times the risk of stroke.
- High blood pressure is more prevalent among less-educated and lower socioeconomic groups.
- High blood pressure is more likely to occur in whites and blacks living in the Southeastern U.S.
- High blood pressure is particularly prevalent in blacks, middle-aged and elderly people, obese people, heavy drinkers, women taking oral contraceptives and people with diabetes.
- Fifty-two percent of people with high blood pressure are not taking medication.
- Only 21 percent of people with high blood pressure receive adequate medical therapy to lower it.
- Uncontrollable risk factors for high blood pressure are age, race, heredity and sex.
- Controllable risk factors include obesity, physical inactivity, sodium intake, alcohol consumption and use of oral contraceptives, appetite suppressants, decongestants and nonsteroidal anti-inflammatory drugs.

Table 5.2
How to Accurately Measure Blood Pressure

1. The subject should be seated in a comfortable position, with the right arm at approximately heart level. Universally, the right arm is used to measure resting blood pressure.

2. The subject should be relaxed and free of distractions.

3. The subject should wear a loose-fitting short-sleeve shirt or blouse. If a shirt sleeve must be rolled or pushed up to access the arm, remove the garment.

4. Determine proper cuff size ahead of time. After measuring arm circumference, refer to Table 5.3. Most blood pressure cuffs are marked with index lines that tell you if the cuff is the proper size (index lines should fall between the two range lines). Note: If the blood pressure cuff is too small, blood pressure will be overestimated; if the cuff is too big, blood pressure will be underestimated.

5. The subject's arm should be rotated outward (anatomical position) and held straight. Place the cuff on the arm so that the lower lip is approximately 1 inch above the antecuital space (the crease in the arm at the elbow joint).

6. Locate the brachial artery by palpating it. Then, firmly place the head (or diaphragm) of the stethoscope over the brachial artery.

7. Inflate the cuff to approximately 160 mmHg, or 20 to 30 mmHg above the expected or known pressure.

8. With the manometer (blood pressure gauge) in good view, adjust the air-release screw so the cuff pressure is reduced by 2 to 5 mmHg per second. Low readings may occur if the rate is too fast, and rapid deflation may cause erroneously high values.

9. Blood pressure is recorded as the first sound heard (systolic blood pressure) and the last sound heard (diastolic blood pressure).

10. Completely deflate the cuff between measurements.

11. Obtain resting blood pressure with the client in the supine, sitting and standing positions. Report large differences between the supine and standing blood pressures to the client's physician. Some individuals have a condition called orthostatic hypotension, which may cause lightheadedness or fainting, especially during exercise.

Source: *American Heart Association High Blood Pressure Fact Sheet* (51-2004-9-96-86-07-141). Dallas: American Heart Association.

prior to clearing an individual for exercise and establishing a training program, the potential benefits of exercise must be weighed against the potential risks. Factors to be considered when recommending exercise for individuals with high blood pressure include:

- Clinical status (stable or unstable hypertension)
- Current medication use (and their effect on exercise)
- Frequency, duration, intensity and mode of exercise that the individual currently is participating in (if any)
- Frequency, duration, intensity and mode of exercise that the individual wants to participate in
- How well the individual manages their hypertension
- Presence of other coronary artery disease risk factors
- Other medical or health conditions directly or indirectly associated with hypertension

Chapter 2 presents a review of general screening and evaluation procedures. In addition, measure resting blood pressure for all new clients (see Table 5.2 for proper technique). If you do not have experience measuring blood pressure, take a class or obtain training at a local hospital. If, during the screening, you detect hypertension, refer the client to their physician for medical clearance to exercise and follow up. If a new client is diagnosed with hypertension and currently is under the care of a physician, it is appropriate to obtain written clearance from the physician's office before the client begins an exercise program (Table 5.4).

During the initial interview, a complete history of the client's hypertension should be obtained. Include:

- At what age hypertension was first diagnosed
- Average resting blood pressure
- Current medications
- Other lifestyle medications that the client is following
- Unusual symptoms during or after exercise

Table 5.3
Guidelines for Choosing a Blood Pressure Cuff

Size (cm) (Upper-arm Circumference)	Type of Cuff	Bladder Size (cm)
33 - 47	Large Adult	33 or 42 x 15
25 - 35	Adult	24 x 12.5
18 - 26	Child	21.5 x 10

Once all of the appropriate information is gathered, decide if you can proceed or if a medical clearance is necessary. A physician's decision to perform an exercise test on a person with suspected hypertension is based on the client's medical history, the severity of the suspected hypertension and the risks versus the benefits of the test.

The benefits of exercise testing in hypertensive individuals include:

- Determining if blood pressure rises appropriately during exercise
- Evaluating the client for symptoms before, during and following exercise
- Recording baseline and exercise blood pressure
- Collection of exercise blood pressure measurements to help determine aerobic exercise intensity to be used during exercise sessions

Exercise Programming and Leadership

A client with clinically stable hypertension should begin an exercise program based on the same criteria used for sedentary individuals. See Table 5.5 for general activity guidelines and recommendations for hypertension.

Mode

The overall exercise training recommendations for individuals with mild to moderate hypertension are similar to those for apparently healthy individuals. Endurance exercise, such as low-impact aerobics, walking and swimming, should be the primary exercise mode. Avoid exercises with an intense isometric component in order to avoid potentially extreme fluctuations in blood pressure. Heavy strength training often has a significant isometric component, as well as most heavy pushing or pulling activities. Weight training can be prescribed, though not initially, using low resistance and high repetition.

Intensity

Low- to moderate-intensity dynamic exercise is recommended over high-intensity, high-impact exercise. High-intensity activities will usually result in both higher heart rates and blood pressures that may well exceed safe ranges and physician guidelines. The exercise intensity level should be near the low end of the heart-rate range (40 percent to 65 percent), and may gradually be increased to 55 percent to 70 percent as the client improves their functional capacity (A.C.S.M., 1995). Other techniques to monitor exercise intensity, such as RPE, breathing rate, and signs and symptoms also should be employed.

Frequency

Encourage hypertensive individuals to exercise at least five to six times per week. Daily exercise may be appropriate for the elderly or individuals with an initial low functional capacity.

Duration

Total exercise duration should gradually be increased, possibly to 30 to 60 minutes per ses-

---

Table 5.4

Client Information to Obtain from Medical Professionals

1) What medications is this client currently taking? How will they affect exercise training?	acceptable blood-pressure range during exercise? At what level should exercise cease?
2) Are there other medical /health conditions of which I should be aware (e.g., other risk factors, CAD, arthritis, etc.)	5) How often should I measure the client's blood pressure during exercise?
3) What are your goals for this client (e.g., reduce blood pressure or other risk factors)?	6) What symptoms, if any, should I watch for while the client is exercising?
4) Do you have any recommendations regarding exercise intensity and an	7) Please provide the results of any clinical exercise tests.
	8) Are any activities contraindicated for this client?

Table 5.5

Typical Activity Guidelines

- Instruct hypertensive individuals to avoid holding their breath and straining during exercise (Valsalva maneuver).

- Weight training should not be used as the primary form of exercise, but as a supplement to endurance training. Circuit training is preferred over free weights. Keep resistance low and repetitions high.

- Because hypertension medication may alter the accuracy of the training heart rate during exercise, intensity may need to be monitored with the RPE scale.

- Be aware of any changes in medications and/or any abnormal signs or symptoms before, during or immediately following exercise.

- The client's physician may have them record their blood pressure before and after exercise.

- Instruct individuals with hypertension to move slowly when making the transition

from floor positions to standing, since they are more susceptible to orthostatic hypotension when beginning to take antihypertensive medication.

- Both hypertensive and hypotensive responses are possible during and after exercise.

- Carefully monitor individuals with severe hypertension initially, and possibly long-term. Such individuals likely are taking one or more antihypertensive medications that can affect the exercise response. A detailed treatment plan, including specific exercise guidelines and blood pressure cut-off points, should be developed with the patient's physician and exercise staff so the exercise training is both safe and effective.

- Individuals with hypertension may have multiple CAD risk factors that should be considered when developing the exercise program.

sion, depending on the client's medical history and clinical status. Signs and symptoms of hyper- and hypotensive responses should be monitored before, during and after exercise.

Rate of Progression

Same as for a sedentary individual.

Conclusion

A well-designed and consistent exercise program can contribute significantly to the quality of life of a client challenged with hypertension. You as a trainer must make sure to complete a thorough assessment in order to determine the appropriateness of exercise training outside of a clinical setting. Specific guidelines from your client's physician and along the results of a maximal graded exercise test will give you important information in order to develop an effective exercise program. And finally, the exercise program should start conservatively and progress gradually, yet with consistent frequency in order to minimize the risk and maximize the benefits of physical activity.

Case Study 1

Medical History/Health History Questionnaire Results

Bob is a 44-year-old construction worker who is mildly overweight, has a history of hypertension and a family history of heart disease, and presently is trying to quit smoking. He had knee surgery one year ago to repair a torn tendon from a work-related injury, and never underwent any rehabilitation.

Previous Exercise/Diet History

Bob has never exercised. In fact, he is only seeking your services for exercising because his wife and doctor have been nagging him. He says, "I don't need to exercise. I work hard all day, and I think that's enough. Besides, when am I going to find time to exercise?"

Bob eats fast food for lunch almost every day, and his wife makes dinner. He does not watch his salt intake, and he does not drink.

Fitness Testing Results

Because Bob has several CAD risk factors, he undergoes an exercise stress test. The results of Bob's treadmill test are as follows.

Exercise Protocol: Bruce
Resting BP: 140/90
Resting HR: 59

STAGE	HR	BP
Stage 1: 1.7 MPH and 10% Grade		
1:00	102	
2:00	116	
3:00	130	148/96
Stage 2: 2.5 MPH and 12% Grade		
4:00	136	
5:00	140	
6:00	146	150/96
Stage 3: 3.4 MPH and 14% Grade		
7:00	150	
8:00	152	
9:00	160	185/102

Patient stopped because of fatigue.
No EKG abnormalities.
Max HR: 160
Max BP: 185/102

Exercise Prescription

Intensity:	40% = 100 bpm
	65% = 124 bpm
Duration:	15 to 20 minutes for
	first few weeks
	20 to 30 minutes
	after one month
Mode:	aerobic exercise
Frequency:	3 to 4 times per week

Other Suggestions for Health Enhancement

Reduce fast food intake, especially the higher-fat foods

Monitor and, if necessary, reduce salt intake.

Consult with a dietitian

Medical History / Health History Questionnaire Results

Sally is a sedentary 62-year-old retired school teacher. Her husband recently passed away and her neighbor has brought her to your facility. Sally's only risk factor for heart disease is her age. Her doctor has recently increased her estrogen intake, and has put her on a calcium supplement. She does have mild, sometimes severe, arthritis.

Previous Exercise / Diet History

Sally walks sometimes, and her diet is excellent. However, she's uncomfortable in a gym setting because she only sees young, fit people, and she's intimidated by the machines. She joined a health club 20 years ago, but only went for two weeks because she was constantly in pain.

Fitness Testing Results

Prior to exercise testing, Sally's resting blood pressure was 150/100. A second measure taken the next day shows 146/94. Based on her initial blood pressure readings, Sally needs to see a physician before participating in an exercise program.

Exercise Protocol: Bruce
Resting BP: 150/92
Resting HR: 80

STAGE	HR	BP
Stage 1: 1.7 MPH and 10% Grade		
1:00	100	
2:00	112	
3:00	120	152/96
Stage 2: 2.5 MPH and 12% Grade		
4:00	130	
5:00	136	
6:00	156	180/104
Stage 3: 3.4 MPH and 14% Grade		
7:00	150	

Patient stopped because of fatigue.
No EKG abnormalities.
Max HR: 156
Max BP: 180/104

Exercise Programming

Intensity:	40% = 110 bpm

	65% = 129 bpm
Duration:	10 to 15 minutes for
	first few weeks
	15 to 25 minutes after 1 month
Mode:	aerobic exercise
Frequency:	3 to 4+ times per week

Other Suggestions for Health Enhancement

Sally must find activities she can participate in away from the club.

Have Sally work out with a friend.

References

American Association of Cardiovascular and Pulmonary Rehabilitation. (1995). *Guidelines for Cardiac Rehabilitation Programs.* (2nd ed.) Champaign, Ill.: Human Kinetics.

American College of Sports Medicine. (1993). ACSM Position Stand: Physical Activity, Physical Fitness and Hypertension. *In Medicine and Science in Sports and Exercise,* 25, 10, i-x.

American College of Sports Medicine. (1995). *ACSM's Guidelines for Exercise Testing and Prescription.* Philadelphia: Williams and Wilkins.

American College of Sports Medicine. (1997). *Exercise Management For Persons with Chronic Diseases and Disabilities.* Champaign, Ill: Human Kinetics.

American Heart Association. *American Heart Association High Blood Pressure Fact Sheet* (51-2004-9-96-86-07-141). Dallas: American Heart Association.

American Heart Association. (1998). *Heart and Stroke Facts and Statistics.* Dallas: American Heart Association.

Duncan, J.J., Farr, J.E., Upton, J., Hagan, R.D., Oglesby, M.E. & Blair, S.N. (1985). The effects of aerobic exercise on plasma catecholamines and blood pressure in patients with mild hypertension. Journal of the *American Medical Association,* 254, 2609-2613.

Fifth Report on the Joint Committee on Detection, Evaluation, and Treatment of High Blood Pressure (JNCV). *Archives of Internal Medicine,* 153,154-183, 1993.

Gordon, N.F. & Scott, C.B. (1991). Exercise and Mild Essential Hypertension. In: Boone, J. L (Ed.) *Primary Care: Hypertension* (pp. 683-695). Philadelphia: W.B. Saunders.

Hagberg, J. M. (1991). Exercise, fitness, and hypertension. In: Bouchard, C., Shepard, R.J., Stephens, T., Sutton, J.R. & McPherson, B.D. (Eds.). *Exercise, Fitness and Health: A Consensus of Current Knowledge* (pp. 455-466). Champaign, Ill.: Human Kinetics.

Kenney, W.L. (1995). *ACSM's Guidelines for Exercise Testing and Prescription* (5th ed.) Philadelphia: Williams and Wilkins.

Tipton, C. M. (1991). Exercise, training, and hypertension: an update. In Hollozy, J.O. (Ed.) *Exercise and Sport Science Reviews* 19, 447-505. Baltimore: Williams and Wilkins.

Trials of Hypertension Prevention Collaborative Research Group. (1992). The effects of non-pharmacologic interventions of blood pressure persons with high normal levels: results of the Trials of Hypertension Prevention, Phase I. *Journal of the American Medical Association,* 267, 1213-1220.

World Hypertension League. (1991). Physical exercise in the management of hypertension: a consensus statement by the World Hypertension League. *Journal of Hypertension,* 9, 283-287.

CHAPTER 6

Coronary Artery Disease

SCOTT O. ROBERTS

Scott Owen Roberts, Ph.D., F.A.A.C.V.P.R., is an assistant professor at Texas Tech University in Lubbock. He has more than 15 years experience as a clinical exercise physiologist, and is a fellow of the American Association of Cardiovascular and Pulmonary Rehabilitation and an ACSM Certified Exercise Program Director. Dr. Roberts has published numerous original scientific articles, trade articles, chapters and books, including Exercise Physiology: Exercise Performance and Clinical Applications *and* Clinical Exercise Testing and Prescription: Theory and Application. *He also served as a section editor for* ACSM's Exercise Management for Persons with Chronic Diseases and Disabilities. *Dr. Roberts has served as a member of ACE's Aerobics Instructor Examination and Personal Trainer Committees.*

Angina
Post Myocardial Infarction

Post Bypass

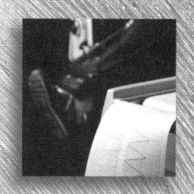

Cardiovascular disease continues to be the leading cause of death in the western world (American Heart Association, 1998). According to 1994 estimates, 57 million Americans have one or more forms of cardiovascular disease. In 1994 alone, cardiovascular diseases claimed more than 950,000 lives, almost half of all deaths in the United States. This year as many as 1.5 million Americans will have a new or recurrent heart attack, and about one-third of them will die as a result. Currently, two out of every five Americans die as a result of cardiovascular disease. The good news is that death rates from cardiovascular disease have been on the decline during the past few years. From 1984 to 1994, death rates from cardiovascular disease declined 22 percent. The reduction in death rates from cardiovascular diseases can be linked to lifestyle changes among Americans and advances in medical treatment. Still, cardiovascular disease is a major killer. Fortunately, it is a disease that is highly preventable.

Overview of
Coronary Artery Disease

Although there are a variety of cardiovascular diseases, including hypertension, stroke, congestive heart failure, etc., the majority of cardiovascular deaths is attributed to coronary artery disease. Coronary Artery Disease (CAD) results from a process known as atherosclerosis. Atherosclerosis occurs when the internal diameter of arteries begins to narrow. This is believed to be caused by injury to the inner lining of the arteries (caused by high blood pressures, high levels of LDL cholesterol, or other chemical agents, such as those from cigarettes). Once the inner lining has been damaged, plaques (consisting of calcified cholesterol and fat deposits) begin to reduce the diameter of the coronary artery.

Arteriosclerosis is a condition that develops as a result of adverse alterations in the arterial vasculature system (mainly in the majority of medium and larger arteries). Such adverse alterations may eventually lead to an inability of the arterial system to meet the demand for oxygen. When atherosclerosis affects the coronary arteries it is called coronary artery disease. When the coronary arteries are unable to meet the heart muscle's demand for oxygen, **myocardial ischemia** (reduced oxygen delivery) occurs. This can lead to **angina pectoris** (chest pain) or myocardial infarction (**heart attack**).

Angina is a symptom of a partial blockage of a coronary artery, while myocardial infarction is the result of a complete blockage. Some individuals suffer from a condition known as **silent ischemia**, which is the diagnosis of coronary artery disease in the absence of classical symptoms, such as chest pain. Such a diagnosis typically occurs following an exercise stress test. Silent ischemia is common among diabetics. There are also two different forms of angina — **stable angina** and **unstable angina**. Stable angina is the typical set of symptoms (discomfort in chest and a heavy, vise-like and/or squeezing pain that often radiates to the shoulders, jaw or neck) that usually occurs at predictable times, such as during stress or exercise (Table 6.1). Once the activity ceases, the pain usually subsides. In contrast, unstable angina occurs in individuals at unpredictable times, or even at rest. Unstable angina is considered a medical emergency, since it has the potential to progress to a myocardial infarction.

Other areas commonly affected by atherosclerosis include the carotid arteries, resulting in a transient ischemic attack (TIA) or cerebral vascular accident (stroke), and the femoral arteries, resulting in claudication. (See Chapters 7 and 20 for further discussions related to exercise in the presence of these disorders.)

Risk Factors for
Coronary Artery Disease

The origin into the study of the causes of CAD in the United States began in a small town in Massachusetts. In the late 1940s, residents of Framingham began to be screened in an effort to determine common characteristics or risk factors that contribute to the development of cardiovascular disease (Dawber, Meadors & Moore, 1951). Since the start of the Framingham study, hundreds of studies have investigated specific causes of coronary artery disease, all of which have led to the development of a list of identified risk factors for CAD (Table 6.2).

Lipid abnormalities, hypertension, diabetes and obesity are considered disease challenges in and of themselves, and are addressed as separate chapters within this text. All exercise programming and leadership for individuals with both CAD and any of these associated pathologies must not exceed the limitations related to CAD. For example, an overweight individual with an otherwise low cardiovascular risk may be able to exercise quite aggressively; however, given a diagnosis of

---

Table 6.1
Signs and Symptoms of Angina and Myocardial Infarction

- An uncomfortable pressure, fullness, squeezing, or pain in the center of the chest that lasts more than a few minutes, or goes away and returns.
- Pain that spreads to the shoulders, neck or arms.
- Chest discomfort with lightheadedness, fainting, sweating, nausea or shortness of breath.
- Chest pressure.

Table 6.2
Risk Factors for Coronary Artery Disease

Modifiable
- Cigarette smoking
- Hypertension
- Diabetes mellitus
- Hypercholesterollemia
- Physical inactivity
- Obesity
- Stress

Non-modifiable
- Age
- Sex
- Family history

CAD, the same individual's exercise program would change quite remarkably.

Smoking

The primary mechanism by which smoking increases CAD risk is through the toxic nature of the smoke, which can cause injury to the inner lining of the artery. In addition, cigarette smoking decreases the oxygen-carrying capacity of the blood and elevates blood pressure, heart rate and myocardial oxygen consumption. Cigarette smoke is linked to undesirable effects on platelet adhesiveness and clotting factors. Cigarette smokers are at greater risk for developing CAD, as well as other diseases. The risk of a heart attack increases with the number of cigarettes smoked per day. There is now evidence linking passive smoke and development of heart disease in non-smokers (Wells, 1988). The good news for smokers is that within a few years of quitting, their risk is reduced to the level of a nonsmoker (Hennekens & Buring, 1985).

Lipid Abnormalities

The association between cholesterol and CAD has been clearly linked. In fact, cholesterol abnormalities continue to be the major preventable risk factors for CAD. Early investigations looking at the association of CAD and cholesterol began with the Framingham study. Since the beginning of the study, numerous observational studies have confirmed that cholesterol is one of the strongest predictors of CAD.

Inactivity

The greater the physical level, expressed by total kcal expended per week, the less the risk of CAD. The exact mechanism relating to a decreased CAD morbidity and mortality with exercise is not entirely clear, but it is probably related to the favorable effects exercise has on blood pressure, obesity, diabetes, blood lipid abnormalities and fibrinolytic activity.

Diabetes

Coronary artery disease and diabetes mellitus are almost synonymous. Diabetes mellitus is often associated with obesity, hypertension, elevated LDL levels and depressed levels of HDL cholesterol. Coronary artery disease is the most common underlying cause of death in diabetic adults in the United States (Kleinman, Donahue & Harris, 1988). The risk of various heart diseases is twofold for diabetic men, and threefold for diabetic women.

High Blood Pressure

Hypertension is a major risk factor for CAD. Chronically elevated blood pressures are believed to alter blood flow patterns, which affects endothelial surfaces and may eventually cause an injury to these inner linings or the arteries, beginning the atherosclerotic process. There is a continuous and direct association between risk of morbidity and mortality from coronary heart disease and increasing levels of blood pressure (MacMahon, Petro & Cutler, 1990). Hypertension also is a major risk factor for stroke.

Obesity

Although not a primary risk factor, obesity is now recognized as an independent risk factor for CAD. Fat distribution is another predictor of CAD risk. The ratio of waist-to-hip circumference ratio correlates more closely with increased risk than do other parameters of obesity. In addition, individuals who carry excessive amounts of fat on their trunks also have greater risk for CAD than individuals who carry fat lower (gynoid obesity).

Treatment of Coronary Artery Disease

When coronary blood flow is unable to meet the heart's demand for oxygen, an individual typically feels chest pressure or chest pain. A temporary blockage or permanent blockage of blood flow can cause this. A temporary blockage is usually due to arterial spasm, whereas permanent blockage is due to stenosis from plaque build-up. A permanent blockage is dangerous because clots can form at these narrowed sections and result in a myocardial infarction.

If a permanent blockage is detected in one or more coronary arteries, typical treatments include medical management, **coronary artery bypass grafting** (CABG) and percutaneous **transluminal coronary angioplasty** (PTCA). Less severe cases of CAD are typically treated with lifestyle modification and medical therapy. Coronary artery bypass grafting is a procedure in which a vein is removed from the patient's leg and sewn from the aorta to the coronary artery, to bypass the blockage. This procedure does appear to prolong life in patients with severe three-vessel disease, but in comparison to medical therapy, it does not seem to prolong life in those patients with less severe disease. However, total relief of angina typically occurs in 60 percent to 75 percent of patients during the first five years following a CABG.

The use of percutaneous transluminal coronary angioplasty (a procedure that uses a small balloon at the tip of a heart catheter to push open plaques) is on the rise. Most patients today who undergo a PTCA have a permanent wire mesh inserted at the point of the angioplasty. This wire mesh device, known as a stent, is expanded within the blockage in order to reduce the potential re-stenosis (old plaque returning to original state) and helps improve recovery.

Some new forms of plaque removal, such as coronary laser (burning the plaque) and high-speed rotational atherectomy (cutting and removing the plaque), are still considered to be experimental.

Diagnostic Testing in Coronary Artery Disease

Diagnostic testing for CAD can be divided into two groups of tests: noninvasive and invasive. Noninvasive tests can be conducted without entering the patient's body. Examples of these tests include the graded exercise test, echocardiogram and myocardial perfusion imaging. In contrast, invasive procedures involve entering the patient's body to gather the information necessary to make a diagnosis. The primary invasive procedure used in the diagnosis of CAD is cardiac catheterization.

Clinical Exercise Testing

Clinical exercise testing has three main uses: a) to diagnose the presence or severity of disease, b) to establish the functional capacity of an individual, and c) to evaluate medical therapy. Diagnostic evaluation of suspected or established cardiovascular disease is perhaps the most common clinical application of clinical exercise testing. The exercise test is probably the best test of the heart because it represents the most common everyday stress that humans experience. Table 6.3 lists common uses of clinical exercise testing.

Before a physician orders a clinical exercise test, sufficient evidence must be present and documented to justify the test. With any kind of exercise testing or exercise prescription, the benefits must outweigh the potential risks. One of the most common reasons for ordering a clinical exercise test is to diagnose and evaluate the status of suspected or known cardiovascular disease. An example of when clinical exercise testing is indicated is when a patient comes to a physician's office for a regular check-up so he/she can begin an exercise program. The physician discovers that the patient is sedentary, overweight, a regular smoker, has high cholesterol and has recently complained of several episodes of chest pain during physical exertion. Because the patient in question is at high risk for CAD, the physician should order a clinical exercise evaluation before allowing the patient to exercise.

Clinical exercise testing is an effective way of evaluating an individual's cardiovascular response to controlled physiological stress (exercise). Regardless if the patient passes or fails the test, both the physician and patient will be better assured of the patient's ability or inability to participate in an exercise program. Thus, clinical exercise testing is useful in diagnosing or quantifying heart and/or other chronic disease conditions.

Clinical exercise testing also is commonly used to determine the functional capacity of healthy, sedentary and/or asymptomatic individuals. For example, after an individual has suffered a heart attack or is recovering from a coronary bypass operation, clinical exercise testing is useful in developing an exercise program. Exercise testing

Table 6.3
Uses of Clinical Exercise Testing

Exercise Testing Apparently Healthy Individuals	Exercise Testing High Risk Individuals	Exercise Testing Individuals With A Known Disease
Determine functional capacity	Diagnostic tool	Determine functional capacity
Screen for disease	Evaluation of suspected heart disease	After myocardial infarction
Motivation	Evaluation of asymptomatic individuals with risk of coronary heart disease	After heart surgery
Develop an exercise prescription	After myocardial infarction	After repair of heart valves or defects
	After coronary angioplasty	Chronic pulmonary disease
	Evaluate dysrhythmias	Chronic renal disease
	Peripheral vascular disease	Diabetes
	Evaluate medical therapy	Evaluate medical therapy

can be used to develop a safe and effective level of exercise for individuals with or without disease. The results of an exercise test can be used to set the initial intensity, duration and frequency of exercise. Follow-up testing can be used to modify an earlier exercise program.

Echocardiogram

An echocardiogram is a safe and painless diagnostic procedure that uses high-frequency sound waves (ultrasound) to take dynamic pictures of the heart. Sound waves, emitted from a transducer, penetrate the patient's chest wall so that various cardiac structures can be observed. From the echocardiogram recordings, it is possible to measure the size of the chambers of the heart, how well the heart valves are working and how forcefully the heart muscle is contracting. Doppler echocardiography is another form of echocardiography that uses sound waves to measure the speed, amount and direction of blood flow. With doppler echocardiography, accurate measurements of cardiac output and stroke volume can be obtained.

Perfusion Imaging

Myocardial perfusion imaging is a diagnostic exam used to evaluate the adequacy of blood supply to the heart. Prior to the start of an exercise test, an intravenous line is inserted into the patient's arm. At peak exercise, a radioisotope is injected into the IV line. The radioisotope is then carried to the heart via the blood. Immediately after the patient ceases exercise, a special camera that can detect radiation visualizes the Thallium-201 as it flows to the heart. If the coronary arteries are clear, Thallium-201 is absorbed evenly throughout the myocardium within a matter of minutes. The first set of pictures taken immediately following exercise determines the adequacy of blood supply to the heart during stress.

If the coronary arteries are normal, the myocardium will receive approximately the same amount of radioactive isotope and the pictures will have a uniform appearance. If one or more of the coronary arteries is blocked, a portion of the myocardium will not receive the isotope and the pictures will show a spot of nonabsorption, sometimes referred to as a "cold spot." After a period of time, the isotope is eventually absorbed into the tissue, and the cold spot disappears. The second set of pictures, taken several hours after exercise, helps to differentiate between exercise-induced ischemia and an area of non-absorbing tissue (usually resulting from a heart attack). Old heart attacks will leave a scar on the heart muscle, and these scars or injuries will not absorb the isotope at all. If the cold spot was caused by exercise-induced ischemia (temporarily reduced isotope absorption), the second set of pictures will be normal. If the cold spot was caused by scar tissue, then the second set of pictures will be abnormal as well. The location of the absorption defects can be used to predict which coronary artery is blocked.

Catheterization

Cardiac catheterization is an "invasive procedure," meaning the body is entered in some way. Cardiac catheterization is the most accurate method of measuring a patient's heart performance and is the only way of determining which coronary arteries are blocked, and to what degree. The entire procedure lasts less than an hour, during which a narrow, flexible tube (catheter) is inserted through the brachial or femoral artery. After the catheter has been inserted into the artery, it is slowly advanced toward the heart while the physician watches its progress on a monitor. During a left ventricular angiogram, the catheter is advanced into the left ventricle. Dye is then injected and a series of pictures is obtained during contraction. During a coronary angiogram, a catheter is inserted into the opening of either the left or right main coronary artery. Dye is injected through the catheter into each coronary artery, and an X-ray camera takes a series of pictures of the coronary arteries. These pictures will detect areas of narrowing (blockages) and assess their severity.

Role of Exercise in Coronary Artery Disease

Clearly, regular physical activity reduces the risk of CAD. How effective is exercise at treating CAD? Initially, extended bed rest was recommended for patients recovering from a myocardial infarction. It was believed that the heart takes approximately six weeks to heal after a heart attack, and that any undue stress might compromise the healing process. Although the heart may be healing OK, the rest of the body is slowly deteriorating. Bed rest results in: a) a decrease in work capacity, b) a decreased adaptability to changes in position, c) a decrease in blood volume, d) a decrease in muscle mass, e) increased risk of thromboembolism, and f) a decrease in respiratory and pulmonary function.

In the early 1940s, physicians began experimenting with early mobilization after a cardiac event, and the results were favorable. Early mobilization of cardiac patients resulted in fewer complications, a faster recovery and a reduction in many of the other related complications of bed rest mentioned above. Today, exercise is a standard therapeutic modality in the treatment of cardiac disease. In almost all cases, individuals recovering from a myocardial infarction, cardiac surgery or other cardiac procedure should benefit from a supervised **cardiac rehabilitation** program and, eventually, outpatient exercise.

The comprehensive rehabilitation of cardiac patients is collectively referred to as "cardiac

---

Table 6.4
Benefits of Exercise in the Prevention and Treatment of Coronary Artery Disease

---

Maintain or Increase Myocardial Oxygen Supply
- Delay progression of coronary artery disease (possible).
- Improve lipoprotein profile (increase HDL-C/LDL-C ratio, decrease triglycerides) (probable).
- Improve carbohydrate metabolism (increase insulin sensitivity) (probable).
- Decrease platelet aggregation and increase fibrinolysis (probable).
- Decrease adiposity (usually).
- Increase coronary collateral vascularization (unlikely).
- Increase epicardial artery diameter (possible).
- Increase coronary blood flow (myocardial perfusion) or distribution (possible).

Decrease Myocardial Work and Oxygen Demand
- Decrease heart rate at rest and submaximal (usually).
- Decrease systolic and mean systemic arterial pressure during submaximal exercise (usually) and at rest (usually).
- Decrease cardiac output during submaximal exercise (probable).
- Decrease circulating plasma catecholamine levels at rest (probable) and at submaximal exercise (usually).

Increase Myocardial Function
- Increase stroke volume at rest and in submaximal and maximal exercise (likely).
- Increase ejection fraction at rest and during exercise (likely).
- Increase intrinsic myocardial contractility (possible). Increase myocardial function resulting from decreased afterload (probable).
- Increase myocardial hypertrophy (probable); but this may not reduce CHD risk.

Increase Electrical Stability of Myocardium
- Decrease regional ischemia or at submaximal exercise (possible).
- Decrease catecholamines in myocardium at rest (possible) and at submaximal exercise (probable).
- Increase ventricular fibrillation threshold due to reduction of cyclic AMP (possible).

Source: Haskell, W.L. (1985). Mechanisms by which physical activity may enhance the clinical status of cardiac patients. In M.L. Pollock & Schmidt (Eds) *Heart Disease and Rehabilitation* (2nd edition). New York: John Wiley & Sons, pp 276-296.

---

rehabilitation." Cardiac rehabilitation is defined as the process by which a person with cardiovascular disease, including but not limited to patients with coronary heart disease, is restored to and maintained at his or her optimal physiological, psychological, social, vocational and emotional status. It is typically divided into three or four phases. Phase One is the period directly following the event up until the patient leaves the hospital. During this period, the focus is on overcoming deconditioning from bed rest and educating the patient about recovery. During Phase Two, the patient attends regular exercise and education classes. During exercise in Phase Two, the patient is generally continually monitored via an ECG telemeter. Phases Three and Four are maintenance phases. Phase Three is usually an outpatient program, while Phase Four is usually considered the exercise a cardiac patient will do on their own or in a community-based facility.

The benefits of exercise for individuals with CAD are numerous (Table 6.4). By getting a patient out of bed as soon as possible following a cardiac event, the deconditioning effects of bed rest are minimized. A progressive exercise program then serves to return an individual to an optimal level of function from not only a physical perspective, but a psychological one as well.

Benefits for Individuals with Angina

Individuals with stable angina generally benefit from exercise training. One of the primary benefits of exercise for individuals with angina is to raise their **ischemic threshold**. This is the point where the symptoms of angina appear recurrently whenever cardiac oxygen demands become too great in relation to the coronary blood flow — during exercise, for example. The ischemia associated with this type of angina generally appears at a reproducible threshold (Figure 6.1). The rate-pressure product (heart rate x systolic blood pressure) is used to determine this threshold. At the beginning of an exercise, a client with stable angina may start to develop anginal symptoms at 7 METS and a rate pressure product of 25,200 (sbp 180 mmHg x 140 bpm). Following an exercise training program, the individual's ischemic threshold is increased to 9 METS at the same double product before he or she begins developing symptoms. Thus, the individual has reduced the oxygen demand on the heart at any given work-

load or oxygen uptake, but the angina occurred at the same rate-pressure product.

Following Myocardial Infarction

Initially, the goal of early mobilization in the hospital for post-MI patients is to overcome the physical and psychological effects of bed rest and to educate the patient and family on the disease process and risk-reduction strategies. The benefits of continued exercise in outpatient settings include: a) improved functional capacity, b) improved oxygen and blood flow, c) thinning of blood, d) improved ventricular performance, and e) relief of anginal symptoms.

Following Bypass Surgery

Initially, the goal of early mobilization in the hospital for post-CABG patients is also to overcome the physical and psychological effects of bed rest. Secondary benefits include: a) overcoming the side-effects of surgery (muscular soreness, stiffness), b) improving functional capacity, and c) secondary prevention of coronary artery disease.

Exercise Assessment Procedures

Proper assessment of a client is critical to designing and leading a safe and effective exercise program. While some clients will come to you as a result of a physician or cardiac rehabilitation referral, most will seek your assistance on their own.

Those who have two or more cardiac risk factors, symptoms, or known disease, must have a physician release and referral to exercise in a community-based setting (Figure 2.2, Chapter 2). Individuals with a history of angina, myocardial infarction or post-CABG all fall into this category. Thus, rarely would submaximal fitness testing prior to entry into an exercise program be appropriate in this group. Once the results of a treadmill test have been completed, the results can be used to establish a safe exercise level. The exact exercise program should be based on the information you gather from your client's physician (Table 6.5).

For a review of general screening and evaluation procedures, see Chapter 2. Standardized exercise testing procedures should be used for persons with angina or myocardial infarction, or following a CABG. All of these conditions place most individuals into the high-risk category and, thus, all exercise testing should be performed in a medical setting. The results can be used to formulate an exercise program. Other fitness testing, such as follow-up fitness testing, may also need to be performed in a medical setting, or in the presence of trained individuals. If a client has been exercising consistently with no symptoms and your client's physician will approve it, submaximal exercise testing may be appropriate for evaluation.

Assessment Guidelines

If your client has been diagnosed with angina, it is important to determine the history of anginal symptoms. This would include: a) how long the symptoms have been present, b) a description of symptoms, c) current medications, d) identification of what triggers the pain, e) identification of what relieves the pain, and f) current medications. Scales are available to subjectively rate anginal pain (Table 6.6).

For the client that is post-MI, explicit physician guidelines are essential. Clients can generally obtain a copy of their discharge activity guidelines to bring to the evaluation appointment. Also, if the client participated in a supervised cardiac rehabilitation program it would be helpful to have those results. Likewise, a current list of all medications is important to review before starting a post-MI client on an exercise program. Post-MI patients must be cleared and released for exercise by their physi-

cian before being permitted to exercise in a community-based setting.

When a potential client comes to you following coronary artery bypass surgery, make sure you obtain a physician referral with specific guidelines. Important assessment questions should involve: a) presence of any residual surgical pain, b) current activity level, c) any medical restrictions, and d) a review of current medications. Most post-CABG patients recovery quickly. Remember that these patients now have additional blood flow to their heart, which theoretically should allow them to exercise harder and longer.

Graded Exercise Test Results

A normal physiological response to graded exercise includes a heart rate that increases linearly with workload. If oxygen consumption is measured it will also increase in the same fashion. Systolic blood pressure also increases linearly with workload, while diastolic blood pressure should stay the same, slightly increase or decrease (within 10 mmHg). There should be no changes in the electrocardiogram that indicates ischemia (Table 6.5). There should be no significant arrythymias.

Responses to Dynamic Exercise

A normal response to exercise is an increase in cardiac output and a decrease in total peripheral resistance (Figure 6.2). When the heart muscle is damaged (due to an infection or myocardial infarction), the ability to respond to the increased demands of exercise may be reduced. The diseased heart has less reserve to respond to an increased demand; thus, cardiac output and stroke volume may not increase in a normal fashion. Another sign of heart failure is a drop in heart rate or a failure of HR to increase during exercise. A drop in or a failure of SBP to rise during incremental exercise is another a sign of a failing heart. **ST segment depression** below the baseline is the classic ECG response to coronary insufficiency, or myocardial ischemia. Myocardial ischemia results from an imbalance between myocardial oxygen supply and demand. The cause of this imbalance is almost always the result of atherosclerotic plaques that narrow and sometimes completely block the blood supply to the heart.

**Figure 6.1
Exercise and the
Ischemic Threshold**

Following exercise training, with or without medical therapy, patients can perform more work before reaching the ischemic threshold.

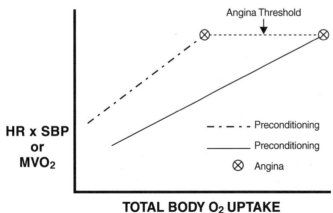

HR x SBP or MVO$_2$

Angina Threshold

- - - - Preconditioning
——— Preconditioning
⊗ Angina

TOTAL BODY O$_2$ UPTAKE WORKLOAD

Graded Exercise Test Summary Sheets

On page 65, you will find an example of a typical summary sheet from a graded exercise test (GXT). Although personal trainers are not expected to have the skills, training and knowledge to interpret a graded exercise test, all personal trainers working with clients with coronary disease should be able to look at a summary sheet and identify key information needed to safely develop an exercise program. Following is an explanation of this summary sheet and key points (as illustrated in Figure 6.3):

1. Evaluating the person for an exercise program, consider why he or she needed the test in the first place. Consider what are normal and abnormal responses for this person.
2. Know what effects various drugs have on the exercise test and exercise prescription (Appendix B).
3. Nonspecific ST changes at rest mean that the ST changes were not clinically significant.
4. Bruce protocol is the most common GXT protocol.
5. Do you think just under five minutes is a good performance for a 65-year-old male?
6. Normal BP and HR response.
7. This confirms a maximal effort for this individual.
8. Double product is maximum heart rate multiplied by maximum blood pressure.

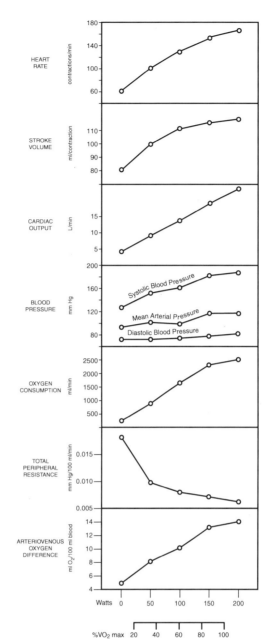

Figure 6.2

Normal Responses to Graded Exercise

Table 6.5

Client Information to Obtain from Medical Professionals

1) What is the diagnosis?
2) Is this person safe to exercise in a community-based exercise setting?
3) What specific guideline do you have regarding the person's maximum heart rate and/or blood pressure during physical activity?
4) What activities do you recommend; what are contraindicated?
5) Do you have specific guidelines related to frequency and duration of activity?
6) Have any signs or symptoms of myocardial ischemia been exhibited?
7) Are symptoms predictable with certain activities, or do they occur anytime?
8) Have any other symptoms been exhibited?
9) Has the client had any other recent surgeries or invasive procedures?
10) Is there any other unassociated medical/health conditions?
11) What medications is the patient taking and what is their effect on exercise testing and training?
12) What are your goals for the patient?

The double product is a good indication of overall myocardial oxygen demand.

9. It looks like this patient did not exercise to his predicted time for his age. What does this tell you (sedentary)?

10. This is a positive treadmill test. This person probably has serious CAD.

This was a positive treadmill test. The client more than likely would not be cleared to exercise until the source of the ischemia (ST-segment depression) was determined.

Fitness Testing for the Personal Trainer

If a client has been explicitly cleared for both submaximal fitness testing and exercise by his/her physician, submaximal fitness testing may by used to track changes in fitness in clients with stable disease. Personal trainers should never perform diagnostic exercise tests or even give the impression that their tests are diagnostic. Fitness tests that are appropriate for personal trainers include body composition assessment and flexibility testing. Muscular strength and endurance testing should be performed only once the client has physician clearance and has established a safe exercise routine under the direction of a qualified trainer.

Exercise Guidelines and Programs

Exercise guidelines are based on the clinical status of the patient. Low-risk cardiac patients should have established stable cardiovascular and physiological responses to exercise. Low risk is generally classified as those patients who:

a) had an uncomplicated clinical course in the hospital

b) have no evidence of resting or exercise-induced ischemia (ST-segment depression)

c) have functional capacities >6 to 8 METS three weeks following the clinical event

d) have normal ventricular function **ejection fraction** (EF) greater than 50 percent, and

e) do not have any significant resting or exercise-induced ventricular arrhythmias.

Following hospital discharge, some patients who are low risk (no complications in hospital and have good functional capacity) may have home exercise prescribed. These patients would

benefit by participating in a moderate exercise program at a fitness facility, in addition to their home exercise regime. Patients following hospital discharge who fall into higher risk categories (complications in the hospital, a large MI, poor functional capacity <4 METS) should be referred to a supervised cardiac rehabilitation program first. Once the cardiac rehab program is completed and the patient meets the criteria in Table 6.7, they are usually cleared to exercise.

Angina

Only clients who have stable angina and who have been cleared to exercise by their physician should be allowed to exercise in a community-based setting. A client with stable angina has reproducible pain during periods of stress or physical exertion. Once the stimulus is removed, the pain stops. The ischemia associated with brief anginal attacks is usually temporary and reversible, and can be relieved by rest and, in severe cases, nitroglycerin. A client with stable angina may experience a sudden increase in the frequency and duration of pain when exercising, or even at rest. When such changes occur, the client's physician should be notified at once. Most often, angina is described as a tightness, heaviness or constriction in the chest. The goal of angina therapy is to improve the patient's quality of life by decreasing the attacks of chest pain and decreasing the possibility of a heart attack. Common medications prescribed for this situation include beta blockers, nitrates, calcium-channel blockers and aspirin.

Clients with stable angina should be able to perform most exercises that apparently healthy individuals can. Trainers must be aware of changes in symptoms. If at any time during exercise a client complains of chest discomfort, stop the exercise immediately. If the pain does not subside, instruct the client to take his/her nitroglycerin. The nitroglycerin should help relieve the pain. If after three

Table 6.6
Angina Scale

1+	Light, barely noticeable
2+	Moderate, bothersome
3+	Severe, very uncomfortable
4+	Most severe or intense pain ever experienced

Hope Hospital • 555 Anystreet • Anycity, Montana 55000
GRADED EXERCISE TEST DATA FORM

| Patient Name: | John Doe | | | Patient Number: | 123456789 |

| Date of Birth: | 10/03/33 | Age: | 65 | Gender: | ☑Male ☐ Female |

② Medications: Propranolol and Aspirin

Referring MD:	B. J. Smith	① Test Indication:	Angina
Resting BP:	120/80	Resting HR:	61
		Predicted MHR:	159

Current Medical History:

④ Test Protocol: Bruce

Stage	Minute	Speed (MPH)	Grade (%)	Heart Rate ⑥	Blood Pressure ⑥
Supine				84	120/80
Standing				109	
I	1	1.7	10	125	
	2			142	
	3			137	125/70
II	4	2.5	12	159 ⑦	
	5			172	142/85

Recovery Minute	Heart Rate	Blood Pressure
1	123	
2	91	130/85
3	104	
4	103	120/80
5	100	114/80
6	93	
7		
8		
9		
10		

Test Results:
1. Total exercise time: 4:45 min. ⑤ Total METS: 6.7
2. Max HR: 182   Max BP: 140/85
3. Max HR achieved/Max HR predicted: 101 percent
4. Predicted HR/target HR: 180/153
5. Double product: 23.6 (thousands) ⑧   ⑨
6. Predicted age/sex exercise duration (minutes): 8.5
Normal heart rate and blood pressure response
Test stopped for ST segment depression (>2mm)
No arrhythmias observed

③ ST Segment Response:
Resting EKG - Nonspecific ST change(s). ST changes inferior leads and V6.

Exercise EKG - Horizontal ST depression 2-3 mm inferior leads and V3-V6. ST elevation 2 mm AVR. ST segment returns to baseline in recovery within 1-5 min.

Impression: ⑩
Positive for ischemia.
Specificity reduced due to resting EKG changes.

Other comments: A Stress Echo was performed and hypokinesis of a small inferior segment was found during exercise, with normal increases in ejection fraction during exercise. Resting ejection fraction was in the 50s and post-exercise in the 60s.

Figure 6.3

Exercise Test Results

nitroglycerin tablets, or 15 minutes, the pain persists, or if symptoms of a heart attack become present, call 911. Hypotension is always a concern following the administration of nitroglycerin; thus, clients should be seated and blood pressure should be monitored during and after administration.

Exercise Guidelines for Angina Clients
1. Clients' CAD risk factors should be well established and documented.
2. Clients should receive clearance from their physician before being allowed to exercise.
3. Monitor exercise intensity closely. Make sure the client is within his/her physician-prescribed exercise heart rate of RPE range. Also monitor signs and symptoms.
4. The client must inform the fitness instructor if he/she has any abnormal signs or symptoms before, during or after exercise.

Table 6.7
Guidelines for Progression to Independent Exercise with Minimal or No Supervision

1. Functional capacity >8 METS or twice the level of occupational demand.
2. Appropriate hemodynamic response to exercise (increase in BP with increasing workload) and recovery.
3. Appropriate ECG response at peak exercise with normal or unchanged conduction, stable or absent arrhythmias, and stable and acceptable ischemic response.
4. Cardiac symptoms stable or absent.
5. Stable and/or controlled baseline HR and BP.
6. Adequate management of risk factor intervention.
7. Demonstrated knowledge of the disease process, signs and symptoms, medication use and side effects.
8. Demonstrated compliance and success with a program or risk intervention.

Kenney, W.L. (1995). *ACSM's Guidelines for Exercise Testing and Prescription,* 5th Edition. Philadelphia, Pa.: Williams & Wilkins.

5. The exercise intensity level should be kept low to start, and gradually increased over time.
6. Clients with angina should be able to define angina, identify their own symptoms and describe the treatment for it.
7. Clients with a history of angina must carry nitroglycerin tablets with them at all times.

Sample Exercise Prescription for Angina

Mode   Dynamic exercise, such as low impact aerobics, walking, etc. Isometric exercises should be avoided. If physician clearance includes it, weight training can be included using low resistance and high repetitions.

Intensity Low-intensity dynamic exercise. The exercise intensity should be set at a low percentage of the individual's maximal heart rate reserve (40 percent to 65 percent). Another method is to set the training heart rate 10 to 25 bpm below the client's ischemic threshold. Trainers should get in the habit of using a variety of methods to monitor clients, such as HR, RPE, signs and symptoms and overall fatigue level.

Frequency Clients should be encouraged to exercise at least 3 to 6 times per week. Clients with low functional capacities may benefit from daily exercise.

Duration Encourage a longer and more gradual warm-up and cool-down (> 10

minutes). Total exercise duration should be gradually increased to 20 to 30 or more minutes.

Myocardial Infarction

Only clients who have stable cardiovascular responses to exercise, are low-risk and who have been cleared to exercise by their physician should be allowed to exercise in an outpatient setting. Clients who are post-MI generally have low functional capacities. A treadmill test should be performed on all patients recovering from a myocardial infarction before beginning an exercise program. Low-risk patients are generally classified as those who: a) had an uncomplicated clinical course in the hospital, b) have no evidence of resting or exercise-induced ischemia (ST-segment depression), c) have functional capacities >6 to 8 METS three weeks following the clinical event, d) have normal ventricular function EF >50 percent, and e) do not have any significant resting or exercise-induced ventricular arrhythmia. Thus, until a client meets these criteria, he or she should not exercise in an outpatient setting, such as a health club.

Exercise Guidelines for Post-Myocardial Infarction

1. Clients' CAD risk factors should be well established and documented.
2. All clients should receive clearance from their physician before being allowed to exercise.
3. Monitor exercise intensity closely. Make sure the client is within his/her physician-prescribed exercise heart rate of RPE range. Also monitor signs and symptoms.

4. The client must inform the fitness instructor if he/she has any abnormal signs or symptoms before, during or after exercise.

5. The exercise intensity level should be kept low to start, and gradually increased over time.

6. Avoid high-intensity exercise.

7. Try and select exercise equipment that allows the intensity level to be set very low (1 to 2 MET level).

8. Monitor the client very closely for signs and symptoms of chest pain and ischemia.

Sample Exercise Prescription for Stable Post-MI

Mode: Dynamic exercise, such as low impact aerobics, walking, etc. Isometric exercises should be avoided. Weight training should be prescribed using low resistance and high repetitions.

Intensity: Low-intensity dynamic exercise is recommended. The exercise intensity should be set at a low percentage of the individual's maximal heart rate reserve (40 percent to 60 percent).

Frequency: Clients should be encouraged to exercise at least 3 to 4 times per week. Clients with low functional capacities may benefit from daily exercise.

Duration: Encourage a longer and more gradual warm-up and cool-down (> 10 minutes). Total exercise duration should be gradually increased to 20 to 40 minutes.

Post PTCA/STENT

Clients recovering from an uncomplicated PTCA with or without a stent placement should for the most part follow the post-CABG guidelines. Unless the patient has had a heart attack prior to the PTCA, the improvement in blood flow to the heart should allow them to do more work than they were able to do before the procedure. Trainers should be aware that in a small percentage of individuals following a PTCA procedure, new clots form or the angioplasty fails. When this occurs, the client will start complaining of chest pain again. Such changes in signs and symptoms should be reported to a physician at once.

Post-bypass Surgery

Only clients who have stable cardiovascular responses to exercise and have been cleared to exercise by their physician should be allowed to exercise in community-based setting. Clients who are post-CABG generally have higher functional capacities than post-MI clients. Clients recovering from open-heart surgery should progress much faster, and with fewer symptoms, than someone recovering from a heart attack. Avoid weight-training activities until the client has been exercising successfully for six to eight weeks and physician clearance has been given.

Exercise Guidelines for Post-CABG

1. Clients' CAD risk factors should be well established and documented.

2. All clients should receive clearance from their physician before being allowed to exercise. See ACSM Risk Stratification chart below.

3. Monitor exercise intensity closely. Make sure the client is within his/her physician-prescribed exercise heart rate of RPE range. Also monitor signs and symptoms.

4. The client must inform the fitness instructor if he/she has any abnormal signs or symptoms before, during or after exercise.

5. The exercise intensity level should be kept low to start, and gradually increased over time.

6. Avoid high-intensity exercise.

7. Try and select exercise equipment that allows the intensity level to be set very low (one to two METS level).

8. Monitor the client very closely for signs and symptoms of chest pain and ischemia.

9. Upper extremity range-of-motion exercises are important.

Sample Exercise Prescription for Stable Post-CABG

Mode Dynamic exercise, such as low impact aerobics, walking, etc. Isometric exercises should be avoided. Weight training should be prescribed using low resistance and high repetitions.

Intensity Low-intensity dynamic exercise versus high-intensity, high impact exercise is recommended. The exercise intensity should be set at a low percentage of the individual's maximal heart rate reserve (40 percent to 65 percent). Other parameters such as RPE, fatigue level and overall signs and symptoms should also be considered.

Frequency Clients should be encouraged to exercise at least 3 to 7 times per week. Clients with low functional capacities may benefit from daily exercise.

Duration Encourage a longer and more gradual warm-up and cool-down (> 10 minutes). Total exercise duration should be gradually increased to 20 to 60 minutes.

Special Precautions

Clients must be aware of their individual risk factors and must recognize signs and symptoms of their disease. The majority of these clients will have a prescription for nitroglycerin. They must always carry it with them and know the proper protocol for taking it. If a client develops chest pain, stop exercise immediately, and follow standardized emergency procedures. All fitness instructors who work with clients must be CPR certified and be knowledgeable of the common effects of cardiac medications on resting, exercise and maximal heart rate and blood pressure.

Conclusion

Perhaps more than any other of the health challenges addressed in this book, the role of exercise in coronary artery disease is the most well understood. While exercise provides numerous well-documented benefits, it also carries with it inherent risks when not properly performed.

The key to working with clients with CAD is to gather explicit guidelines from the client's physician and to progress conservatively. Be knowledgeable of your client's "normal" symptoms and be sensitive to any symptom changes. The referring physician must be informed at the outset of the type of exercise setting in which you will be working. The exercise program you design for your client must never exceed the guidelines given by the

client's physician. If you are unable to obtain the necessary guidelines from your client's physician you should delay your involvement until the information is available.

With proper information collection, conservative programming and leadership, you can help clients with coronary artery disease begin or return to regular physical activity and optimal quality of life.

Case Studies

Case Study #1 (Post-CABG)

Medical History / Health History Questionnaire Results

Bob is a 36-year-old construction worker. He is mildly overweight, has hypertension, a family history of heart disease and is presently trying to quit smoking. One month ago, he complained of chest pain at work, and was subsequently rushed to hospital. A coronary angiogram confirmed that he had two blocked arteries. Physicians tried to do angioplasty to open his clogged arteries, but the procedure did not work. Subsequently, as a preventive measure, Bob had open-heart surgery. His recovery in the hospital was excellent. His follow-up test results are below (Figure 6.5).

Previous Exercise / Diet History

Never exercised before. Only reason he is exercising is because his wife and doctor have told him he needs to. Eats fast food for lunch every day. Only good meal is dinner.

Summary of Client Interview

Thinks he gets enough exercise at work. "Hey I work hard all day, isn't that enough!" "When am I going to possibly find the time to exercise?"

Exercise Program

Mode Need to find out what he will be willing to do. Perhaps walking will be best. Weight training should be prescribed using low resistance and high repetitions as soon as possible because of the nature of his work.

Intensity RHR = 60

MHR = 176

Heart-Rate Reserve Method: HR 130 (60 percent) to 141 (70 percent).

(His physician recommends that he exercise at a bit higher intensity than the usual post-

GRADED EXERCISE TEST DATA FORM

Patient Name:	Bob		Patient Number:	123456789
Date of Birth:		Age: 35	Gender: ☑Male ☐ Female	
Medications:	ADA, Coumadin and Procardia			

Referring MD:	B. J. Smith	Test Indication:	Angina, post-CABG
Resting BP:	140/90	Resting HR:	59

Current Medical History: This 36-year-old male had one episode of chest pain one month ago. Coronary angiography revealed that he had two narrowed arteries. A double bypass operation was performed without any complications.

Figure 6.4

Exercise Test Results

Test Protocol: Bruce

Stage	Stage Time	Speed (MPH)	Grade (%)	Heart Rate	Blood Pressure
Supine				60	120/80
Standing				80	
I	1:00	1.7	10	86	
	2:00			102	
	3:00			120	125/76
II	4:00	2.5	12	136	
	5:00			140	
	6:00			146	140/80
III	7:00	3.4	14	150	
	8:00			152	
	9:00			160	156/82
IV	10:00	4.2	16	170	
	10:30			176	TERMINATION

Recovery Minute	Heart Rate	Blood Pressure
1:00	166	
2:00	140	130/85
3:00	120	
4:00	108	120/80
5:00	102	114/80
6:00	96	

Treadmill Results:
1. Total exercise time: 10:30 min. Total METS: 13
2. MAX HR: 176   MAX BP: 156/80

Physiological Response to Exercise
Normal heart rate and blood pressure response.

Test Stopped for:
Fatigue

Arrhythmias
None noted.

ST Segment Response
< 1 mm at peak exercise.

Impression
Normal test response
ASA - anti-coagulant, no effect on the test.
Coumadin: Anti-coagulant, no effect on test.
Procardia: Nifedipine - increases exercise capacity in patients with angina, decreases rest and exercise BP. May increase or have no effect on resting and exercise HR.

bypass patient, because he is younger than the average, will be returning to a physically active occupation and because he had such a successful follow-up graded exercise test.)

Frequency Should be encouraged to exercise at least three to four times per week. Main thing is to keep him motivated!

Duration Total exercise duration should be gradually increased from to 20 to 60 minutes.

Case Study #2 (Post MI)
Medical History / Health History Questionnaire Results

Sally is a sedentary 59-year-old retired schoolteacher. Her husband recently passed away. She has a

Figure 6.5

Exercise Test Results

GRADED EXERCISE TEST DATA FORM

Patient Name: Sally		Patient Number: 123456789	
Date of Birth:	Age: 59	Gender: ☐ Male	☑ Female
Medications: Premarin, Baby Aspirin and Propranolol.			
Referring MD: B. J. Smith		Test Indication: Post-cardiac rehab discharge test.	
Resting BP: 130/85		Resting HR: 68	

Current Medical History: This is a 59-year-old female with a history of heart disease. She had her second heart attack two months ago. She had successful angioplasty with stent implant. Otherwise, she is in good health.

Test Protocol: Bruce

Stage	Stage Time	Speed (MPH)	Grade (%)	Heart Rate	Blood Pressure		Recovery Minute	Heart Rate	Blood Pressure
Supine				76	136/90		1:00	140	
Standing				82			2:00	136	130/85
I	1:00	1.7	10	86			3:00	104	
	2:00			102			4:00	90	120/80
	3:00			120	125/76		5:00	90	114/80
II	4:00	2.5	12	136			6:00	82	
	5:00			140					
	6:00			146	140/80				
III	7:00	3.4	14	150	TERMINATION				

Treadmill Results:
1. Total exercise time: 7 min.   Total METS:
2. MAX HR: 150   MAX BP: 130/85

Physiological Response to Exercise
Normal heart rate and blood pressure response.

Test Stopped for:
Fatigue. Plus some chest tightness at max exercise (1 to 2 on a 4-point angina scale).

Arrhythmias
None

ST Segment Response
1.5 mm at max. exercise.

Impression
Positive for ischemia

ASA - anti-coagulant, no effect on the test.
Premarin - estrogen replacement, no effect on test.
Propranolol - increases exercise capacity in patients with angina, decreases resting and exercise BP, and may decrease rest and exercise HR.

history of heart disease, and is recovering from her second heart attack. She completed cardiac rehabilitation two weeks ago (Figure 6.5) and her neighbor has brought her down to your fitness center. Her doctor has recently increased her estrogen intake, as well as putting her on a calcium supplement.

Previous Exercise / Diet History

Irregular walking. Her diet is excellent.

Summary of Client Interview

"I'm really uncomfortable here, especially around all these young, healthy people;" "I don't think I can use any of these machines, they are for young people" "Last time I joined a health club (20 years ago) I only went for two weeks because I hurt all of the

time;" "I'm also scared about having chest pains again."

Exercise Prescription

Mode   Need to find out what she will be willing to do at the health club. Don't bring her into the club at the busiest times. Given her age and strength, an activity that allows for good stabilization is important (stationary cycling). Water exercises also might be good.

Intensity   RHR = 76

MHR = 150

Heart-rate Reserve Method: HR 113 (50 percent) to 120 (60 percent).

This training heart rate is well below her ischemic threshold.

Frequency Clients should be encouraged to exercise at least three to four times per week.

Main thing is to keep her motivated!

Duration Total exercise duration should be gradually increased to 20 to 30 minutes.

She may need multiple sessions per day to start out with (10 minutes/day).

References

American College of Sports Medicine. (1997). *Exercise Management For Persons With Chronic Diseases and Disabilities.* Champaign, Ill.: Human Kinetics.

Blair, S.N., Kohl, H.W., Paffenbarger, R.S., D.G., Clark, K.H. Cooper & Gibbons, L.W. (1989). Physical fitness and all-causes mortality: A prospective study of healthy men and women. *Journal of the American Medical Association.* 262, 2395.

Dawber, T. R., Meadors, G.F. & Moore, F.E., (1951). Epidemiological approaches to heart disease: The Framingham Study. *American Journal of Public Health,* 41, 279-286.

Gibbons, R.J., Balady, G.J., Beasley, J.W., Bricker, J.T., Duvernoy, W.F.C., Froelicher, V.F., Mark, D.B., Marwick, T.H., McCallister, B.D., Thompson, P.D, Winters, W.L., Jr. & Yanowitz, F.G. (1997). ACC/AHA guidelines for exercise testing: A report of the American College of Cardiology/ American Heart Association Task Force on Practice Guidelines (Committee on Exercise Testing). *Journal of the American College of Cardiology,* 30, 260-315.

Haskell, W.L., Alderman, E.L., Fair, J.M., et al. (1994) Effects of intensive risk factor reduction on coronary atherosclerosis and clinical events in men and women with coronary artery disease. *Circulation,* 89, 975-990.

Haskell, W.L. (1985). Mechanisms by which physical activity may enhance the clinical status of cardiac patients. In M.L. Pollock & Schmidt (Eds): *Heart Disease and Rehabilitation* (2nd edition). New York: John Wiley & Sons, pp 276-296.

Hennekens, C.H., and Buring, J.E. (1985). Smoking and coronary heart disease in women. *Journal of the American Medical Association,* 253, 3003-4.

Jennings, G., Nelson, L., Nestel, P., et al. (1986). The effects of changes in physical activity on major cardio-vascular risk factors, hemodynamics, sympathetic function, and glucose utilization in man: a controlled study of four levels of activity. *Circulation,* 73, 1, 30-40.

Kenney, W.L. (1995) *ACSM's Guidelines For Exercise Testing and Prescription,* 5th Edition. Philadelphia, Penn.: Williams & Wilkins.

Kleinman, J.C., Donahue, R.P., Harris, M.I., et al. (1988). Mortality among diabetics in a national sample. *American Journal of Epidemiology,* 128, 389-401.

Lilly, L.S. (1998). *Pathophysiology of Heart Disease* 2nd edition. Philadelphia, Penn.: Williams & Wilkins.

MacMahon, S., Petro, R., Cutler, J., et al. (1990). Blood pressure, stroke, and coronary artery disease. I. Prolonged differences in blood pressure — prospective observational studies corrected for the regression dilution bias. *Lancet,* 335, 765-74.

Ockene, I. & Ockene, J. (1992). *Prevention of Coronary Heart Disease.* Boston, Mass.: Little, Brown and Company.

Ornish, D., Brown, S.E., Scherwitz, L.W., et al. (1990). Can lifestyle changes reverse coronary heart disease? The Lifestyle Heart Trial. *Lancet,* 336, 129-133.

Powell, K. E., Thompson,P.D., Caspersen, C.J. & Kendrick, J.S. (1987). Physical activity and the incidence of heart disease. *Annual Review of Public Health,* 8, 253.

Stein, R.A., Michielli, D.W., Glantz, M.D., et al. (1990). Effects of different exercise intensities on lipoprotein cholesterol fractions in healthy middle-aged men. *American Heart Journal,* 119, 277-83.

Wells, A. (1988). An estimate of adult mortality in the United States from passive smoking. *Environ. Int.,* 14, 249-65.

Will, P.M., et al. (1996). Prescribing Exercise for Health. *AFP,* 53, 579-585.

CHAPTER 7

Peripheral Vascular Disease

BRAD A. ROY

Brad A. Roy, Ph.D., F.A.C.S.M., is the director of The Summit, Kalispell Regional Medical Center's facility for health promotion and fitness in Kalispell, Mont. Dr. Roy has more than 20 years experience working with clinical patients in the rehabilitation setting and has successfully consulted with numerous world-class athletes. He received his master's degree in exercise physiology from San Diego State University and his doctorate in the same subject from Columbia Pacific University.

Common Symptoms
Special Concerns

Contraindications

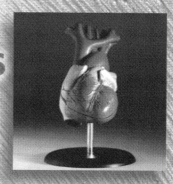

A painful and often debilitating condition, peripheral vascular disease (PVD) is characterized by atherosclerotic narrowing of the peripheral arteries, most predominately in the lower extremities. The resulting decreased blood flow through the aorta and its branches results in an impaired ability to appropriately increase blood flow during physical activity to meet the oxygen demand of the working muscles. This imbalance between supply and demand leads to the symptoms of PVD and concurrent activity limitations.

It is estimated that approximately 12 percent of the general population, and up to 20 percent of seniors, are affected by PVD. Nearly 35 percent of individuals diagnosed with PVD also have coronary artery disease (CAD). In fact, it is not uncommon for individuals with CAD to experience symptoms of PVD following coronary artery bypass surgery, which improves their cardiac function and subsequent ability to exercise. The overall survival rate at five years is 73 percent for individuals with PVD, compared to 93 percent for normal-age matched controls (Hammond, Merli & Zieler, 1993). Generally, mortality related to PVD results from arterial disease of either a cardiac or cerebral etiology. During the 24-year Framingham study, five percent of the population developed lower-extremity arterial disease (Drawber, 1980; Kannel, Skinner & Schwartz, 1970). Prevalence estimates for PVD are most likely low. A number of subjects are asymptomatic while others gradually decrease activity levels when symptoms arise rather than report them to their physician. Some deny the existence of the disease process and simply attribute the symptoms to deconditioning or aging.

Etiology and Pathophysiology

PVD affects the medium and large arteries serving the body. The most common sites for atherosclerotic lesions include the iliac, femoral and popliteal arteries. Risk factors for PVD are similar to those of CAD, such as hyperlipidemia, smoking, hypertension, diabetes, family predisposition, physical inactivity, obesity and stress. The most prominent of these are smoking and diabetes. As with CAD, one or more risk factors can trigger a cascade of events that eventually lead to plaque formation and subsequent narrowing of the arteries.

Arteries are composed of three layers: 1) the outer layer, the adventitia; 2) the middle layer, the media (muscular layer); and 3) the innermost layer, the intima. Atherosclerotic plaques form in response to injury of the intima. When chronically exposed to irritants (e.g., tobacco) and other injury-producing mechanisms, a repair process is triggered within the endothelial lining of the intima that eventually results in plaque formation. The resulting decrease in blood flow can cause ischemia and its associated pain. Additionally, plaque typically is unstable and can spontaneously rupture, causing thrombosis formation, which can rapidly cut off blood supply and cause ischemia and even death of the affected tissue.

Aging also produces arteriosclerotic changes in the arteries, such as intimal thickening and loss of elasticity. Often referred to as hardening of the arteries, the arteriosclerotic process is compounded by the effects of atherosclerotic plaque formation. These two processes result in arterial narrowing and the ischemic symptoms of PVD. Symptoms of PVD also can result from, or be accentuated by, arterial spasm.

It is estimated that 90 percent of individuals with PVD are smokers. Tobacco use not only impacts the arterial wall, but the effects of nicotine and carbon monoxide also reduce oxygen supply to the musculature. Nicotine stimulates the sympathetic nervous system, resulting in increased peripheral resistance and vasoconstriction. The subsequent decreased blood flow reduces the available oxygen to the tissues, compounding the already compromised muscular blood flow. In addition, nicotine promotes clot formation by increasing platelet aggregation. Further adding insult to injury is the effect of carbon monoxide binding with hemoglobin in place of oxygen. Therefore, smoking should be treated aggressively in individuals with PVD.

Research also indicates that PVD occurs 11 times more frequently in diabetic than nondiabetic individuals. Diabetes accelerates the process of arteriosclerosis and atherosclerosis, affecting both the large vessels and microcirculation through the arterioles, venules and capillaries. Diabetics with PVD have been shown to have a greater involvement of the smaller and more distal arteries than those individuals without diabetes. Gangrene, a major complication of PVD, is estimated to be 40 times greater in diabetics. The incidence of limb amputation also is significantly greater in diabetics than nondiabetics. Other lesser causes of PVD are infectious processes, vasospastic disorders and congenital malformations.

Because progression of PVD is slow, many patients remain asymptomatic for years before significant narrowing occurs and produces symptoms. When symptoms begin to develop, most individuals significantly curtail their physical activities before complaining to their physician. Unfortunately, the resulting deconditioning dramatically reduces the individual's functional capabilities and places them at increased risk for developing other chronic disease conditions.

Common Symptoms

The most predominant symptom of PVD is pain during weight-bearing activities such as walking. This pain is caused by a limited arterial supply that cannot meet the increased metabolic demand of the working muscle. The sequence of pain, aching or burning in the calf, thigh and/or buttocks that is relieved by rest is referred to as intermittent claudication. In most individuals symptoms are reproducible at a given exercise workload. Many individuals with PVD can only walk a limited distance before needing to rest. Positional change is not required to bring symptomatic relief, and following a brief rest period the individual usually is able to walk another short distance before stopping again. A subjective rating of pain can be made with the following four-point scale (ACSM, 1991):

Grade I: Definite discomfort or pain, but only at initial or modest levels (established, but minimal)

Grade II: Moderate discomfort or pain from which the patient's attention can be diverted by a number of common stimuli (e.g., conversation)

Grade III: Intense pain (short of Grade IV) from which the patient's attention cannot be diverted except by catastrophic events (e.g., fire, explosion)

Grade IV: Excruciating and unbearable pain

In severe cases, pain is not rapidly relieved by terminating the activity, and in very severe cases, pain is present even at rest. Pain at rest results when blood flow no longer meets the resting metabolic demands of the extremity, and is described as a persistent dull pain and numbness. Other signs and symptoms include edema, weakness and fatigue, numbness, cold extremities, diminished or absent arterial pulses, paresthesia, skin color changes, bruits, atrophy of the toes and, in severe cases, gangrene (Hammond, 1993; Barnard & Hill, 1989). Of particular concern is the diabetic individual with PVD who may not be aware of symptoms because of decreased sensation resulting from peripheral neuropathy.

Symptoms of PVD may be worsened by a variety of factors that affect arterial blood flow. Individuals should be cautioned not to dangle their legs in an effort to reduce discomfort as this results in edema that further reduces flow. Smoking, infection, injury and/or trauma, and cold temperatures also may accentuate symptoms.

Because of pain, individuals with PVD have a markedly impaired functional capacity (average peak oxygen uptake of 14 ml/kg/min) and ability to participate in physical activities, especially those requiring ambulation (Hiatt, Regensteiner, Hargarten, Wolfel & Brass, 1990). Individuals with PVD typically have an exercise capacity that is even lower than individuals with CAD. Quality of life is dramatically altered as normal occupational, personal and social activities are impacted.

Diagnostic Criteria

PVD is diagnosed through findings from a detailed history and physical exam, along with information gathered from both noninvasive and invasive diagnostic tests. Physical exam findings indicate diminished or absent peripheral pulses, decreased skin temperature, and trophic skin changes such as dusky color, hair loss, thin/shiny skin and abnormal nails (Hammond, 1993).

Noninvasive diagnostic tests that assess resting (and frequently exercise) blood flow and/or blood pressure are utilized in evaluating PVD. Typically, ankle and arm systolic pressures are measured at rest and post-exercise using a pneumatic cuff and doppler ultrasonic flow detector. The ratio of ankle to arm systolic pressure (ankle/brachial index or ABI) is a simple and reliable tool for evaluating the severity of arterial narrowing and occlusion. The normal ABI is greater than 0.9, while an index of 0.7 to 0.9 indicates mild disease, 0.4 to 0.7 moderate claudication and less than 0.4 severe disease.

Historically, diagnostic exercise testing for PVD has consisted of walking on a treadmill at a standardized workload of 2 mph, 12-percent grade. Prior to the exercise test, resting bilateral ankle and arm blood pressures are measured in the supine position and ABIs are calculated. Following measurement of resting pressures, the individual ambulates on the treadmill at the prescribed workload for five minutes or until symptoms cause termination of the activity. Because many individuals with PVD also have CAD, it is important that brachial blood pressure and ECG be monitored during exercise and that the testing session be physician-supervised. Both cardiac and lower-extremity symptoms can be monitored by a four-point scale with termination occurring at two-point angina or two-point leg pain. After the exercise test, the patient immediately lies down, and left brachial and left and right posterior tibial artery pressures are taken and repeated each minute until pressures return to normal. Individuals with PVD will typically have decreased tibial artery pressures compared to their resting levels. The resulting decreased ABI indicates significantly reduced blood flow distal to the occlusive lesions.

While the constant-load treadmill test is well accepted by physicians, it does have limitations. Individuals with PVD have different ranges of functional capacity, so while the test is ideal for some, the standardized workload may be too difficult or too easy for others. Therefore, a number of clinicians have proposed graded treadmill protocols that utilize a standard velocity with periodic changes in elevation (Hiatt, Nowaz, Regensteiner & Hossack, 1988; Gardner, Skinner, Cantwell & Smith, 1991; Gardner, Skinner, Vaughn, Bryant & Smith, 1992). Since graded tests have been shown to improve reproducibility and provide more specific information regarding functional limitations, they may be an important alternative to constant-load tests.

Other methods commonly used in diagnosing and evaluating severity of PVD include ultrasound dublex scans that frequently are enhanced by color-flow imaging and arteriography (an invasive study of the arteries). Non-weight-bearing activities such as cycle ergometry are not recommended in PVD evaluations as the lower leg muscles are not sufficiently challenged. When treadmill exercise is not available, evaluations can be conducted by utilizing a toe-raise exercise or flexion-extension as described by Carter (1972).

Medical Management

Treatment of PVD with various medications has been only marginally effective. Pentoxifylline (Trental) has been effective in increasing the exercise capacity of people with PVD. Pentoxifylline improves the flow properties of blood by decreasing its viscosity, thus enhancing tissue oxygenation. Pentoxifylline has no effect on the heart-rate or blood-pressure response to exercise. Anti-platelet agents such as aspirin also have been helpful in some individuals and are commonly prescribed. Vasodilating medications have been shown to increase symptoms in some individuals with PVD. This is due to the medications' effects on normal vessel segments that shunt blood away from the inadequately perfused diseased vessels (arterial "steal").

Exercise Benefits for Individuals with PVD

Exercise consistently has been shown to be effective in improving ambulation distances in individuals with PVD. In fact, all randomized and nonrandomized exercise training studies to date have documented improved exercise performance. Hiatt and co-workers randomly assigned 20 PVD subjects to either a three-month supervised treadmill program or a nonexercising control group. The exercise intervention group walked for one hour three times per week with progressive intensity increases over the 12-week program. Maximal walking time was increased by 123 percent and VO_2max by 30 percent in the intervention group. Treadmill walking speed also was significantly improved (Hiatt, 1990). Hiatt and Regensteiner also reported significant exercise improvements in 29 patients who were randomized either to a treadmill walking program, treadmill walking and resistance training, or control group. Both intervention groups were found to have significantly improved exercise performance compared to the control group. However, the addition of resistance training to the treadmill walking program did not further augment the response (Hiatt, Wolfel, Meier & Regensteiner, 1994).

Williams and co-workers (1991) found that a vascular rehabilitation program resulted in significant reductions in cardiovascular risk factors along with improvement in exercise tolerance in 45 PVD subjects who completed their study. The program consisted of 24 supervised exercise sessions, 12 educational lectures and development of a home exercise program. Reducing cardiovascular risk factors is extremely important in the PVD population as many individuals also have CAD. Significant improvements in blood pressure, lipids, body weight and metabolic control serve to lower risk for cardiovascular complications such as stroke and myocardial infarction. Exercise plays an important role in controlling each of these risk factors.

While all published training studies to date have documented significant improvements in exercise performance, the mechanism for this improvement has not been clearly explained.

Animal studies have documented increases in collateral flow following arterial occlusion and exercise training, while results in humans have shown mixed results. A few researchers have associated improvements in human exercise performance with increased blood flow, although little scientific evidence currently exists to support this enticing theory. A number of other mechanisms also may play a significant role in stimulating exercise performance improvements following training. Changes in blood viscosity and capillary and mitochondrial density, along with increases in oxidative and glycolytic enzymes, all of which improve oxygen utilization, may improve exercise performance.

Improvements in walking mechanics and pain perception also significantly influence exercise performance. Hiatt et al. (1990, 1994) found that oxygen consumption for a constant submaximal workload significantly decreased following training (a lower VO_2 for a given submaximal workload suggests improved walking economy).

Client Assessment

Community-based exercise programs are not appropriate for all individuals with PVD. Those with symptomatic and/or unstable CHD, CHF, diabetes and/or resting pain should be referred to medically supervised programs. Therefore, prior to initiating an exercise program for clients with PVD, gather a comprehensive medical history, including clinical exercise test results, cardiac risk factors, symptomology, current medications, and information regarding other acute and chronic health problems (e.g., CAD, CHF and diabetes). This information will assist you in developing an appropriate individualized exercise program, and in determining which individuals should be referred to medically supervised programs. See Table 7.1 for a list of questions that may be helpful when speaking with the client's physician.

Unlike CAD, in which severe ischemia results in a myocardial infarction and possibly death, there is no evidence that severe peripheral ischemia during exercise results in tissue damage in the legs (Barnard & Hall, 1989). However, since many individuals with PVD have concurrent CAD, strict attention must be focused on cardiac symptoms and risk factors. Clients with PVD should undergo a complete medical evaluation by their physician prior to beginning the exercise program. It is recommended that the evaluation include a physician-supervised exercise test. Carefully review the medical history and stress test results, and seek physician input on potential exercise limitations and specific intensity recommendations for eligible clients.

Knowledge of the client's current CAD risk factors is critical, as risk reduction should be an important goal of the therapeutic program. While uncontrolled hypertension results in arterial damage, aggressive treatment can exacerbate claudication symptoms if pressures fall too low and hinder peripheral blood flow. Assist the physician in evaluating therapy by reporting changes in and/or new occurrences of symptoms. Tobacco use should be stopped immediately, as continued smoking promotes progression of both PVD and CAD. Overweight individuals should receive nutritional counseling to assist in controlling body weight, and to encourage good hydration habits, especially as physical activity is increased.

Table 7.1

Client Information to Obtain from Medical Professionals

1) Is there any underlying cardiac disease? If so, does the client require ECG monitoring?

2) What are the client's symptoms?

3) What other risk factors does this client have (e.g., smoker, diabetic, etc.)?

4) Has the client undergone an exercise test? What were the results?

5) What medications does the client take?

6) What are your activity/intensity recommendations? If the client is diabetic, what is your recommendation regarding the timing of exercise around meals/medications?

7) What are your specific goals for this client?

Give special attention to the diabetic client with PVD to ensure safe participation in the exercise program. Meticulous foot care is important for all PVD clients, especially those who are diabetic, as associated peripheral neuropathy places them at increased risk for foot lesions, infection and subsequent development of gangrene. Feet should be inspected and washed daily, and nails carefully manicured. Wearing appropriate footwear to reduce friction and trauma from ambulatory activities also is important.

You should know the signs and symptoms that suggest a worsening metabolic state that might precipitate a hypoglycemic reaction. Carbohydrate snacks should be available during and following activity sessions, and exercise during peak insulin activity should be avoided. The optimal time for exercise is one to two hours after a light meal, and activity should be promptly discontinued at first suspicion of a worsening metabolic state. Most diabetic clients have their own glucometer. They should be encouraged to check blood sugar prior to and following exercise and report the results.

Your primary role is to prescribe and monitor therapeutic exercise. You also should provide adjunctive education and encouragement to assist the client in reducing risk factors and maintaining appropriate foot/skin hygiene. Work closely with the client's physician and other health professionals (e.g., clinical exercise physiologist, physical therapist, dietitian and nurse) to develop and implement an appropriate individualized program. Some PVD clients may be recent graduates of cardiac, vascular or physical rehabilitation programs, and you should meet with the clinical staff to gather additional information that will assist in planning the exercise program.

Absolute and Relative Contraindications to Exercise

Absolute contraindications for exercise testing and training in PVD are similar to those presented in Chapter 6 for CAD. These include unstable angina, uncontrolled hypertension, orthostatic hypotension, severe aortic stenosis, acute illness/fever, uncontrolled atrial or ventricular dysrhythmias, CHF, thrombophlebitis, recent embolism and uncontrolled diabetes. Other contraindications include pain at rest and ischemic ulcerations with which weight-bearing activities should be avoided. Also of concern is the hypothesis that exercise may reduce cutaneous oxygen delivery to a degree that local wound healing is impaired. Therefore, exercise training should be carefully considered when localized wounds are apparent. Exercise should be terminated if the client experiences cardiac signs/symptoms (angina, excessive shortness of breath or fatigue, lightheadedness, pallor, cyanosis), hypoglycemic symptoms and/or foot trauma.

Fitness Testing for Individuals with PVD

While constant-load treadmill testing is commonly used to measure pre- and post-exercise ankle/brachial indexes to document the severity of PVD, such tests are of limited value in determining functional capacity. Studies suggest that hemodynamic severity as defined by ABI does not correlate well to treadmill exercise performance (Barnard, 1989). Therefore, graded exercise protocols that measure VO_2, along with other types of treadmill walking and field tests, may be better protocols for measuring exercise capacity.

Two easily conducted, common treadmill tests measure either the walking distance to initial claudication symptoms or the absolute distance before claudication symptoms cause the individual to stop walking. Protocols are designed so that individuals walk at a constant velocity of 2 to 3 mph with 2 percent to 3.5 percent grade increases every two to three minutes. Reproducibility is significantly greater with graded exercise than with the constant-load protocols (Barnard, 1989), as tests cover various walking ability ranges. Therefore, it is recommended that graded treadmill protocols be used to evaluate exercise performance and document therapeutic improvement in individuals with PVD. Because many clients with PVD will have underlying CAD, and because graded exercise protocols induce higher exercise intensities, exercise tests should be physician-supervised and ECG and blood pressure responses monitored.

Submaximal field testing, although used infrequently, may be applicable in estimating functional capacity and documenting therapeutic improvement. The six-minute walk, during which you measure the maximum distance the client can ambulate in six minutes, is commonly used with pulmonary patients and the elderly and may be practical for use with patients with PVD. The six-minute walk test has the advantage of requiring little equipment other than a stop watch, a calibrated measuring wheel and a walking track or hallway. Clients should be encouraged to walk as far and as fast as they can in six minutes and symptoms should be carefully monitored. Those who have been medically cleared by their physician can be tested in the community setting without direct physician supervision.

Exercise Programming for Individuals with PVD

The goal of exercise for individuals with PVD is to improve arterial flow, increase oxygen extraction and improve walking mechanics that ultimately serve to decrease oxygen demand at a given workload. Additional goals include modifying underlying risk factors, such as smoking, and educating the client about PVD (symptoms, foot care, nutrition, etc.). To maximize training results and lower risk of complications, an appropriate exercise program is essential.

Generally, walking is the exercise of choice because it uses the lower-leg muscles, effectively producing ischemia in the affected limb(s). This is important as ischemia may be the primary stimulus for development of collateral circulation and other improvements in oxidative metabolism (Scheel, 1981; Mathien & Terjung, 1986; and Mannarino, Pasqvalini, Menna, Maragoni & Orlandi, 1989). To improve exercise capacity, it is important to encourage PVD clients to walk to the point of severe pain (three to four on a five-point scale) before stopping. The client should then rest until the pain subsides and repeat the ambulatory activity, once again walking to the point of severe limb pain. This process should initially be repeated for a total of 20 to 30 minutes. Gradually progress to 40- to 60-minute sessions. The client can use a walking track, hallway or even outdoor walking paths. The initial workload intensity should stimulate claudication pain within two to six

minutes of walking. When eight to 12 minutes of continuous walking can be tolerated, increase the walking pace or progress the total activity time.

Treadmill walking provides a controlled environment for training PVD clients and is the activity of choice for CAD patients who require close monitoring. Initial treadmill velocity is generally set at 2 mph and gradually advanced in 0.2 mph increments to 3 mph. Once the client has achieved a walking pace of 3 mph, introduce changes in elevation to achieve the desired stimulus.

Clients can progress by increasing their continuous walking time without resting and/or increasing velocity and elevation. As mentioned, clients are generally advanced when eight to 12 minutes can be achieved without reaching moderate claudication pain (Regensteiner, 1995).

Select clients also may benefit by gradually adding other activities that challenge the cardiopulmonary system, such as bicycle ergometry, various cross trainers and aquatic activities. However, the upright posture is preferable to the horizontal as it enhances lower-extremity perfusion. Aquatic activities should consist of shallow-water exercises and/or deep-water aerobics utilizing a flotation device to maintain an upright posture (Hammond, 1993). Caution should be taken during shallow-water activities to not injure the feet; it is recommended that some type of footwear be worn to protect the client from scrapes, cuts and bruises.

Light upper-extremity resistance training also may be of benefit. However, extreme caution should be taken to ensure that clients are free of cardiovascular symptoms, stay within moderate intensities (RPE 11 to 13) and are taught appropriate lifting techniques. Obtain physician clearance before advancing clients with PVD into these more intense activities. While daily walking should be encouraged, clients should participate in adjunct training activities two to three times per week.

Carefully document the results of each exercise session including activity data (e.g., mode, intensity, distance walked), client symptoms and precipitating events, and any physiologic measurements that are taken (e.g., blood sugar, blood pressure). Also document the treatment for any symptoms and the response, and record all test results and other outcome measures. Careful documentation will provide information for reporting outcomes and investigating any change in symptomology.

Emergency Procedures

You should be well versed in basic life support (CPR) because PVD clients frequently suffer from underlying CAD. Also, become familiar with the signs and symptoms associated with diabetes-induced hypoglycemia and be prepared to respond to such emergencies. Develop and practice using an emergency response plan prior to training clients.

Special Concerns

After participating in exercise for a few weeks, a number of individuals with PVD will develop CAD symptoms. These individuals are asymptomatic at first because low initial workloads do not significantly challenge the cardiopulmonary system. However, when improved walking abilities allow clients to walk at higher intensities, cardiac symptoms may result. Therefore, you should be familiar with the signs and symptoms of CAD, and should stop the exercise session if symptoms arise. Immediately refer the client to their physician. Because subtle, seemingly minor symptoms can be the precursor of major catastrophic events, symptoms should not be taken lightly and immediately should be reported to the client's physician.

As has previously been stressed, proper foot care is essential. Pay close attention to your clients' feet, especially those who are diabetic. If infection, wounds and/or ulcerations appear, immediately refer the client to their physician.

Finally, every exercise session should be preceded by a short interview with the client to unveil any new or worsening symptoms. The interview assesses the appropriateness of the exercise training session and allows you to make necessary modifications. Regular exercise can dramatically improve PVD clients' ambulatory abilities and can safely be accomplished when special precautions and attention to detail are adhered to. Many individuals with PVD are able to delay, and in some cases avoid, major surgical procedures with consistent exercise training and successful risk factor modification.

Case Study

A 57-year-old male railroad engineer complains to his physician of dyspnea and severe leg pain while walking, and states that he is only able to walk about two blocks before having to stop and rest. Following a brief rest period, he is able to continue walking for another short distance before stopping again. The patient has a 40-year history of smoking two packs of cigarettes per day. He denies any symptoms of chest, neck, jaw or arm pain/tightness. His resting heart rate is 98 b/min and blood pressure is 148/92. At 67 inches tall and 154 pounds, the patient is overweight and his physical activity has been reduced progressively over the past year because of leg pain.

Pulmonary function testing produced the following results that were interpreted as indicative of mild obstructive airway disease:

Table 7.2

Typical Activity Guidelines

- Encourage walking to the point of severe limb pain, followed by rest. Repeat the walking bout for a specified number of repetitions. Exercise should be undertaken on a daily basis.

- Initial intensity should stimulate claudication pain within two to six minutes of walking.

- Walking is the activity of choice for individuals with concurrent cardiac disease who require close monitoring.

- Teach individuals to recognize the warning signs/symptoms of heart problems and instruct them on what to do should such symptoms arise.

- Stress proper foot care and instruct individuals to see their physician immediately if infection, wounds and/or ulcerations appear.

Measure	Predicted	Actual
Vital Capacity	3.50L	3.30L
FEV1	2.75L	2.42L
DLCO	22.8 ml/mHg/min	23.6 ml/mHg/min

A duplex ultrasound evaluation identified arterial narrowing and reduced blood flow in the lower extremity, predominately on the right. A doppler treadmill exercise test was ordered to document the severity of the patient's limitations. Because of his smoking history, the treadmill test was physician-supervised with continuous 12-lead ECG monitoring. The exercise protocol began at 2 mph at a 2-percent grade that increased two percent every two minutes. The patient was able to walk 21 seconds at a 6-percent elevation for a total exercise time of four minutes and 21 seconds. The test was stopped because of severe leg cramping that was rated four on a scale of one to four. Peak heart rate was 154 beats/min, blood pressure was 178/90 and no symptoms or ECG changes suggested cardiac ischemia.

Following cessation of exercise, the patient immediately was placed in the supine position and brachial and tibial pressures were taken. Pressure measurements were repeated at one-minute intervals during the 10-minute recovery. Results are shown in Table 7.3 and suggest moderate claudication severity and physical deconditioning.

Based on the patient's history, physical exam and test results, the following diagnosis was made: 1) PVD of moderate severity, predominately affecting the lower right extremity; 2) mild hypertension; 3) physical deconditioning; 4) overweight. A decision is made to treat the patient medically with exercise, nutrition counseling and smoking cessation. He is referred to you for development of an exercise program.

Prior to the initial meeting with the client, carefully review the medical history and seek input from the referring physician regarding the exercise training plan. Since the client underwent a supervised exercise test, it is not necessary to conduct a separate fitness evaluation. Information from the graded clinical test can be used as the baseline functional ability, and a repeat test under physician supervision can be arranged following three months of consistent training. Additionally, the client should be supported in his efforts to stop smoking, as this will be critical in slowing the disease's progression and in avoiding future cardiopulmonary complications.

During the initial meeting with the client, assess current symptoms, activity levels and nutritional habits. Discuss exercise benefits with the client (such as increased walking capacity, blood pressure control, weight loss and reduced risk of CAD) and encourage exercise consistency. Make the client aware of the symptoms of CAD and emphasize the importance of immediately reporting symptoms should they arise. Stress the importance of walking to the point of severe pain before stopping and explain that claudication symptoms, unlike cardiac symptoms, do not result in damage to the affected limb. Review appropriate foot care and evaluate walking shoes.

Begin the exercise training program with level-ground walking at approximately 2 mph to the point of severe claudication pain. The client should rest until the pain eases before undertaking another walking bout. Continue this exercise-rest sequence until the client has walked for 25 to 30 minutes. Increase session length in five-minute increments up to 45 to 50 minutes of activity. Once the client can walk for eight to 12 minutes without stopping, increase the walking

Table 7.3
Exercise Doppler Results

TIME	BRACHIAL		TIBIAL		AAI	
	Left	Right	Left	Right	Left	Right
Resting	148	150	142	134	0.96	0.91
Immed. Post	190		155	120	0.82	0.63
Post 1 min	188		154	120	0.82	0.64
Post 2 min	174		152	124	0.87	0.71
Post 5 min	162		144	124	0.89	0.71
Post 10 min	146		138	130	0.94	0.89

pace. The goal is to achieve a normal walking pace of 3 mph. The initial two to three sessions should be conducted on the treadmill where the work rate can easily be controlled and the client carefully monitored for symptoms and responses. Subsequent sessions can continue on the treadmill or utilize a walking track or path.

The primary goal of the training program is to improve function and quality of life by increasing the pace and distance walked before the occurrence of symptoms that limit activity. Additionally, the walking program will assist in achieving successful weight reduction. The combination of fitness adaptations with weight loss is critical in reducing blood pressure, another potential benefit of the exercise program.

Once improvement is documented on the follow-up test, consider adding light upper-extremity resistance training to the program and possibly other forms of aerobic exercise that will augment functional capacity. Carefully instruct the client on proper lifting techniques. One set of eight to 12 repetitions is adequate to stimulate a training response, and heavier weights and additional sets should be discouraged.

References

American College of Sports Medicine. (1995). *ACSM's Guidelines for Exercise Testing and Prescription.* (5th ed.) Baltimore: Williams and Wilkins.

Barnard, R.J. & Hall, J.A. (1989). Patients with Peripheral Vascular Disease. In: Franklin, B.A. (Ed.) *Exercise in Modern Medicine.* Baltimore: Williams & Wilkins.

Carter, S.A. (1972). Response of ankle systolic pressure to leg exercise in mild or questionable arterial disease. *New England Journal of Medicine,* 287, 578-582.

Drawber, T.R. (1980). *The Framingham Study: The Epidemiology of Atherosclerotic Disease.* Cambridge: Harvard University Press.

Gardner, A.W., Skinner, J.S., Cantwell, B.W. & Smith, L.K. (1991). Progressive vs. single-stage treadmill tests for evaluation of claudication. *Medicine and Science in Sports and Exercise,* 23, 402-408.

Gardner, A.W., Skinner, J.S., Vaughn, N.R., Bryant, C.X. & Smith, L.K. (1992). Comparison of three progressive exercise protocols in peripheral vascular occlusive disease. *Angiology,* 43, 661-671.

Hammond, M.C., Merli, G.J. & Zieler, R.E. (1993). Rehabilitation of the Patient with Peripheral Vascular Disease of the Lower Extremity. In: Delisa, J.A. *Rehabilitation Medicine, Principles and Practice.* (2nd ed.) Philadelphia: J.B. Lippincott Co.

Hiatt, R.H., Wolfel, E.E., Meier, R.H. & Regensteiner, J.G. (1994). Superiority of treadmill walking exercise versus strength training for patients with peripheral arterial disease: Implications for the mechanism of the training response. *Circulation,* 90, 1866-1874.

Hiatt, R.H., Regensteiner, J.G., Hargarten, M.E., Wolfel, E.E. & Brass, E.P. (1990). Benefit of exercise conditioning for patients with peripheral arterial disease. *Circulation,* 81, 602-609.

Hiatt, W.R., Nawaz, D., Regensteiner, J.G. & Hossack, K.F. (1988). The evaluation of exercise performance in patients with peripheral vascular disease. *Journal of Cardiopulmonary Rehabilitation,* 12, 525-532.

Kannel, W.B., Skinner, J.J. Jr., Schwartz, M.J., et al. (1970). Intermittent claudication incidence in the Framingham study. *Circulation,* 41, 875-883.

Mannarino, E., Pasqualini, L., Menna, M., Maragoni, G. & Orlandi, O. (1989). Effects of physical training on peripheral vascular disease: A controlled study. *Angiology,* 40, 5-10.

Mathien, G.M. & Terjung, R.L. (1986). Influence of training following bilateral stenosis of the femoral artery in rats. *American Journal of Physiology,* 250, H1050-H1059.

Scheel, K.W. (1981). The stimulus for coronary collateral growth: Ischemia or mechanical factors? *Journal of Cardiopulmonary Rehabilitation,* 1, 149-153.

Williams, L.R., Ekers, M.A., Collins, P.S. & Lee, J.F. (1991). Vascular rehabilitation: Benefits of a structured exercise/risk modification program. *Journal of Vascular Surgery,* 14, 320-326.

CHAPTER 8

Selected Cardiovascular Disorders

BRAD ROY
DEAN MACCARTER

Brad A. Roy, Ph.D., F.A.C.S.M., is the director of The Summit, Kalispell Regional Medical Center's facility for health promotion and fitness in Kalispell, Mont. Dr. Roy has more than 20 years experience working with clinical patients in the rehabilitation setting and has successfully consulted with numerous world-class athletes. He received his master's degree in exercise physiology from San Diego State University and his doctorate in the same subject from Columbia Pacific University.

Dean MacCarter, Ph.D., has extensively studied and published information on cardiac pacing and assessment procedures for appropriate exercise-rate response for people with pacemakers. In addition to the more standardized techniques for appropriate pacemaker-patient programming, his contributions to cardiac pacing include rate-response algorithm development for pacemakers capable of restoring an individual's chronotropic response to exercise. He also is an active member of the North American Society of Pacing and Electrophysiology (NAPSE).

Exercise Testing
Program Initiation
Follow-up

Valvular Heart Disease

Blood flow through the heart is regulated by four cardiac valves that allow blood to move from the atria to the ventricles or from the ventricles into the pulmonary or systemic circulation. The valves consist of an opening (orifice), leaflets that function to open and close the valve, and chordae tendineae and papillary muscles that assist in the process. Some or all of the components can become dysfunctional, obstructing flow or allowing blood to leak through the valve orifice.

Valvular heart disease generally results from one of four primary causes: 1) acute rheumatic fever; 2) infection; 3) degenerative changes frequently associated with congenital abnormalities; and 4) myocardial ischemia/infarction that results in papillary muscle dysfunction. Typically affecting all three layers of the heart, rheumatic carditis frequently leads to permanent deformity and impairment of the cardiac valves. The mitral and aortic valves are most commonly affected, although the tricuspid and pulmonary valves also can be involved. The good news is that acute rheumatic fever has significantly waned over the past half-century in the United States.

Diseased valves generally are classified as stenotic and/or regurgitant. Stenotic valves result from a narrowed orifice, and thickening and calcification of the valve leaflets or chordae tendineae. As stenosis gradually develops and progresses, the heart compensates by thickening the muscular walls of the affected chamber(s) to maintain cardiac output. This cardiac muscular hypertrophy results in increased myocardial oxygen demand, as the heart works hard to overcome the increased resistance caused by the narrowed valve opening.

Valvular leakage or regurgitation can have an acute onset or develop gradually over time. Regurgitation results in volume overload in the affected chamber(s) as blood continues to flow through the valve following closure or is pumped backward during systole. Over time, as the affected chamber(s) compensate for the additional blood, the regurgitant valve causes dilation and thickening of the chamber walls.

Mild degrees of valvular stenosis or regurgitation generally produce no symptoms, and individuals can safely participate in physical training at moderate-to-vigorous intensities. Moderate-to-severe valve disease produces symptoms and limits an individual's exercise capabilities. These individuals are candidates for reconstructive or replacement surgery. Valve replacement, once reserved for individuals with severe disease, is now encouraged at moderate levels to prevent damage to the myocardium (heart muscle). The most common symptoms are dyspnea, fatigue and weakness, especially with exertion. In severe cases of valvular stenosis, angina, syncope and pulmonary edema (lung congestion) may be present.

Diagnosis

Diagnosis of valvular disease is based on symptoms, physical findings and colorflow doppler echocardiography. Murmurs are usually the first and most common physical finding. Murmurs are extra heart sounds heard during auscultation of the heart. The location on the chest, the specific time in the cardiac cycle that a murmur is heard, and the sound characteristics of the murmur provide clues as to its type and potential severity.

Echocardiography images combined with color-flow doppler velocity measurements provide accurate assessments of the valve area and disease severity. Velocity of blood flow increases as blood moves through a narrowed valve. Doppler echocardiography is used to estimate velocity changes by measuring the pressure drop across a valve and converting it to a velocity $P=4V^2$. The velocity information is then superimposed on a color-coded display of blood flow through the valve, providing the clinician with numerical data and a visual image to assess the severity of disease.

Treatment

Treatment of valvular disease consists of medical management and/or surgical valve repair or replacement. Medical management generally focuses on antibiotic prophylaxis to prevent further damage from infective endocarditis, and medications to treat symptoms of pulmonary vascular congestion, control rhythm abnormalities, augment cardiac output and protect the individual from embolic events. The most common medications prescribed are:

diuretics — used to treat symptoms of vascular congestion

Digoxin — used to control atrial fibrillation and augment left-ventricular function

beta blockers and calcium channel blockers — used to slow heart rate and augment diastolic flow

anticoagulants — provide protection against embolic events

vasodilators — used to reduce systemic vascular resistance

It is important that you are familiar with the various effects that medications may have on the exercise response of patients with valvular heart disease. Briefly, beta blockers reduce resting and exercise heart rate and blood pressure, and serve to lower myocardial oxygen demand. The reduced heart rate also increases diastolic filling time, augmenting myocardial oxygen supply. Beta blockers can worsen symptoms of claudication in individuals with peripheral vascular disease, and may precipitate bronchospasms in individuals with reactive airway disease. Some calcium channel blockers also may reduce heart rate and blood pressure, so be aware of possible post-exercise hypotension. This also is true with peripheral vasodilators. Diuretics can cause fluid and electrolyte abnormalities that can precipitate hypotension and rhythm abnormalities. Digoxin, which is often used to control the ventricular rate in atrial fibrillation, can cause exercise-induced ST depression on the electrocardiogram. A detailed review of pharmacologic factors in exercise can be found in the *Resource Manual for Guidelines for Exercise Testing and Prescription* (American College of Sports Medicine, 1993).

Types of Valvular Heart Disease

Aortic Stenosis

Aortic stenosis, or narrowing of the aortic valve, is caused by gradual calcification and fibrosis of the valve orifice. The obstruction of flow from the left ventricle into the aorta during systole causes a significant increase in systolic left-ventricular blood pressure (the pressure in the left ventricle that drives blood into the aorta). This increase in left-ventricular systolic pressure results in increased velocity across the valve area and, ultimately, increased myocardial oxygen demand. Over time, the left ventricle becomes hypertrophied (Lilly, 1993). Such left-ventricular hypertrophy tends to stiffen the ventricle, which then increases ventricular diastolic pressure and stimulates left-atrial hypertrophy as well. Left-atrial hypertrophy is an important adaptation that augments forward flow from the atrium to the ventricle during atrial contraction.

Generally, individuals with aortic stenosis remain asymptomatic for years until the valve deformity is severe. Symptoms of aortic stenosis are CHF (due to elevated left-atrial and pulmonary pressures that result from left-ventricular contractile dysfunction), angina (related to the imbalance between myocardial demand and supply) and exertional syncope. Syncope is caused by an inability to increase cardiac output during exercise because of the narrowed opening and vasodilation of the peripheral muscle beds, which result in reduced cerebral blood flow.

Once symptoms develop, surgery is the only effective treatment option. Individuals with symptomatic aortic stenosis are at increased risk for sudden death, and are not candidates

for exercise-training programs prior to surgical intervention.

Aortic Regurgitation

Aortic regurgitation is characterized by leakage of blood into the left ventricle during diastole. Acute aortic regurgitation results in a markedly elevated left-ventricular diastolic pressure that is transmitted to the left atrium and pulmonary circulation. The result is severe dyspnea and, in some cases, pulmonary edema. Acute aortic regurgitation usually requires immediate surgical intervention.

In chronic aortic regurgitation, the ventricle dilates and hypertrophies to accommodate the increased blood volume and elevated diastolic pressure. Symptoms of exertional and nocturnal dyspnea and exertional angina gradually occur over a period of years as the ventricle fails to meet the progressively increasing overload (Lilly, 1993). Asymptomatic individuals may be medically treated with diuretics and vasodilators, which reduce afterload (blood remaining in the chamber following contraction). Symptomatic individuals are candidates for surgical intervention.

The etiology of aortic regurgitation may result from rheumatic fever, endocarditis, aortic aneurysm/dissection, syphilis and Marfan's Syndrome. All individuals with Marfan's or syphilitic aortitis are at increased risk for sudden death due to weakening of the aortic wall, and should avoid strenuous exercise.

Individuals with mild-to-moderate aortic regurgitation usually can participate in recreational activities without undue harm because the volume workload of the heart muscle demands less oxygen than the pressure work associated with aortic stenosis. Since aortic regurgitation occurs during diastole, regurgitation may be reduced during exercise as the heart rate increases and the total diastolic time is shortened (Cumming, 1993).

Mitral Stenosis

Mitral stenosis primarily is of rheumatic etiology and is characterized by fibrous thickening of the valve leaflets. The narrowed passageway from the left atrium to the left ventricle results in decreased blood flow through the valve during ventricular diastole and elevated atrial pressures. This rise in pulmonary resistance results in increased myocardial oxygen demand. In severe mitral stenosis, angina and potentially fatal pulmonary edema can occur (Cumming, 1993). Common symptoms are dyspnea and muscular fatigue, especially with exertion. Muscular fatigue is caused by the right ventricle's inability to overcome elevated pulmonary vascular pressures and the subsequent fall in left-ventricular stroke volume and cardiac output. Heart rate is generally rapid, even at low work levels, in an attempt to compensate for the reduced stroke volume. The decreased cardiac output results in significantly lower VO_2max values, which range from 12 to 20 ml/kg/min (Cumming, 1993; Weber & Janicki, 1986). Because of the potential for fatal pulmonary edema, intense exercise should be avoided in symptomatic individuals with mitral stenosis, and physician clearance should be obtained before training these individuals.

Mitral Regurgitation

Mitral regurgitation permits retrograde blood flow from the left ventricle into the left atrium, as a result of incomplete valve closure during systole. Similar to aortic regurgitation, mitral regurgitation places a volume load on the left ventricle as the regurgitated blood is returned to it during diastole. Both the left atrium and ventricle undergo marked chamber dilation, and left-ventricular stroke volume is reduced as blood is returned to the left atrium. In mild mitral regurgitation, heart rate, blood pressure and ECG responses are usually normal, as is cardiac output during exercise.

Common causes of mitral regurgitation are: 1) myxomatous degeneration; 2) myocardial infarction; 3) mitral valve prolapse; and 4) bacterial destruction of the leaflets. Mitral regurgitation overloads the left ventricle, and can slowly cause contractile impairment and eventually CHF. Therefore, the timing of surgical intervention is critical to preserve the myocardium. Unfortunately, the long-term outlook for individuals with artificial mitral valves is poor, so surgery typically is delayed as long as possible (Lilly, 1993). Prognosis is better in individuals who undergo mitral valve repair. Medical treatment typically consists of diuretics and vasodilators, such as ACE inhibitors.

While mild regurgitation produces no symptoms, more severe cases result in dyspnea (due to increased left-trial pressures) and exercise-induced fatigue (from reduced cardiac output). Individuals with severe mitral regurgitation should be monitored closely, as hypotension and arrhythmias can occur. It is not uncommon for individuals with mitral regurgitation to develop atrial fibrillation.

Mitral Valve Prolapse

Affecting about 7 percent of the population, and more common in females than males, mi-

Table 8.1

Client Information to Obtain from Medical Professionals

1) What exercise intensity level is currently appropriate for this client? What rate of progression do you recommend?

2) What exercises, if any, are contra-indicated?

3) What medication is the client taking, and what possible adverse effects should I be aware of?

4) What warning signs and symptoms should I be aware of, and how should they be treated?

5) Are there any rhythm abnormalities? Does the client require ECG monitoring?

If so, would they be better served in a formal cardiac rehabilitation program?

6) What other medical conditions does this client have (e.g., musculoskeletal problems)?

7) What are the long-term goals for this client?

8) What kind of progress can I expect from this client?

9) What pacemaker does the client have? How is it programmed (e.g. upper-rate limits, etc.)?

tral valve °prolapse is characterized by bulging of the valve leaflets into the left atrium during ventricular systole (Lilly, 1993). Mitral valve prolapse is one of the leading causes of mitral regurgitation; however, the regurgitation generally is of little clinical significance. Of greater concern is the tendency for individuals with mitral valve prolapse to develop ventricular ectopy and associated accelerated atrial and ventricular rhythms. Though caution should be used when designing exercise programs for individuals with uncontrolled arrhythmias, most individuals with mitral valve prolapse can participate in recreational and sport activities.

Individuals with any degree of left-ventricular dysfunction at rest should not participate in competitive sports, and those on anticoagulation therapy should avoid body-contact activities. Those with one or more of the following criteria should participate only in low-intensity competitive sports and/or exercise training. Individuals who meet none of these criteria may engage in all forms of competitive sports and exercise training (Joy, 1996).

1. history of syncope, documented to be arrhythmogenic in origin
2. family history of sudden death associated with MVP
3. repetitive forms of sustained and nonsustained supraventricular arrhythmias, especially when exaggerated by exercise
4. moderate-to-severe mitral regurgitation
5. prior embolic event

Exercise Testing for Clients with Valve Disease

Clinical exercise testing primarily is used to assess ventricular function, measure exercise capacity, evaluate symptoms (e.g., angina and dyspnea), observe cardiac rhythm and chronotropic capacity, and quantify disability. Additionally, serial exercise tests serve to monitor improvement or deterioration over time, and adjust therapy as needed. Clinical exercise testing has little diagnostic value in predicting coronary artery disease in valvular heart disease.

Objective measurements of exercise capacity can assist you in counseling clients regarding appropriate recreational, occupational and physical-training activities, as well as possible limitations. However, you must understand how medications affect exercise-testing results and your client's ability to perform physical activity.

Digoxin can cause ischemic-looking ST-T wave changes on the resting and/or exercise electrocardiogram, and these ECG changes should be considered nondiagnostic. Additionally, electrocardiographic change that suggests reduced cardiac blood flow is a common finding in valvular heart disease, despite the fact that a large number of individuals have normal coronary arteries on angiography (Aronow & Harris, 1975). Therefore, ST depression is not a reliable indicator of myocardial ischemia in valvular heart disease, and other forms of exercise testing should be used to evaluate coronary circulation.

Beta blockers and some calcium channel blockers blunt heart rate. You should consider this effect when testing and/or prescribing exercise intensity. Fitness tests that rely on heart rate for VO_2 predictions are inaccurate for individuals on beta blockers, and direct measurements of VO_2 are preferred. During clinical evaluations, the reduced heart-rate response may not allow the heart muscle to work hard enough to provoke ischemia. Therefore, individuals who are being evaluated for possible ischemia should undergo exercise testing with nuclear or echo imaging. Additionally, RPE, rather than heart rate, should be used to monitor exercise intensity.

Exercise testing of clients with valvular disease is not without risk, so the possible benefits must be carefully weighed against these risks. Of particular concern are individuals with aortic stenosis who are at increased risk of developing ventricular arrhythmias and exertional syncope. Aortic stenosis is a relative contraindication for exercise testing. Signs and symptoms of an abnormal response to exercise in individuals with valvular disease are similar to those of coronary artery disease (i.e., excessive fatigue, weakness, pallor, dyspnea and angina). In individuals with mitral stenosis, excessive exercise can result in pulmonary edema and symptoms of dyspnea and/or coughing (Cumming, 1993). Individuals with mitral stenosis should not be pushed to intense levels of exertion, and the evaluation should be immediately terminated if symptoms of dyspnea and/or cough develop.

Chest pain, another exertional symptom of concern, may indicate myocardial ischemia or pulmonary hypertension, or may be a benign symptom not related to the heart muscle, but may be of chest-wall orientation. Additionally, dizziness, confusion, facial pallor and unsteady gate may be signs of reduced cerebral blood flow. Symptoms of angina and/or reduced cerebral blood flow should be taken seriously, and the exercise test or session should be terminated immediately.

Along with ventricular rhythm abnormalities (e.g., ventricular tachycardia), individuals with valve disease may develop other exertional arrhythmias such as atrial fibrillation, atrial flutter and supraventricular tachycardia. Consider terminating the test if these arrhythmias develop, especially if the ventricular response is rapid. Many individuals with valvular heart disease also have resting arrhythmias, such as atrial fibrillation and frequent PVCs. These are not necessarily a contraindication for exercise testing or training, as long as the ventricular rate is well controlled. Frequently, resting PVCs decrease with exertion (Cumming, 1993).

Exercise testing of individuals with valve disease is highly recommended prior to initiating an exercise-training program and should be conducted under physician supervision. Submaximal fitness tests, such as the six-minute-walk test, may be safely conducted once your client has been medically cleared by their physician. Clients who have undergone recent clinical exercise testing generally do not require an additional fitness evaluation, as clinical data can be utilized to develop the exercise program.

Exercise Training for Clients with Valvular Heart Disease

Nonsurgical Clients

Little scientific evidence supports the thesis that exercise training improves the mechanical function of an abnormal cardiac valve. Therefore, improvement in valve function is not one of the primary objectives of exercise training for individuals who have not undergone surgical intervention. In fact, exercise training is not recommended for individuals with moderately severe to severe symptoms.

Since physical inactivity leads to other chronic health problems and exercise training improves muscloskeletal working capacity, there is merit in maintaining the functional status of the individual prior to surgical intervention. However, the physician must weigh the benefits against the potential risks prior to recommending exercise programming.

Ensure that clients with valve disease (who have not undergone surgical intervention) obtain physician clearance prior to participating in an exercise-training program. This is especially critical for clients who are symptomatic with exertion. Physicians may prefer that these patients initially exercise in a monitored setting (e.g., cardiac rehabilitation) and, in some cases, that exercise be abstained from until surgery is performed.

Table 8.2

Typical Activity Guidelines

Specific guidelines will depend on the type and severity of the valvular disease, which must be determined by the cardiologist. Generally, strenuous exercise should be avoided until the extent of the disease is determined.

- Clients should participate in aerobic activities of mild-to-moderate intensity and duration.
- Stress proper breathing and lifting techniques during resistance training, which may be contra-indicated in some clients.
- Discuss adverse responses to exercise (e.g., angina, shortness of breath, etc.). If they occur, the client should cease exercise and contact their physician.
- Emphasize proper hydration, especially for clients taking diuretics.
- Encourage gentle stretching exercises to improve mobility/flexibility.

Generally, individuals with valvular heart disease are classified in one of the following categories recommended by the American Heart Association exercise standards (Fletcher, Balady, Froelicher, Hartley, Haskell & Pollock, 1995):

Class B: These individuals have a known, stable cardiovascular disease with low risk for vigorous exercise, but slightly greater risk than for class A (apparently healthy individuals). Generally, this group has an exercise capacity greater than 6 METs, no evidence of heart failure or angina, no abnormal ventricular rhythms and an appropriate hemodynamic response to exercise. Class B individuals also are able to satisfactorily self-monitor exercise intensity. Activity should be individualized and prescribed by qualified personnel trained in basic CPR. Exercise training should be initiated under medical supervision and then may be continued in non-medical settings once the individual understands how to monitor intensity.

Class C: These individuals are at moderate-to-high risk for cardiac complications during exercise and/or are unable to self-regulate activity or to understand recommended intensity parameters. This includes individuals with valvular heart disease with 1) an exercise capacity less than 6 METs; 2) symptoms; 3) abnormal hemodynamic response to exercise; and/or 4) life-threatening disease. Medical supervision with ECG and blood pressure monitoring is recommended during all exercise sessions until safety is established.

Only a limited number of studies on the effects of exercise training on individuals with nonsurgical valve disease have been published, and the results have not been overly impressive. Unfortunately, many reported studies have suffered from methodological problems, such as small numbers, nonrandomization and short training duration (one to six weeks). Scordo (1991) evaluated 38 women (mean age = 34) with symptomatic mitral valve prolapse who were randomly assigned to either exercise or control groups. Subjects in the exercise group participated in 12 weeks of aerobic exercise training three times per week for 45 to 60 minutes each session. Intensity was maintained between 60 percent and 85 percent of the maximum achieved heart rate, and a perceived effort of "somewhat hard" on the Borg RPE Scale. Exercise capacity, quantified from peak exercise time and peak workload, achieved on pre- and post-exercise testing was significantly improved following training. It is unfortunate that VO_2 was not directly measured to control for treadmill familiarization, which may influence estimated VO_2 values. Additionally, it would have been helpful if the ventilatory threshold was measured as a submaximal marker of improvement. However, it must be noted that general well-being was rated higher on the post-test compared to the pre-test scores, suggesting that participation in exercise training results in greater confidence and quality of life. No major complications were associated with exercise training, which indicates that individuals with mild-to-moderate mitral valve prolapse can safely participate in exercise-training programs.

When working with pre-surgery valvular heart disease patients, it is critical that you communicate closely with your client's physician to ensure a safe and appropriate training program. Generally, mild to moderate exercise intensities are prescribed, and aerobic activities are encouraged. Resistance training must be applied with caution, and proper technique and breathing stressed. Review the resistance-training program with your client's physician prior to implementing it. Also, carefully monitor your client for adverse exercise responses such as angina, shortness of breath, blood pressure changes and associated symptoms, such as lightheadedness and color changes. Be prepared to respond to emergency situations.

Exercise Training Following Surgery

Generally, there is an immediate improvement in exercise capacity and exercise-induced symptoms following valve repair or replacement surgery. The degree of improvement depends on the presence and severity of valve-induced myocardial changes (e.g., cavity size, hypertrophy, stiffness), rhythm abnormalities, other valve involvement and the degree of physical deconditioning prior to surgery. Many individuals successfully return to occupational and leisure-time activities without participating in formal rehabilitation programs. Physicians frequently encourage post-valve-surgery patients to begin walking programs, starting with short durations of five to 10 minutes, two to three times per day. Gradually, the length of each walking bout is increased to 20 to 30 minutes and the sessions are reduced to one per day, four to five times per week.

Because valve disease only recently has become a recognized diagnosis for cardiac rehabilitation programs, very little outcome data exists on the effects of chronic exercise training on individuals with this disease. As previously discussed, many individuals only need a few sessions of monitored exercise before moving to an unmonitored setting, while others require no ECG monitoring at all. However, a number of post-surgery individuals have rhythm abnormalities and/or are noncompliant regarding exercise-intensity limits and, thus, benefit from monitored exercise sessions. Guidelines for exercise-training program development for individuals with valve disease are similar to those for participants in cardiac rehabilitation programs. It is important that you receive physician clearance prior to initiating a training program for a client with valvular heart disease.

Your role in the continuum of care for individuals with valve disease is generally in the post-rehabilitation setting and with pre- and post-intervention clients who are stable, asymptomatic and cleared by their physician for participation in physical-activity programs. Symptomatic individuals, especially those who have not undergone surgical repair or replacement and those with rhythm abnormalities, should be referred to their physician with the recommendation that they initially be enrolled in a supervised cardiac rehabilitation program.

Moderation is the key to exercise training for valve-disease clients. Strive for consistency, not intensity. While some clients may be able to work at higher intensities and strive to improve performance, the primary goal of the majority is to improve health-related fitness. Therefore, intensity should be set at easy-to-moderate levels. Because many individuals may be on anti-coagulants, have prosthetic valves that may cause mechanical hemolysis during exercise-induced tachycardia, and have limited valve openings, caution is urged in recommending moderate-to-high exercise training intensities (Moir, 1989).

The RPE scale is an ideal tool for monitoring intensity in valve-disease clients. Intensity should be set at an RPE between 10 and 13 for most individuals. It may be necessary to work with your client for a few sessions to help them accurately judge intensity and monitor their response (e.g., symptoms, fatigue levels, aches/pains, etc.). This will assist you in making appropriate adjustments. It is always best to take a conservative approach and to strive for consistency over time.

Dynamic exercise, such as walking, bicycling and the use of other cardiovascular machines, generally serves as the foundation of the training program. Isometric and upper-extremity exercises that use small portions of the muscle mass are more intense and result in increased myocardial oxygen demands. Resistance training can be an important part of the exercise program, but proper technique and breathing must be emphasized. Use of light-to-moderate weights is recommended for one set of 10 to 12 repetitions for each specific exercise.

While the formal exercise program can be carried out three to four times per week, 30 minutes of daily physical activity also should be encouraged. In other words, encourage clients to live a physically active lifestyle and look for opportunities to physically move during the course of each day. Walking is an excellent activity for most clients, especially those just beginning an activity program. Deconditioned clients should begin with short durations (five to 10 minutes, two to three times a day) and gradually progress to one 30- to 45-minute session of continuous aerobic conditioning three to four times per week. Better-conditioned individuals can begin with longer durations.

The program should be tailored to each individual based upon their current level of conditioning, disease status, risk factors and other health problems. Additionally, carefully assess your client's likes and dislikes, and set realistic goals and objectives. Individualizing the program is critical in developing adherence over time and, thus, stimulating conditioning adaptations. The goal is to make physical activity a part of your client's lifestyle. Help your client identify barriers to physical activity, and point out strategies to overcome each identified barrier.

Special Concerns

Because only a limited number of studies have been published, the effects of chronic exercise training on valve disease are unknown. Be careful to obtain physician clearance prior to starting an exercise training program for clients who have not undergone valve repair or replacement. Also, be cognizant of the acute problems that can arise, and be well versed in basic life support (CPR) and emergency procedures. Be alert for symptoms of ischemia (e.g., chest, arm, neck or jaw discomfort), faintness, nausea or lightheadedness, shortness of breath and excessive fatigue (clients should not feel exhausted). Additionally, monitor your client's ability to carry on a conversation during exercise to ensure appropriate intensity. Should symptoms occur, terminate the exercise session and immediately notify your client's physician. Also be aware of the signs of heart failure (ankle edema, mild nocturnal dyspnea, sudden weight gain and unusual fatigue). Should such signs appear, postpone exercise and refer your client to their physician for further evaluation.

There still are a number of unanswered questions regarding chronic exercise training. For this reason, generally keep intensities at low-to-moderate levels. The long-term effect of exercise training on the already overloaded heart is unknown. Will the rate of valve fibrosis/calcification increase? Will the heart enlarge at a more rapid rate, inducing atrial fibrillation or excessive dilation of the chamber (Moir, 1989)? In addition, the optimal amount of exercise is not yet known. Some individuals probably are better off doing no exercise, while others may be able to safely participate in more vigorous activities. Because of these unanswered questions, it is best to work closely with your client's physician and/or cardiac rehabilitation staff to develop a conservative and safe training program.

Case Study

A 68-year-old retired male photographer is referred to you for development of an ongoing exercise training program. He recently has completed a phase II cardiac rehabilitation program following replacement of his mitral valve. Your client has a longstanding history of mitral regurgitation that was first identified as a heart murmur at age 18. Prior to surgery, he experienced symptoms of fatigue and shortness of breath with mild-to-moderate exertion. He experienced no chest pain and no evidence of heart failure was present. Thallium exercise-testing results were normal except for a resting and exercise rhythm of atrial fibrillation. The client has led a fairly active life, except for the three months prior to surgery when his symptoms worsened. He enjoys golfing, skiing and walking, and current medications include coumadin and vitamins. Table 8.3 presents data from his pre- and post-cardiac rehabilitation exercise tests.

Prior to meeting with your client, gather his medical history and meet with the cardiac-rehabilitation staff to review the rehab exercise-training program and past responses, and to receive input regarding long-term recommendations.

Note that your client is on coumadin, so contact sports are not recommended. With the underlying cardiac rhythm of atrial fibrillation, RPE rather than heart rate should be used to monitor exercise intensity. According to the rehabilitation staff, your client's goals are to improve his endurance and overall muscular strength in order to continue enjoying golf and skiing. A fitness evaluation is not necessary as your client has just undergone his post-rehabilitation treadmill test

Table 8.3

Variable	Pre-test	Post-test
Height/Weight	70"/160lbs	70"/158lbs
Resting BP	116/66	118/70
Peak Exercise		
Exercise duration	7:00 min	7:00 min
Peak Wk load	3 mph/ 14.5%	3.6 mph/ 16.5%
Peak HR	155	157
Peak BP	130/60	152/78
Peak VO$_2$	1560 ml/min	1827 ml/min
	21.5 ml/kg/min	25.5 ml/kg/min
Ventilatory Threshold		
Heart Rate	110	112
RPE	13	13
VO$_2$	1092 ml/min	1327 ml/min

and this data is adequate for developing the exercise program.

During your initial meeting with the client, discuss the results of the cardiac-rehabilitation program and ask your client to restate his long-term goals and objectives. He relates that he also would like to participate in day hikes this summer to take scenic wilderness and wildlife photographs, so the training program should prepare your client for the varied terrain of wilderness areas. The following program is mutually agreed upon between you and your client, and a copy of the program is forwarded to the cardiac-rehabilitation staff for their follow-up records.

Aerobic Training

Mode: Walking with short, hill intervals, both on a treadmill and outdoors when weather permits. A stair climber and elliptical cross trainer are recommended one to two times per week to add variety and cross training.

Intensity: Set the average intensity at an RPE of 11 to 13, based on the ventilatory threshold of "somewhat hard" identified on the post-rehabilitation exercise test. Intensity may rise as high as 15 for short, three- to five-minute periods during hill-climbing intervals. Conduct interval sessions once per week.

Frequency: Four to five times per week with three sessions of steady walking, one session of hill intervals and one session of cross training.

Duration: Initially, set duration at 30 minutes of aerobic conditioning, and progress in five-minute increments to a maximum of 40 to 60 minutes.

Resistance Training

Encourage participation in two resistance-training sessions per week that emphasize light weights, appropriate technique and one set of 10 to 12 repetitions for each activity. Exercises should consist of four lower-extremity exercises, five upper-extremity exercises and one abdominal exercise.

Mobility/Flexibility

Continue lower- and upper-extremity stretching exercises, which were learned in the cardiac-rehabilitation program, as part of the warm-up and cool-down phases of aerobic conditioning. Emphasize slow, controlled movements and take care to stretch only to the point of tension.

Follow-up

Ask your client to maintain a log of daily activities and responses to the training program. Review the log weekly and check for symptoms and adherence to the recommended training program, especially intensity guidelines. Meet with your client once per week for training; the other sessions are self-directed. Additionally, assist your client in planning his day hikes by providing accurate information regarding food, hydration, rest periods, clothing, shoes and first aid. Arrange a follow-up exercise test with the cardiac rehabilitation staff in four months, just prior to the beginning of the summer hiking adventures.

Pacemakers

Since the first cardiac pacemaker implant 40 years ago, the incidence of permanent pacemaker implants in the U.S. has grown to approximately 110,000 annually. Eighteen percent of these are replacement pacemakers for already-existing systems. Worldwide, about 300,000 pacemakers are implanted each year (Goldschlager, Ludmer & Creamer, 1995).

In the U.S. today, a majority of implanted pacemakers are dual-chambered (rate-adaptive) devices. These devices sense and/or pace in both the right atrium and ventricle with an appropriately adjusted or programmed A-V delay to facilitate atrial contribution to ventricular diastolic filling. These pacemakers are called either DDD or DDDR devices. Letter codes refer to the chamber(s) paced, sensed and the response to sensing, respectively. The "D" refers to double chamber (e.g., both right atrium and right ventricle being paced and sensed) and to a dual-triggered or inhibited means of pacing response. The letter "R" refers to programmable rate response, which is driven by a specific sensor, such as body activity or acceleration, ventilation, temperature, QT intervals or other metabolically related signals. Generally, dual-chambered pacemaker leads are placed in the right-ventricular apex and right-atrial appendage for ventricular and atrial stimulation, respectively. Other patients may have single-chamber (rate-responsive) pacemakers called AAIR or VVIR units. These pacemakers only sense and pace (according to a sensor signal) in the right atrium or right ventricle, respectively, via an inhibitory (I) mode.

The heart muscle contracts and pumps blood when stimulated by action potentials (electrical signals) that sweep across the muscle cell membranes. Cardiac muscle consists of two types of specialized cells: contractile cells, which do the mechanical work, and autorhythmic cells, which specialize in initiating and conducting action potentials. The cardiac cells responsible for autorhythmicity are found within the heart in the following locations:

- *the sinoatrial node (SA node):* found in the right atrium near the opening of the superior vena cava
- *the atrioventricular node (AV node):* found at the base of the right atrium near the septum
- *the bundle of His (AV bundle):* a tract of cells originating at the AV node that span to the interventricular septum where they divide into the right and left bundle branches
- *the purkinje fibers:* small terminal fibers that extend from the bundle of His and spread throughout the ventricular myocardium.

Normal rhythmic conduction originates in the SA node and spreads throughout both atria. Two special pathways assist in this process: the interatrial pathway, extending from the SA node to the left atrium, and the internodal pathway, extending from the SA node to the AV node. Once the impulse arrives at the AV node, conduction is slowed and delayed about .1 second to enable the atria to contract and empty their contents into the ventricles. Following the AV nodal delay, the impulse rapidly travels down the bundle of his and throughout the ventricular muscle via the purkinje fibers.

Approximately 40 percent to 60 percent of pacemaker patients exhibit defects in their sinus node's ability to modulate heart rate, in accordance with metabolic demand during exercise (Sutton, 1995). This is the result of various conduction system defects or blocks in impulse conduction that result from aging and/or heart disease. Therefore, more patients are receiving rate-adaptive devices to correct for what is termed chronotropic incompetence or insufficiency. The cardiac pacemaker serves as a substitute impulse source that provides appropriate excitation of cardiac tissues upon demand.

It is these patients — who are, for the most part, deconditioned — who present a challenge for designing and assisting in effective exercise training programs to improve functional capacity. However, recent data (Greco, Guardini & Citelli, 1998) indicates that rate-adaptive pacemaker patients can benefit from aerobic exercise training. Eleven patients (seven males and four females) with rate-adaptive pacemakers underwent aerobic exercise training according to ACSM guidelines. Significant improvement was noted in ventilatory threshold, peak oxygen uptake and total exercise time following the training program.

Required Follow-up Equipment for Pacemaker Clients

It is mandatory that immediate access be available to the required pacemaker programmer provided by the manufacturer. You must have pacemaker-programming support and device "read out" or monitoring prior to the start of any pacemaker-client training program. You should clearly understand what type of pacemaker device your client has, the mode of pacemaker programming (e.g., chambers sensed or paced, fixed-rate or rate-response), and the lower- and upper-programmed rates. It also is important to know what type of rate-response sensor, if any, the pacemaker utilizes, and whether rate response is activated and to what degree.

Many pacemaker patients, with or without rate-adaptive sensors, are programmed prior to patient discharge according to the manufacturer's recommendations. However, you must always bear in mind that your client may not be appropriately programmed for their fitness level and/or their cardiac or pulmonary disease condition. *Upon review of your client's current pacemaker settings, it is important to either review these parameters with your client's current follow-up physician, or to arrange for their physician's presence during the first training session.*

In addition, be aware of any medications your client is currently taking, such as anti-arrhythmic inotropic agents or other drugs used to treat cardiac disease or metabolic disorders. Clients with brady/tachy syndrome, a type of sick sinus disease, may be taking beta blockers to suppress supraventricular tachycardia, especially during exercise. Pacemaker clients on beta blocker medication may be even more dependent on the pacemaker device for appropriate chronotropic response due to the negative effects of the medication.

Testing Prior to Training — Program Initiation

Before exercise training can be performed at a specific workload on the bicycle, treadmill or any other piece of exercise equipment, your client's rate-response level must be assessed (e.g., whether there is a normal match of paced rate or intrinsic rhythm to metabolic demand). Since many dual-chambered pacemaker clients have sick sinus syndrome (SSS) with intermittent brady/tachycardia, beta blocker medication may have been prescribed to reduce overall sinus node rate. In such situations, your client may become more dependent on the pacemaker's stimulation rate during exercise. A majority of VVIR clients and many DDDR clients also have advanced A-V block as a conduction defect and are, therefore, dependent on the pacemaker for ventricular activation. Chronotropic incompetence (defined as an attained heart rate at peak exercise of less than 100 beats per minute (bpm) or at a rate of less than 60 percent of age-predicted maximum heart rate at anaerobic (ventilatory) threshold may be present during early exercise or exercise onset, or later during higher intensities above the client's anaerobic (ventilatory) threshold. It is important that you know whether your client's rate response to exercise is intrinsic or paced, and at which exercise levels. This can be achieved by standard telemetry methods or review of actual pacemaker "data log" files following exercise.

To ensure that your client's paced rate is matched to their metabolic demand, a low-intensity treadmill exercise test called the LITE protocol should be performed (Lewalter, Mac-Carter, Jung, Bauer, Schimpf, Manz & Luderitz, 1995). The LITE protocol is a six-minute, constant workload test at 35 external watts of work or approximately 65 watts of work on the bicycle. The treadmill elevation is set at 8-percent grade, and the speed adjusted between 1.0 and 1.5 mph, depending on the client's body weight. As a general rule, heavier patients who weigh approximately 85 to 90 kg will walk on the treadmill at speeds close to 1.0 to 1.2 mph, while patients in the range of

60 to 75 kg will walk at faster speeds of 1.4 to 1.5 mph. The average heart rate attained during the LITE protocol is 102 ±19 bpm (Lewalter, Jung, Bauer, Schimpf, Manz & Luderitz, 1995; Lewalter, Jung, MacCarter, Bauer, Schimpf, Manz & Luderitz, 1994).

LITE Protocol by Individual Body Weight

Weight lbs. (kg)	Treadmill Grade	Treadmill Speed (mph)	Watts
100 (45.2)	8%	2.2	35
110 (49.7)	8%	2.0	35
120 (54.2)	8%	1.8	35
130 (58.7)	8%	1.7	35
140 (63.2)	8%	1.6	35
150 (67.8)	8%	1.5	35
160 (72.3)	8%	1.4	35
170 (76.8)	8%	1.3	35
180 (81.3)	8%	1.2	35
190 (85.8)	8%	1.2	35
200 (90.3)	8%	1.1	35
210 (94.9)	8%	1.1	35
220 (99.4)	8%	1.0	35
230 (103.9)	8%	1.0	35
240 (108.4)	8%	1.0	35

The heart-rate-to-work-rate relationship (HR/WR ratio) during exercise has been reported in normal subjects to average .37 ± .13 beats/min/watt. However, the HR/WR ratio is slightly greater in women (.43 ±.15), as compared to men (.32 ± .09) (Lewalter, MacCarter, Jung, Schimpf, Manz & Luderitz, 1995). Usually, using the known average relationship, you can expect a four- to five-beat increase in paced heart rate (ppm) for every 10-watt increment of work performed.

Exercise Training for Clients with Pacemakers

Let's review the following example. A 60-year-old male patient with SSS and an ELA medical rate-adaptive, ventilation sensor-driven pacemaker (Chorus RM, Model 7034) has sinus bradycardia and third-degree AV block. He has no evidence of myocardial ischemia or structural heart disease. His age-predicted maximum heart rate is 160 bpm. Recently, upper rates for rate-adaptive pacemakers have been programmed to 90 percent of the client's age-predicted maximum heart rate to adequately restore heart-rate reserve. Therefore, the upper programmable rate could be set at approximately 140 to 145 bpm.

This upper rate allows your client to exercise at higher exercise intensities above the anaerobic threshold, which is estimated to occur at 70 percent of age-predicted maximum heart rate or at approximately 115 bpm. Often, pacemaker clients are programmed to upper rates of 120 bpm, which may limit their functional capacity and rate response at anaerobic levels of exercise. However, for the purpose of implementing effective aerobic training programs, an observed training rate in the range of 110 to 120 bpm, or at approximately 50 percent to 60 percent of VO_2max, is sufficient for most older patients (Skinner, 1993).

Monitor systolic blood pressure to make certain there is not an inadequate rise or a marked decrease during exercise training. In general, a normal systolic blood pressure rise from rest to peak exercise is 60± 25 mmHg for men and women between the ages of 40 and 65 years (Froelicher & Pashkow, 1993). Also, monitor the level of perceived exertion (RPE) using the 15-point Borg scale during your client's training program. Do not train your client at an RPE level higher than 13 or 14, or above MET levels of four to six (Skinner, 1993; Froelicher & Pashkow, 1993).

It is understood that more athletically trained pacemaker subjects can exercise at higher heart-rate and MET levels. If your client is younger and athletically inclined, the follow-up physician should program upper pacemaker rates closer to 90 percent of age-predicted maximum or 145 ppm for more effective exercise-program design and training.

If your 60-year-old client in the preceding example was to exercise at 80 watts of external treadmill work, an attained heart rate of 4-5 beats per 10-watt increments of work, or a 32-40 bpm increase in heart rate above the standing resting rate is expected, which is typically 75 to 80 bpm for normal control subjects. Therefore, your client's expected exercise heart rate is approximately 115 ppm, which agrees closely with the predicted heart rate at the anaerobic threshold. As you know, clients can benefit significantly from exercising at close to their anaerobic threshold for the purposes of optimizing fat metabolism and enhancing functional capacity. Therefore, designing a program for your client in this heart-rate range for 20 to 30 minutes, three times a week,

may provide both cardiac and fitness benefits. For example, training pace rates in the 150 to 155 bpm range may be programmed for the pacemaker in a 50-year-old woman with a ventilation-driven DDR pacemaker (META 1252) who participates in marathon and triathlon events.

If your client has a history of ischemic heart disease or has suffered from myocardial infarction, limit the upper-programmed rate closer to 85 percent of their age-predicted maximum heart rate or the 110 to 120 bpm level. This is especially important if your client demonstrates an ischemic anginal threshold at rates slightly above the 120 ppm range. Remember, the true ST segment depression cannot be easily assessed during paced activity unless intermittent intrinsic rhythm is observed.

Take caution when exercising pacemaker clients with congestive heart failure, class II and below. Upper-paced rate or intrinsic rates should not occur above 110 to 115 bpm, in order to optimize stroke volume output. Programming appropriate A-V delays for patients with DDD or DDDR devices enhances diastolic function and facilitates the contribution of atrial contraction to ventricular filling. However, as stated earlier, programming of A-V delays should be performed by your client's physician.

Summary

Be aware of the type of pacemaker implanted in your client. Rate-adaptive devices offer advantages over rate-responsive VVI, AAI and DDD devices, especially if your client has heart disease or is chronotropically incompetent. Aging clients with left-ventricular dysfunction become ever more rate-dependent to increase cardiac output during exercise. The rate-response factor or slope of rate response reflects how effectively the pacemaker can change its paced rate in response to detected changes in the sensor signal and in accordance with your client's metabolic demand. The pacemaker rate should be programmed according to your client's age, fitness level and cardiac status, and should not be a limitation to exercise training. Proper testing is necessary to establish appropriate rate response prior to implementation of the exercise training program. In addition to perceived exertion and systolic blood pressure, all training sessions and routine warm-up and cool-down periods should be monitored. Care also should be taken for immediate cardiac resuscitation or cardioversion of life-threatening ventricular tachyarrhythmias, if necessary.

References

American College of Sports Medicine. (1993). *Resource Manual for Guidelines for Exercise Testing and Prescription* (2nd ed.) Philadelphia: Williams and Wilkins.

Aronow, W.S. & Harris, C.N. (1975). Treadmill Exercise Test in Aortic Stenosis and Mitral Stenosis. *Chest,* 68, 507.

Cumming, G.R. (1993). Valvular and Congenital Heart Disease in Adults. In S.S. Skinner, (Ed.) *Exercise Testing and Exercise Prescription for Special Cases: Theoretical Basis and Clinical Application* (2nd ed.), 317-338, Philadelphia, Pa.: Lea and Febiger.

Fletcher, G.F., Balady, G., Froelicher, V.F., Hartley, H., Haskell, W.L. & Pollock, M.L. (1995). *Exercise Standards: A statement for health professionals from the American Heart Association.* AHA Medical/Scientific Statement.

Fletcher, G.F., Balady, G., Blair, S.N., Blumenthal, J., Caspersen, C., Chaitman, B., Epstein, S., Sivarajan-Froelicher, E.S., Froelicher, V.F., Pina, I.L. & Pollock, M.L. (1996). Statement on exercise: Benefits and recommendations for physical activity programs for all Americans. A statement for health professionals by the Committee on Exercise and Cardiac Rehabilitation of the Council on Clinical Cardiology, American Heart Association. *Circulation,* 94, 4, 857-862.

Froelicher, V. & Pashkow, F. (1993). *Clinical Cardiac Rehabilitation.* Baltimore, Md.: Williams and Wilkins.

Goldschlager, N., Ludmer, P. & Creamer, C. (1995). *Clinical Cardiac Pacing.* Philadelphia, Pa.: W.B. Saunders Co.

Greco, M.E., Guardini, S. & Citelli, L. (1998). Cardiac Rehabilitation in Patients with Rate Responsive Pacemakers. *Pace,* 21, 568-575.

Joy, E. (1996). Mitral Valve Prolapse in Active Patients: Recognition, Treatment and Exercise Recommendations. *The Physician and Sportsmedicine,* 24, 7.

Lewalter, T., Jung, W., MacCarter, D., Bauer, W., Schimpf, R., Manz, M. & Luderitz, B. (1994). Heart Rate During Exercise: What is the Optimal Goal of Rate Adaptive Pacemaker Therapy? *American Heart Journal,* 127, 1026-1030.

Lewalter, T., MacCarter, D., Jung, W., Bauer, T., Schimpf, R., Manz, M. & Luderitz, B. (1995). The "Low Intensity Treadmill Exercise" Protocol for Appropriate Rate Adaptive Programming of Minute Controlled Pacemakers. *Pace,* 18, 1374-1387.

Lewalter, T., MacCarter, D., Jung, W., Schimpf, R., Manz, M. & Luderitz, B. (1995). Heart Rate to Work Rate Relation Throughout Peak Exercise in Normal Subjects as a Guideline for Rate-Adaptive Pacemaker Programming. *The American Journal of Cardiology,* 76, 812-816.

Lilly, L.S., Chan, E., Duh, E. & Stidham, B. (1993). Valvular Heart Disease. In L.S. Lilly (Ed.) *Pathophysiology of Heart Disease,* 130-146. Philadelphia, Pa.: Lea and Febiger.

Moir, W.T. (1989). Nonischemic Cardiovascular Disease. In B.A. Franklin, Gordon, S. & Timmis, G.C. (Eds.) *Exercise in Modern Medicine* 81-106. Baltimore, Md.: Williams and Wilkins.

Scordo, D.A. (1991). Effects of Aerobic Exercise Training on Symptomatic Women with Mitral Valve Prolapse. *American Journal of Cardiology,* 67, 863-868.

Skinner, J.S. (1993). *Exercise Testing and Exercise Prescription for Special Cases: Theoretical Basis and Clinical Application* (2nd ed.) Philadelphia, Pa.: Lea and Febiger.

Sutton, R. (1995). *Sinus Node Disease.* Philadelphia, Pa.: W.B. Saunders Co.

Weber, K.T. & Janicki, J.S. (1986). *Cardiopulmonary Exercise Testing: Physiological Principles and Clinical Applications.* Philadelphia, Pa.: W.B. Saunders Co.

Section Three

Pulmonary Diseases

Chapter 9
Asthma

Chapter 10
Chronic
Obstructive
Pulmonary
Disease

CHAPTER 9

Asthma

CHRISTINE CUNNINGHAM

Christine "CC" Cunningham, M.S.,
is an NATABOC-certified athletic
trainer with extensive experience
as a personal trainer. Formerly the
director of programming for First
Fitness Inc., she is now a private
consultant specializing in fitness
program development and
education. She is a frequent
lecturer and writer and an
American Council on Exercise
Master Practical Trainer.

Asthma Triggers
Prophylactic Medications
Diaphragmatic Breathing

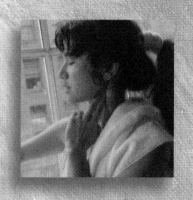

Asthma affects an estimated 14 million Americans. Considered a restrictive lung disease because it can be reversed spontaneously or with medication, asthma can develop at any age. Many asthmatics outgrow the disease while others are affected throughout their lives. Genetics play a large part in determining who will develop asthma. However, there are currently no reliable means for predicting who will develop asthma or how long the disease will affect them.

Asthma attacks are a lung reaction causing breathing difficulty. Treatment focuses on reducing the severity and frequency of attacks. With proper treatment, asthmatics can lead a normal life and suffer no lung damage. Untreated asthma can lead to lung damage and even death. Asthma can effectively be controlled with proper exercise programming, use of medication and trigger control. You should not work with an asthmatic who does not have control of their asthma. Untreated asthma can be dangerous, and those individuals who do not seek proper intervention are unsuitable for involvement in community-based exercise programs.

Benefits of Exercise

Regular exercise offers asthmatics the same benefits as their nonasthmatic counterparts, including increased functional capacity, decreased fear of experiencing asthma symptoms and improved self-image. Generally, asthmatics participate less in sports and are found to be less physically conditioned than their nonasthmatic peers. A study performed by Emtner et al. (1996) showed that asthmatics were deterred from participating in a regular exercise program because they felt anxiety about incurring an attack during exercise and they lacked instruction on how to exercise appropriately. But with proper medication and exercise programming, asthmatics can improve their fitness level and excel to the highest levels of athletic competition.

What is Asthma?

Asthma is an increase in resistance to airflow through the bronchiole tubes in response to exposure to a trigger. Common asthma triggers are allergens, irritants and exercise. An asthmatic's lungs are hypersensitive to triggers. Exposure to a trigger causes the smooth muscles surrounding the bronchioles to constrict, thus reducing the size of the airways. The cells lining the tubes also become inflamed and produce a clear mucus that further clogs the airways. Air has difficulty passing through the bronchiole tubes to and from the alveolar sacs (where the exchange of gas with blood takes place) thus reducing oxygen availability. Because asthma is an air-trapping disease, exhalation is affected more severely than inhalation.

Symptoms of asthma include:
➤ coughing
➤ wheezing
➤ chest tightness
➤ shortness of breath

A prolonged asthma attack may lead to an alteration in blood gases, increasing the concentration of CO_2 due to the difficulty in removing the gas through exhalation.

Asthma is diagnosed through a combination of patient reporting and testing. A patient may notice the onset of symptoms when in the presence of triggers. If the triggers are allergens, allergy testing can confirm the sensitivity of the patient to that substance. During lung function tests, asthmatics demonstrate a reduction in their **FEV1** (volume of air forcibly expired in one second) and **peak expiratory flow rate** (PEFR).

Asthma can vary in its severity. Infrequent sufferers may experience intermittent symptoms with no evidence of the condition demonstrated between episodes. Those who suffer more severe symptoms risk a chronic reduction in lung function that can lead to impaired functional capacity and difficulty performing activities of daily living. Despite the severity of symptoms, asthma can effectively be controlled through medication and patient education.

Asthma Triggers

The three most common asthma triggers are allergens, irritants and exercise. Other triggers include infection, emotions and stress. One or more of these may cause the onset of asthma symptoms.

Allergens

Not all asthmatics have allergic triggers, although allergens are frequent offenders. The most common allergens are food, pollen, dust, molds and pets. When allergic asthmatics come in contact with an allergen, their airways react with bronchospasm. Allergy testing provides allergic asthmatics with a list of allergens to be avoided. The list is not comprehensive, however, as allergies can develop and change over time. Some allergens may be seasonal or more prevalent in a specific environment, such as indoor dust. Avoiding offending allergens is the best way to reduce the likelihood that they will lead to an asthma attack.

Irritants

Irritants such as secondhand smoke, pollution, perfume and cold air also can trigger bronchospasm. Like allergens, avoiding exposure is the best method for dealing with irritants. The effects of cold air can be reduced by wearing a scarf or mask over the mouth and nose to warm the air before it enters the lungs. Other potential irritants, such as cleaning chemicals and construction dust, may be introduced to an environment unexpectedly. Always be aware of the possibility that previously unidentified irritants may be present and cause asthma symptoms.

Exercise

When exercise triggers an asthma attack, it is called exercise induced asthma (EIA). During exercise of moderate to high intensity, the increase in ventilatory rate allows insufficiently warmed and humidified air to enter the lungs. This causes the lungs to react with bronchospasm. The reaction generally occurs within the first six to 12 minutes of exercise or five to 10 minutes after exercise has stopped. A proper warm-up and cool-down are critical to controlling EIA. Exercise may be the only asthma trigger for some individuals who have no symptoms when exposed to other suspected triggers. However, it is estimated that up to 90 percent of asthmatics have EIA in conjunction with other triggers (McFadden & Gilbert, 1994).

Other Triggers

Illness, such as colds and sinus infections, can exacerbate asthma symptoms. Although asthma is not a psychological disorder, emotion and stress can increase the sensitivity of the airways. Both laughter and crying can trigger an asthma attack. During an attack, fear or panic can make the symptoms worse, so it is important to reassure and calm the client while taking the proper steps to resolve the attack.

Asthma Medications

Asthma is controlled through a combination of trigger avoidance and medication. A wide variety of medications are available for use with asthma, and new medications are being developed to further increase the ease and effectiveness of asthma treatment. Physicians prescribe medication combinations specific to the severity and triggers of an individual's asthma.

Medications can be classified into two major categories: rescue and prophylactic. Both types assist in reducing the frequency and severity of asthma attacks. Rescue medications can be used prior to exposure to a trigger or during an attack to alleviate symptoms. Prophylactic medications taken over a period of time are used to reduce the sensitivity of the airways to triggers.

Rescue Medications

Rescue medications include beta-agonists, short-acting theophylline and adrenaline. The most commonly used medications are beta-agonist inhalers such as albuterol (Ventolin or Proventil). These inhalers act quickly to relax the smooth muscles and are prescribed for use in the event of an attack. Beta-agonist inhalers also are used prior to exposure to triggers, especially exercise, to reduce the chance of an attack. Used 15 to 30 minutes prior to exercise, the inhalers can eliminate EIA symptoms for up to two hours. Side effects include increased heart rate and shakiness, although shakiness subsides over time. The magnitude of these side effects varies greatly with each user.

Short-acting theophylline helps relieve symptoms within one to two hours after taking the medication, and its side effects are similar to beta-agonists. Adrenaline generally is reserved for hospital use due to its significant effects on heart rate and blood pressure.

Prophylactic Medications

Prophylactic medications are not designed to provide immediate relief from bronchospasm. Prescribed by a physician, they are designed to block the specific mechanisms that precipitate an asthma attack, such as histamine release in the presence of an allergen. Long-acting theophylline, cromolyn sodium, leukotriene inhibitors and corticosteroids are members of this group.

Theophylline side effects may include nausea, headache and shakiness. Cromolyn sodium and leukotriene inhibitors cause no significant side effects. Corticosteroids differ from the other three medications in that there are many known side effects that vary depending on the form. In some asthma situations, the benefits of steroid use far outweigh the potential side effects. Corticosteroids come in both oral and inhaled forms. Inhaled steroids are the preferred treatment because they are associated with little or no side effects. The potential side effects associated with long-term oral steroid use include osteoporosis, weight gain, high blood pressure, muscle weakness and mood changes. Corticosteroids used to treat asthma are not the same steroids used to build muscle mass. Muscle building steroids are anabolic steroids and should not be confused with corticosteroids.

Before You Begin Training

Prior to working with an asthmatic client, you must gather necessary information from the client or client's physician (see Table 9.1). Use this information when determining exercise environment, when scheduling and when determining exercise intensity.

What to Do During an Asthma Attack

During physical activity, an asthma attack may be triggered by the exercise or exposure to an allergen or irritant. In the event that the trigger is not exercise, the workout may have to be postponed or moved to another location. Always make sure the client has rescue medications handy before beginning exercise.

Use the following procedure whenever an asthmatic experiences symptoms during exercise:

1) Reduce exercise intensity to allow for easy administration of medication. Do not attempt to have the client "run through" an attack or stop the exercise abruptly.

2) Provide assistance in retrieving the medication and creating an environment where it easily can be taken by the client. At no time should you administer any medication to the client.

3) Provide calm support and reminders for the client to control their breathing rate using the diaphragmatic breathing technique detailed on page 108.

If symptoms do not subside, completely stop the exercise and seek medical attention.

Once asthma symptoms have been relieved, exercise can resume. After resolution of an attack, an asthmatic may experience a period within which they are less likely to experience asthma symptoms. This is called a refractory period. Exercise programming for the asthmatic must be flexible enough to accommodate a possible attack during a session and to maximize the opportunity provided by a refractory period.

Fitness Testing

Fitness testing for asthmatics may require modifying existing test protocols to accommodate environment and intensity. The chosen test should be conducted in the environment least likely to cause an asthma trigger. In addition, the presence of triggers should be controlled for each test in order to compare the results. Indoor testing is recommended because outdoor triggers are more difficult to control. During testing, use the Borg scale for Rating of Perceived Exertion (RPE) and the Dyspnea scale (Table 9.2) to allow clients to assess their level of fatigue and breathlessness. Also use the client's usual program of medication prior to testing. Testing protocols that include a warm-up period, such as the Rockport Fitness Treadmill Test, are best suited for asthmatics.

Table 9.1

Client Information to Obtain from Medical Professionals

1) What are the identified asthma triggers?

2) What rescue medication should be used in the event of an asthma attack?

3) What medications, if any, should be taken prior to exercise, and how much time should be allotted for the medication to take effect?

4) What are the potential side effects of the prescribed rescue and prophylactic medications?

5) What is the client's previous exercise history?

6) What are the client's long- and short-term goals?

7) Are there any known limitations for exercise?

8) Are there any confounding medical conditions that may limit exercise?

Table 9.2
Dyspnea Scale

0.5	– very, very slight
1	– very slight
2	– slight
3	– moderate
4	– somewhat severe
5	– severe
7	– very severe
10	– very, very severe

Testing may not be appropriate initially in an exercise program for asthmatics unfamiliar with exercise and apprehensive about attacks. Postpone testing until the client becomes comfortable exercising with asthma. Use conservative intensities to prescribe the exercise until testing is conducted.

Exercise Programming

Exercise programming for the asthmatic is relatively simple if the disease is effectively controlled. Programming must be changeable based on the asthmatic's condition. Symptom-free days allow for intense training, while other days may require a reduction in intensity. You should discuss the client's current condition at the beginning of each session and be prepared to make necessary modifications. Pre-exercise medication should be taken before every exercise session as prescribed by their physician. For additional guidelines see Table 9. 3.

Asthmatics may have a reduced functional capacity due to their asthma, as well as a previous lack of participation in physical activity. Considerations for determining exercise intensity include the client's state of deconditioning, psychological preparedness for exercise and severity of the disease. Training at intensities of 50 percent to 60 percent of predicted maximal heart rate has been shown safe for asthmatics and effective at increasing functional capacity. Deconditioning or severe asthma may necessitate programming at lower intensities. Emtner et al. (1996) demonstrated that adult asthmatics can safely exercise at intensities of 80 percent to 90 percent predicted maximal heart rate. Intervals of moderate intensity alternated with high intensity have been shown to be the best-tolerated method of high-intensity training for asthmatics (Morton et al., 1981). Intervals as short as one or two minutes may be necessary early in an exercise program for deconditioned or severe asthmatics. Child asthmatics also have been successful with high-intensity activity (Varray et al., 1991). Children may require increased supervision during exercise to ensure early symptoms of an attack are identified and treated. Follow the American College of Sports Medicine guidelines for cardiovascular training to determine the desired training effect and necessary intensities for success. Emphasize a gradual introduction to exercise, and frequently reassess and modify programming according to the client's response to the program.

Special consideration for psychological barriers to exercise may have to be accommodated in

Table 9.3

Typical Activity Guidelines

- Avoid asthma triggers during exercise.
- Always have rescue medication nearby for use in the event of an attack.
- Establish a flexible program that can accommodate fluctuations in exercise capacity due to asthma symptoms.
- Utilize an extended warm-up and cool-down.
- Emphasize hydration before, during and after exercise.
- Practice diaphragmatic breathing.
- Determine exercise intensity according to the client's state of deconditioning, psychological preparedness for exercise and asthma severity.
- Incorporate intervals for high-intensity training.
- Closely monitor the client for early signs of an asthma attack and respond immediately. Get medical help if symptoms do not subside.
- Use perceived exertion and the Dyspnea scale to communicate with the client regarding symptoms.
- Choose exercise testing that accommodates a warm-up period.

the early phases of an exercise program. Intensities may have to be reduced until the asthmatic is comfortable with exercise and can distinguish between the breathlessness of asthma and exercise. The RPE scale is a valuable tool for asthmatics to learn during this period.

The following special program considerations minimize the likelihood of an attack from exercise.

Extended Warm-up and Cool-down

Warm-ups and cool-downs should be extended for the asthmatic. A warm-up of at least 15 minutes has been shown to reduce the probability of an attack (Morton et al., 1981). During this period, the exercise intensity is gradually increased to 50 percent to 60 percent of predicted maximal heart rate. It is thought that the extended warm-up allows the lungs to get past the early period of six to 12 minutes when an attack is likely to occur. The longer, lower intensities allow the lungs to better accommodate the change in breathing rate.

The second most likely period for an attack is five to 10 minutes after the exercise has stopped. For this reason, an extended cool-down is as important as the extended warm-up for preventing the onset of symptoms. Suddenly stopping exercise may induce an attack.

Controlled Environment

Environment can make a big difference in the presence and concentration of asthma triggers. Outdoor running has been found to be the most difficult for asthmatics, most likely due to the presence of allergens and pollution triggers. Indoor exercise also can present a challenge if the asthmatic's triggers include mold and dust. The warm, humid environment of swimming is considered the most asthma-friendly. During swimming, warm, moist air just above the water line is inhaled. This reduces the exposure of the lungs to cool, dry air—the suspected cause of EIA.

While water is the preferred environment for the asthmatic, not everyone enjoys swimming. Exercise in other environments is acceptable for asthmatics. Exercise intensity may have to be modified to keep breathing rates lower, and active participation in an asthma-management program with a physician is essential. In the event that an asthma trigger is encountered, exercise capacity may

be reduced. Modify the exercise program for that session to reflect the severity of the symptoms.

Adequate Hydration

Proper hydration assists the asthmatic in reducing the consistency of the mucus produced by the bronchiole tubes in response to a trigger. Thinner mucus is more easily expelled, reducing the blockage of the bronchiole tubes. Mucus blockage, called plugs, can lead to lung infections such as bronchitis if left in the lungs too long. Asthmatics should hydrate sufficiently before, during and after exercise.

Diaphragmatic Breathing

Diaphragmatic breathing, also called pursed-lip or belly breathing, is recommended for asthmatics. You can incorporate practice of this technique into exercise sessions. Diaphragmatic breathing assists with air exchange by involving the muscle contraction. The proper method for diaphragmatic breathing is:

1) Inhale deeply through the nose, extending the belly, allowing the diaphragm to drop down.

2) Exhale through the mouth, drawing in the belly. The lips can be pursed slightly if desired.

Case Study 1

Anna is a 45-year-old, lifelong asthmatic who has come to you to begin an exercise program for weight loss. During the initial interview, you discover that Anna has never exercised before because she felt it was unsafe for asthmatics. Her physician has recommended she try a supervised program of exercise to assist with her weight-loss goals. Through further questioning, Anna reveals that she experiences asthma symptoms when climbing stairs or chasing after her grandchildren. She knows she is allergic to pollen, grass, mold, dust and pets. Cigarette smoke also bothers her. Anna uses an albuterol inhaler when she experiences symptoms and is on a regular program of inhaled corticosteroids.

Begin by addressing Anna's fear of exercise. She is not wrong to be concerned and needs to be reassured that every attempt will be made to avoid a serious attack. Discuss how she can identify her symptoms and communicate them to you at their onset. Any sensation of chest tightness, coughing or wheezing should immediately be responded to. Introduce the Dyspnea and RPE scales to provide a communication tool, as well as to start Anna thinking about the differences between exercise and asthma breathlessness. Explain to Anna that her weight-loss program may take a little longer to get into full swing, and set her program goals accordingly.

Anna may or may not have received advice on how to use her inhaler prior to exercise. If she is not 100 percent sure of the proper timing and dosage, postpone her exercise until her physician has given these instructions. Schedule the sessions so Anna has the time to use her inhaler appropriately before each session.

Case Study 2

Jacob, a 22-year-old college student, recently has been diagnosed with exercise-induced asthma (EIA). He is an avid runner. During the past few years, Jacob has noticed that he has had increasing difficulty training; some days are better than others. His diagnosis of EIA may explain the problem, but he wants to know how to go about training for a 10K race. His physician prescribed a cromolyn sodium inhaler for use three times a day (one time is 20 minutes prior to running) in combination with an albuterol inhaler.

Begin by talking to Jacob about early identification of asthma symptoms. Jacob's years of training with the problem may make him likely to ignore early signs like chest tightness and a slight cough. Encourage Jacob to use his rescue inhaler when symptoms are first recognized. Jacob also may want to keep a log of each workout, noting the environmental conditions and his asthma symptoms, to identify other triggers, such as cold air, that can be dealt with. Jacob should discuss this log with his physician.

Begin Jacob's program with fitness testing. Be sure Jacob uses his inhaler prior to the test to obtain the best results. Educate him on the importance of proper hydration, and enforce fluid intake during training sessions. Drinking while running takes practice and may initially cause Jacob some distress. He should prepare his system for consuming water during training so he is prepared on race day.

An extended warm-up is essential for Jacob. When calculating training mileage, the warm-up is not included, however Jacob will need to incorporate the extended warm-up into every workout and pre-race routine. The most difficult part of integrating the pre-race warm-up is perfecting the gradual intensity increase without stopping and standing around during race line-up. Jacob should develop a plan and practice his transition from warm-up to race intensity to determine how long and how hard his warm-up has to be.

Base prescribed exercise intensities on the results of the fitness test and Jacob's daily condition. With practice, the medication and warm-up routine should allow Jacob to train at high intensities and progress without difficulty. If Jacob frequently experiences asthma attacks during the workout, he should discuss his medication and pre-exercise procedure with his physician. If Jacob finds he can tolerate a given exercise intensity one day, and not another, asthma most likely is the cause. If his intensity intolerance is consistent day to day reassess his program and make the same modifications you would for a healthy runner who experiences a training plateau.

References

Emtner, M., Herala, M. & Stalenheim, G. (1996). High-intensity physical training in adults with asthma: A 10-week rehabilitation program. *Chest*, 109, 2, 323-31.

Garfinkel, S., Kesten, S., Chapman, K., et al. (1992). Physiologic and nonphysiologic determinants of aerobic fitness in mild to moderate asthma. *American Review of Respiratory Disorders*, 145, 741-45.

Mc Fadden, E.R. & Gilbert, I.A. (1994). Exercise-induced asthma. *The New England Journal of Medicine*, 330, 19, 1362-68.

Morton, A., Fitch, K. & Hahn, A. (1981). Physical activity and the asthmatic. *The Physician & Sports Medicine*, 9, 51-64.

Varray, A., Mercier, J., Terral, C., et al. (1991). Individualized aerobic and high-intensity training for children in an exercise re-adaptation program. *Chest*, 99, 579-86.

Recommended Reading

Adams, F.V. (1995). *The Asthma Source Book*. Los Angeles: Lowell House.

Altman, N. (1991). *What You Can Do about Asthma*. New York: Dell Publishing.

National Heart Lung Blood Institute. (1991). *The Guidelines for the Treatment of Asthma*. Bethesda, Md.: National Asthma Education Program.

Weinstein, A.M. (1987). *Asthma: The Complete Guide to Self-Management of Asthma and Allergies for Patients and Their Families*. New York: Fawcett Crest.

CHAPTER 10

Chronic Obstructive Pulmonary Disease

ZEBULON V. KENDRICK
JOSEPH LEBZELTER

Zebulon Kendrick, Ph.D., F.A.C.S.M., is a professor in the Department of Physical Education at Temple University and the director of the Biokinetics Research Laboratory at Temple University. Dr. Kendrick has an extensive list of both applied and basic science publications. His research interests include human metabolism and the biology of aging.

Joseph Lebzelter, Ph.D., is the Research Director of the Exercise Physiology Unit of the Pulmonology Department, Rabin Medical Center, Beilinson Campus, Tel-Aviv, Israel. Dr. Lebzelter's research areas include unsupported arm exercise, exercise training in lung volume reduction surgery and heart-lung transplant patients and outcomes in heart recipients and patients with end-stage chronic obstructive pulmonary disease.

Pulmonary Function

The Exercise Program

Environmental Considerations

Chronic Obstructive Pulmonary Diseases (COPD) are airway disorders including bronchitis, emphysema and asthma, characterized by the presence of airflow obstruction which may be accompanied by airway hyperactivity (American Thoracic Society [ATS], 1995). The prevalence of chronic bronchitis and emphysema has increased 60 percent since 1982. They are estimated to occur in 16 million people and are the fourth leading cause of death (96,000 deaths in 1994) in the United States. About 14 percent of males and 12 percent of females between 65 and 74 years of age have developed features of COPD (American Lung Association [ALA], 1998). Asthma, which is an allergy-, exercise- or infection-induced bronchospasm, is addressed in Chapter 9.

Although not all individuals with COPD are cigarette smokers (82 percent of the cases), those who smoke or who have smoked are at the greatest risk for developing COPD (ALA, 1998). The impact of cigarette smoking on lung function likely depends upon the intensity of the environmental exposure, the timing of the exposure during growth and baseline lung function. Cigarette smoke may increase the release of the proteolytic enzyme elastase from inflammatory cells attracted into the lungs and may inactivate ∂-1 antitrypsin which protects the lungs from elastase. The imbalance between elastase production and the diminution of ∂-1 antitrypsin is particularly important in the development of emphysema. Persons with COPD who stop smoking should slow the disease's progression. Bacterial and viral infections, air pollution and industrial dusts are often implicated as causes of COPD.

Bronchitis is an inflammatory disorder of the small airways characterized by a chronic cough, excessive sputum production and thickened airways, which affects 5 percent of the population in the United States (ALA, 1998). The retention of mucous secretions associated with bronchitis provides an organically rich medium for bacterial colonization of the airways. Emphysema is characterized by increases in the normal air spaces from either dilation of the alveoli or progressive permanent destruction of the alveoli wall and alveolar-capillary membrane. This destruction results in **hypoxemia** during exercise and, with advanced disease, hypoxemia during both rest and exercise.

Arterial hypoxemia in COPD is due to the mismatching of **ventilation to perfusion**

ratio of the lungs because of high airway resistance (i.e., underventilated lungs) and normal or reduced perfusion of the lungs. Since hypoxemia is a stimulus of pulmonary arteriole constriction, pulmonary vascular resistance increases. This may lead to pulmonary hypertension and additional stresses on the right ventricle of the heart and, in severe COPD, leads to secondary polycythemia via production of erythropoietin.

The multiple and complex pathophysiological relationships among COPD and the cardiovascular and muscular systems add to the difficulty in elucidating and understanding the effects of diagnostic and therapeutic strategies for COPD. Alterations in mechanical properties of the lungs, such as hyperinflation, diminution of the volume of the pulmonary capillary bed and arterial hypoxemia produce hemodynamic changes that stress the cardiovascular system and limit its ability to deliver oxygen (O_2) to exercising muscles. Moreover, the COPD patient is usually deconditioned and may be malnourished and underweight (Schols, Mostert, Soeters, Greve, & Wouters, 1989). These characteristics are more significant with end-stage, intensive care patients. Ambulatory COPD patients may have low levels of anabolic hormones (i.e., growth hormone and sex hormones) which result in muscle atrophy during deconditioning (Casaburi, Carithers, Tosolini, Phillips, & Bhasin, 1997). In addition, some medications (i.e., corticosteriods) used in the treatment of COPD may also weaken skeletal muscle (Casaburi, 1998; Decramer, Lacquet, Fagard, & Rogiers 1994).

Progressive deconditioning associated with inactivity in COPD is characterized by decreases in O_2 uptake, cardiac output, stroke volume and **Arteriovenous O_2 Difference** which may initiate a vicious cycle where **dyspnea** (i.e., dyssynchronous breathing leading to shortness of breath) occurs at lower and lower physical demands (Figure 10.1) (Kelsen & Criner, 1991).

Although improvements in lung or cardiovascular function in COPD with exercise training are significantly limited, exercise has been recognized as an important diagnostic and therapeutic tool in the evaluation and predication of intervention outcomes in COPD patients as

Figure 10.1

Influence of exertional dyspnea on inactivity and deconditioning

Dyspnea with Moderate Exertion

↓

Fear Resulting in Less Activity and Deconditioning

↓

Dyspnea with Mild Exertion

↓

Fear Resulting in Further Inactivity and Deconditioning

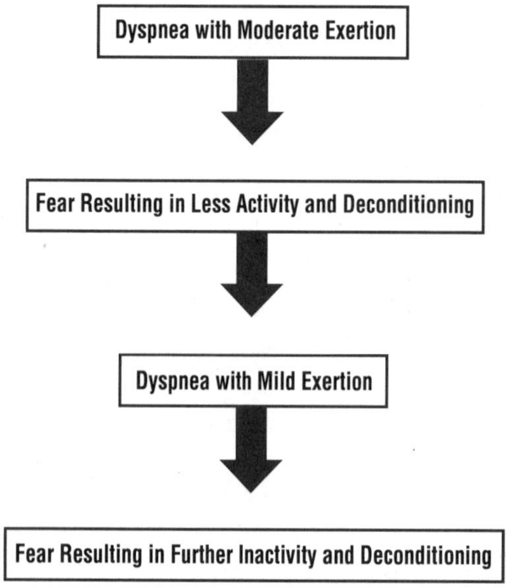

candidates for procedures such as lung volume reduction surgery and lung transplantation. Exercise is also used as a modality to desensitize the COPD patient to dyspnea, slow the rate of deconditioning and subsequently improve the patient's quality of life.

Most of the existing literature concerning exercise responses of COPD patients is based on lower body exercise. This is surprising since many with severe COPD demonstrate poor tolerance and early onset of dyspnea during upper-body exercise (Celli, 1994). Because of the close anatomical associations between the musculature of the arms, upper torso and rib cage as well as the increases in respiratory workload, performance of unsupported arm exercise during upper body **activities of daily living** (ADL) becomes progressively more difficult, even to the point that these activities may be terminated.

Pulmonary Function and Gas Exchange at Rest and During Exercise

Responses of Clinically Normal Persons

Minute ventilation can increase about 20-fold above resting values to supply suitable oxygen during high intensity exercise in a fit individual (Dempsey & Fregosi, 1985). An abrupt increase in minute ventilation occurs at the initiation of exercise with increases in both **tidal volume** and respiratory rate. Minute ventilation at low power outputs is mainly increased through an increase in tidal volume. Once tidal volume has reached a maximal value (about 2/3 of the vital capacity), further increases in ventilation occur mainly by increasing the frequency of breathing. Minute ventilation increases linearly with increasing O_2 uptake and work level up to about 60 percent of one's maximal work capacity (Wasserman, 1978). The **ventilatory equivalent** (i.e., VE/VO_2) is about 20 to 30 L for every liter of O_2 uptake in normals (Wasserman, Hansen, Sue, & Whipp, 1987) and increases linearly until the compensation point (i.e., anaerobic threshold).

Minute ventilation (80 to 120 L/min) does not reach the maximal ventilatory capacity (150 to 200 L/min) in normals. The efficiency of ventilation (i.e., **VD/VT ratio**) declines from values of 20 percent to 30 percent at rest to values of 5 percent to 20 percent during exercise when CO_2 production is above 1.0 L/min (Shepard, Campbell, Martin, & Enns, 1955; Whipp & Wasserman, 1969). Therefore, the volume of wasted ventilation during exercise in normals decreases for two reasons. First, with larger tidal volumes there is a reduction in **dead space**. Second, the relatively overventilated apical area of the lungs is better perfused when stroke volume and pulmonary artery pressure increase with exercise, thereby reducing physiological dead space.

The cardiac output rises immediately with exercise and may rise five- to six-fold of its rest-

Table 10.1.
Impairments in Ventilatory, Gas Exchange, Cardiopulmonary Responses and Work Performance in COPD

Ventilation
Increased airway resistance, especially in expiration.

Hyperinflation leading to muscle weakness of ventilatory muscles.

Increased VD/VT leading to a decrease in the efficiency of ventilation.

Reduced tidal volume
Decrease in maximal minute ventilation (breathing capacity), and a decrease in ventilatory reserve.

Increased effort (work) of breathing.

Increased incidence of dyspnea due to inability of the respiratory system to meet the metabolic demands of the exercise effort. Since exercise tidal volume is reduced in COPD, more energy is expended in increasing the frequency of breathing for all submaximal exercise efforts.

Gas Exchange
Destruction of the alveolar-capillary membrane, reducing diffusion capacity, resulting in arterial hypoxemia

Inequality in the ventilation : perfusion ratio resulting in arterial hypoxemia

Cardiopulmonary Changes
Decrease in maximal cardiac output.

Decrease in maximal heart rate.

Decrease in hemoglobin saturation of O_2 leading to arterial hypoxemia.

Increase in pulmonary artery pressure.

Increase in right-ventricular afterload.

Work Capacity
Decrease in maximal O_2 uptake.

Decrease in maximal work capacity

ing value in well-trained persons. At an O_2 uptake of 3 L/min, cardiac output increases about four-fold. The increase in blood flow causes a rise in venous return to the right side of the heart, leading to an increase in pulmonary blood flow. This increase in pulmonary blood flow is accompanied by an increase in pulmonary artery pressure and a fall in pulmonary vascular resistance.

Responses of COPD Patients

Reductions in maximal exercise capacity and maximal O_2 uptake in patients with severe airflow limitation are related to the reduction in **forced expiratory volume in one second (FEV1)** and loss of elastic recoil (Table 10.1). Patients with COPD adapt by increasing the total time of inspiration and expiration. Also, the marked increases in total lung volume and **residual volume** associated with hyperinflation in COPD are also associated with an expansion of the thoracic cage resulting in inefficient inspiratory muscle action and a decreased maximal inspiratory flow.

Resting O_2 uptake is usually greater in individuals with COPD than in normals (Lanigan, Moxham, & Ponte, 1990) because of the increased work of breathing. Although one may expect that O_2 uptake for a given exercise intensity is greater in COPD patients, this does not appear to be the case (Jones, Jones, & Edwards, 1971; Levinson & Cherniack, 1968; Nery et al., 1982). An increase in work rate below the anaerobic threshold in normals results in an initial and rapid increase in O_2 uptake followed by an exponential rise until a plateau is reached. The O_2 uptake to work rate relationship usually does not approach a plateau in COPD patients because they have greater difficulty in removing CO_2 than in delivery of O_2 to working muscle. Many COPD patients demonstrate worsening

hypoxemia and increases in alveolar to arterial O_2 gradient. Interestingly, individuals with chronic bronchitis have lower arterial O_2 than those with emphysema both at rest and exercise. Since hypoxemia results in a reduction in O_2 delivery to the working muscles and an impairment in metabolic responses to exercise, **hypoxia** can stimulate ventilation at lower work rates than would occur in the absence of hypoxemia. Oxygen supplementation has been shown to reduce the work of breathing; relieve tachypnea; and improve exercise tolerance, right ventricular function, pulmonary hypertension, and both the length and quality of life (Criner & Celli, 1988).

Exercise O_2 desaturation is usually observed in severe COPD patients with a FEV1 <35 percent of age- and sex-matched predicted values. Alveolar partial pressure of CO_2 may increase during exercise as the VD/VT ratio increases (Killian, Mahutte, Howell, & Campbell, 1980), which is in contrast to the large reduction to the VD/VT ratio observed in normals.

The ability of the COPD patient to maintain elevated ventilation for prolonged periods is diminished due to reduced inspiratory muscle strength resulting in a mechanical derangement of the respiratory muscles. Although minute ventilation at peak exercise may approach or reach maximal voluntary ventilation, it cannot be sustained (Clark, Freedman, Campbell & Winn, 1969; Mahler & Harver, 1988).

Respiratory Muscle Function

Breathing is exquisitely tuned to meet metabolic needs. As breathing is augmented, the inspiratory muscles of the chest wall are stimulated to produce more forceful contractions. The major inspiratory muscle during quiet breathing is the diaphragm, which shortens by about

Figure 10.2

Pathophysiology of exertional dyspnea

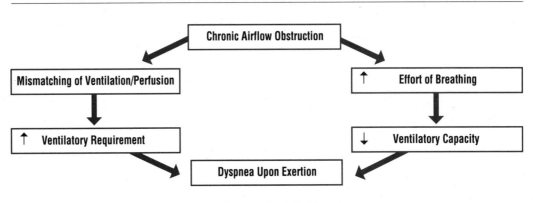

40 percent in normals. When minute ventilation increases to about 30 percent of its maximum, accessory respiratory muscles are utilized. In COPD when breathing is inefficient due to airflow obstruction and hyperinflation, intercostal and accessory muscles are recruited at lower levels of ventilation, increasing the work of breathing.

The complex mechanical actions of inspiratory muscles permit inspiration to occur under a variety of conditions that may otherwise seriously interfere with breathing. In upright postures, vigorous contraction of the diaphragm during high levels of ventilation produces negative intrapleural pressure, which tends to collapse the upper rib cage. This collapse is prevented by simultaneous contraction of the intercostal and accessory muscles (Goldman, Grassiano, Mead & Sears, 1978). If diaphragm excursion is curtailed by posture, or abdominal muscle contraction, intercostal and scalene muscles become the primary movers, with diaphragmatic contractions serving to stabilize the lower chest wall.

The pulmonary impact of COPD may be broadly categorized as an increased demand on respiratory muscles (increased effort of breathing and increased ventilatory requirement), a mismatching in the ventilation-to-perfusion ratio resulting in arterial hypoxemia, and a reduction in the functional capability of these muscles (reduced strength and endurance). Alone or in combination, these changes may lead to alterations in breathing pattern, a heightened sense of dyspnea or even respiratory failure (Figure 10.2).

Resting ventilation constitutes about 40 percent of maximum ventilatory capacity of COPD patients as compared to about 5 percent of capacity in normals (Pardy, Hussain & Macklem, 1984; Rochester, Arora, Braun & Goldberg, 1979). The COPD patient usually exhibits an increase in minute ventilation with an energy cost of breathing that is markedly elevated because of the increased airway resistance and hyperinflation (Tobin et al., 1983a, 1983b). The patient must generate greater inspiratory pressures to provide similar ventilation as normals. Severe COPD patients de- pend upon the activation of muscles of the upper thorax, shoulder girdle and neck because of limited diaphragmatic contractions and require an O_2 uptake greater than that for normals.

During exercise, the ability of the respiratory muscles to generate force is seriously impaired. Since increases in lung volume reduce the force output of inspiratory muscles for a given level of activation, hyperinflation compromises the ability of inspiratory muscles to generate pressure and increases expiratory demand (Grimby, Elgefors & Oxhoj, 1973). Geometric changes in the chest wall with COPD make the inspiratory muscles operate at shorter than normal lengths and thereby reduce their ability to significantly lower intrathoracic pressure. During expiration, the use of accessory musculature increases O_2 utilization of the expiratory muscles, further reducing the overall efficiency of breathing in COPD patients. When patients with moderate-to-severe COPD attempt to exercise, they produce expiratory pressures in excess of those required to achieve maximal flow. An increase in pleural pressure during prolonged expiration can impede venous return to the heart and impair cardiac output (Scharf, 1989).

Breathing Pattern During Exercise

During exercise, healthy individuals maintain an end-expiratory lung volume below their normal **functional residual capacity** and an end-inspiratory volume near the total lung capacity. As the intensity of the exercise increases to near maximal efforts, tidal volume may reach 50 percent of total lung capacity, with end-expiratory lung volume remaining between functional residual capacity and residual lung volume (Younes & Kivinen, 1984). The inspiratory time increases while the expiratory time decreases during exercise in normals and in patients with mild to moderate COPD (Bradley & Crawford, 1976; Schaaning, 1978). With severe COPD, there is little or no change in the inspiratory time during exercise. Initially, this response may be beneficial because a greater expiration time may facilitate further increases in ventilation (Dodd, Brancatisano & Engel, 1984; Younes, 1990). This facilitation of ventilation occurs at the expense of an increased load on the inspiratory muscles.

When normal subjects exercise, end-expiratory lung volume is reduced because of increased activation of expiratory musculature of the abdomen and the rib cage (Younes & Kivinen, 1984). In contrast, COPD patients usually demonstrate increases in end-expiratory lung volume and develop positive end-expiratory pressures during exercise (Dodd et al., 1984; Grimby et al., 1973). This increase in end-expiratory pressure is primarily related to the increase in breathing frequency, which diminishes the expiratory time and limits the volume of expired gas.

Cardiac and Pulmonary Vascular Response to Exercise

Maximal exercise heart rate is usually less than 80 percent to 85 percent of predicted in COPD patients (Belman, 1993; Dillard, Piantadosi & Rajagopal, 1985; Make & Buchholtz, 1991) (Table 10.1) while submaximal exercise heart rates are usually higher when compared to the responses of age-matched normals (Spiro, Hahn, Edwards & Pride, 1975). Cardiac output and O_2 uptake increase with increasing exercise intensity in normals, however, these responses are attenuated in COPD patients.

The slope of the rise in heart rate to exercise O_2 uptake in COPD patients may be comparable to normals (Nery, Wasserman, French, Oren & Davis, 1983; Spiro et al., 1975) or may be depressed (Gallagher & Younes, 1986; Jones et al., 1971). These relationships are dependent upon the severity of underlying airflow obstruction (Matthews, Bush & Ewald, 1989). Because the fractional reduction in the maximal heart rate during exercise is less than that of the peak O_2 uptake, the **O_2 pulse** is lower in COPD patients, suggesting that using heart rate to estimate the intensity of the exercise may be erroneous for this population (Belman, 1993). Although maximal values of the O_2 pulse may be reduced, O_2 pulse usually rises with increasing work rate in COPD patients.

Pulmonary vascular dynamics and associated cardiac function during exercise differ from the patterns seen in normals. In patients with emphysema, loss of vascular surface area, alveolar hypoxia and acidemia induces pulmonary vasoconstriction. As airway obstruction and hypoxemia increase during exercise, pulmonary vascular resistance and pulmonary artery pressure rise and thus increase the **afterload** on the right ventricle.

Interdependence of the Right and Left Ventricles in Heart Function in COPD

Since the right and left ventricles of the heart are tightly coupled, each side of the heart can act directly upon the other through the compliant interventricular septum (Glantz et al., 1978). The enlargement or increased wall tension of the right ventricle which occurs with COPD may lead to a mechanical impairment of the left ventricle (Pinsky, 1994; Robotham, 1981; Scharf, 1989; Weber, Janicki, Sharoff & Fishman, 1981).

Destruction of the pulmonary vascular bed and arterial hypoxemia in COPD results in pulmonary hypertension and right-ventricular distention which, in turn, may decrease the filling of the left ventricle (Bove & Santamore, 1981; Janicki & Weber, 1980). Distention of the right ventricle leads to an increase in left-ventricular filling pressure, which can exacerbate pulmonary vascular congestion.

Right-ventricular Dysfunction During Exercise

Right-ventricular dysfunction during exercise occurs in the majority of patients with COPD (Mahler, Brent, Loke, Zaret & Matthay, 1984; Matthay et al., 1980). The expected increase in right-ventricular **ejection fraction** of at least 5 percent during exercise may not occur in patients with COPD and right-ventricular dysfunction (Matthay & Berger, 1984). The lack of an increase in ejection fraction during exercise may be due to the restricted, relatively nonrecruitable pulmonary vascular bed which typically has an inordinately high pulmonary artery pressure. An increase in pulmonary artery pressure is common during exercise in COPD patients and may be due to a failure of the pulmonary vascular bed to vasodilate as pulmonary blood flow increases. This may produce a fall in right-ventricular ejection fraction, leading to an increase in right-ventricular end-diastolic volume (Slutsky, Hooper, Ackerman & Moser, 1982).

Maximal O_2 uptake correlates to right-ventricular ejection fraction in COPD patients (Morrison et al., 1987). The increase in right-ventricular ejection fraction during exercise is inversely correlated with increases in total pulmonary resistance but not with pulmonary artery pressure, suggesting that right-ventricular function could, along with decreased ventilatory capacity, limit exercise in COPD patients.

Left-ventricular Dysfunction

Patients with severe COPD often manifest cardiac dyspnea, orthopnea, jugular venous distension, ankle edema and rales, which suggest impairment of left-ventricular function (Wise, 1991). Autopsy reports have indicated left-ventricular hypertrophy in COPD patients with right-side heart failure (Murphy, Boger, Adamson & Rubin, 1977; Rao, Cohen, Eldridge & Hancock, 1968; Unger et al., 1975). Left-ventricular dysfunction during exercise has also been observed in COPD patients who have no evidence of primary cardiac disease (Brown et al., 1984; Matthay &

Berger, 1984). It is important to note, however, that severely impaired left-ventricular function is uncommon in COPD, even when decompensation is present (Steele et al., 1975).

Pharmacologic Agents and Exercise Interaction

A major goals of pharmacologic interventions for the COPD patient are to induce bronchodilation, improve pulmonary function, decrease inflammation, and facilitate expectoration of sputum. Although pharmacologic intervention does not alter the progression of COPD, such intervention may alleviate symptoms associated with dyspnea and may improve pulmonary function and exercise tolerance (Celli, 1996). To date, most of the drug-exercise interactions cited in the literature have been concerned with cardiopulmonary interactions (Table 10.2). The following will briefly outline drug-exercise interactions of selected

Table 10.2
Effects of Pharmacological Agents on Cardiopulmonary Responses of COPD Patients

Agent	Cardiovascular Effects	Pulmonary Effects
ACE inhibitors	Decrease peripheral resistance Reduce preload and afterload Increase cardiac output Reduce cardiac size	May reduce pulmonary vascular resistance
Calcium Channel Blockers	Depress myocardium contractility Dilate coronary arteries Reduce afterload	May reduce pulmonary vascular resistance.
Digitalis	Increases cardiac output Improve left ventricular filling pressure and ejection fraction	Promotes diuresis, alleviating venous congestion, edema, dyspnea and orthopenia
Diuretics	Reduce preload in patients with systolic dysfunction Increase excretion of sodium and chloride Reduce edema	Decrease pulmonary edema and work of breathing
Nitrates	Induce smooth muscle relaxation dilating arterial and venous beds Reduce preload and afterload Reduce blood pressure and systemic vascular resistance	Reduces pulmonary vascular resistance May reduce pulmonary hypertension
Nitroprusside	Relaxes vascular smooth muscle and dilates vessels Reduces afterload	Reduces pulmonary vascular resistance
Phosphodiesterase Inhibitors	Exert positive inotropic effect resulting in vasodilation Increases cardiac output	Reduces peripheral vascular resistance and pulmonary wedge pressure

Adapted from Galiber, D.P., & Dunn, M.I. (1994). *Journal of Respiratory Disease*, 15, 565-577.

classes of drugs used in therapies for COPD. Other chapters in this book will provide a more in-depth discussion of the cardiopulmonary interactions of many of these drugs at rest and during exercise.

Supplemental Oxygen

Supplemental oxygen in severe COPD patients improves right-ventricular function, thoracoabdominal compliance and airway resistance. The beneficial effects of administering supplemental oxygen during exercise in severe COPD patients relate to a decreased effort of breathing, a delay in diaphragmatic fatigue and an alteration in the pattern of ventilatory muscle recruitment (Eden & Turino, 1986; Kelsen & Criner, 1991).

ß2-Selective Bronchodilators

The ß2-selective bronchodilators (ß-agonists) are potent medications (Ferguson & Cherniak, 1993) (Table 10.3). Some COPD patients exhibit measurable improvement in FEV1 and functional **vital capacity** following a metered dose of ß-agonists. Short-acting medications (i.e., albuterol, pirbuterol, metaproterenol, isoetharine and terbutaline) are often used as a prophylaxis prior to exercising. Tremor, headache, nervousness, tachycardia, tachyphylaxis and insomnia are commonly reported side effects of these drugs. Both the COPD patient and the exercise technician need to be aware of untoward responses to this class of drugs during exercise or exercise testing (Table 10.4).

Anticholinergic Agents

Anticholinergic agents may exert clinically significant bronchodilator effect in patients with airflow obstruction. Patients with chronic bronchitis may benefit from anticholinergic therapy because of the induced bronchodilation and reduction in mucus production. Aerosolized anticholinergic medications are effective and are free of the many side effects that are observed with oral administration of these agents (Table 10.3).

Theophylline

Theophylline is considered a third-line medication because its bronchodilation effect is limited and its therapeutic range is narrow. Theophylline enhances ventilatory responses to hypoxia and improves ventilatory endurance, presumably through its beneficial effects on diaphragmatic contractility. The diuretic effects of theophylline may also improve cardiac performance (Jenne et al., 1984) (Table 10.4).

Calcium Channel Blockers

Calcium channel blockers (antagonists) such as oral nifedipine (20 mg three times daily) have failed to produce significant improvement in pulmonary function. However, calcium channel antagonists have been consistently effective in protecting against exercise-induced bronchoconstriction (Table 10.2). Nifedipine has been found to inhibit hypoxic pulmonary vasoconstriction. Sublingual nifedepine and inhaled verapamil have been demonstrated to attenuate exercise-induced bronchospasm as well as eucapnic **hyperventilation** with cold air (Ahmed & Abraham, 1985).

Leukotriene Inhibitors

Leukotrienes are a family of lipid mediators that can impair mucocilliary clearance, enhance mucus secretion, chemotactically attract leuko-

Table 10.3
Meter-Dose Inhaler Vasodilating Agents Used for COPD

Agent	ß1	*Relative Level of Activity* ß2	Anticholinergic
Beta agonists			
Albuterol	Mild	High	None
Bitolterol	Mild	High	None
Isoproterenol	Moderate	Moderate	None
Metaproterenol	Mild	Moderate	None
Pirbuterol	Mild	Moderate	None
Terbutaline	Mild	Moderate	None
Anticholinergic			
Ipratropium	None	None	High

Adapted from Ferguson G.T, & Cherniack, R.M, *New England Journal of Medicine*, 66, 181-186

cytes to the airways and facilitate pulmonary vascular permeability. Two approaches have been developed to decrease the action of leukotrienes. One is by blocking leukotriene synthesis and the other is to interfere with the binding of a leukotriene to its receptor (Busse, 1998; Manning et al., 1990; O'Byrne & Daahlem, 1997).

Several leukotriene antagonists have been evaluated in subjects with exercise-induced bronchospasm. In eight asthmatic patients administered 20 mg of zafirlukast two hours prior to exercise, the post-exercise FEV1 was reduced by 22 percent as compared to 36 percent with placebo treatment (Finnerty, Wood-Baker, Thomson & Holgate, 1992). In another study, 24 asthma patients received 2.4 g/day of zileuton for two days. The administration of zileuton inhibited the incidence of exercise-induced bronchospasm by 41 percent when compared to the placebo treatment. The FEV1 was 86 percent of baseline values at five minutes of recovery from exercise, while FEV1 was 74 percent of baseline values for the placebo treatment (Meltzer, Hasday, Cohn & Bleeker, 1996). On the basis of these studies, 5-lipoxygenase inhibitors and leukotriene D4 antagonists appear equally effective in the treatment of patients with exercise-induced bronchospasm or asthma.

Arrhythmias During Exercise in COPD Patients

COPD patients may develop arrhythmias during exercise. A single (modified V5) lead is typically used to measure heart rate and monitor for arrhythmias or ischemic changes for exercise testing. If available, a recent resting 12-lead electrocardiogram should be reviewed before exercise testing but is not necessary unless ischemic heart disease is suspected (Ries, 1994). It is important to note that Chenog and colleagues (1990) found that 87 percent (98 of 122) COPD patients did not exhibit any significant exercise-induced arrhythmias during maximal exercise if they were without arrhythmias at rest. However eight patients without coronary artery disease and without arrhythmias at rest had significant exercise-induced arrhythmias (defined as six or more ventricular premature beats per minute), bigeminy, multiform couplets or nonsustained ventricular tachycardia (Table 10.4). Therefore, it may be prudent to suspect that

Table 10.4
Potential Systemic and Cardiovascular Effects of ß-Adrenergic Agonists and Theophylline

Effect	ß-agonists	Theophylline
Systemic Effects		
Nausea	Yes	
Vomiting	Yes	
Anxiety	Yes	Yes
Tremors	Yes	
Seizures	Yes	
Palpitations	Yes	
Cardiovascular Effects		
Reduced peripheral vascular resistance	Yes	
Diuresis	Yes	
Positive inotropism	Yes	
Increase perfusion	Yes	
Sinus tachycardia	Yes	Yes
Supraventricular tachycardia	Yes	Yes
Premature ventricular contractions	Yes	Yes
Sustained ventricular tachycardia	Yes	Yes
Atrial fibrilation	Yes	
Multifocal atrial tachycardia		Yes

These effects are usually not as pronounced with inhaled agents.

ischemic disease may be present in COPD patients. Additionally, COPD patients who are administered theophylline may be more sensitive to its arrythmogenic effects than normals (Levine, Michael & Guarnieri, 1985).

Upper- and Lower-body Exercise Responses

Exercise Responses of Normals

Physiologic responses to upper-body exercise are often more dramatic than for lower-body exercise (Astrand, Guharay & Wahren, 1968; Bevegard, Freyschuss & Strandell, 1966; Davies & Sargeant, 1974) (Table 10.5). Submaximal arm exercise is usually performed at a higher O_2 uptake than leg exercise regardless of body position (Berg, Kanstrup & Ekblom, 1975; Bevegard et al.; Stenberg, Astrand, Ekblom, Royce & Saltin, 1967). Because of differences in muscle mass, lower-body exercise usually elicits greater peak oxygen uptake than upper-body exercise. At a given submaximal power output, heart rate, systolic and diastolic blood pressures, rate-pressure product (product of heart rate and systolic blood pressure), minute ventilation, respiratory exchange ratio, and blood lactate content are higher, and stroke volume and anaerobic threshold are lower during arm than during leg exercise (Astrand, Ekblom, Messin, Saltin & Stenberg, 1965; Bevegard et al.).

Cardiac output at a given submaximal O_2 uptake has been found to be similar for arm cranking and leg cycling exercises with a strong association between cardiac output and metabolic demand (Clausen, 1976; Miles et al., 1984). The mechanisms that influence each mode of exercise are distinctly different with exercise heart rate and stroke volume consistently higher for arm exercise as compared to leg exercise. Total peripheral resistance is greater at workloads of 1.0 L O_2/min during arm than leg exercise (Astrand et al., 1965; Bevegard et al., 1966). Blood pressure increases linearly with increasing workload for both modes of exercise, with mean arterial pressure often 20 to 25 mmHg higher during arm exercise, mostly because of elevation of diastolic pressure. Stabilizing the torso and grasping the hand-crank of the arm exercise machines may

result in an isometric-like effect, which may produce a **pressor reflex** that elevates the mean arterial pressure (Rowell & Sheriff, 1988; Sawka, 1986). Arm exercise performed with elevated arms results in greater increases in mean arterial pressure than with lowered arms, particularly during high-intensity exercise (Astrand et al., 1968).

A greater elevation in heart rate is observed with increasing exercise intensity during arm cranking than during leg cycling. This is likely due to greater sympathetic stimulation with little or no increase in stroke volume (Blomqvist, 1985; Davies & Sargeant, 1974). Stroke volume during leg cycling increases by 40 percent to 60 percent and plateaus at approximately 60 percent of peak work capacity (Miles et al., 1984; Sawka, 1986). The lack of increase in stroke volume during arm exercise is attributed to the lower venous return when compared to leg cycling.

A greater mechanical compression of the vasculature may occur during arm exercise than leg exercise since the smaller muscle mass of the upper body will have to develop a greater muscle tension for any given submaximal workload (Sawka, 1986). As intramuscular pressure exceeds perfusion pressure, vascular resistance increases and blood flow is reduced. The viscosity of the blood may also increase, thereby increasing peripheral resistance during arm exercise (Miles, Cox & Bomez, 1989).

Exercise Responses of COPD Patients

Marked mechanical and metabolic responses to gravity occur in COPD patients who perform complex purposeful arm movements. In fact, performing simple or seemingly trivial unsupported arm ADL such as tying shoes, combing hair and brushing teeth often results in dyspneic breathing because of impaired respiratory muscle function (Celli, Criner & Rassulo, 1988; Celli, Rassulo & Make, 1986; Criner, Rassulo & Celli, 1985).

Under conditions in which the diaphragm is impaired, accessory muscle use is increased. The upper and lower trapezius, latissimus dorsi, serratus anterior, subclavian, and pectoralis minor and major have extrathoracic and thoracic anchoring points. These muscles assist in the positioning of the arms and shoulders during arm exercise and provide an extrathoracic fulcrum that exerts a pulling force on the rib cage during unsupported arm exercise. Because of their use in upper torso stability, shoulder girdle muscles decrease their participation in ventilation when performing unsupported arm exercise. The competition between ventilatory and nonventilatory tasks placed upon these muscles may cause respiratory muscle function derangement and early fatigue.

Ventilatory responses to unsupported arm exercise and unloaded leg cycling in patients with severe COPD have been previously studied (Celli et al., 1986). Significant dyspnea occurs during arm exercise, causing termination of the exercise in severely obstructed patients. The dyspnea is most likely due to progressive hyperinflation, which places the diaphragm at a mechanical disadvantage and requires a greater contribution of accessory inspiratory muscles for ventilation. Some patients with less severe COPD are able to perform unsupported arm exercise for several minutes without experiencing dyspnea. When unsupported arms are extended, muscles of the rib cage reduce their ventilatory activity, requiring other muscles to assume a greater portion of the ventilatory burden.

The pattern of ventilatory muscle recruitment during both supported and unsupported arm exercise in severe COPD patients has been compared (Criner et al., 1985). Endurance time for unsupported arm exercise was shorter than that for supported arm exercise, even though the latter was more stressful, as reflected by greater heart rates, minute ventilations and O_2 uptakes. Unsupported arm exercise elicited greater differences between end-inspiratory and end-expiratory transdiaphragmatic pressures. Leg exercise, unsupported arm exercise and supported arm exercise all lead to increases in metabolic demand and ventilation. Submaximal unsupported arm exercise leads to greater increases in O_2 uptake, CO_2 production and minute ventilation than supported arm and leg exercise (Celli et al., 1988). In normals, the rise in minute ventilation is associated with increases in tidal volume during unsupported arm exercise, whereas the increase in minute ventilation is secondary to an increase in respiratory rate for COPD patients (Martinez, Couser & Celli, 1991).

Many patients with severe COPD intuitively perform arm tasks while resting elbows on a firm surface. Diaphragm recruitment is usually less with supported arms than with elevated unsupported arms, and recruitment of abdominal, thoracic and accessory muscles during exhalation is reduced with arm support. Clearly, respiratory muscle function is maintained for longer periods of time when elbows are supported compared to when the arms are unsupported (Banzett, Topulos, Leith & Nations, 1988; Criner & Celli, 1988).

Table 10.5
Comparison of Normal Submaximal and Maximal Exercise Responses to Upper- and Lower-body Exercise

Variable	Response(s)
Submaximal Exercise	
O_2 Uptake	Upper body > Lower body exercise
Heart Rate	Upper body > Lower body exercise
Stroke Volume	Lower body > Upper body exercise
Cardiac Output	Upper and lower body responses are similar
Mean Arterial Pressure	Upper body > Lower body exercise
Mean Arterial Pressure With Elevated Arms	Elevated arms > Lower arms > Lower body exercise
Minute Ventilation	Upper body > Lower body exercise
Anaerobic Threshold	Lower body > Upper body exercise
Maximal Exercise	
O_2 Uptake	Lower body > Upper body exercise
Maximal Heart Rate	Upper and Lower body exercise are similar
Cardiac Output	Lower body > Upper body exercise

Management of COPD: General Strategies

Clinical, educational and exercise strategies should be used in the management of COPD. Clinically, healthcare professionals work to identify and eliminate the source(s) of bronchopulmonary inflammation, identify and treat reversible airway narrowing with appropriate medications, and prevent exacerbations of COPD by routine vaccinations against infectious agents and prophylactic administration of antibiotics (Hsia, 1998). Educational programs should address COPD and its progression and rehabilitation with instructions on how to administer medications, instructions on how to use devices for inspiratory muscle training (if required), information about dyspnea, and information about exercise adherence and positive effects of exercise on reducing or desensitizing the COPD patient to dyspnea. Because of the significant deconditioning that occurs in COPD, the exercise phase of the rehabilitation program should be designed to slowly and progressively integrate physical activity to improve the quality of the patient's life.

Deconditioning of COPD patients may be due to a sedentary lifestyle; other comorbid conditions or medications to treat those conditions; learned techniques to conserve energy when performing activities; and malnutrition from recurrent infections and poor nutritional intake. Moreover, patients with COPD are also generally older adults.

It has been reported that almost 85 percent of older adults are suffering from at least one chronic disease such as arthritis, diabetes, coronary heart disease, hypertension, peripheral vascular disease and obesity (Jette & Branch, 1981) [many of these comorbid conditions are addressed in other chapters of this book]. In COPD, the reductions in muscular strength and the presence of one or more of these comorbid conditions may have a profound impact on the performance of ADL, exercise tolerance and compliance with the exercise prescription.

Remediation of Exertional Dyspnea

When the COPD patient experiences dyspnea, it may be prudent for the COPD patient to stop exercise and rest in a comfortable position. Often the most comfortable position is sitting with the head down and leaning forward. While in this position, the patient inhales and exhales through the mouth. Initially, the patient may be breathing rapidly, but as recovery begins, breathing should become more deliberate, with longer but not forcible exhalations. Pursed lip breathing may be desired as the patient becomes more comfortable. Once the breathing has slowed, nose breathing should be used followed by diaphragmatic breathing.

For pursed lip breathing, the COPD patient should inhale through the nose for one count, purse the lips and breathe out slowly for two counts. It is important that the patient does not forcibly exhale.

Diaphragmatic breathing is a strategy whereby a person consciously expands their abdominal wall during inspiration. Diaphragmatic

Table 10.6
Training Modalities and Exercise Prescription for Lower- and Upper-body Exercise

Variable	Leg Exercise	Arm Exercise	Unsupported Arm Exercise
Training Intensity	60% of achieved work capacity	60% of achieved work capacity	Anterior arm elevation to shoulder level for 2 min
Exercise Volume	increase work every 5th session as tolerated	Increase work every 5th session as tolerated	Increase weight (250 g every 5th session as tolerated
Monitor	Heart rate and dyspnea	Heart rate and dyspnea	Heart rate and dyspnea
Cycling Frequency	60 rpm	50 rpm	As tolerated by breathing
Exercise Frequency	3 to 5 times/week	2 times/week	2 times/week
Exercise Duration	At least 30 min	At least 15 min	At least 10 min
Program Length	24 to 30 sessions	24 to 30 sessions	24 to 30 sessions

breathing may be felt by having the COPD patient place one hand on the upper chest and one hand on the abdomen below the waist. As the patient inhales through the nose and exhales through the pursed lips, only the hand on the abdomen should feel movement.

One benefit of a regular exercise for the COPD patient is desensitization of exertional dyspnea, (Haas, Salazar-Schicci & Axen, 1993). The desensitization to exertional dyspnea is in part based upon the premise that successful participation in exercise programs provides suitable feedback that difficult tasks can be mastered. Another outcome may be a lessening of the feeling of helplessness and despair that is often associated with deconditioning. Moreover, social interactions are established in group exercise programs, and these interactions provide a calming of unrealistic fears about COPD and exercise tolerance. This hypothesis is particularly relevant because participation in group exercise usually provides better results than a home exercise program. Since the COPD patient may become socially isolated as the symptoms of the disease become more severe, group exercise programs are also important to lessen the extent of social isolation. Finally, distraction stimuli such as group exercises, listening to music when exercising and mental imagery may also lessen the dyspneic sensations of the COPD patient.

Psychological Impacts of COPD

Deconditioning, increased dyspnea, limitations on performance of ADL, and changes in social interactions can result in significant anxiety and depression in COPD patients (Agle & Baum, 1977; McSweeny, Grant, Heaton, Adams & Timms, 1982) as well as impaired cognitive function (Grant et al., 1987; Prigatano, Parsons, Wright, Levin & Hawryluk, 1983).

Episodes of dyspnea as well as other symptoms of COPD can be frightening and may result in chronic anxiety. Becoming anxious about performing physical activity may lead to intense hyperventilation prior to or during activity (Cooper, 1997). A second manifestation of anxiety may be inappropriate or hysterical breath holding, which is easily recognized by observing the patient's facial expressions. Exercise programs may reduce anxiety and lessen the fear of performing physical activities (Cooper; Emery, Schin, Hauck &

MacIntyre, 1998), desensitize the COPD patient to exertional dyspnea (Haas et al., 1993), and improve self-concept (Cooper, 1997).

The Exercise Program

Exercise programs should be personalized and "prescriptive," be a part of the pulmonary rehabilitation strategy, and provide regular updates on client progress. The environment should be free of air pollutants, industrial dusts and smoke, and the exercise program should not be performed in a cold environment. Goals of the exercise program for the COPD patient should include improvement of flexibility to increase the range of motion; improvement of balance, gait and breathing efficiency; reduction of excessive body mass and increases in lean body mass; and enhancement of body image (Cooper, 1997).

Preferably, the COPD patient should be evaluated with a symptom-limited cardiopulmonary exercise tolerance test. Medications should be taken as usual so that appropriate responses to the exercise tolerance test can be obtained. Since dyspnea and other symptoms of COPD are more likely to occur in the early morning, both the exercise tolerance test and exercise program should be performed in the late morning or early afternoon. Patients who exhibit marked hypoxemia during the exercise tolerance test are poor candidates for an exercise program and may benefit from O_2 supplementation. Supplement O_2 is effective in reducing the ventilatory effort at a given intensity of work, improves arterial O_2 saturation during exercise and increases exercise tolerance (Mahler, 1998). Since supplementation of O_2 has been shown to reduce dyspnea, it may be particularly beneficial during the initial exercise sessions, especially with clients who experience anxiety (ATS, 1995).

A major goal of aerobic exercise for rehabilitation of COPD patients is for cardiovascular reconditioning. This goal may be achieved by performing intervals of large-muscle activities such as walking or cycling. Shorter episodes of higher intensities of aerobic exercise may be used as long as intensity does not evoke episodes of dyspnea (Cooper, 1997). Generally, exercise guidelines for patients with mild emphysema should be similar to those of normals as long as the COPD patient is informed that they will likely experience more fatigue with exertion which will lessen with improved exercise tolerance. With moderate to severe emphysema, the onset of fatigue levels is earlier, and these patients are more likely to experience exercise-related dyspnea.

The perceived intensity of exercise should be somewhere between fairly light to somewhat hard (RPE between 11 and 13). This intensity of exercise should allow the COPD patient to increase the duration of exercise and to reduce or become desensitized to dyspnea. Initial patient tolerance to exercise will most likely be low, with a low fatigue level, especially with moderate to severe COPD. As exercise tolerance improves and desensitization to dyspnea occurs, exercise may be performed one or two sessions a day for at least 30 minutes.

Although there is little information on outcomes of resistive training of the COPD patient, it is reasonable to assume that resistive training and strengthening of the upper extremity may reduce dyspnea associated with the asynchronous breathing during unsupported arm exercise. Improving general body muscular strength may assist the COPD patient in many other areas, such as attaining performance goals for ADL, lessening the incidence and severity of injury from falls (Tinetti et al., 1994; Tinetti & Powell, 1993), improving ambulation and gait (Gryfe, Amies & Ashley, 1977; Tinetti & Powell), improving ease of changing body positions (Fiatarone & Evans, 1993), and lessening the dependence upon others for the performance of ADL.

General guidelines of resistive training for maneuvers performed by normals with free weights and/or machines should be appropriate for COPD patients. A 3-RM instead of a 1-RM test may be used to reduce the exercise stress of determining the appropriate exercise intensity and to prevent or minimize an episode of exertional dyspnea. In establishing the resistive training program, the number of repetitions performed for a given resistance should be emphasized more than the amount of weight being lifted (Cooper, 1997).

Water exercise has been used as an exercise modality to improve musculoskeletal and cardiorespiratory functions in special populations (Danneskiold-Samsoe, Lyngberg, Risum & Telling, 1987; Gehlsen, Grigsby & Winant, 1984; Routi, Troup & Berger, 1994). Since water is approximately 1,000 times denser than air, the movement of body segments or the entire body through water creates sufficient drag (resistance) to develop muscular strength and endurance (Costill, Maglischo & Richardson, 1992). This modality for resistive training may be excellent for persons with musculoskeletal limitations or contraindications for performing land exercise.

Table 10.7

Client Information to Obtain from Medical Professionals

1) Is this patient classified with mild, moderate or severe COPD? What symptoms of COPD does the patient exhibit?

2) What comorbid conditions and risk factors does this patient have? What symptoms of comorbid conditions does the patient present?

3) What is the nutritional status of the patient?

4) What medications is the patient taking for COPD, and do any of these have interactions with exercise tolerance? What other medications is the COPD patient taking for comorbid conditions and do any of these have interactions with exercise or with medications taken for COPD?

5) Does the patient need to take any medications (such as inhalers) prior to exercising?

6) Does the patient need supplemental oxygen during exercise?

7) What are the activity (exercise) contradindications of the patient?

8) What are the results of previously performed pulmonary function and exercise tolerance test? What are the recommended limits of exercise tolerance of this patient?

9) Should the patient's exercise program be based more on resistive training or aerobic training? What is the recommended intensity of training for the patient.

Whenever performing resistive exercise, one must be aware of the potential of a pressor effect, including elevated heart rate and blood pressure. As a result of the pressor effect, the exercise heart rate during resistive training may not accurately reflect the true intensity of training. In addition, the pressor effect may be more profound for unsupported arm exercise than for supported arm exercise.

Guidelines for Exercise Programming

Flexibility Exercises

Stretching of the major muscle groups of both upper and lower extremities is essential. Stretching should be incorporated as part of the warm-up before aerobic training and as part of the cool-down after aerobic training.

Aerobic Exercises

The exercise activity or mode of training should incorporate large muscle groups that can be continuous and rhythmic in nature. Types of exercise include walking, cycling, rowing, and water exercises or swimming. An indoor exercise activity is an important option for most clients with respiratory disease in case of inclement weather.

The recommended minimal frequency of formal physical activity is three to five days/week (Table 10.6). An alternate day schedule approximates this goal. Eventually, exercise should become part of the daily routine of the COPD patient. The minimal intensity of exercise should be at least 50 percent of peak O_2 uptake or the symptom-limited exercise tolerance. The duration of each exercise session should be at least 20 to 30 minutes of continuous exercise.

Intervals of exercise and rest may be necessary for some COPD clients, especially those with severe disease. The initial exercise session may include several five-minute walks with two-minute rest intervals. As the severity of COPD increases, clients may need several weeks to months to be able to walk continuously for more than 20 minutes.

Supplemental oxygen should be prescribed based on standard criteria (i.e., $PaO_2 < 55$ percent or arterial oxygen saturation of 88 percent). The appropriate flow rate for O_2 should be adjusted to maintain arterial oxygen saturation >90 percent as monitored by oximetry.

The Exercise Program

Since no standard exercise programming format exists, it must be individually tailored for the COPD client. Clients eligible for an exercise program should have their respiratory disability evaluated, have had no recent exacerbation of disease, and be receiving appropriate bronchodilator therapy (Clark, 1994; Patessio & Donner, 1995). Efficacy of exercise training is related to basic exercise physiology principles. These include specificity of training for improvement of ADL and general exercise tolerance. The appropriate exercise frequency, intensity and duration need to be established to elicit positive training effects and maintenance of work capacity, and to prevent detraining. Since training effects are transient, it is essential to involve the COPD client in satisfying physical activities so that a long-term commitment to exercise will be realized.

Two distinct modes of training should be implemented: aerobic/mobility training and resistive training. Both modes of training should include activities to develop endurance and strengthen the musculature of the lower and upper extremities. The optimal training program should combine an adapted choice of activity, a precise definition of training intensity, the consideration of training improvement and evaluation of training effect (Varry & Prefaut, 1995).

A cardiopulmonary exercise test should be performed to determine external mechanical load (work), presence of lactic acidosis, hypoxemia, hypercapnia (by arterial blood gases), incidence of arrhythmias, blood pressure, rating of perceived exertion or visual analog scale for dyspnea. Because dyspnea is the most common complaint and primary cause of exercise limitation, one may want to use the onset of dyspnea instead of heart rate to establish the intensity of exercise.

Most training and testing techniques recommend that the exercise prescription include repeated intervals of walking until dyspnea occurs. For example, a six-minute walk distance test can be used as a reference criteria for clients with severe COPD. In cases of less severe COPD, a 12-minute walk distance may be more appropriate. Stair climbing, step climbing, treadmill walking and leg cycle ergometry are all appropriate modalities for aerobic training. Since muscles of the shoulders and chest participate both in ventilation and in arm positioning during ADL, training of the musculature of the arms and chest for development of strength and endurance is important (Casaburi et al., 1997; Cooper, 1997). General body resistive training may include wrist curls, arms curls, partial leg squats, calf raises and supine dumbbell press with free-weights. It is not unusual for COPD clients with mild to moderate emphysema to perform eight to 10 repetitions at a resistance that is 50 percent to 80 percent of their 1- or 3-RM. For severe emphysema, the initial resistance for some of the maneuvers may be as little as 4 kg for 10 repetitions. The resistance should be increased when the patient can successfully complete 10 to 12 repetitions without dyspnea, breath holding or undue fatigue. A minimum standard of lifting 10 kg may be desirable to impact ADL.

Endurance training at a work rate associated with lactic acidosis is more effective for a training effect in COPD clients than a less intense work rate. Imposing exercise sessions of durations greater than 30 minutes may influence patient motivation to continue to exercise.

Training of Respiratory Muscles

Respiratory muscles can be trained to improve strength and the ability to endure a respiratory load. Respiratory muscle strength training should include high intensity, low frequency stimuli such as a resistive load, while endurance training should include low intensity, high frequency stimuli. There are three types of endurance training approaches — threshold loading, flow resistive loading and voluntary isocapnic hyperpnea. The pulmonary rehabilitation team will provide the personal trainer with suitable information concerning the recommended method of respiratory muscle training.

Flow resistive loading has been demonstrated to improve muscle strength and endurance (Belman & Shadmehr, 1988; Larson, Kim & Sharp, 1988) as well as reduce the incidence of dyspnea to the inspiratory load and during exercise (Falk et al., 1985). In studies using flow resistive loading, COPD patients breathed through devices with decreasing lumen (hole)

sizes to increase resistance. Decrease in the size of the lumen increases the resistance to breathing as long as tidal volume, frequency of breathing and time are held constant.

Special Consideration

Exercise Precautions

The COPD client's exercise session should be terminated and/or the exercise program should be changed if any of the following events occur:

1. The client experiences chest, neck, arm pain that is unusual or of unknown origin.
2. Breathing becomes so difficult that the client is gasping for air or dyspnea occurs during recovery from exercise.
3. The client experiences dizziness or nausea.
4. The patient develops unusual or increased ankle swelling.
5. The heart rate of the client becomes noticeably faster or slower than the prescribed heart rate for the exercise being performed.
6. The client experiences excessive fatigue lasting one to two hours following exercise.

Breathing During Exercise

Three basic principles for economical breathing during exercise should be stressed:

1. Avoid breath-holding during exertional activities.
2. Exhale through pursed lips during exertion.
3. Try to control respiratory frequency by slowing a fast rate of breathing.

Relaxation training may assist in learning better control of breathing during exercise and at rest. Relaxation will also reduce the resting energy cost, thereby lessening the metabolic demand.

Environmental Considerations

Smoking avoidance: Avoidance of smoking usually results in decreased airway irritation, sputum production and coughing.

Air pollution: COPD clients should be encouraged to consider moving away from a polluted environment. If pollution levels are particularly high, the COPD patient should be counseled to avoid outdoor physical activity. Inhalation of airway irritants such as dust, toxic fumes and pollens should be avoided. The house and particularly the bedroom should be kept dust free as much as possible. High-efficiency particulate air, activated charcoal or electrostatic filters to remove particles and pollutants should be considered.

Infection: The COPD patient should avoid exposure to persons with respiratory tract infections. Influenza may precipitate a rapid respiratory deterioration in COPD. Annual immunization may decrease the likelihood of contracting influenza.

Weather and Altitude: Sputum production and bronchial obstruction may be aggravated by either excessively hot or cold environments or by abrupt changes in these conditions. In hot weather, the use of an air conditioner may be very helpful in lessening the incidence of dyspnea in COPD clients. High altitude should be avoided because of lower arterial oxygen levels, exacerbation of hypoxemia-induced pulmonary hypertension and possibly **cor pulmonale**. Air travel exposes persons to high altitude, even in pressurized cabins. Thus, if air travel is planned, the COPD patient should be encouraged to use supplemental oxygen. if necessary which will be provided upon request by the commercial carrier.

High fluid intake: Water is the best expectorant available for liquefying sputum. Clients who have difficulties in clearing thick sputum should be encouraged to drink from 10 to 12 glasses of water daily.

Nutrition: Dyspnea and medications that may produce nausea commonly result in severe loss of appetite and subsequent weight loss of the COPD patient. A high-protein diet with multiple small feedings will help improve caloric intake and counteract weight loss in the COPD patient. Clients should avoid foods that will lead to abdominal discomfort. Supplemental vitamins should be considered. In some cases, the use of supplemental oxygen while eating may be beneficial.

Antireflux program: The COPD patient should eat small dry meals and drink fluids between meals rather that during mealtime to help to prevent reflux. The COPD patient should remain in an upright position for at least one hour following a meal. Spicy foods and alcohol should be avoided. Tight clothing should be avoided so there is no additional pressure on the abdomen.

Oxygen Supplementation: Similar to any drug, oxygen has both beneficial and potentially deleterious effects. The physical risks associated with oxygen supplementation include fire hazard or tank explosion, trauma from a catheter or masks, and drying of mucous membranes because of the dry (dehumidified) gas and the high gas flow rates. In some clients, oxygen supplementation may also result in increased CO_2 retention and absorptive atelectasis. (Mahler, 1998).

Case Studies

Case Study 1

B.M. is a 42-year-old Caucasian woman who has experienced exertional dyspnea during the last two years, which has limited her ability to perform household ADL. Her body mass index was 24 m²/kg and her hip/waist ratio was within normal range. She is a smoker (20 **pack-years**).

Recently, she has experienced increase in the episodes and duration of colds associated with chest tightness, wheezing, paroxysmal nocturnal dyspnea and orthopnea. She had chronic congestion seven years ago, and for two years she was treated for her allergies. She denied any previous history of chronic sputum production, hemoptysis chest pain or cardiac arrhythmia. Physical examination revealed wheezes during quiet breathing and during forced expiration. Hematological examination was within normal limits. Her chest film revealed the presence of granulomatous disease, but otherwise was normal. Pulmonary function test indicated that her FEV1 (1.6 L) was significantly reduced and the presence of airway obstruction pattern consistent with asthma was noted, which was reversible following bronchodilator therapy.

She achieved a peak heart rate of 186 bpm, peak blood pressure of 160/80 mmHg, breathing frequency of 25 breaths/min, minute ventilation of 48 L/min with a breathing reserve of 74 L, peak O_2 uptake of 25 mL/kg/min, and an O_2 saturation of 95 percent at rest and 90 percent at peak exercise on her cardiopulmonary exercise test. The exercise test indicated no major respiratory abnormalities, but the oxygen uptake indicated deconditioning and mild hypoxemia. There was no apparent exertional dyspnea. Based on an ADL questionnaire, her energy expenditure was estimated to be between five and METS. She was placed on theophylline and prednisone (20 mg/b.i.d.), terbutaline sulfate (t.i.d.), and an anticholinergic bronchodilator inhaler.

She was referred to a pulmonary rehabilitation program for improving overall body conditioning. She attended classes two to three times per week for 45 minutes/session for three months. The prescribed exercise intensity was at 50 percent of her achieved peak O_2 uptake, with perceived exertion between 11 and 13 by Borg's scale. Her exercise training consisted of indoor walking, bicycling, treadmill walking and resistive training with free weights. Her O_2 saturation was monitored by oximetry before, during and following exercise. Warm-up and cool-down periods were for seven to 10 minutes. Her program compliance was good. She returned to the laboratory after three months for reevaluation.

The results of the pulmonary function test were unchanged on post-test evaluations. The peak O_2 uptake improved significantly with adequate arterial O_2 saturation, which suggested an improvement in the ventilation-to-perfusion ratio. She remained active for the next six months and was able to maintain household ADL without experiencing dyspnea or undue fatigue.

Case Study 2

N.L is a 57-year-old longshore shipyard retiree who was evaluated for exacerbation of dyspnea that worsened in the last month. He was originally evaluated in 1982. His smoking history was 80 pack-years. His current medications include oral corticosteroids and both short- and long-acting bronchodilators.

During the last 15 years he has had recurrent hospitalization due to his severe emphysema (most recent FEV1 = .86 L (28 percent of the predicted value, improving to 38 percent after bronchodilator therapy). His functional status during household ADL is severely reduced despite his drug therapy. Recent chest radiographic findings indicate marked hyperinflation. The pattern of emphysema was predominately upper lobe (peripheral), and the presence of discrete bulle was noted. Physical examination indicated distant bilateral breath sounds. Heart sounds revealed an S4 gallop in the cardiac apex. No evidence of cyanosis, clubbing or congestive heart failure was found. Recent pulmonary function test result indicated a total lung capacity of 140 percent and residual volume 240 percent of the predicted. His single breath **diffusion capacity** was severely reduced by 27 percent of the predicted. In room air, arterial blood gases analyses revealed hypoxemia (pH = 7.41, PaO_2 = 64.4 mmHg and $PaCO_2$ = 42.4 mm Hg).

In order to improve the functional status of Mr. N.L., a bilateral lung volume reduction surgery was scheduled for three months later. He participated in a hospital-based outpatient pulmonary rehabilitation program to condition his respiratory muscles and to improve his ADL. Prior to beginning the pulmonary rehabilitation program, he underwent preoperative baseline tests. His peak O_2 uptake was 10.1 mL/kg/min; peak heart rate was 125 bpm; and O_2 saturation was 83 percent). Mr. N.L. was able to walk 325 m in six minutes, and he reported that he had a chronic daily phlegm production.

His exercise prescription included treadmill walking (2.0 mph with 0 percent elevation) three days/week for the first two weeks which was increased to 2.5 mph for the next 10 weeks. Exercise duration was initially 15 minutes with rests for dyspnea and was increased to 20 minutes for weeks six to 12. Respiratory muscle retraining was accomplished using an inspiratory muscle trainer initially set for 15 percent of his achieved maximal inspiratory pressure, which was progressively increased to 50 percent of the achieved maximal inspiratory pressure by the end of the 12th week. Leisure walking for 20 minutes (with rest break every five minutes of walking) was recommended as home training on days he did not report to the hospital for weeks five to 12. Pulmonary function tests and performance of ADL revealed significant improvement following the pulmonary rehabilitation program.

Twenty-one days following the bilateral lung volume reduction surgery, Mr. N.L. was discharged from the hospital. He continued to perform his home exercise. Pulmonary function tests performed at his three-month post-surgery follow-up revealed an improvement in FEV1 (40 percent) and functional vital capacity (21 percent). His tolerance to perform ADL also continued to significantly improved.

Suggested Readings

American Thoracic Society Statement. (1995). Standards for the diagnosis and care of patients with chronic obstructive pulmonary disease. *Respiratory and Critical Care Medicine*, 152, 5, S84-S96.

Belman, M.J. (1993). Exercise in patients with chronic obstructive pulmonary disease. *Thorax*, 48, 936-946.

Breslin, E.H. (1995). Breathing retraining in chronic obstructive pulmonary disease. *Journal Cardiopulmonary Rehabilitation*, 15, 25-33.

Celli, B.R., Rassulo, J. & Make, B.J. (1986). Dyssynchronous breathing during arm but not leg exercise in patients with chronic airflow obstruction. *New England Journal of Medicine*, 314, 1485-1490.

Clark C.J. (1994). Setting up a pulmonary rehabilitation programme. *Thorax,* 49, 270-278.

Cooper, C.B. (1997). Pulmonary disease. In: *ACSM's Exercise Management for Persons with Chronic Diseases and Disabilities (*pp 74-80). Champaign, Ill.: Human Kinetics.

Haas, F. Salazar-Schicchi, J. & Axen, R. (1993). Desensitization to dyspnea in chronic obstructive pulmonary disease. In: Casaburi. R., & Petty, L. (Eds). *Principals and practice of pulmonary rehabilitation.* (pp. 241-251). Philadelphia, Pa., W.B. Saunders.

Hsia, C.C.W. (1998). Pathophysiology of lung disease. In: *ACSM'S Resource Manual for Exercise Testing and Prescription,* 3rd edition, J.L. Reitman (Ed.), (pp 314-325. Baltimore, Md.). Williams and Wilkins,

Patessio A. & Donner C.F. (1995). The role of exercise training in pulmonary rehabilitation. *European Respiratory Review,* 5, 25, 47-50.

Varray A., & Prefaut C. (1995) Exercise training in patients with respiratory disease: procedures and results. *European Respiratory Review,* 5, 25, 51-58.

References

Agle, D.P. & Baum, G.L. (1977). Psychological aspects of chronic obstructive pulmonary disease. *Medial Clinics of North America,* 61, 749-758.

Ahmed, T. & Abraham, W.M. (1985). Role of calcium-channel blockers in obstructive airway disease. *Chest,* 88, 2, S142-S151.

American Lung Association. (1998). http://www.lungusa.org/index2.html

American Thoracic Society Statement. (1995). Standards for the diagnosis and care of patients with chronic obstructive pulmonary disease. *Respiratory and Critical Care Medicine,* 152, 5, S84-S96.

Astrand, P.O., Ekblom, B., Messin, R., Saltin, B. & Stenberg, J. (1965). Intra-arterial blood pressure during exercise with different muscle groups. *Journal of Applied Physiology,* 20, 253-256.

Astrand, I., Guharay, A. & Wahren, W., Jr. (1968). Circulatory responses to arm exercise with different arm positions. *Journal of Applied Physiology,* 25, 528-532.

Banzett, R.B., Topulos, G.P., Leith, D.E. & Nations, C.S. (1988). Bracing arms increases the capacity for sustained hyperpnea. *American Review of Respiratory Disease,* 138, 106-109.

Belman, M.J. (1993). Exercise in patients with chronic obstructive pulmonary disease. *Thorax,* 48, 936-946.

Belman M. & Shadmehr, R. (1988). Targeted resistive ventilatory muscle training in chronic obstructive pulmonary disease. *Journal of Applied Physiology.* 65, 2726-2735.

Berg, U., Kanstrup, L. & Ekblom, B.E. (1975). Maximal oxygen uptake during exercise with various combinations of arm and leg work. *Journal of Applied Physiology,* 41, 191-196.

Bevegard, S., Freyschuss, U. & Strandell, T. (1966). Circulatory adaptation to arm and leg exercise in supine and sitting position. *Journal of Applied Physiology,* 21, 37-46.

Blomqvist, C.G. (1985). Upper-extremity exercise testing and training. In N.K. Wenger (Ed.) *Exercise and the Heart* (2nd ed.) (pp. 175-183). Philadelphia, Pa.: F.A. Davis.

Bove, A.A. & Santamore, W.P. (1981). Ventricular interdependence. *Progressive in Cardiovascular Disease,* 23, 365-388.

Bradley, G.W. & Crawford, R. (1976). Regulation of breathing during exercise in normal subjects and in chronic lung disease. *Clinical Science in Molecular Medicine,* 51, 575-582.

Brown, S.E., Parkon, F.J., Miline, N., Linden, G.S., Stansbary, D.W., Fischer, C.E. & Light, R.W. (1984). Effect of digoxin on exercise capacity and right ventricular function during exercise in chronic airflow obstruction. *Chest,* 85, 187-191.

Busse, W.W. (1998). Leukotrienes and inflammation. *American Journal Respiratory and Critical Care Medicine,* 157, 6, S210-S213.

Casburi, R. (1998). Special considerations for exercise training testing and prescription. In: J.L. Reitman (Ed.). *ACSM's Resource Manual for Guidelines for Exercise Testing and Prescription* (pp. 334-338), Baltimore, Md., Williams and Wilkins.

Casaburi, R. Carithers, E., Tosolini, J., Phillips, J. & Bhasin,S. (1997). Randomized placebo controlled study of growth hormone in severe COPD patients undergoing endurance exercise training. *American Journal of Respiratory Critical Care Medicine,* 155, A498.

Celli, B.R. (1994). The clinical use of upper extremity exercise. *Clinics in Chest Medicine,* 15, 339-349.

Celli B.R. (1996). Current thoughts regarding treatment of chronic obstructive pulmonary disease. *Medical Clinics of North America,* 80, 589-609.

Celli, B.R., Criner, G.J. & Rassulo, R. (1988). Ventilatory muscle recruitment during unsupported arm exercise in normal subjects. *Journal of Applied Physiology,* 64, 1936-1941.

Celli, B.R., Rassulo, J. & Make, B.J. (1986). Dyssynchronous breathing during arm but not leg exercise in patients with chronic airflow obstruction. *New England Journal of Medicine,* 314, 1485-1490.

Cheong, T., Magder, S., Shapiro, S., Martin, J.G., & Levy, R.D. (1990). Cardiac arrhythmias during exercise in severe chronic obstructive pulmonary disease. *Chest,* 97, 793-797.

Clark C.J. (1994). Setting up a pulmonary rehabilitation programme. *Thorax,* 49, 270-278.

Clark, T.J.H., Freedman, S., Campbell, E.J.M. & Winn, R. (1969). The ventilatory capacity of patients with chronic airway obstruction. *Clinical Science,* 36, 307-316.

Clausen, J.P. (1976). Circulatory adjustments to dynamic exercise and effect of physical training in normal subjects and in patients with coronary artery disease. Progress in Cardiovascular Disease, 18, 459-495.

Cooper, C.B. (1997). Pulmonary disease. In: *ACSM's Exercise Management for Persons with Chronic Diseases and Disabilities* (pp. 74-80). Champaign: Ill., Human Kinetics.

Costill, D.L., Maglischo E.W. & Richardson A.B. (1992). *Swimming.* Oxford, England:Blackwell Scientific

Criner, G.J. & Celli, B.R. (1988). Effect of unsupported arm exercise on ventilatory muscle recruitment in patients with severe chronic airflow obstruction. *American Review of Respiratory Disease,* 138, 856-861.

Criner, G.J., Rassulo, J. & Celli, B.R. (1985). Respiratory muscle recruitment during unsupported and supported arm exercise in patients with severe chronic obstructive pulmonary disease. *Chest,* 85, 14S.

Danneskiold-Samsoe B., Lyngberg K., Risum T., & Telling M. (1987). The effect of water exercise therapy given to patients with rheumatoid arthritis. *Scandanavian Journal of Applied Physiology,* 19, 31-35.

Davies, C.T.M. & Sargeant, A.J. (1974). Physiological responses to standardized arm work. *Ergonomic,* 17, 41-49.

Decramer, M., Lacquet, L.M., Fagard, R. & Rogiers, P. (1994). Corticosteriods contribute to muscle weakness in chronic airflow obstruction. *American Journal of Respiratory Critical Care Medicine,* 150,11-16.

Dempsey, J.A. & Fregosi, R.F. (1985). Adaptability of the pulmonary system to changing metabolic requirements. *American Journal of Cardiology,* 55, 59D-67D.

Dillard, T.A., Piantadosi, S. & Rajakopal, K.R. (1985). Prediction of ventilation at maximal exercise in chronic airflow obstruction. *American Review of Respiratory Disease,* 132, 230-235.

Dodd, D.S., Brancatisano, T. & Engel, L.A. (1984). Chest wall mechanics during exercise in patients with severe chronic airflow obstruction. *American Review of Respiratory Disease,* 129, 33-38.

Eden, E., Turino G.M. (1986). Therapeutic applications to pulmonary circulation in chronic obstructive lung disease. *Seminar in Respiratory Medicine,* 8, 2, 184-194.

Emery, C.F., Schein, R.L., Hauck, E.R. & MacIntyre, N.R. (1998). Psychological and cognitive outcomes of a randomized trail of exercise among patients with chronic obstructive pulmonary disease. *Health Psychology,* 17, 232-240.

Falk, P., Eriksen, A.M., Kolliker, K., et al. (1985). Relieving dyspnea with an inexpensive and simple method in patients with severe chronic airflow limitation. *European Journal of Respiratory Disease,* 66, 181-186.

Ferguson, G.T. & Cherniack R.M. (1993). Current Concepts: Management of Chronic Obstructive Pulmonary Disease. *New England Journal of Medicine,* 328, 181-186.

Fiatarone, M.A. & Evans, W.J. (1993). The etiology and reversibility of muscle dysfunction in the aged. *Journal of Gerontology* [Special Issue], 48, 77-83.

Field, S., Kelly S.M. & Macklem P.T. (1982). The oxygen cost of breathing in patients with cardiorespiratory disease. *American Review Respiratory Disease,* 126, 13.

Finnerty, J., Wood-Baker, R., Thomson, H. & Holgate, S. (1992). Role of leukotrienes in exercise-induced asthma. *American Review Respiratory Disease,* 145, 746-749.

Galiber, D.P. & Dunn, D.P. (1994). Managing left ventricular failure in patients with COPD. *Journal of Respiratory Disease,* 15, 565-577.

Gallagher, C.G. & Younes, M. (1986). Breathing pattern during and after maximal exercise in patients with chronic obstructive pulmonary disease, interstitial lung disease, and cardiac disease, and in normal subjects. *American Review of Respiratory Disease,* 133, 1152-1158.

Gehlsen G.M., Grigsby S.A. & Winant D.M. (1984). Effects of an aquatic fitness program on the muscular strength and endurance of patients with multiple sclerosis. *Physical Therapy,* 64, 653-657.

Glantz, S.A., Misbach, G.A., Moores, W.Y., Mathey, D.G., Levken, J., Stowe, D.F., Parmley, W.W. & Tyberg, J.V. (1978). The pericardium substantially affects the left ventricular diastolic pressure-volume relationship in the dog. *Circulation Research,* 42, 171-180.

Goldman, M.D., Grassiano, A., Mead, J. & Sears, T.A. (1978). Mechanics of the human diaphragm during voluntary contraction: Dynamics. *Journal of Applied Physiology,* 44, 840.

Grant, I., Prigatano, G.P., Heaton, R.K., McSweeny, A.J., Wright, E.C. & Adams, K.M. (1987). Progressive neuropsychologic impairment and hypoxemia. *Archives of General Psychiatry,* 44, 999-1006.

Grimby, G., Elgefors, B. & Oxhoj, H. (1973). Ventilatory levels and chest wall mechanics during exercise in obstructive lung disease. *Scandinavia Journal of Respiratory Disease,* 54, 45-52.

Gryfe C.I., Amies A. & Ashley M.J. (1977). A longitudinal study of falls in an elderly population. *Aging,* 6, 201-210.

Haas, F. Salazar-Schicchi, J. & Axen, R. (1993). Desensitization to dyspnea in chronic obstructive pulmonary disease. In: Casaburi. R. & Petty, L. (Eds). *Principals and Practice of Pulmonary Rehabilitation* (pp. 241-251). Philadelphia, Pa.: W.B. Saunders.

Hsia, C.C.W. (1998). Pathophysiology of lung disease. In J.L. Reitman (Ed.), *ACSM'S Resource Manual for Exercise Testing and Prescription,* 3rd edition (pp. 314-325). Baltimore, Md.: Williams and Wilkins.

Idell, S. & Kronenberg, R.S. (1986). Drug therapy for chronic obstructive pulmonary disease. *Seminar in Respiratory Medicine,* 8, 2, 129-139.

Janicki, J.S. & Weber, K.T. (1980). Factors influencing the diastolic pressure volume relation of the cardiac ventricles. *Federation Proceedings,* 39, 133-140.

Jenne, J.W., Sievere, J.R., Druz, W.S., Solano, J.V., Cohen, S.M. & Sharp J.T. (1984). The effect of maintenance theophylline therapy on lung work in severe chronic obstructive pulmonary disease while standing and walking. *American Review Respiratory Disease,* 130, 600-605.

Jette, A.M. & Branch, L.G. (1981). The Framingham disability study: II. Physical disability among the aging. *American Journal of Public Health,* 71, 1211-1216.

Jones, N.L., Jones, G. & Edwards, R.T.H. (1971). Exercise tolerance in chronic airway obstruction. *American Review of Respiratory Disease,* 103, 477-491.

Kelsen, S.G. & Criner, G.J. (1991). Rehabilitation of patients with COPD. In N.S. Cherniack (Ed.), *Chronic Obstructive Pulmonary Disease* (pp. 520-534). Philadelphia, Pa.: W.B. Saunders.

Killian, K.J., Mahutte, C.K., Howell, J.B.L. & Campbell, E.J.M. (1980). Effect of timing, flow, lung volume, and threshold pressures on resistive load detection. *Journal of Applied Physiology,* 49, 958-963.

Larson J.L., Kim, M.J. & Sharp J.T. (1988). Inspiratory muscle training with a pressure threshold breathing device in patients with chronic obstructive pulmonary disease. *American Reviews of Respiratory Disease,* 138, 689-96.

Lanigan, C., Moxham, J. & Ponte, J. (1990). Effect of chronic airflow limitation on resting oxygen consumption. *Thorax,* 45, 388-390.

Levine, J.H., Michael, J.R. & Guarnieri, T. (1985). Multifocal atrial tachycardia: a toxic effect of theophylline. *Lancet,* 1,12-13.

Levinson, H. & Cherniack, R.M. (1968). Ventilatory cost of exercise in chronic obstructive pulmonary disease. *Journal of Applied Physiology,* 25, 21-27.

Mahler, D.A. (1998). Pulmonary rehabilitation. *Chest,* 113, 263S-268S.

Mahler, D.A., Brent, B.N., Loke, J., Zaret, B.L. & Matthay, R.A. (1984). Right ventricular performance and central circulatory hemodynamics during upright exercise in patients with chronic obstructive pulmonary disease. *American Review of Respiratory Disease,* 130, 722-729.

Mahler, D.A. & Harver, A. (1988). Prediction of peak oxygen consumption in obstructive airway disease. *Medicine and Science in Sports and Exercise,* 20, 574-578.

Make, B. & Buchholz, J. (1991). Exercise training in COPD patients improves cardiac function. *American Review of Respiratory Disease,* 143, A80.

Manning, P.J., Watson, R.M., Margolskee, D.J., Williams, V.C., Schwartz, J.I. & O'Byrne, P.M. (1990). Inhibition of exercise induced bronchoconstriction by MK-571, a potent leukotriene D4-receptor antagonist. *New England Journal of Medicine,* 323, 1736-1739.

Martin, B.J., Powell, E., Shore, S., Emrich, J. & Engel, L.A. (1980). The role of respiratory muscles in the hyperinflation of bronchial asthma. *American Review of Respiratory Disease,* 121, 441-447.

Martinez, F.J., Couser, J.I. & Celli, B.R. (1991). Respiratory response to arm elevation in patients with chronic airflow obstruction. *American Review of Respiratory Disease,* 143, 476-480.

Matthay, R.A. & Berger, H.J. (1984). Radionuclide angiocardiographic assessment of right and left ventricular performance. In L.J. Rubin (Ed.), *Pulmonary Heart Disease* (pp. 223-245). Boston, Ma.: Martinus Nijhoff.

Matthay, R.A., Berger, H.J., Davies, R. A., Loke, J., Mahler, D., Gottschalk, A. & Zaret, B.L. (1980). Right and left ventricular exercise performance in chronic obstructive pulmonary disease: Radionuclide assessment. *Annals of Internal Medicine,* 93, 234-239.

Matthews, J.I., Bush, B.A. & Ewald, F.W. (1989). Exercise responses during incremental and high intensity and low intensity steady state exercise in patients with obstructive lung disease and normal control subjects. *Chest,* 96, 11-17.

McSweeny, A.J., Grant, I., Heaton, R.K., Adams, K.M. & Timms, R.M. (1982). Life quality of patients with chronic obstructive pulmonary disease. *Archives of Internal Medicine,* 142, 473-478.

Meltzer, S.S., Hasday, J.D., Cohn, J. & Bleeker, E.R., (1996). Inhibition of exercise induced bronchospasm by zileuton: a 5-lipoxygenase inhibitor. *American Journal Respiratory and Critical Care Medicine,* 153, 931-935.

Miles, D.S., Cox, M.H. & Bomze, J.P. (1989). Cardiovascular responses to upper body exercise in normal and cardiac patients. *Medicine and Science in Sports and Exercise,* 21, 5, S126-S131.

Miles, D.S., Sawka, M.N., Hanpeter, D.E., Foster, J.E., Doerr, B.M. & Frey, M.A.B. (1984). Central hemodynamics during progressive upper and lower-body exercise and recovery. *Journal of Applied Physiology,* 57, 366-370.

Morrison, D.A., Adcock, K., Collins, C.M., Goldman, S., Caldwell, J.A. & Schwartz, M.I. (1987). Right ventricular dysfunction and the exercise limitation of chronic obstructive pulmonary disease. *Journal of the American College of Cardiology,* 9, 1219-1229.

Murphy, M.L., Boger, J., Adamson, J.S. & Rubin, S. (1977). Evaluation of cardiac size in chronic bronchitis and pulmonary emphysema. *Chest,* 71, 712-717.

Muller, N., Bryan, A. C. & Zamel, N. (1980). Tonic inspiratory muscle activity as a cause of hyper-inflation in histamine-induced asthma. *Journal of Applied Physiology,* 49, 869-874.

Nery, L.E., Wasserman, K., Andrews, J.D., Huntsman, D.J., Hansen, J.E. & Whipp, B.J. (1982). Ventilatory and gas exchange kinetics during exercise in chronic airway obstruction. *Journal of Applied Physiology,* 53, 1594-1602.

Nery, L.E., Wasserman, K., French, W., Oren, A. & Davis, J. A. (1983). Contrasting cardiovascular and respiratory responses to exercise in mitral valve and chronic obstructive pulmonary disease. *Chest,* 83, 446-453.

O'Byrne, P.M. & Daahlem, S.E. (Eds.). (1997). New oral preventive therapy in asthma and oral leuko-triene receptor antagonist. *European Respiratory Review,* 7(46), 251-280.

Pardy, R.L., Hussain, S.N.A. & Macklem, P.T. (1984). The ventilatory pump in exercise. *Clinical Chest Medicine,* 5, 35-49.

Patessio A., Donner C.F. (1995). The role of exercise training in pulmonary rehabilitation. *European Respiratory Review* 5, 25, 47-50.

Pinskey, M.R. (1994). Heart-lung interactions during positive-pressure ventilation. *New Horizons,* 2, 443-456.

Prigatano, G.P., Parsons, O., Wright, E., Levin, D.C. & Hawryluk, G. (1983). Neuropsychological test performance in mildly hypoxemic patients with chronic obstructive pulmonary disease. *Journal of Consulting and Clinical Psychology,* 51, 108-116.

Rao, B.S., Cohn, K.E., Eldridge, F.L. & Hancock, E.W. (1968). Left ventricular failure secondary to chronic pulmonary disease. *American Journal of Medicine,* 45, 229-241.

Reid, W.D. & Warren, C.P. (1984). Ventilatory muscle strength and endurance training in elderly subjects and patients with chronic airflow limitation: A pilot study. *Physiology Canada,* 36, 305-311.

Ries, A.L. (1994). The importance of exercise in pulmonary rehabilitation. *Clinics Chest Medicine,* 15, 327-337.

Robotham, J.L. (1981). Cardiovascular disturbances in chronic respiratory insufficiency. *American Journal of Cardiology,* 47, 941-949.

Rochester, D.F. (1992). Nutritional repletion. *Seminar in Respiratory Medicine,* 13, 44-52.

Rochester, D.F., Arora, N.S., Braun, N.M.T. & Goldberg, S.K. (1979). The respiratory muscles in chronic obstructive pulmonary disease (COPD). *Bulletin European Physiopathology Respiration,* 15, 951-975.

Ruoti R.G., Troup, J.T. & Berger, R.A. (1994). The effects of nonswimming exercise on older adults. *Journal of Orthopedic Sports Physical Therapy,* 19, 140-145.

Rowell, L.B. & Sheriff, D.D. (1988). Are muscle "chemoreflexes" functionally important? *News in Physiological Science,* 3, 250-253.

Sawka, M.N. (1986). Physiology of upper body exercise. *Exercise and Sports Science Reviews,* 14, 175-211.

Schaaning, J. (1978). Respiratory cycle time duration during exercise in patients with chronic obstructive lung disease. *Scandinavia Journal of Respiratory Disease,* 59, 313-318.

Scharf, S.M. (1989). Effects of normal and stressed inspiration on cardiovascular function. In S.M. Scharf & S.S. Cassidy (Eds.), *Heart-Lung Interactions in Health and Disease* (pp. 427-461). New York: Marcel Dekker.

Schols, A.M., Mostert, R., Soeters, P.B., Greve, L.H. & Wouters, E.F.M. (1989). Nutritional state and exercise performance in patients with chronic obstructive pulmonary disease. *Thorax,* 44, 937-941.

Shephard, R.J., Campbell, E.J.M., Martin, H.B. & Enns, T. (1955). Factors affecting pulmonary dead space as measured by single breath analysis. *American Journal of Physiology,* 183, 661.

Slutsky, R.A., Hooper, W., Ackerman, W. & Moser, K. (1982). The response of right ventricular size, function, and pressure to supine exercise: A comparison of patients with chronic obstructive lung disease and normal subjects. *European Journal of Nuclear Medicine,* 7, 553-558.

Spiro, S.G., Hahn, H.L., Edwards, R.H.T. & Pride, N.B. (1975). An analysis of the physiological strain of submaximal exercise in patients with chronic obstructive bronchitis. *Thorax,* 30, 415-425.

Steele, P., Ellis, J.H., Van Dyke, D., Sutton, F., Creagh, E. & Davis, H. (1975). Left ventricular ejection fraction in severe chronic obstructive airways disease. *American Journal of Medicine,* 59, 21-28.

Stenberg, J., Astrand, P.O., Ekblom, B., Royce, J. & Saltin, B. (1967). Hemodynamic response to work with different muscle groups sitting and supine. *Journal of Applied Physiology,* 22, 61-70.

Tinetti M.E., Baker, D.I., McAvay, G., Claus, E.B., Garrett, P., Gottschalk, M., Koch, M.L., Trainor, K. & Horwitz, R.I. (1994). A multifactoral intervention to reduce the risk of falling among elderly people living in the community. *New England Journal of Medicine,* 331, 821-827.

Tinetti, M.E., Powell, L. (1993) Fear of falling and low self-efficacy: A cause of dependence in elderly persons. Journal of Gerontology, [Special Issue], 48, 35-38.

Tobin, M.J., Chadha, T.S., Jenouri, G., Birch, S.J., Gazeroglu, H.B. & Sackner, M.A. (1983a). Breathing patterns: 1. Normal subjects. *Chest,* 84, 202-205.

Tobin, M.J., Chadha, T.S., Jenouri, G., Birch, S.J., Gazeroglu, H.B. & Sackner, M.A. (1983b). Breathing patterns: 2. Diseased subjects. *Chest,* 84, 286-294.

Unger, K., Shaw, D., Karliner, J.S., Crawford, M., O'Rourke, R.A. & Moser, K.M. (1975). Evaluation of left ventricular performance in acutely ill patients with chronic obstructive lung disease. *Chest,* 68, 135-142.

Varray A. & Prefaut C. (1995) Exercise training in patients with respiratory disease: procedures and results. *European Respiratory Review,* 5, 25, 51-58.

Wasserman, K. (1978). Breathing during exercise. *New England Journal of Medicine,* 298, 780-785.

Wasserman, K., Hansen, J.E., Sue, D.Y. & Whipp, B.J. (1987). *Principles of exercise testing and interpretation.* Philadelphia, Pa.: Lea & Febiger.

Weber, K.T., Janicki, J.S., Sharoff, S. & Fishman, A.P. (1981). Contractile mechanics and interaction of the right and left ventricles. *American Journal of Cardiology,* 47, 686-695.

Whipp, B.J. & Wasserman, K. (1969). Alveolar-arterial gas tension differences during graded exercise. *Journal of Applied Physiology,* 27, 61-65.

Wise, R.A. (1991). Chronic obstructive pulmonary disease and the peripheral circulation. In N.S. Cherniack (Ed.), *Chronic Obstructive Pulmonary Disease* (pp. 167-177). Philadelphia, Pa.: W.B. Saunders.

Younes, M. (1990). Determinants of thoracic excursions during exercise. In B.J. Whipp & K. Wasserman (Eds.), *Pulmonary Physiology and Pathophysiology of Exercise: Lung Biology in Health and Disease* (pp. 1-65). New York: Marcel Dekker.

Younes, M. & Kivinen, G. (1984). Respiratory mechanics and breathing pattern during and following maximal exercise. *Journal of Applied Physiology,* 57, 1773-1782.

Section Four

Metabolic Diseases

Chapter 11
Diabetes
Mellitus

Chapter 12
Obesity

Chapter 13
Blood Lipid
Disorders

CHAPTER 11

Diabetes Mellitus

LARRY S. VERITY

Larry S. Verity, Ph.D., F.A.C.S.M., is
a professor of exercise physiology in
the Department of Exercise and
Nutritional Sciences at San Diego
State University. He is a Fellow of
the American College of Sports
Medicine and is certified as an
Exercise Specialist. He has served as
a writing consultant with the
American Council on Exercise, and
has published reviews and original
manuscripts on diabetes and exercise
in peer-reviewed publications. He has
had Type 1 diabetes for 22 years and
is without complications.

Pathophysiology

Exercise Benefits

Lifestyle & Habits

O nly two decades ago, physical exercise for diabetics was frowned upon. In fact, diabetes was used as an excuse to avoid exercise. Today, questions continue to be asked regarding whether a diabetic can exercise safely. Does exercise actually help diabetics or does it hamper the condition? Can exercise control diabetes? Is it safe for diabetics to exercise any time? Do complications from diabetes affect one's ability to regularly participate in exercise? To answer these questions, you must know about the disease. In this chapter, I will discuss what you may do to assess a diabetic's capabilities and design a safe and effective exercise program.

You may interact with a variety of clients, including those with diabetes. Physical exercise plays an important role in the management of diabetes. It promotes a variety of health-related benefits. Among them, it improves the body's cardiovascular function and its ability to metabolize glucose.

Physical activity appears to play a pivotal role in preventing Type 2 diabetes in men (Helmrich, Ragland, Leung & Paffenbarger, 1991) and women (Manson et al., 1991). Still, you should realize that exercise is not an answer for all metabolic problems related to diabetes. Under certain conditions, exercise can lead to abnormally high levels of blood glucose and ketone bodies in

Type 1 diabetes, and can increase the risk of low blood glucose responses in diabetics. Given the benefits and risks of exercise for diabetics, you need to understand this disease; identify practical aspects of physical activity for diabetics; and design and modify exercise programs to improve disease management and health outcomes.

Definition of Diabetes Mellitus

Diabetes is a disorder that disrupts glucose, protein and fat metabolism. Typically, persons with diabetes have an elevated blood glucose level [called **hyperglycemia**] that results from deficient insulin secretion, insulin action, or both (ECDCDM, 1997). In diabetics, fasting and pre-meal blood glucose levels are usually in the range of 80 - 115 mg/dl. Diagnosis of diabetes requires that blood glucose level meets a minimum value of 126 mg/dl or greater on at least two separate occasions (ECDCDM, 1997). You should understand the acceptable limits of blood glucose for diabetics.

Classification and Etiology of Diabetes Mellitus

Diabetes is a metabolic syndrome composed of four classifications; however, this chapter will review the two primary classes of diabetes that account for 95 percent of the diabetic population, including Type 1 and Type 2 diabetes mellitus (ADA, 1996).

Both Type 1 and Type 2 diabetes have distinct causes and clinical characteristics. Each requires different strategies for disease management. Table 11.1 presents an overview of differences between Type 1 and Type 2 diabetes.

Type 1 Diabetes Mellitus. Type 1 diabetes requires insulin administration (e.g., via injections or pump) to control elevated blood glucose levels. This type of diabetes occurs in about 5 percent to 10 percent of the diabetic population, and in persons less than 30 years of age (ADA, 1994b). Risk factors for this type of diabetes include genetic, autoimmune and environmental elements (ECDCDM, 1997). Usually, a central defect, or deficient release of insulin [insulin is a hormone produced, stored and released from the pancreatic beta-cells] is the principal cause of hyperglycemia in Type 1 diabetes. An autoimmune response selectively destroys the pancreatic beta-cells. That stops insulin production and creates hyperglycemia. Because insulin is an essential hormone that regulates glucose, fat and protein metabolism, the Type 1 diabetic must inject insulin daily at regular intervals to maintain as normal a metabolism as possible.

Insulin action in Type 1 diabetes is directly related to the degree of glucose control (Reaven, 1988). Usually, good glucose control yields normal insulin action, while poor control reduces insulin's action. Thus, therapeutic strategies focus on achieving as near-normal blood glucose control as possible to improve insulin's action and lessen the likelihood for long-term complications associated with this type of diabetes.

Type 2 Diabetes Mellitus. Type 2 diabetes may require dietary intervention, oral drugs and/or insulin injections to control blood glucose levels. This type of diabetes occurs in 90 percent to 95 percent of the diabetic population and usually affects persons over 30 years of age. You must identify risk factors for Type 2 diabetes, including

Table 11.1
Distinguishing Characteristics Between Type 1 and Type 2 Diabetes Mellitus

Type 1		Type 2
Insulin requiring (formerly: juvenile onset)	Synonyms	Non-insulin requiring (formerly: adult onset)
IDDM	Former Abbreviation	NIDDM
< 30 years	Age of Onset	> 30 Years
5-10%	Cases of Diabetes in US (%)	90-95%
Autoimmune deficiency	Pathological Factor	Family History
100%	Insulin Use	40%
Recent weight loss	Body Weight History	Weight gain
Uncommon	Obese at Diagnosis	Common (80% obese)
None	Insulin Production	Deficient
Common	Ketoacidodic Episodes	Uncommon
Absent	Response to Diet Alone	In some mild forms
May be present	Insulin Resistance	Common

obesity, older age, family history of diabetes and physical inactivity (ADA, 1994a). In addition, minority populations have greater susceptibility to Type 2 diabetes, as the risk for diabetes is higher in Native Americans, African Americans, Hispanic Americans, and Asian and Pacific Island Americans compared to Non-Hispanic whites (CDC, 1997). Clinically, Type 2 diabetics report recent vision problems and slow-healing wounds (ADA, 1991). Most Type 2 diabetics produce insulin, yet suffer from a "peripheral defect" in insulin action (e.g., skeletal muscle) resulting in poor insulin action, or **insulin resistance**, which is primarily responsible for **hyperglycemia**.

Although insulin resistance is common in peripheral tissues (e.g., skeletal muscle, liver) and a universal feature of Type 2 diabetes, lifestyle changes that focus on diet and physical activity to promote weight loss can favorably modify insulin action (Bourn et al., 1995). Therefore, a primary strategy for managing Type 2 diabetes is to improve insulin action through a reduction in body weight/fat and an increase in physical activity, as insulin resistance has been linked not only with hyperinsulinemia and hyperglycemia, but also with an increased prevalence of hypertension and hyperlipidemia (Reaven, 1988). Insulin resistance also contributes to the progression of cardiovascular and peripheral vascular disease in Type 2 diabetics and increases both morbidity and mortality. Weight loss improves the quality of life and reduces the morbidity related to insulin resistance.

You must realize that both types of diabetes are associated with serious complications and premature death. Additionally, you must encourage your diabetic clientele to adopt healthy lifestyle habits and perform regular Self-Blood Glucose Monitoring (SBGM) to reduce such adverse health outcomes.

Pathophysiology of Diabetes Mellitus

Diabetes leads to a variety of metabolic and physiologic problems. The disease affects both the macrovascular (e.g., cardiovascular disease, peripheral vasculature, cerebral vasculature) and microvascular (e.g. retina, kidney and peripheral nerves) systems. Yet the onset of problems is less likely to occur in physically active Type 1 (LaPorte et al., 1986)

and Type 2 (Schneider, Vitug & Ruderman, 1986) diabetics. Moreover, good metabolic control is associated with a significant reduction in diabetic complications.

Macrovascular, microvascular and nerve disease complications are commonly linked to hyperglycemia and diabetes. You should know whether a client has complications because these reflect the severity and duration of the disease, and may contribute to accelerated morbidity and excessive mortality in diabetics. Diabetes affects 5 percent to 6 percent of the United States population (CDC, 1997) and is a common cause of premature onset of macrovascular diseases (Colwell, et al., 1989).

Macrovascular Disease. Large vessel disease, or macrovascular disease, is common in persons with diabetes. One type of macrovascular disease, coronary heart disease, is accelerated in people with glucose intolerance and hyperglycemia (Kannel & McGee, 1979). That leads to premature morbidity and mortality. Additionally, diabetes contributes to accelerated atherogenic processes in other large vessels, including those to the lower extremities (peripheral vasculature) and to the brain (cerebral vasculature). Lower extremity complications usually limit the weight-bearing tolerance of afflicted individuals, and contribute to a greater risk of nontraumatic amputations. Cerebral vascular disease, another serious complication, is worsened by high blood pressure, and increases the risk of stroke in diabetics. Consequently, you must know whether a diabetic client has any macrovascular disease. If this is the case, you must modify the assessment, programming and leadership accordingly.

Multiple risk factors for macrovascular disease in the nondiabetic population are well established, and are commonly present in Type 1 and Type 2 diabetics (ADA, 1991). For nondiabetic populations, modification of smoking, elevated lipid levels, high blood pressure and physical inactivity are independently related to the risk of macrovascular disease and are prevalent in persons with diabetes (ADA, 1993). Moreover, obesity is independently linked to an increased risk for macrovascular disease and is characteristic of most Type 2 diabetics.

Physiological and metabolic abnormalities of diabetes that are believed to exacerbate the macrovascular atherogenic process are glucose

Table 11.2
Benefits of Regular Physical Activity on Health-Related Parameters in Type 1 and Type 2 Diabetes

	Change		Change
Cardiovascular-Related		**Body Composition**	
• aerobic capacity, or fitness level	↑	• body fat, especially in obese	↓
• resting heart rate	↓	• fat free mass	↑
• blood pressure in mild-moderate hypertensives	↓	• body fat distribution	favorably ↑
• work of the heart at submaximal loads	↓	**Metabolic Aspects**	
• abnormal thickening of the heart	favorably ↓	• insulin sensitivity	↑
Lipid/Lipoprotein Alterations		• glucose metabolism	↑
• HDL	↑	• thermic effect of food	↑
• LDL	↓/↔	• basal and postprandial insulin needs	↑
• VLDL/Triglycerides	↓	**Psychological Aspects**	
• Total Cholesterol	↔	• self-concept/self-esteem	↑
• Risk Ratio [Total cholesterol/HDL]	↓	• depression	↑
		• stress response to psychologic stimuli	↑

intolerance, hyperglycemia and insulin resistance (Reaven, 1988). Though there may be different mechanisms responsible for the pathogenesis of atherosclerosis in Type 1 and Type 2 diabetes, no clinical trials have found that modification of any individual risk factor for either type of diabetes lessens the risk of atherosclerotic vascular disease (ADA, 1993). Given the current knowledge regarding nondiabetic populations and atherosclerotic disease, diabetics should modify existing risk factors to lower their risk for macrovascular disease.

Microvascular and Neural Complications. Small vessel diseases, or microvascular complications, and nerve diseases are common outcomes of long-standing diabetes. Usually, the onset of microvascular disease progressively contributes to failure of the target tissue involved. The three different types of microvascular complications include retinopathy (eye disease), nephropathy (kidney disease) and neuropathy (nerve disease). Respectively, these complications of diabetes are the leading cause of new blindness and end-stage renal disease in adults, and contribute to nervous system damage in 60 percent to 70 percent of diabetics (ECD-CDM, 1997). Moreover, these complications can affect work tolerance, as well as the mode and intensity of work performed. You must know whether microvascular complications exist to safely and effectively program exercise for diabetics.

A recent study (ADA, 1993) reported that near-normalization of blood glucose reduced the risk for onset and/or progression of microvascular disease in Type 1 diabetics by more than 50 percent, and suggests similar outcomes for Type 2 diabetics (ADA, 1994a). Compelling data links diabetes complications with poor blood glucose control, and affords diabetes healthcare professionals persuasive evidence about the importance of maintaining metabolic control through self-blood-glucose monitoring [SBGM] to prevent or delay progression of complications. Thus, you can help in diabetes management by encouraging clients to maximize glucose control and lessen the progression of small vessel complications.

Therapeutic Interventions for Diabetes Mellitus

The core elements of diabetes therapy include insulin, diet and exercise, and focus on blood glucose regulation (e.g., diet and insulin). The primary goal of treating diabetes is not only to normalize glucose metabolism, but also to delay or prevent disease complications common to diabetes. More recently, diabetes treatment has expanded to include behavioral strategies to enhance self-care management of the disease (Figure 11.1). You are now part of the diabetes management team and can motivate clients to participate safely and regularly in physical activity. Also, you must be proactive in communicating with other members of the diabetes treatment team (e.g., personal physician, nurse educator) to ensure the safety and effectiveness of a physical activity program.

Exercise Benefits: Its Role in Diabetes Management

Regular physical activity and/or exercise spurs fitness benefits for both Type 1 and Type 2 diabetics (Table 11.2). Mild to moderate exercise may assist with daily glucose regulation on a short-term basis for both Type 1 and Type 2 diabetes, which may explain the role of regular exercise to favorably alter metabolic functions related to glucose metabolism. Regular exercise helps lessen cardiovascular risk factors, such as mild to moderate hypertension, insulin resistance and abnormal lipid profiles. Regular exercise affects not only metabolic control, but also factors related to cardiovascular and psychological health in diabetes.

Short-term Benefits of Exercise in Type 1 Diabetes Mellitus

Although circulating insulin is derived from an exogenous injection site, or through a continuous infusion pump, exogenous insulin absorption does not mimic the normal insulin secretory pattern, especially during physical exercise. Consequently, insulin administration poses a potential problem for Type 1 diabetics to sustain near-normal glucose levels while exercising. Yet some medical professionals believe that exercise is not appropriate for Type 1 diabetics. They identify the risks for diabetics to participate safely in physical activities.

Insulin therapy for most Type 1 diabetics typically consists of multiple-dose exogenous insulin injections. Exogenous insulin absorption is not well regulated and results in varying degrees of insulin excess or deficiency in the peripheral blood. Insulin levels are very important during the increased metabolic demands of physical exercise. In Type 1 diabetics, several factors influence the blood glucose response to exercise, including the time of the insulin injection; location of insulin injection (i.e., active versus nonactive muscle sites); pre-exercise glucose; pre-exercise nutrition; intensity and duration of the exercise session; and the novelty of the exercise performed.

Given so many factors to regulate, it is not surprising that physical exercise brings about unpredictable blood glucose responses in Type 1 diabetes. Because of the dependency upon exoge-nous insulin and an inability to regulate the absorption of insulin, Type 1 diabetics commonly oscillate between insulin excess and insulin deficiency. Hence, the degree of "insulinization" and the level of blood glucose before the start of exercise determine the blood glucose response during and after exercise for Type 1 diabetics. In well-controlled or well-insulinized Type 1 diabetics, a single session of moderate exercise brings about normal metabolic responses. Under certain conditions, blood glucose may increase or decrease, depending on insulin levels.

Hypoinsulinemia. Hypoinsulinemia, or insulin deficiency, results in elevated blood glucose and ketone bodies before exercise. Insulin-deficient diabetics rely heavily upon free fatty acids [FFA] as a primary energy source, which leads to elevated ketones in the blood and urine.

What happens when an insulin-deficient diabetic exercises? As work increases, there is an increase in metabolic functions to provide adequate fuel for the body. Unfortunately, a person with inadequate insulin is not able to adequately regulate blood glucose levels, and experiences an increase in blood glucose, along with an increase in FFA use and ketone production. Exercise seems to worsen **hyperglycemia** in an insulin-deficient state because insulin action does not promote normal metabolic functions. Diabetics should use SBGM before exercise, as this is the safest way to determine whether exercise will help improve insulinization action and lower glucose levels.

Figure 11.3

Diabetes treatment requires a team approach

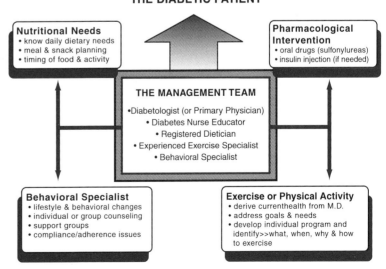

Hyperinsulinemia. Hyperinsulinema, or high insulin levels, usually occurs when exogenous insulin absorption is accelerated by increased muscle contraction and blood flow. This can cause exercise-induced **hypoglycemia**. Insulin injection into nonactive muscle is recommended on exercising days, although the strict use of nonactive muscle as an injection site may not prevent hypoglycemia during exercise in Type 1 diabetes.

Elevated insulin levels suppress hepatic glucose production, which causes an imbalance between the rate of peripheral glucose use and production, and results in lowering of blood glucose. Although a decrease in blood glucose is a beneficial short-term effect of exercise, prolonged exercise can bring about hypoglycemia. Consequently, blood glucose lowering is dependent upon such factors as pre-exercise levels of blood glucose and insulin, antecedent nutrition, and exercise duration and intensity. Regular SBGM, as well as modifying food intake and insulin dose on exercise days are useful strategies to prevent hypoglycemia in Type 1 diabetes.

Post-exercise Hypoglycemia. Although hypoglycemia can occur during exercise, low blood glucose can develop many hours after an acute exercise bout in Type 1 diabetes. Short-lived, post-exercise metabolic adjustments increase the risk for hypoglycemia in the first few hours following an exercise bout. To prevent acute- and late-onset hypoglycemia, strategies should combine aggressive post-exercise SBGM with adjustment of pre-

and post-exercise insulin and caloric intake, as changes in insulin dose and caloric intake are not totally effective.

Postprandial (after a meal) Exercise Responses. The majority of Type 1 diabetics exercise after a meal, rather than in a postabsorptive or fasted state. Usually, persons with Type 1 diabetes have glucose fluctuations with each meal, due to the relative timing of insulin injection and rate of insulin absorption from the injection site. Mild exercise after breakfast blunts glucose elevations throughout the course of a day in Type 1 diabetes. It may also prove valuable because of a reduced risk for hypoglycemia during and following exercise. However, postprandial exercise in Type 1 diabetes is quite variable, and is dependent upon the pre-exercise glucose level, timing of insulin injection with nutrition before activity, and exercise intensity and duration.

Long-term Benefits of Exercise in Type 1 Diabetes Mellitus

Our current knowledge about the long-term benefits of regular exercise on various health aspects offers a persuasive rationale for persons with Type 1 diabetes to participate in physical activities. Effective exercise programming is based upon an understanding of both short- and long-term benefits, as well as the related risks.

Glucose Metabolism. A single session of exercise acutely lowers blood glucose in Type 1 diabetics for a variable amount of time. The syner-

Table 11.4

Client Information to Obtain from Medical Professionals

1) How well controlled is my client's diabetes?

2) How often has my client been into your office over the past two years?

3) Does my client have any other co-existing conditions (e.g., hypertension or high cholesterol) or health challenges that I should pay close attention to?

4) My client has indicated that s/he is taking medications. Will these medications influence the ability to control his/her diabetes and/or engage in regular physical activity?

5) Does my client have any evidence of macrovascular complications, especially

coronary-, cerebro- and peripheral-vascular diseases?

6) Does my client have any evidence of small vessel disease, especially retinopathy and nephropathy, or neuropathy?

7) Are there any precautions or considerations that I should be aware of before beginning my client on a regular physical activity program?

8) If my client has any events or problems that I am concerned about, is it okay to contact your office for advice or recommendations regarding how to handle this situation?

gistic effect of exercise + insulin on lowering blood glucose is well established, and a reason that exercise should be part of disease management strategy. In Type 1 diabetics, physical training improves aerobic capacity (e.g., VO_2 max), which is related to glucose uptake and glycemic control (Arslanian, Nixon, Becker & Drash, 1990). However, regular exercise is not effective for improving blood glucose control of Type 1 diabetes and should not be a sole means of controlling blood glucose. You should recommend regular physical exercise for cardiovascular conditioning and modification of cardiovascular risk factors in Type 1 diabetes, rather than as a single means for better glucose control.

Although regular exercise improves metabolic control in those with poor control, it does not facilitate a level of metabolic control that is desirable for children, adolescents or Type 1 diabetic adults. You should educate clients on daily use of SBGM, insulin adjustment and nutritional needs combined with regular exercise to facilitate near-normalization of glucose control.

Insulin Sensitivity. Physical training enhances the sensitivity of peripheral tissue to insulin action in Type 1 diabetes, as reflected by reduced daily insulin dosage (Koivisto et al, 1986).

While physical activity augments insulin-mediated glucose disposal into skeletal muscle and improves insulin action, physical inactivity facilitates the reversal of important glucose transport activities. Physical activity has a transient effect on glucose transport because insulin sensitivity is lessened for several days after physical activity ceases (Koivisto et al., 1986). Thus, physical inactivity may be responsible for increased **insulin resistance**.

Lipids and Lipoproteins. Physical training favorably alters lipids and lipoproteins in Type 1 diabetics (Schneider et al., 1986). An improved aerobic fitness is also related to favorable lipid profiles in Type 1 diabetics (Austin, Warty, Janosky & Arslanian, 1993), which lessens the likelihood for accelerated atherosclerosis. Lipid profiles are most effectively altered when regular exercise is combined with nutritional modifications.

Psychological Health Issues. The psychological benefits of regular exercise in nondiabetics has been rigorously substantiated; however, such benefits for Type 1 diabetics have received little attention. The rigors of diabetes management are emotionally stressful, particularly for young children and adolescents, and can adversely influence glycemic control (Lustman, Carney & Amado, 1981). Given that regular exercise lessens physiological reactivity to mental stressors (Kelley & Seraganian, 1984), it may help reduce stress by enhancing psychological well-being, and improving the quality of life for Type 1 diabetics (Vasterling, Sementilli & Burish, 1988).

Short-term Benefits of Exercise in Type 2 Diabetes Mellitus

Type 2 diabetics may suffer from abnormal insulin secretion, and hepatic and peripheral insulin resistance. Their obesity, hyperglycemia, hyperinsulinemia and physical inactivity also contribute to insulin resistance.

Glucose Levels. An acute bout of mild-moderate exercise lowers blood glucose levels, but not to hypoglycemic levels for Type 2 diabetics. The amount of the decrease is related to the duration of physical activity, and is attributed to an attenuation of hepatic glucose production; meanwhile, muscle glucose uptake increases in a normal manner. Sustained insulin levels during exercise are primarily responsible for reducing hepatic glucose production.

Blood glucose levels of Type 2 diabetics who perform higher intensity exercise respond much differently than to low intensity exercise. When obese, Type 2 diabetics exercise at a high intensity for short durations, blood glucose levels increase in the presence of hyperinsulinemia, and may persist for up to one hour post-exercise. Thus, mild to moderate exercise is more appropriate to lower glucose in Type 2 diabetes.

Insulin Sensitivity. Insulin insensitivity — or insulin resistance — is the universal abnormality of Type 2 diabetes with or without fasting hyperglycemia. It significantly reduces insulin-mediated glucose uptake. Since insulin-mediated glucose uptake occurs primarily in skeletal muscle, the rate of insulin-mediated glucose uptake relates directly to the amount of muscle mass, and inversely to fat mass (Yki-Jarvinen & Koivisto, 1983).

The short-term effect of exhaustive exercise can increase insulin sensitivity, or its action, for 12 to 16 hours post-exercise in most, but not all, Type 2 diabetics. Thus, the benefit of a single bout of exercise is short-lived.

Long-term Benefits of Exercise in Type 2 Diabetes Mellitus

Recently, the National Institutes of Health [NIH] (1987) formulated a consensus regarding the impact of diet and exercise on metabolic control and quality of life issues for persons with Type 2 diabetes. The pathogenesis of hyperinsulinemia, hypertension, hyperlipidemia and hyperglycemia, which are direct precursors for coronary heart disease, have been linked with insulin resistance (Reaven, 1988). Thus, therapy must focus on lessening insulin resistance and its health consequences.

Therapies to control glucose levels and reduce long-term complications in Type 2 diabetes, especially of macrovascular origin, should feature behavioral interventions that promote: 1) prudent nutritional regimes for weight reduction; 2) compliance to prescribed oral agents and/or insulin injections, if required; and 3) a physically active lifestyle. The major premise of physical exercise as a part of managing this disease is its potential to improve insulin sensitivity and glucose metabolism. Hence, the role of regular exercise on health in Type 2 diabetes is important.

Metabolic Control: Glucose Control and Insulin Sensitivity. Regular exercise improves the aerobic capacity in Type 2 diabetes and is linked with modest glucoregulatory changes in HbA1 and/or glucose tolerance, while consistent improvements in insulin sensitivity occur with or without a change in body composition (Koivisto et al., 1986). Usually, the most favorable change in glucose control accompanies regular exercise and dietary regimentation. Although improved glucose tolerance and insulin sensitivity can be achieved in mild Type 2 diabetes with seven days of exercise alone, such changes are relatively short-lived and usually deteriorate within 72 hours of the last exercise bout. Thus, glucose tolerance and insulin sensitivity are a reflection of the last individual exercise bout, rather than training per se. Type 2 diabetics may achieve metabolic control through a combination of physical activity and dietary regimes.

Lipids and Lipoproteins. The atherogenic nature of diabetes is largely known, and elevated lipids and lipoproteins contribute to cardiovascular disease risk in Type 2 diabetes (Ruderman & Haudenschild, 1984). Increased aerobic capacity in Type 2 diabetes is related to a more favorable lipid profile, which lessens the likelihood for accelerated atherosclerosis and its related mortality. The lipid-altering effect of exercise appears to be maximized when combined with a diet program and loss of weight (Wallberg-Henricksson, 1992).

Certainly, the intensity, duration and frequency of exercise training influence lipid and lipoprotein changes. Moreover, dietary advice, counseling and behavioral intervention aid in lowering fat intake and body weight. The effect of exercise on lipid and lipoprotein may depend on body weight.

Table 11.5

Typical Activity Guidelines

- Make sure that blood glucose is monitored before and after physical activity and take recommended action if blood glucose is too high or too low.

- Know whether macrovascular and/or microvascular complications exist — these require special attention and can modify physical activity.

- Always wear a medical ID bracelet or necklace.

- If insulin injection is required for diabetes management, make injections into a nonactive muscle site on the days of physical activity.

- Report any uncomfortable perceptions or problems you are having.

- If you have co-existing heart disease you should have a stress test and obtain physician approval prior to beginning an exercise program.

For Type 2 diabetes:

- Participate in low level activity (e.g., home or walks) every other day.

For Type 1 diabetes:

- Participate in physical activity according to tolerance at least three times per week.

Body Weight Reduction. Obesity is common in four out of five Type 2 diabetics (CDC, 1997). It also contributes to insulin resistance (NIH, 1987), while excess abdominal fat increases poor diabetes control, lipids levels and cardiovascular complications (Van Gaal et al., 1988). Weight loss is recommended for obese persons with diabetes, especially those with upper body obesity, as blood pressure, insulin resistance, glucose levels and lipid profiles can be favorably altered. However, most obese clients with diabetes do not lose weight, and those that are moderately successful regain it. Thus, effective therapy must address long-term weight loss and improved glucose control for obese persons with diabetes.

Although various programs promote weight loss, combining behavioral modification with low calorie diets have produced the most encouraging long-term weight loss results in Type 2 diabetics (Wing, 1989). A strategy for obese people with diabetes to achieve and maintain weight loss includes a low calorie diet, physical activity and behavioral modification. Any single therapy is less effective in producing long-term weight loss (Zierath & Wallberg-Henricksson, 1992).

The addition of exercise may not significantly add to the rate of weight loss; however, physical activity augments insulin sensitivity, which has marked effects on other metabolic functions and macrovascular risk factors. You may emphasize the long-term maintenance of dietary and exercise behaviors to manage weight and glucose control in Type 2 diabetics. Certainly, management strategies using self-reporting of behavior, relapse prevention training and spousal/family support systems may also help sustain weight loss in people prone to regain the lost weight.

Psychological Issues. The impact of diabetes on lifestyle and health and the psychosocial adjustments to complications later in life may have important consequences on perceived stress, glucose control and psychological health. With prolonged duration of diabetes, complications are more prevalent (ADA, 1996) and require greater psychosocial adjustments (Wulsin, Jacobsen & Rand, 1993). Long-term outcomes of diabetes add to perceived stress of disease management (Surwit & Feinglos, 1988) and affective disorders, especially depression (Gavard et al., 1993).

Given that diabetes management is emotionally stressful, particularly in elderly Type 2 diabetics, and that this stress can adversely influence glycemic control (Lustman et al., 1981), regular physical activity may play an important role in reducing stress, enhancing psychological well-being and augmenting the quality of life for Type 2 diabetics (Vasterling et al., 1988).

Pre-Exercise Screening and Client Assessment

The diabetes management team must encourage clients to participate in physical activity. While regular exercise carries significant benefits, the risks are also undeniable. It is best to proceed cautiously. You must acquire information about each diabetic client to ensure safe and effective participation in physical activity. Assessment of clients with diabetes includes the following important areas:
- Medical information
- Physician approval
- Lifestyle and habits questionnaire
- Pre-test screening
- Health-related fitness assessment

Medical Information and Physician Approval

Diabetic clients must receive physician approval to begin an exercise program. You should determine whether vascular and/or neural complications exist (Gordon, 1995). You should learn about a client's health and clinical status. How long has the client suffered from diabetes? How long has he or she taken medication? Are other co-existing conditions present (e.g., hypertension, elevated lipids, smoking habits, obesity)?

Because diabetes is a potentially progressive disease, you should develop a continuing-care plan that requires clients to have periodic (i.e., at least one physician visit per year) medical evaluations. These follow-up visits may identify the onset or progression of complications.

Depending on the client and amount of time he or she has suffered from diabetes, a stress test may be advisable before the start of an exercise program (ACSM, 1995). Stress tests are advisable for Type 1 diabetics who have had the disease for more than 15 years and are older than 30, and Type 2 diabetics older than 35.

A stress test is needed to assess cardiorespiratory integrity — as heart disease risk is increased with both Type 1 and Type 2 diabetes (ADA, 1996) — and to identify safe exercise heart rate limits for persons with or without neural complications (e.g., autonomic neuropathy). A stress test can also identify a hypertensive response to exercise. You may then design a safe program.

You must ask your clients about current medication(s) for diabetes and other conditions. All Type 1 diabetics and some Type 2 diabetics use insulin to aid in lowering blood glucose. Prior to initiating any exercise program, the client pinpoints the daily dose(s) of insulin and location of the insulin injection. You must also keep a ready supply of simple sugar (e.g., candy bar, snacks) to counter the likelihood of low blood glucose, or hypoglycemia. In some clients who require insulin injections, physical activity combined with close monitoring of blood glucose may contribute to a lowering of the daily insulin requirement. However, any adjustment of insulin dosage must be carefully balanced with nutritional needs and close glucose monitoring. It must also be discussed thoroughly with the client's physician, diabetes educator or nurse practitioner. Under no circumstances should you recommend an unusual lowering of daily insulin dosage.

Oral medications are commonly prescribed for Type 2 diabetics. About 40 percent are prescribed insulin (CDC, 1997). The purpose of oral drugs is to lower blood glucose by augmenting insulin release and insulin action, or sensitivity. Once again, you should ask clients to identify the daily dosage of oral medications. Oral agents to lower blood glucose for Type 2 diabetics include: Glucotrol XL (glipizide extended release); Prandin (repaglinide); Amaryl (glimepiride); Rezulin (troglitazone); Glucophage (metformin); and Micronase (glyburide).

Medication dosage can be reduced following a period of weight loss and/or physical activity; however, only the client's physician should make changes in oral medications. You should encourage clients who are taking oral medications to regularly monitor and record their blood glucose, and provide this information to the physician. This may help a physician in determining dosage.

Are there other types of medications that you should anticipate in clients with diabetes? About 60 percent to 65 percent of all persons with diabetes develop hypertension (CDC, 1997). Hypertensive medications are outlined in the hypertension chapter of this book. Drugs commonly prescribed to treat high blood pressure can adversely elevate blood glucose. These include diuretics, beta blockers and calcium

Figure 11.2

Factors to consider when designing an exercise program for a diabetic

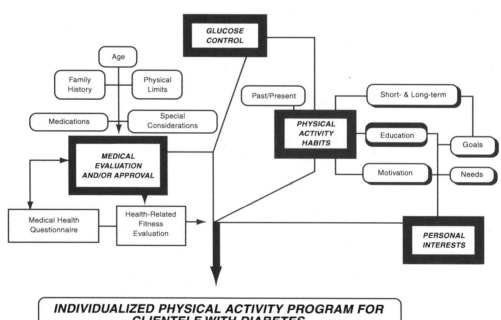

INDIVIDUALIZED PHYSICAL ACTIVITY PROGRAM FOR CLIENTELE WITH DIABETES

channel blockers. Furthermore, beta blockers are known to mask the symptoms related to low blood glucose. Other hypertensive medications may actually lower blood glucose, including ACE inhibitors and alpha-adrenergic antagonists (Ganda, 1995). The varying effects of hyperintensive medications is further reason to monitor blood glucose.

You should follow standard fitness screening procedures (ACSM, 1995; Van Camp, 1993). Using a questionnaire (e.g., PAR-Q) is appropriate. If the client responds positively to a question, you must ascertain its significance through a follow-up with the client's physician. Also, if any client with diabetes has been diagnosed with coronary heart disease, or has suffered a heart attack, then this is a contraindication to exercise. The advanced personal trainer should refer the client to a clinical setting for supervised exercise.

Lifestyle and Habits Questionnaire

You should consider a number of factors before developing an exercise program for diabetics (Figure 11.2). Based on limitations identified by the physician, you can devise a safe and effective individualized exercise program. To motivate the client, you should devise an exercise program that considers personal interests and past and/or present exercise habits. Because more than 70 percent of diabetics do not engage in regular physical activity (Ford & Herman, 1995), you must develop an activity program that motivates clients to participate and develop long-term habits. The program should address a client's personal goals.

Identifying personal goals and needs in a physical activity program to maintain the Type 2 diabetic's interest is crucial. Additionally, past exercise habits can provide important information regarding present exercise habits. Previous habits and interests can also provide you with information about the client's awareness and knowledge of his/her disease, and about his or her effort in trying to control blood glucose. Glucose control is a life long habit and helps ensure that exercise is safe and effective.

Education about the role of SBGM before and after each exercise session is usually presented in diabetes education classes. If your client has not participated in a series of diabetes education classes, you should encourage your client to do so. This will aid his/her understanding of the disease and the importance of regular glucose monitoring. You may also provide your client with a list of diabetes educators and other resources.

Pre-test Screening

You should administer the PAR-Q, review and sign informed consent and possible release forms, and measure the resting heart rate and blood pressures. The diabetic should bring his/her glucose meter on the day of the health-related fitness assessment and on subsequent exercise days for glucose monitoring before and after each exercise session.

Resting heart rate and blood pressure assessment are commonly used as a screening aid for apparently healthy persons to partake in physical activity (Verity, 1993). About 60 percent to 65 percent of persons with diabetes have high blood pressure or hypertension. Medications used to treat hypertension may actually lower the resting heart rate; however, resting blood pressure may remain elevated. Consequently, diabetics may have a normal resting heart rate but elevated blood pressure.

A resting heart rate of > 120 bpm, or resting blood pressure exceeding 180/105 mmHg, are contraindications to exercise (Gordon, 1995). Other contraindications to exercise follow previously established guidelines (ACSM, 1995).

Health-related Fitness Assessment

Fitness assessments are integral to effective exercise programming. You can chart client progression and set goals to motivate clients. Fitness evaluations include body composition, cardiorespiratory fitness and musculoskeletal fitness tests. Although fitness assessments can be administered, you may have to adapt the procedure for some diabetics. If any testing procedures are changed, you should record the modifications of the client's initial test so that you are consistent in your subsequent evaluations.

Body composition. Excessive body weight and/or body fat is common in diabetics. More than 80 percent of persons with diabetes are overweight or obese (ADA, 1996). Skinfold and circumference measures are the preferred methods to determine body fat. However, it is acceptable to use the same generalized equations that have established norms for age and gender of apparently healthy persons for Type 1 diabetics. The determination of body fat is not very useful for Type 2 diabetics, because most are obese. More importantly, fitness appraisers can measure and record skinfold thicknesses, as well as circumferences, on Type 2 diabetics. These have far greater practical outcomes and can be easily compared with previous assessments.

Cardiorespiratory Fitness. Diabetics tend to participate less frequently in regular physical activity (Ford and Herman, 1995). Moreover, scientific research suggests that Type 2 diabetics who perform a graded exercise test consume a lower amount of oxygen than nondiabetics throughout low level to high level work (Regensteimer et al., 1995). Fitness appraisers are encouraged to use standard submaximal testing protocols to assess cardiorespiratory fitness in persons with diabetes. Also, you should include heart-rate data, as well as ratings of perceived exertion [RPE] information in a cardiorespiratory assessment. However, diabetics can pose difficulties in administering a valid submaximal test.

Many diabetics are hypertensive and take heart-rate altering medications, which make a submaximal test to assess cardiorespiratory fitness an invalid assessment. In some diabetics, you may opt for a bicycle protocol (e.g., YMCA protocol). A neural condition, autonomic neuropathy, slows the heart rate and limits the validity of submaximal protocols that assess heart-rate responses to submaximal work.

Fitness appraisers may find field tests (e.g., 12-minute walk/run test) to be suitable for the diabetic client. Yet performance in this type of test requires motivation to achieve a near-maximal effort and knowledge of pacing oneself. Because many diabetics are not physically active, the use of a field test may only be useful for those who have a recent history of regular exercise.

Many diabetics will have to undergo a stress test. It is always a good idea to obtain a copy of this report for your records through client consent. In case the cardiorespiratory fitness assessment cannot be administered, you may use the information from a stress test to aid in developing an aerobic program for your client.

Musculoskeletal Fitness. Administration of tests to assess muscle endurance, muscle strength and joint flexibility in diabetics is appropriate only in those who do not have diagnosed complications, especially microvascular (ACSM, in press; Hornsby, 1995; Vitug et al., 1988). Ensure medical health status prior to initiating any portion of the musculoskeletal fitness battery. Fitness appraisers are encouraged to use standard testing protocols that do not use 1-RM to assess musculoskeletal fitness in persons with diabetes (e.g., YMCA).

Guidelines for Exercise Programming

Diabetics are less active than nondiabetics. About 70 percent of persons with diabetes are sedentary (Ford and Herman, 1995). Diabetics are older, perceive their health more poorly, and identify physical or orthopedic limitations four times more frequently than their nondiabetic counterparts (Ford and Herman, 1995). You should keep these distinguishing factors in mind when devising an exercise plan.

The acronym FITT has commonly focused upon cardiorespiratory programming aspects, where F=frequency of activity per week; I=intensity of the exercise session; T=time of each exercise session; and T=type of activity or mode. Developing an exercise plan by using the FITT acronym is commonplace. But you should incorporate RPE to identify exercise intensity, as disease progression and complications (e.g., autonomic and peripheral neuropathy) can limit the ability to accurately assess heart rate. Additionally, the FITT program differs for Type 1 and Type 2 diabetics (Figure 11.3).

In this chapter, I will introduce the acronym FIRST for a musculoskeletal fitness program, where F=frequency of resistance training per week; I=intensity of each lift; R=repetitions performed for each muscle group; S=number of sets performed; and T=type of exercise performed by muscle group. Just as FITT programming depends on the type of diabetes, so does FIRST programming (Table 11.4).

When developing the FIRST program, you should ensure that clients do not possess complications that might prevent safe and effective outcomes. You may need to lower the intensity of each lift, require higher repetitions, forego lifting to exhaustion and limit isometric contractions to lessen exercise-induced blood pressure elevations.

Exercise Programming for Type 1 Diabetes

For Type 1 diabetics, daily aerobic exercise has been recommended to better regulate insulin dosage and diet needs for glucose control (ACSM, 1995). Yet improving glucose control for Type 1 diabetes is best achieved through intensive insulin therapy combined with SBGM. Thus, Type 1 diabetics are best served by following the FITT principle in Figure 11.3 and exercise three to five days per week to improve aerobic capacity and accrue other health-related benefits. You should know that exercise is not recommended for glucose control in Type 1 diabetics, and that daily exercise is unrealistic. Moreover, higher intensity activity can in-crease the risk of elevating blood glucose and suffering musculoskeletal injuries (Gordon, 1995; Hornsby, 1995). Type 1 diabetics who do not have complications should exercise between 55 percent to 75 percent of functional capacity, or an RPE of 3-5 (using the 1-10 scale). Each activity session should be about 20-30 minutes to spur improved aerobic fitness and health-related benefits.

Finally, strength training in Type 1 diabetics may increase aerobic capacity along with increased muscle mass and improved glucose control by increasing insulin sensitivity (Soukup & Kovaleski, 1993). Type 1 diabetics who do not have complications can participate in a moderate strength-training program that mimics a program that nondiabetics use (Table 11.5). A Type 1 diabetic should seek physician approval and heed strict limits on participation.

Exercise Programming for Type 2 Diabetes

Type 2 diabetics can follow an exercise program adopting FITT principles (refer to table 11.3). The focus of such programming is to burn calories and lose weight (ACSM, 1995). Physical activity of 40 to 60 minutes in duration at a low intensity of 40 percent to 65 percent of functional capacity is appropriate for overweight/obese

persons to burn an adequate number of calories. A recent study revealed that low intensity walking improved insulin action and glucose control, and lowered body weight in Type 2 diabetics (Yamanouchi et al., 1995). It confirmed that moderate physical activity is helpful for Type 2 diabetics (USDHHs, 1996). Because obesity is a problem for Type 2 diabetics, more moderate exercise reduces the likelihood of foot irritation and/or musculoskeletal injury.

Exercising 5 to 6 days per week maximizes caloric expenditure necessary for weight management. Although walking is the most convenient activity, persons with claudication pain may have to perform low- or non-weight-bearing activity (e.g., swimming, aquacize, stationary cycling), or alternate between different types of weight-bearing versus non-weight-bearing activities. Moreover, peripheral neuropathy, which may lead to foot irritation, may preclude weight-bearing activities, due to the possibility of foot irritation.

Finally, it may also benefit Type 2 diabetics to engage in light-to-moderate resistance training (Table 11.4), which increases muscle mass and lowers basal insulin levels. Resistance training is safe and effective to provide cardiovascular and metabolic benefits for persons with diabetes (Hornsby, 1995). However, it is important for Type 2 diabetics to participate regularly in a FITT program before the start of a FIRST program. Most of these clients are severely decondi-

---

Table 11.7

F.I.T.T.
Physical Activity Program for Cardiovascular Improvements in Diabetes

Variable	Exercise Nondiabetic	Exercise Type 1	Exercise Type 2
Frequency	3-5 d/wk	3-5 d/wk	5-6 d/wk
Intensity*	55-90% HR max 3-6 RPE	55-70% HR max 3-5 RPE	40-70% HR max 2-5 RPE
Time	20-30 min/session	20-30 min/session	40-60 min/session
Type**		dynamic movement	bicycle; walk walking the dog house & yard work grocery shopping mall walking water aerobics

*Note: Specific heart rate may not be appropriate for persons on HRAM or those with autonomic neuropathy.

**(Persons may require non-weight-bearing activity or alternating with weight-bearing activities, due to peripheral vascular disease (claudication pain).

Table 11.8

F.I.R.S.T.
Physical Activity Program for Musculoskeletal Improvements in Diabetes*

Variable	Type 1	Type 2
Frequency	2-3 d/wk	1-2 d/wk
Intensity**	40-60% 1 RM	lower level activity
Repetitions	8-12/exercise	15-20/exercise
Sets	2-3 sets/exercise	1-2 sets/exercise
Type of exercise	8-12 muscle groups	u. ext.: 4-5 exercises
		l. ext.: 4-5 exercises
		ADL; house & yard work

*Persons with microvascular disease, especially proliferative retinopathy, should refrain from vigorous strength-training activities.

**Complications may limit activity and/or intensity

tioned. Dynamic, whole body activity through the FITT program will enhance their ability to accommodate the strength and endurance requirements of FIRST.

Guidelines for Exercise Leadership

Diabetics should consider numerous factors before starting an exercise program.

Safety before, during and after exercise is of paramount importance (Table 11.5).

You should ensure that clients learn certain practical information before exercising.

Documenting each exercise session helps you when communicating with a client's physician about cardiovascular adaptations and metabolic changes resulting from regular exercise. A daily log may be a particularly efficient way to record vital information — both quantitative and qualitative.

In fact, a qualitative assessment of the client's ability and performance is essential. You may evaluate the client's self-concept, self-esteem, motivation to exercise regularly and other quality-of-life issues. You should report noticeable dysfunctional changes immediately to a physician. They may include:

- an inability to accurately palpate and obtain a heart rate
- a loss of sensation in the feet or toes during weight-bearing activities
- increasing pain in the legs during weight-bearing activities
- deterioration in reading the RPE chart
- unusual forgetfulness or memory problems

- persistent fatigue

You must evaluate the client on a daily basis and report both quantitative and qualitative information regarding the exercise session. Barring more immediate problems, you should offer written documentation to the client's physician on an annual basis. This documentation may compare fitness assessments to those from the previous year. They may include the frequency and amount of daily submaximal work and heart rate; medication doses; glucose levels before and after sessions (averaged weekly or monthly); and any qualitative assessments previously described.

Risks of Exercise in Clients with Diabetes

As the diabetic engages in regular physical activity, are there risks associated with participation, or will s/he develop problems? If so, what are the signs and symptoms of these problems?

The most common problem encountered by diabetics subsequent to physical activity is low blood glucose, or hypoglycemia. Hypoglycemia can occur at any time (before, during or after exercise) and is defined as blood glucose < 80 mg/dl. A client may be experiencing hypoglycemia, or an insulin reaction, when they sweat profusely; are clammy and pale-looking; get shaky; have difficulty answering specific questions; slur their speech; seem exhausted; or become light-headed and may pass out.

It is important then for the client to ingest a simple sugar snack (e.g., candy bar) or drink (e.g., orange juice). After five minutes, blood glucose should be checked to determine whether more carbohydrates are needed. This cycle should be repeated until a client's blood glucose returns close to 100 mg/dl. You should also terminate the exercise session.

Is there any way to prevent the occurrence of an insulin reaction? Hypoglycemia is not totally preventable. Exercise-induced hypoglycemia most commonly occurs in insulin-requiring diabetics. To minimize the occurrence of low blood glucose, you should link each exercise session to: (1) the timing and site of insulin injection; (2) the antecedent and post-exercise nutrition; (3) the time of day; and (4) the pre- and post-exercise blood glucose monitoring.

The insulin injection should occur at least one hour before exercising, and preferably in a non-exercising area. Some insulin-requiring diabetics reduce the dosage of intermediate insulin by 30 percent, or omit the short-acting insulin dose before exercising. For persons on insulin pumps, a reduction in insulin dosage is recommended before, during and after mild to moderate exercise to minimize the risk of acute and late-onset hypoglycemia (Sonnenberg et al., 1990).

Consumption of carbohydrates is critical for Type 1 diabetics to avoid low blood glucose levels. Between 15 and 30 grams of carbohydrates should be consumed for every 30 minutes of moderate exercise (ADA, 1994b). A complex carbohydrate snack helps lessen post-exercise reductions in blood glucose and late-onset hypoglycemia.

When the diabetic exercises is also key in avoiding hypoglycemia. Depending on insulin administration and nutrient intake, the best time for Type 1 diabetics to exercise is one to two hours after breakfast, or at least in the morning hours. Postprandial exercise aids in mitigating glucose excursions throughout the day and is not as susceptible to dramatic decrements in blood glucose, as is the case at other times.

Yet it is also important to individualize an exercise regime. A program must fit into a diabetic's schedule.

Table 11.9
Practical Recommendations When Participating in Physical Activity for Persons with Type 1 and Type 2 Diabetes

Check with your Physician:
- You may need to limit the intensity of physical activity, especially if any disease complications are present;
- You may want to join a supervised program for guidance and assistance, especially if you have not been physically active for a long period of time.

Self-blood Glucose Monitoring [SBGM:
Perform before and after each physical activity session. Excellent cognitive training for diabetics to understand individual glucose response to physical activity. It is important to ensure that your blood glucose is in relatively good control before beginning higher intensity physical activity. If your blood glucose is:
- > 250 mg/dl, then higher intensity physical activity should be postponed;
- < 100 mg/dl, then eat a snack consisting of carbohydrates;
- between 100-250 mg/dl, then physical activity can be performed.

Keep a Daily Log:
Record value and time of day the SBGM is performed and amount/timing of any pharmacologic agent (e.g., oral drugs or insulin). Also, include approximate time (mins), intensity (heart rate) and distance (miles or meters) of each activity session. This will aid the diabetic in understanding the type of response to possibly expect from specific physical activity bouts.

Plan for an Exercise Session:
- how much (e.g., time and intensity) activity is anticipated?;
- if needed, carry extra carbohydrate feedings

Exercise with Partner:
Affords a "support system" for the physical activity habit. Initially, diabetics should exercise with a partner until glucose response is known. Ideally, a partner who accompanies the physically active diabetic is a source of social support, and encourages continued participation in this healthy lifestyle.

Wear a Diabetes I.D.:
Never leave home without it. Hypoglycemia or other problems can arise that require an understanding of the condition.

Wear Good Shoes:
Proper-fitting and comfortable footwear can minimize foot irritations and sores, and reduce the occurrence of orthopedic injuries to the foot and lower leg.

Practice Good Hygiene:
Always take extra care to inspect feet for any irritation spots to prevent possible infection. Tend to all sores immediately. Report hard-to-heal sores to your physician. Prevent irritations when physically active by using Vaseline on feet and wearing socks inside-out.

Modify Caloric Intake Accordingly:
Through frequent SBGM, caloric intake can be regulated more carefully on days of and following physical activity. For insulin-requiring diabetics, blood glucose can drop after physical activity and latent post-exercise hypoglycemia can be prevented. Also, in consultation with your physician, a decrease in insulin dosage may be necessary.

Self-blood glucose monitoring is essential for Type 1 diabetics and is strongly recommended for Type 2 diabetics. Glucose monitoring is appropriate before and after exercising. Given the understanding of glucose levels, diabetics can take more appropriate routes of action to lessen the frequency of severe glucose shifts.

What about high blood glucose levels? Elevated blood glucose occurs in diabetics who are not well insulinized because of excessive caloric intake and/or not enough insulin. Exercise will only worsen the hyperglycemia and ketone levels when pre-exercise glucose levels are elevated. Pre-exercise glucose levels exceeding 250 mg/dl indicate poor control and necessitate postponement of exercise. A log enables a management team to evaluate glycemic excursions and prevent a reccurrence. When the blood glucose is high, an appropriate dosage of insulin is necessary for the diabetic. Exercise is not recommended until the blood glucose is < 250 mg/dl.

High intensity exercise has been found to elevate blood glucose from a normal to hyperglycemic level. It is believed that the role of counter-regulatory hormones on glucose production plays a major part in this type of glycemic excursion. Moderate intensity exercise is recommended to facilitate more normal glucose levels and lessen the likelihood of musculoskeletal injury.

Progression of Program

The progression of the FITT and FIRST program is determined by several factors, including age, functional capacity, medical and disease complications, and personal preferences and goals (ACSM, in press; ACSM, 1995; Gordon, 1995). Initial changes in FITT programming for diabetics should focus on the duration of the exercise session rather than the intensity. That can prevent blood glucose increases; provide a safe and effective exercise that is not unduly taxing; and increase the likelihood that someone sticks with a program.

For clients without complications, initial levels of abilities are quite different between types of diabetes. For example, Type 1 diabetics follow a similar FITT program to that of apparently healthy persons. They can initially engage in continuous, moderate physical activity for 20 minutes, while Type 2 diabetics may only be able to engage in low level physical activity for five to 10

minutes before fatiguing. The initial phase of FITT programming for Type 2 diabetes requires low intensity and short duration (e.g., < 15 minutes) activity at least three times per week, and preferably five times per week (ACSM, in press; USDHHS, 1996). But the Type 1 diabetic may not require significant modifications in the initial phase of FITT programming. You must closely observe client response to a program, modifying it to prevent fatigue and enhance the enjoyment.

Progression of the program after the initial phase should be approached with caution, especially in Type 2 diabetes. For both types of diabetes, the duration of an activity should be increased before the intensity. The duration should be gradually increased to accommodate the ability and clinical status of each client. Because diabetics are likely to be obese and older, they may require a longer period of time to adapt to program changes. Once the client is able to last for a desired amount of time, programmatic changes should be small and approached with caution to lessen the risk of undue fatigue, musculoskeletal injuries and/ or relapse.

Some well-controlled Type 1 diabetics may set a goal to participate in competitive athletics (e.g., 10K, marathons, triathlons, biathlons, etc.). A small number of these clients may require higher intensity, longer duration workouts. Successful participation in competitive athletics by a Type 1 diabetic is dependent upon rigorous SBGM, appropriate insulinization, proper nutrient intake and regular medical visits. Still, most diabetics will not strive to compete in athletics. They will need to improve functional aspects that relate to quality of life. Because diabetes onset is related to older age, obesity and dysfunction of physiologic and neurologic processes, the most valuable aspect of any program should relate to functional outcomes specific to each client and his/her limitations.

Medical Concerns and Disease Complications

Are there other medical concerns that advanced personal trainers should understand? YES!! Although complications are common in diabetes (ADA, 1996), their existence does not preclude physical activity. Rather, there are physical activity precautions and limitations for diabetics who have one or more types of microvascular and/or neural complications. The options for diabetics with disease complications are discussed below. You should familiarize yourself with diabetic complications.

Diabetics with the following complications should be referred to a clinical setting where close supervision and monitoring can occur.

Retinopathy. Although exercise increases systemic and retinal blood pressure, there is no evidence that physical activity acutely worsens the retinopathy present in diabetes (Vitug et al., 1988). Diabetics with proliferative retinopathy who engage in low intensity exercise can significantly improve cardiovascular function. However, systolic blood pressure should be monitored during each exercise session and limited to 20-30 mmHg above resting. Clients with retinopathy may exercise safely when they are properly supervised.

Clients with retinopathy should not engage in such activities as strength training or those that require them to raise their arms over their heads. These may cause systolic blood pressure to rise dramatically. Under such circumstances, increased blood pressure may increase the likelihood of retinal hemorrhaging when proliferative retinopathy is present (Vitug et al., 1988).

Nephropathy. Increased blood pressure is a common precursor to worsening of this microvascular disease (Graham & Lasko-McCarthey, 1990); however, it remains to be proven if exercise-induced blood pressure changes exacerbate the progression of nephropathy. It is prudent to avoid activities that cause systolic blood pressure to rise to 180-200 mmHg (e.g., performing Valsalva maneuver, high intensity aerobic or strength exercises), as systemic pressure increases could potentially exacerbate the progression of this disease. Persons with progressive nephropathy or end-stage renal disease may benefit from lower intensity physical activities. Most clients with nephropathy should be referred to a clinical setting where their fragile metabolic condition may be carefully monitored. In many cases, clients with this disease participate in physical activity sessions while undergoing renal dialysis.

Neuropathy. Neuropathy is a nerve disorder. The two main **nerve diseases** related to diabetes are autonomic neuropathy [AN] and peripheral neuropathy [PN]. When this disease affects the autonomic nerves to the heart, it is called cardiac autonomic neuropathy [CAN]. The heart rate is altered. The maximal heart rate drops, and the resting heart rate increases (e.g., HR rest > 100 bpm). This causes hypertension and hypotension, and increases the risk for exercise-induced hypotension after strenuous activity (Vinik, 1995). Persons with AN have impaired sweating and thermoregulatory abilities and impaired hypoglycemia awareness. Persons with CAN exhibit a lower fitness level and fatigue at relatively low workloads due to the disruption in nerve innervation to the heart (Vitug et al., 1988). Consequently, physical activity for these persons should focus upon low-level daily activities, where mild changes in heart rate and blood pressure can be accommodated. Any exercise program for persons with AN or CAN should require physician approval and proceed cautiously.

Peripheral nerve disease affects the extremities, especially the lower leg and feet. Repeated weight-bearing activities on insensitive feet can lead to chronic irritation, open sores and musculoskeletal injuries, especially fractures. Persons with PN are susceptible to overstretching due to loss of sensation, as well as infection, particularly when daily hygiene is lacking. Proper footwear for any weight-bearing activity is important to prevent undetectable sores, which may turn into infections. However, people with PN should participate in non-weight-bearing activities (Graham and Lasko-McCarthey, 1990). Such interventions may include aquatics, recumbent cycling, chair exercises and upper extremity exercises. Additionally, activities requiring a full range of joint motion are highly effective in reducing stiffness due to muscle contractures.

Case Studies

Case Study 1. Jim is a Type 1 diabetic. He is 35 years old and has had diabetes since the age of 13. He is 5'10" and weighs 165 pounds. He currently injects insulin and monitors his blood glucose twice each day. He visits his doctor each year and reports his health as "good." He reports no diabetes-related complications. Jim's goal is to begin an aerobic program so that he can run a 10K with his son who is 13 years old. He has come to you for professional assistance.

You must obtain more information about Jim's health before developing an exercise program. According to established guidelines (ACSM, 1995), Jim is classified as "diseased" and must obtain physician's approval before exercising. I recommend having Jim complete a comprehensive medical health history questionnaire to ascertain any known cardiovascular or diabetes-related complications; assess his exercise history; and obtain information about his usual meal times and insulin injections.

From this screening, you should probably recommend that Jim enroll in a diabetes education class. His two daily insulin injections are probably not adequate to control his blood glucose levels. He should try to do better. The SBGM before and after each exercise session is a requirement for you to work with him. Jim was heavily involved in high school and college sports, but has not been regularly active for about 12 years.

To develop an appropriate exercise regime, you should conduct a fitness assessment (Verity, 1993). Results from the submaximal YMCA bicycle protocol found Jim's aerobic fitness to be average for his age and gender. His body composition from skinfold assessment was 17 percent, while his musculoskeletal fitness was good. Results from the fitness and exercise habits assessments suggest that Jim can immediately participate in aerobic activity. A program should be individualized and focus on the lower-end range for each FITT element. His desire to participate in a 10K does not preclude alternative activities (e.g., recumbent cycle ergometer, upright cycle ergometer, stair stepping). You should record each blood glucose reading, and if his pre-exercise blood glucose is > 250 mg/dl, postpone the session. If Jim's pre-exercise blood glucose is < 80 mg/dl, he should consume about 15-20 grams of carbohydrates for every 30 minutes of anticipated exercise.

When initiating the FIRST program, begin at the lower range of recommended frequency, intensity, repetitions and sets. It is essential to learn proper lifting techniques and breathing cues (e.g., breath on effort) before starting a FIRST program. If Jim does the FIRST program following the FITT regime, he should check his blood glucose after completing his resistance training. If there is a long delay (e.g., several hours) between the aerobic and resistance training programs, then he should do the SBGM before and after each respective regime.

Case Study 2. Jane is 50 years old and was diagnosed with Type 2 diabetes five years ago. Jane is 5'2"

and weighs 180 lbs. She is currently taking an oral medication (troglitazone) for her diabetes and an anti-hypertensive medication (beta blocker) for her stage 1 high blood pressure, and does not monitor her blood glucose. Jane reports that her health is okay. She does not suffer from complications, but gets easily fatigued doing housework and cleaning. Furthermore, she reports that taking a stroll with her husband at the local mall makes her knees and hips uncomfortable after about 15 to 25 minutes. She has not seen her doctor in over a year; however, her diabetes educator has encouraged her to participate in regular physical activity. She has asked you to assist in the development of an activity regime. Her goals are to improve her endurance and lose about 45 lbs.

Jane requires her recommended annual check-up on the clinical status of her diabetes (e.g., the evaluation of the presence/absence/progression of disease complications). She must receive her physician's approval to begin an exercise program with a personal trainer.

Because Jane is 50 years old and has had Type 2 diabetes for more than five years, she should undergo a stress test prior to engaging in an exercise program. Her discomfort while walking requires further evaluation. The lack of regular blood glucose monitoring must be addressed. You must require SBGM before and after each exercise session as a prerequisite to your work together.

Once physician approval, information from the stress test and disease status are obtained, you can develop an exercise regime. Of greatest importance are a client's personal interests and goals. Because Jane has difficulty with short-term weight-bearing activity, you should choose activities that are less wearing on her joints. You should help her identify enjoyable activities that she would be likely to do regularly. You should encourage her to seek out weight management professionals to advise her about losing weight.

Jane should exercise wherever the social stigma of obesity and overweight issues is minimized. Jane must feel comfortable in her exercise surroundings. This is an important issue because the exercise environment can cripple Jane's motivation to maintain her physical activity program.

What health-related fitness assessments can be administered? Jane's heart rate-altering medication (e.g., beta blocker) eliminates the use of a cardiorespiratory fitness assessment using submaximal protocols that base aerobic capacity on heart-rate determinations. A field test requiring a weight-bearing exercise (e.g., 1.5 mile walk/run test or 12-minute walk/run test) is inappropriate. The stress test conducted by her physician is an excellent starting point. From the stress test, resting and maximum parameters, including heart rate, blood pressure and RPE, can be identified. Jane's physician can determine the upper limit of exercise intensity. Based on this information, she should not exercise at more than 70 percent of her maximum heart rate.

You can devise a FITT program for Jane. You should individualize the program and focus it at the lower range for each FITT element. The program must be safe, effective, reasonable and prudent for this type of client. The FITT should look as follows: F = 4-6 days per week; I = 50-60 percent of maximal heart rate, or RPE 2-3 (on 1-10 scale); T (time) = 15-30 minutes; T (mode) = alternate between weight-bearing (e.g., walking) and non-weight-bearing (e.g., aquacize; recumbent ergometer; chair exercises) activities.

Is it necessary to assess a person who is already known to be obese? What will be gained? Body composition is not essential but you should do some sort of physical assessment. You should initially measure body weight, selected skinfold site thickness and circumferences. They provide a good baseline for serial assessments. Jane's measurements were as follows: body weight -184 lbs.; abdominal skinfold - 36 mm; iliac skinfold - 32 mm; thigh skinfold - 40 mm; tricep skinfold - 34 mm; chest skinfold - 28 mm; waist circumference - 42 in; hip circumference - 48 in; upper arm circumference - 18 in; and thigh circumference - 22 in. From these measurements, it is obvious that weight loss will have a favorable impact on her anthropometric measurements. They can also be motivating for Jane as she strives to improve her fitness and lose weight.

Should you assess Jane's musculoskeletal fitness? No. Jane has enough to do at this point. Incorporating an additional routine into her activity regime is not appropriate at the outset. As previously indicated, start with FITT before proceeding to FIRST.

You should record each blood glucose reading before and after the activity session. Jane cannot exercise if her pre-exercise blood glucose is > 250 mg/dl. If her pre-exercise blood glucose is < 80 mg/dl, then she should consume about 15-20 grams of carbohydrates for every 30 minutes of anticipated exercise. Jane's beta blocker for hypertension can mask hypoglycemia so you should periodically check her blood glucose, especially at the start of a program.

Jane is willing to come to your fitness facility two or three days each week. You should recommend that she exercise on two additional days. You should

instruct her on the correct use of RPE to ensure a safe and effective exercise environment when she is not supervised.

Always encourage clients to drink adequate amounts of water, especially clients prone to dehydration. Discourage them from exercising when the temperature is above 80 degrees.

During the first activity session, you should instruct Jane on a designed program. Jane should be comfortable when exercising. You should not downplay the intensity level. She should expend energy. Also, she must accurately monitor her blood glucose. In order for Jane to last the recommended 30 to 60-minute exercise period, you may have to alternate a circuit of five-minute aerobic activities with 10-minute rest intervals, or initiate a low-level aerobic interval program of similar work and rest intervals. Keep in mind that the Type 2 diabetic must be constantly monitored and given prompt feedback about accomplishments and progress. Also, ensure that blood glucose levels are normal when the client leaves your facility to minimize the risk of low glucose or hypoglycemia problems.

References

ACSM [American College of Sports Medicine] (in press). ACSM Position Stand: Physical Activity and Type 2 Diabetes. *Medicine and Science in Sports and Exercise.*

ACSM [American College of Sports Medicine]. (1995). *Guidelines to Exercise Testing and Exercise Prescription* (5th ed.). Media, Pa.: Williams & Wilkins.

ADA [American Diabetes Association]. (1993). Position statement: Implications of the diabetes control and complications trial. *Clinical Diabetes*, 11, 91-6.

ADA [American Diabetes Association]. (1994a). *Medical Management of Non-insulin-dependent (Type 2) Diabetes*, 3rd ed. Alexandria, Va.: Author.

ADA [American Diabetes Association]. (1994b). *Medical management of insulin-dependent (Type 1) diabetes*, 2nd ed. Alexandria, Va.: Author.

ADA [American Diabetes Association]. (1996). *Diabetes: 1996 Vital Statistics.* Alexandria, Va.: Author.

Arslanian, S., Nixon, P., Becker, D. & Drash, A. (1990). Impact of physical fitness and glycemic control on in vivo insulin action in adolescents with IDDM. *Diabetes Care*, 13, 9-15.

Austin, A., Warty, V., Janosky, J. & Arslanian, S. (1993). The relationship of physical fitness to lipid and lipoprotein(a) levels in adolescents with IDDM. *Diabetes Care*, 16, 421-25.

Bourn, D.M., J.I. Mann, B.J. McSkimming, M.A. Waldron & J.D. Wishart. (1995) Impaired glucose tolerance and NIDDM: does a lifestyle intervention program have an effect? *Diabetes Care*, 17, 1311-1319.

Campaigne, B.N. & Gunnarsson, R. (1988). The effects of physical training in people with insulin-dependent diabetes. *Diabetic Medicine: A Journal of the British Diabetic Association,* 5, 429-433.

Campaign, B.N. & R. M. Lampman (1994). *Exercise in the Clinical Management of Diabetes.* Champaign, Ill.: Human Kinetics.

CDC (1997). *National Diabetes Fact Sheet: National estimates and general information on diabetes in the United States.* Atlanta, Ga.: US Department of Health and Human Services, Centers for Disease Control and Prevention.

Eastman, R.C., R. Silverman, M. Harris, J.C. Javitt, Y.P. Chiang & P. Gorden (1993). Lessening the burden of diabetes: Intervention strategies. *Diabetes Care,* 16, 1095-1102.

ECDCDM [Expert Committee on the Diagnosis and Classification of Diabetes Mellitus] (1997). A report of the expert committee on the diagnosis and classification of diabetes mellitus. *Diabetes Care,* 20, 1183-1197.

Ford, E.S. & W.H. Herman (1995). Leisure-time physical activity patterns in the U.S. diabetic population: Findings from the 1990 national health interview survey — health promotion and disease prevention supplement. *Diabetes Care,* 18, 1, 27-33.

Ganda, O.P. (1995). Patients on various drug therapies. In: *The Health Professional's Guide to Diabetes and Exercise* (pp. 235-240). Alexandria, Va.: American Diabetes Association.

Gavard, J.A., Lustman, P.J. & Clouse, R.E. (1993). Prevalence of depression in adults with diabetes. *Diabetes Care,* 16:1167-78.

Gordon, N. (1995) The exercise prescription. In: *The Health Professional's Guide to Diabetes and Exercise* (pp. 71-82). Alexandria, Va.: American Diabetes Association.

Graham, C. & Lasko-McCarthey, P. (1990). Exercise options for persons with diabetic complications. *Diabetes Educator,* 16, 212-20.

Helmrick, S.P., Ragland, D.R., Leung, R.W. & Paffenbarger, R.S. (1991). Physical activity and reduced occurrence of non-insulin-dependent diabetes mellitus. *The New England Journal of Medicine,* 325, 147-52.

Hornsby, W.G. (1995). Resistance Training. In: *The Health Professional's Guide to Diabetes and Exercise* (pp. 85-88). Alexandria, Va.: American Diabetes Association.

Kelley, S. & Seraganian, P. (1984). Physical fitness level and autonomic reactivity to psychosocial stress. *Journal of Psychosomatic Research,* 28, 279-87.

Koivisto, V.A., Yki-Jarvinen, H. & DeFronzo, R.A. (1986). Physical training and insulin sensitivity. *Diabetes/Metabolism Reviews,* 1, 445-81.

LaPorte, R.E., Dorman, J.S., Tajima, N., Cruickshanks, K.J., Orchard, T.J., Cavender, D.E., Becker, D.J. & Drash, A.L. (1986). Pittsburgh insulin-dependent diabetes mellitus morbidity and mortality study: Physical activity and diabetic complications. *Pediatrics,* 78, 1027-33.

Lustman, P., Carney, R. & Amado, H. (1981). Acute stress and metabolism in diabetes. *Diabetes Care,* 4, 658-9.

Manson, J.E., Rimm, E.B., Stampfer, M.J., Colditz, G.A., Willett, W.C. & Krolewski, A.S. (1991). Physical activity and incidence of non-insulin dependent diabetes mellitus in women. *Lancet,* 338, 774-78.

National Institutes of Health [NIH]. (1987). Consensus development conference on diet and exercise in non-insulin-dependent diabetes mellitus. *Diabetes Care,* 10, 639-44.

Reaven, G.M. (1988). Banting Lecture 1988: Role of insulin resistance in human disease. *Diabetes,* 37, 1595-607.

Regensteiner, J., J.Sippel, E. McFarlang, E. Wolfel & W. Hiatt. (1995). Effects of non-insulin dependent diabetes on oxygen consumption during treadmill exercise. *Medicine and Science in Sports and Exercise,* 27, 875-81.

Ruderman, N. & Haudenschild, C. (1984). Diabetes as an atherogenic factor. *Progress in Cardiovascular Diseases,* 26, 373-412.

Schneider, S.H., Vitug, A. & Ruderman, N.B. (1986). Atherosclerosis and physical activity. *Diabetes/Metabolism Reviews,* 1, 4, 513-33.

Sonnenberg, G.E., Kemmer, F.W. & Berger, M. (1990). Exercise in type 1 (insulin-dependent) diabetic patients treated with continuous subcutaneous insulin infusion. *Diabetologia,* 33, 696-703.

Soukup. J.T. & Kovaleski, J.E. (1993). A review of the effects of resistance training for individuals with diabetes mellitus. *The Diabetes Educator,* 19, 4, 307-312.

Surwit, R.S. & Feinglos, M.N. (1988). Stress and autonomic nervous system in type II diabetes: A hypothesis. *Diabetes Care,* 11, 83-85.

USDHHS [U.S. Department of Health and Human Services] (1996). *Physical activity and health: A report of the Surgeon General.* Atlanta, Ga.: US Department of Health and Human Services, Centers for Disease Control and Prevention.

Van Camp, S. (1993). Health screening. In: *Aerobics Instructor Manual* (pp. 146-155). San Diego, Calif.: American Council on Exercise.

Van Gaal, L., Rillaerts, E., Creten, W. & De Leeuw, I. (1988). Relationship of body fat distribution pattern to atherogenic risk factors in NIDDM: Preliminary results. *Diabetes Care,* 11, 2, 103-06.

Vasterling, J.J., Sementilli, M.E. & Burish, T.G. (1998). The role of aerobic exercise in reducing stress in diabetics patients. *The Diabetes Educator,* 14(3):197-201.

Verity, L.S. (1993). Fitness testing and aerobic programming. In: *Aerobics Instructor Manual* (pp. 156-195). San Diego, Calif.: American Council on Exercise.

Vinik, A.I. (1995). Neuropathy. In: *The Health Professional's Guide to Diabetes and Exercise* (pp. 183-197). Alexandria, Va.: American Diabetes Association.

Vitug, A., Schneider, S.H. & Ruderman, N.B. (1988). Exercise and type I diabetes mellitus. In K. Pandolph (Ed.). *Exercise and Sports Science Reviews* (Vol. 16) (pp. 285-304). New York: MacMillan Publishing Company.

Wallberg-Henricksson, H. (1992). Exercise and diabetes mellitus. In J.O. Holloszy (Ed.). *Exercise and Sport Science Reviews* (vol. 22) (pp. 339-368). Philadelphia, Pa.: Williams & Wilkins.

Wing, R.R. (1989). Behavioral strategies for weight reduction in obese type II diabetic patients. *Diabetes Care,* 12, 139-44.

Wulsin, L.R., Jacobsen, A.M. & Rand, L.I. (1993). Psychosocial adjustment to advanced proliferative diabetic retinopathy. *Diabetes Care,* 16, 1061-66.

Yamanouchi, K., T. Shinozaka, K. Chikada, T. Nishikawa, K. Ito, S.Shimizu, N. Ozawa, et al. (1995). Daily walking combined with diet therapy is a useful means for obese NIDDM patients not only to reduce body weight but also to improve insulin sensitivity. *Diabetes Care,* 18, 775-778.

Yki-Jarvinen, H. & Koivisto, V.A. (1983). Effects of body composition on insulin sensitivity. *Diabetes,* 32,965-69.

Zierath, J.R. & Wallberg-Henricksson, H. (1992). Exercise training in obese diabetic patients: Special considerations. *Sports Medicine,* 14, 3, 171-89.

Suggested Readings

ADA [American Diabetes Association]. (1998). American Diabetes Association: Clinical Practice Recommendations 1998. *Diabetes Care,* 21(Suppl. 1).

Gordon, N.F. (1993). *Diabetes: Your Complete Guide.* Champaign, IL: Human Kinetics.

CHAPTER 12

Obesity

ROSS ANDERSEN
SHAWN FRANCKOWIAK

Ross Andersen, Ph.D., F.A.C.S.M., is an assistant professor of medicine in the division of geriatric medicine and gerontology at the Johns Hopkins University School of Medicine. He is a fellow of the American College of Sports Medicine, and has served for two years as the associate director of exercise science at the Johns Hopkins Weight Management Center. Dr. Andersen has authored an extensive list of both applied and basic publications. He has served as the chair of the ACE Lifestyle and Weight Management Consultant Certification Committee and sits on the ACE Board of Directors.

Shawn Franckowiak is a consultant in exercise science for the Johns Hopkins Weight Management Center. He has designed hundreds of exercise programs for obese patients and has authored various papers published in medical and weight-control journals. Franckowiak serves as study coordinator, exercise specialist and group leader for medical trials for weight reduction focusing on behavior change and nutrition awareness for the Johns Hopkins School of Medicine.

Limitations
Weight
Maintenance

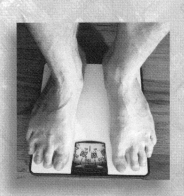

Program Design

Obesity is associated with several health risks such as hypertension, hyperlipidemia and coronary artery disease. Obesity also can have an adverse effect on quality of life by limiting mobility, impairing physical capacity and reducing an individual's capacity to perform activities of daily living. These findings have prompted the American Heart Association to add obesity to its list of risk factors for the development of coronary artery disease (Eckel et al., 1998).

Obese individuals are more likely to face social, academic and career discrimination. Unfortunately, Americans and individuals residing in other developed countries are becoming increasingly more overweight. Kuzmarski et al. (1997) recently reported that 33.3 percent of adult men and 36.4 percent of adult women in America are overweight. Furthermore, 14.4 percent of men and 16.2 percent of women are now considered severely overweight. We have recently reported a similar trend in American children that shows 26 percent of American children currently are overweight and 10 percent are severely overweight (Crespo et al., 1998).

The economic cost of **obesity** in the United States alone is substantial, estimated at 6 percent of our national health expenditure (Wolf, 1998a). Wolf and Colditz recently have reported that the annual direct costs of disease attributable to obesity in the United States exceeds $51 billion per year (Wolf et al., 1998b).

A critical question of great concern to both clinicians and researchers is "Why has the prevalence of overweight increased so dramatically over the past 10 years?" Genetics can play a key role in determining how people metabolize calories. However, the gene pool in western countries has not changed substantially in the past 30 years. Many people believe that the increased prevalence of overweight is simply due to the fact that overweight people eat too much. Surprisingly, many reports suggest that Americans are actually eating less food and have reduced **fat** consumption in recent years. However, when we look at trends in physical activity, we see that very few Americans are regularly active. In fact, only 22 percent currently are active enough to derive health benefits from their activity, and 25 percent are completely **sedentary**.

Prentice and Jebb recently reported that the prevalence of obesity has doubled in England over the past 10 years (Prentice et al., 1995). This trend was mirrored by increases in the number of cars and televisions per household.

We recently investigated the relationship between physical activity and television watching with body weight and level of fatness in American children (Andersen et al., 1998) and found a very strong relationship between television watching and fatness. We also found that 26 percent of American children watched four or more hours of television each day, and that rate was much higher in Mexican-American (30 percent) and African-American (43 percent) children. Finally, we reported that children who watched the most television tended to be significantly fatter than those who watched little television. Furthermore, boys and girls who watched the most television and who were not regularly active were fatter than children who watched little television and who were highly active. These findings have important implications for fitness professionals working with overweight clients. You must realize the importance of regular exercise in helping people manage their weight.

Though we know physical inactivity plays a major part in the obesity epidemic, we also are conscious of other factors that contribute to the rise in our nation's overweight population. Complex factors involving endocrine abnormalities, medication, hypothalamic problems or simply overeating (behavioral) cause individuals to seek assistance for weight loss. Medications such as corticosteroids for treatment of certain medical conditions and an endocrinologic disease like **hypothyroidism** may alter metabolic rate or cause lethargic behavior, limiting

Table 12.1
Annual Direct and Indirect Costs of Disease Attributable to Obesity in the United States (1995 dollars)

Disease	Direct cost (billions)	Indirect Cost (billions)
type 2 diabetes	$32.4	$30.74
CHD	6.99	—
hypertension	3.23	—
gallbladder disease	2.59	0.151
breast cancer	0.840	1.48
endometrial cancer	0.286	0.504
colon cancer	1.01	1.78
osteoarthritis	4.3	12.9
Total	**$51.64**	**$47.56**

Source: Wolf, A.M., Colditz, Calif. (1998) Current estimates of the current economic cost of obesity in the United States. *Obesity Research*, 6, 97-106

overall mobility and exercise. Furthermore, at a recent Presidential Lecture at the 1998 National American College of Sports Medicine Conference, Dr. Kelly Brownell, a leading researcher on behavioral issues relating to obesity at Yale University, suggested that the everyday "toxic environment" in which we live makes it easy to obtain high-fat, highly palatable foods for a reasonable price just by going to the drive-thru at the nearest fast-food restaurant. The environment that Brownell mentions makes it difficult for health professionals to educate individuals on appropriate food choices for weight control. While the many causes of obesity are complex, researchers indicate that physical activity is one of the leading interventions for successful treatment.

It also is important to help overweight people reduce the number of sedentary activities in which they participate. Sedentary activities, such as television watching, playing computer games, "surfing" the Internet, playing board games and talking on the phone are activities that can be targeted for reduction. All of these activities are low in energy expenditure and also may be associated with, or even prompt, eating.

State-of-the-Art Treatment for Obesity

Anyone who has treated overweight people knows there are no simple answers to successful-

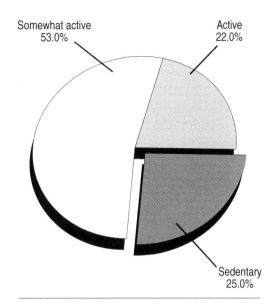

Source: *Report of the Surgeon General*

Figure 12.1

Physical activity patterns among americans

ly treating this complex problem. Unfortunately, most people who lose weight ultimately regain it. Therefore, state-of-the-art weight-management programs are increasingly placing a strong emphasis on the prevention of weight regain.

Dietary modification is the most common method used to lose weight. Most expert panels have agreed that a balanced calorie-deficit diet of 1,000 to 1,500 kcal/day is a relatively safe level of restriction for healthy adults (National Task Force on the Prevention and Treatment of Obesity, 1994). While restricting calories, it also is helpful to reduce fat consumption. In addition, it is common to encour-

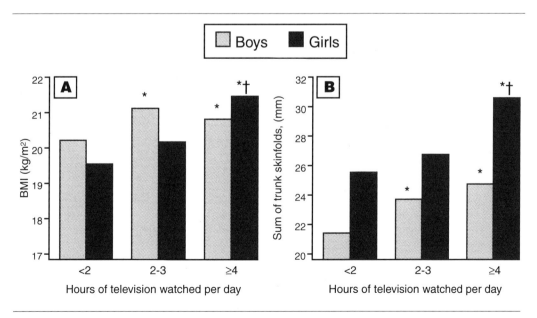

Results from the Third National Health and Nutrition Examination Survey. *Journal of the American Medical Association.*

Figure 12.2

Mean body mass index (BMI) (A) and the mean sum of the subscapular and suprailiac skinfolds (B) in relation to hours of television watched daily among U.S. children aged 8 to 16 years, 1988 through 1994. Asterisk indicates significantly greater (<.001) than the less-than-2-hour group; dagger indicates significantly greater (P<.001) than the 2- to 3-hour group.

age overweight people to increase their consumption of fruits and vegetables. This may help increase feelings of satiety and ensure the RDAs for vitamins and minerals are met. Details on helping clients select a healthy meal plan can be found in the *ACE Lifestyle and Weight Management Consultant Manual*. Fitness professionals without training in the food sciences should understand that only registered dietitians can safely develop diets for clients. Therefore, it will be helpful to look for dietitians in your area to whom you can refer clients for meal planning.

Most commercial weight-loss programs acknowledge that exercise is important. However, these programs usually do not offer facilities or experts to help clients begin an exercise program. Simply increasing levels of exercise without restricting calories is a relatively poor way to lose weight. However, when combined with a healthy diet, increasing physical activity may result in optimal changes in **body composition** by contributing to a negative **energy balance** and preserving lean body mass. In addition, exercise has been shown to positively enhance mood and psychological well-being (Institute of Medicine, 1995).

Pharmacotherapy has been used to treat serious obesity for more than 40 years. The incidence of prescribed medications has increased dramatically, as has the public interest in this mode of treatment. Generally, medications are used to treat persons whose weight is causing obesity-related disease (e.g., diabetes, hypertension, insulin resistance, hypercholesteremia) and who have not been successful with less-aggressive treatment (e.g., commercial weight-loss programs or clinic/support groups). Recently, fenfleuramine and dexfenfleuramine were found to be associat-ed with memory loss and functional damage to cardiac valves and quickly were withdrawn from the market. This has left many patients and physicians with negative attitudes toward pharmacologic therapy for the treatment of obesity.

A compound initially targeted to treat depression, sibutramine hydrochloride (Meridia, Knoll Pharmaceutical), recently has been approved to assist obese people in losing weight and keeping it off. Sibutramine usage is associated with significant reductions in food intake. Thus, it appears to affect the brain's appetite centers.

Other drugs are currently being developed to decrease metabolic efficiency or to inhibit the uptake of fatty acids into adipocytes. As a clinical exercise specialist, it often may be easy to fall into the trap of thinking that the only way to lose weight is with a healthy, self-selected meal plan and a tailored exercise program. Given the complexity of obesity, you should be aware that pharmacotherapy, in addition to a sensible diet and exercise program, may be appropriate for some individuals, and that pharmacotherapy may offer an ideal opportunity to work closely with the medical community.

Weight Maintenance

Klem et al. (1997) recently reported the results of the **National Weight Control Registry**, the largest study of individuals who are successful at long-term weight-loss maintenance. This database includes 629 women and 155 men who have lost an average of 30 kg and maintained a minimum weight loss of 13.6 kg for five years. Approximately 55 percent of this study's sample reported they had used a formal program or had sought professional assistance to lose weight. More

---

Table 12.2

Client Information to Obtain from Medical Professionals

1) Does the client have exercise clearance? If not, what are the restrictions on their participation in a traditional exercise program?

2) If the client has existing disease conditions or is taking medications, what modifications for exercise should be implemented?

3) Are there contraindications involving any modes of exercise for this client (e.g., avoidance of high-impact exercise for an obese client with osteoarthritis)?

4) Do you have any recommendations for increasing exercise adherence for the referred client? (May involve asking about previous exercise history or investigating the client's goals and needs.)

Recommendations
and Position Stands
on Developing
Exercise Programs
for the Obese
Population

women (60 percent) than men (37 percent) used a formal program or professional assistance for weight loss. Interestingly, 89 percent of the sample modified both their dietary intake and physical activity levels to lose weight. Only 1 percent reported increasing only their activity level.

To keep weight off, members of the registry reported consuming smaller portions of food approximately five times per day. They also reported being active. On average, they walked 28 miles per week. The men expended more energy each week through heavy-intensity activities. The study's authors concluded that the long-term maintenance of weight loss is facilitated by regular physical activity.

An active lifestyle plays a central role in helping people maintain weight loss. Exercise is probably the strongest predictor of long-term success in weight management. This stresses the need for adding exercise to each phase of the weight-management program.

Recommendations and Position Stands on Developing Exercise Programs for the Obese Population

The first federal guidelines on the identification, evaluation and treatment of overweight and obesity in adults were released in 1998 by the National Heart, Lung and Blood Institute (NHLBI), in cooperation with the National Institute of Diabetes and Digestive and Kidney Diseases (NIDDK). The guidelines were developed by a 24-member expert panel chaired by Dr. F. Xavier Pi-Sunyer, director of the Obesity Research Center, St. Luke's/ Roosevelt Hospital Center in New York City.

Based on an extensive review of the scientific literature on overweight and obesity, these clinical practice guidelines for healthcare professionals present a new approach for the assessment of overweight and obesity, and also establish principles of safe and effective weight loss. According to the guidelines, assessment of overweight involves evaluation of three key measures: **body mass index (BMI)**, waist circumference, and a patient's risk factors for diseases and conditions associated with obesity.

The expert panel has defined overweight as a BMI of 25 to 29.9 and obesity as a BMI of 30 or more, which is consistent with the definitions used in many other countries. BMI describes body weight relative to height and is strongly correlated with total body fat in adults. It is recommended that BMI be determined in all adults. People of normal weight should have their BMI reassessed every two years. The guidelines recommend weight loss to lower high blood pressure and total cholesterol and to raise low levels of HDL cholesterol. Furthermore, they suggest that weight loss can lower elevated blood glucose in overweight persons with two or more cardiovascular risk factors and in obese persons who are at increased risk. Finally, they recommend that overweight patients without known risk factors focus efforts on weight maintenance.

Healthcare professionals also are advised to determine waist circumference, which is strongly associated with abdominal and or visceral fat. Excess visceral fat is an independent predictor of disease risk. The panel concluded that waist circumference is a better marker of abdominal fat and a better predictor of disease risk than the **waist-to-hip ratio**. A waist circumference of more than 40 inches in men and more than 35 inches in women signifies increased risk for heart disease in those who have a BMI of 25 to 34.9.

The new guidelines stress that there are no simple or easy cures for weight loss. The most successful weight-loss strategies include calorie restriction, increased activity and behavior change designed to improve eating and physical-activity habits. The guidelines advise physicians to have their patients try lifestyle therapy for at least six months before embarking on physician-prescribed drug therapy.

Traditional Exercise

Traditional exercise-program design focuses on exercise needed to optimize fitness. Such traditional exercise prescriptions have been developed, with modifications made for the obese populations, to ensure safety with close monitoring by a trained exercise professional. Guidelines set forth by the American College of Sports Medicine (ACSM, 1995) for exercise prescription suggest the inherent need for adaptations of traditional exercise prescriptions when developing exercise programs for the obese population. These guidelines mention a primary goal of exercising to increase energy expenditure of at least 200 to 300 kcal per exercise session. Walking, usually offered initially because it tends to be less intimidating for the client, is an easy **low-impact**, low-skill activity that works well as an energy-expending aerobic exercise. The exercise program for the obese individual involves not only cardiorespiratory fitness, but also strength training and daily physical activity. Modifications are suggested to ensure that cardiovascular intensity is at the low end of the appropriate target-heart-rate range (low end of 60 percent to 90 percent of heart-rate maximum) (ACSM, 1995). It is your responsibility to design exercise programs that effectively meet goals of weight loss and **fat-free mass** preservation to prevent the onset of disease or worsening of the current status of the client.

Recommendations on Physical Activity

The alarming statistics on the increasing prevalence of obesity in the United States, coupled with evidence that physical activity can favorably affect body-fat distribution (U.S. Department of Health and Human Services, 1996), have inspired certain organizations, such as the Centers for Disease Control and Prevention, American College of Sports Medicine and the National Institutes of Health, to make recommendations on how much and what type of activity is necessary to produce physical-activity benefits. Researchers find that inactive persons are at an increased risk of becoming obese (Brownell, 1995), and that previous exercise prescriptions by organizations focus on set-

ting guidelines for proper frequency, intensity and duration of exercise to optimize fitness. On the other hand, new physical activity recommendations focus on promoting lifelong physical activity for attaining health benefits and weight control. The current recommendations of these organizations advocate that people attempt to accumulate 30 minutes or more of moderate-intensity physical activity on most, and preferably all, days of the week (National Institutes of Health, 1996; Pate et al., 1995; U.S. Department of Health and Human Services, 1996).

The aim of these recommendations is to promote a wide variety of activities that are acceptable for increasing energy expenditure. Creating outlets for physical activity throughout the day thereby leads to increased daily energy expenditure. Experts believe that caloric restriction (which exceeds caloric intake) and physical activity remain the most successful form of treatment for obesity (Brownell et al., 1992). These short bouts of activity done at the convenience of the obese client may be even more important when we realize that the resting energy expenditure typically declines with dieting and weight reduction (Wadden et al., 1990). This suggests that energy expenditure via physical activity becomes very important in the latter phases of weight reduction and during weight maintenance after weight loss.

Physical Activity as a Safe Alternative to Traditional Exercise for the Overweight Client

Safety is a constant concern when beginning an exercise program, and the various physical activities that are offered within physical-activity recommendations offer low-impact, non-invasive ways of expending calories in conjunction with, or as an alternative to, the traditional cardiovascular exercise program. By promoting physical activity, you allow the client to prog-

Table 12.3

Typical Activity Guidelines

- After obtaining exercise clearance, design an exercise program based on limitations for the specific diseases associated with obesity.

- Develop exercise programs to produce safe weight loss and achieve client goals.

ress from participating in small amounts of light activity to engaging in more challenging exercises, such as treadmill walking or other modes of traditional exercise. These new recommendations differ from previous traditional guidelines in that research indicates that similar conditioning benefits are produced from engaging in noncontinuous bouts of moderate-intensity physical activity at various times throughout the day (Donnelly et al., 1994; DeBusk et al., 1990). Three 10-minute bouts of moderate-intensity walking have been shown to be comparable to a continuous 30-minute bout of exercise. Following are a few examples of activities that increase energy expenditure:

- parking at the far end of the parking lot and walking to the entrance
- yard activities, such as gardening, raking leaves and mowing the lawn
- housework, such as cleaning, vacuuming, dusting and dishwashing
- taking stairs whenever possible, rather than elevators and escalators
- walking at lunch breaks, and to and from offices at the workplace
- using fewer labor-saving devices, such as cordless phones and remote controls
- playing with, and babysitting, toddlers

Lifestyle Physical Activity Can Be a Preferable Mode of Exercise

Increased lifestyle activity can be an excellent form of exercise for those who previously have had bad experiences participating in exercise programs, who have had medical problems that require abstinence from traditional exercise, or who have had difficulty finding time to exercise. Traditional exercise programs have been devised to optimize fitness levels, but obese individuals often find it too difficult to comply with a vigorous exercise regimen. Obesity typically is associated with low levels of leisure-time physical activity (Crespo et al., 1995), and beginning a moderate or vigorous exercise routine may be threatening and intimidating to an obese client who feels winded by simply climbing one flight of stairs. This fear of vigorous exercise is often cited as a barrier to engaging in physical activity, and it has been found that exercise-program dropout rates could even be twice that of those engaging in

less-threatening moderate-intensity activities (Sallis et al., 1986). These physical activity recommendations also warn that individuals exercising at vigorous levels should not decrease their intensities to adhere to these new physical activity guidelines.

Physical Activity Offers a Variety of Options

While some clients may find intensity to be a barrier for becoming physically active, others mention lack of time as a reason for abstaining from exercise (U.S. Department of Health and Human Services, 1996). Promoting physical activity to your client can be a welcome alternative and may be a terrific means of increasing energy expenditure or supplementing a banner exercise program. When working with obese clients, a primary goal should be to produce a daily negative energy balance and, consequently, weight loss. However, guidelines promoting energy expenditure through intermittent bouts of physical activity instead of a traditional exercise program (vigorous activity for 20 to 60 minutes three times a week), offer a wider variety of activity options to a client who may be fairly deconditioned, or who lacks the time to devote to exercise.

It may be important to evaluate activity levels of the client and determine where improvements in energy expenditure can be made. Ideally, you and your client must devise a plan for increasing activity levels and progressing toward the adoption of an active lifestyle. The new physical activity recommendations provide more options for the obese individual who may not enjoy exercise. Continuing to stay physically active has been found to be a very powerful tool to decrease body weight, and to predict whether long-term weight reduction is maintained (Kayman et al., 1990).

Evaluation of the Program: Participation, Safety and Effectiveness

The American Heart Association recommends that the following data be collected in standardized face-to-face interviews with participants at the time of program initiation and again at follow-up. The data, compiled in aggregate form by gender, should include:

1. Definitions for the length of the weight-loss and weight-maintenance phases of the program
2. Percentage of all participants who completed the program
3. Percentage of those completing the initial weight-loss phase of the program who achieve various degrees of weight loss and weight gain, including the mean and range of weight-loss values for the program
4. Percentage of participants who began and completed the weight-maintenance phase of the structured program (self-reported data are not acceptable)
5. Percentage of participants who maintain weight loss at one, two and five years
6. Percentage of participants with improved cardiovascular-disease **risk factor** status at one, two and five years
7. Percentage of participants who experience adverse medical or psychological effects, and the nature and severity of these effects
8. Reasons for dropping out
9. Percentage of participants who meet their goals

Additional information about a program's characteristics should include:

1. Relative emphasis on the diet, exercise and behavior components
2. Frequency, duration and kinds of contacts
3. Nature and duration of the structured maintenance phase
4. Flexibility of food choices and suitability of food types being promoted

Ideas for Helping the Overweight Client Adhere to Exercise

Adherence is an important issue in maintaining exercise compliance for your overweight client. Some common ideas that have been suggested to produce long-term adherence in the overweight client are (Andersen et al., 1992):

- scheduling a convenient exercise appointment
- being a caring role model
- providing a variety of exercises that are not only safe, but also enjoyable
- encouraging input from your client when designing their exercise program
- striving to reduce boredom through theme exercise classes or holiday programs
- educating clients with literature, bulletin boards or newsletters
- providing incentives
- moderation

It is important that your client does not feel uncomfortable about either the fitness center's environment or clientele (your client should not feel embarrassed about their weight, and should be comfortable using all areas of the training facility).

Client Assessment

Information from the Physician

Seek clearance from your obese client's physician before they embark on their exercise program. Chapter 4 details the information you must seek from physicians. Specifically, it will be important to request information on the potential limitations that your client may have, as well as medications that may affect exercise performance. It also is important to ask about any modes of activity that should be excluded.

Fitness Assessments for Obese Individuals

A fitness evaluation for an overweight person can be an intimidating experience. Many people are frightened that they will fail their evaluation, so to explain to the overweight individual that the purpose of a fitness assessment is to help develop a safe but challenging program that best meets their needs, and to provide a baseline for future comparison.

Blood Pressure

Participants should sit quietly and calmly with feet resting on the ground before taking their blood pressure. If you are working with a large person, you will need to use a large-adult cuff to ensure accuracy (using a normal cuff on a very large arm will produce erroneous results).

Normal blood pressure is considered to be a systolic pressure less than 130 mmHg and a diastolic pressure less than 85 mmHg. High normal pressures are systolic pressures of 130 to 139 mmHg and diastolic pressures of

85 to 89 mmHg. Mild hypertension is considered to be systolic pressures of 140 to 159 mmHg or diastolic pressures of 90 to 99 mmHg. When systolic or diastolic pressures fall into different categories, select the higher value. Modest weight loss can often ameliorate blood pressure problems in overweight people (Anonymous, 1993).

Body Composition

The primary objective of overweight people joining a weight-loss program is to lose fat. With this in mind, it will be tempting for you to perform body composition assessments on your overweight clients. For a detailed explanation of assessing body composition in overweight people, refer to the *ACE Lifestyle and Weight Management Consultant Manual.*

Circumference measures offer a low-cost way to estimate body composition and show clients how they are shrinking as they lose weight. Furthermore, the waist-to-hip ratio may be calculated and compared to nationally available norms. Most generalized skinfold equations poorly predict percent fat in overweight people. It is often very difficult to reproduce **skinfold measures** in overweight people, and they also may be embarrassed by having large folds of fat pinched.

If you are assessing body composition with bioelectric impedance, use the fatness-specific equations of Segal (See the *ACE Lifestyle and Weight Management Consultant Manual* Body Composition Chapter). We do not feel that NIR (Futrex) machines offer the sensitivity or accuracy required to give overweight people feedback on their changing body composition.

Aerobic Testing

Many tests have been developed to assess or predict **VO$_2$max**. Since overweight people are at a greater risk for developing medical complications during an assessment, maximal testing should be avoided unless it is physician-supervised. Take clients through a thorough warm-up before the test. Having clients work up to approximately 75 percent of their exercise capacity also demonstrates that you do not subscribe to the no-pain-no-gain mentality. Monitor patients for shortness of breath, chest pain or severe discomfort during any aerobic test.

A graded treadmill test is probably the best way to estimate aerobic endurance in overweight people who do not have knee pain, since they often use walking as a mode of aerobic exercise. Cycle ergometry also can be used to test aerobic capacity in overweight persons.

Most sedentary overweight people have low aerobic endurance when they begin a program. Therefore, initial workloads and progressions should be lower than those for a leaner, fitter population. Asking clients their rate of perceived exertion at the end of each workload can assist you in prescribing initial exercise intensities that they find comfortable.

Exercise Programming and Leadership for the Overweight Client

Disease-Specific Limitations Associated with Obesity

Various limitations may be associated with or exacerbated by obesity. Obesity is related to an increase of imposed risk of diseases such as non-insulin-dependent diabetes mellitus, hypertension, cardiovascular disease, gallbladder disease and cholecystectomy (Colditz, 1992). While it may be unclear whether metabolic, behavioral, genetic or nutritional issues solely contribute to the development of obesity, it is realized that the overweight client must be handled safely and effectively. Diseases associated with obesity indicate that certain precautions must be taken when working with this population.

Set realistic weight-loss goals based on preventing disease and improving your client's current condition. Often, clients have lofty goals of unrealistic weight loss of 100 to 150 pounds. It may be important to focus on setting smaller goals to initiate weight loss if you believe the client is setting themselves up for failure. Developing goals that focus on modest weight-loss improvements is associated with substantial health benefits. Researchers believe that even a 10-percent weight loss can lead to substantial health improvements (Blackburn et al., 1992). These small weight losses may be adequate enough to ameliorate disease attributable to obesity. In any case of disease-specific limitations, it is important to devise modified exercise programs to safely meet the needs of your client. Three of the more common diseases associated with obesity are diabetes, hypertension/cardiovascular disease and arthritis.

Prescribing Exercise for Disease-specific Limitations

Safety Considerations

Diseases have debilitating effects on your client's capability to exercise. Safety considerations such as current CPR certification, active communication of feelings during exercise between you and your client, and understanding disease conditions and adaptations with exercise and weight gain ensure the best possible care. It also may be appropriate to refer your client to a physician if it is suspected that exercise is unsafe. Ultimately, exercise for obese individuals with disease limitations should be designed to improve such existing conditions, countering the onset of disease in the future and enhancing **quality of life**.

Special Concerns and Contraindications

Keep in mind that the typical overweight client is not seeking exercise guidance to become an athlete. The self-confidence and physical-ability levels of your overweight client may be much lower than that of a normal-weight individual. Therefore, pay close attention to possible problems that may occur during exercise. Excess weight may predispose your overweight client to poor coordination or flexibility, and irritation or chafing of skin by inadequate seat positioning of certain pieces of equipment. Furthermore, obesity is associated with poor balance, which thereby increases chances of injury by falls from a stationary bike or treadmill. Obese individuals are at increased risk of joint or ligament damage and are more likely to suffer from dehydration from increases in perspiration or physical activity. Choosing the appropriate exercises and monitoring the overweight client is essential to reduce the adverse conditions that may be produced by exercise in this population.

Diabetes Mellitus

Exercise Benefits

Studies show a direct beneficial effect of regular exercise on glucose tolerance, peripheral insulin sensitivity and carbohydrate **metabo-lism** (American Diabetes Association, 1998). Exercise can be an excellent therapeutic intervention for this population. However, make sure your diabetic client has had a medical examination prior to beginning an exercise program.

Possible Exercise Modifications

Weight-bearing Activity

An increase in weight-bearing exercise may pose a problem for your overweight diabetic client. Of special concern are those with a history of peripheral neuropathy or diabetic foot ulcers. Unfortunately, they will have increased formation of, and reduced sensitivity to, the onset of blisters or trauma produced by sudden increases in weight-bearing activities, such as brisk walking and jogging. Physicians often recommend having the client check their feet after performing exercise to monitor whether any trauma has occurred without their awareness. If possible, gradually increase the duration of the activity, avoid hard surfaces, and have the client wear supportive footwear and inspect their feet daily. If any wounds, pain or discomfort occur in response to exercise, refer your client to their physician.

Intensity

The American Diabetes Association recommends that exercise-program design be dictated by medical status. Activities that drastically elevate blood pressure or are strenuous, such as power lifting, boxing, heavy competitive sports, weightlifting, jogging, high-impact aerobics and racquet sports, are mentioned as activities that should be discouraged, along with activities producing the **Valsalva Maneuver** (forced exhalation against a closed glottis) (American Diabetes Association, 1998). In conjunction with your client's physician, the design of their training program should involve light-to-moderate-intensity activities in controlled environments. Other medical conditions must also be taken into account when choosing these activities. Particularly, diabetes is a major risk factor for cardiovascular disease. Most likely, the obese diabetic client is deconditioned. This limitation, along with being overweight, makes the exercise challenging, and should necessitate gradual progression of duration and intensity of all modes of exercise. If your client has goals entailing competition in sports involving vigorous exercise, consult their physician to receive input on safe training for the specific sport.

Resistance Training

The acceptability of strength training for the obese diabetic individual should be dictated by your client's physician and medical status (American Diabetes Association, 1998). It is very important to make your overweight diabetic client aware of the importance of breathing and form during strength training. Power-lifting activities can be dangerous and should be avoided. However, activities such as circuit training with medium weights, medium-to-high repetitions and low-to-medium volume are advantageous to safe lean-body-mass development.

*Awareness of Temperature
and Thermoregulation*

Adequate fluid intake should occur before, during and after exercise if possible to avoid dehydration, and pay close attention to exercising in the extreme heat and cold. Train your client during mornings or evenings when outdoor conditions are cooler and less humid, or have your client perform indoor activities in a temperature-controlled environment. Chapter 11 covers disease specifics of diabetes in more detail.

Hypertension and Cardiovascular Disease

While many hypertensive individuals use medications to control their disease, established recommendations for these persons include weight loss (more specifically decreased body mass index) and exercise (Bakris et al., 1996). Ideally, successful treatment for this disease would be to decrease blood pressure to less than 140 mmHg - Systolic and 90 mmHg - Diastolic (Atkinson, 1993). Successful aerobic exercise in hypertensive clients who also are diabetic has been shown to improve metabolic abnormalities and decrease blood pressure (Bakris et al., 1996). So, while exercise has been established as a non-pharmacological method of treating hypertension, what is appropriate exercise for the client should be considered.

Similar to the exercise program for the diabetic client, lower-intensity endurance exercises

should be developed for your obese hypertensive client. The ACSM (1995) recommends 40 percent to 70 percent of VO$_2$max, a light-to-moderate-intensity exercise that seems optimal for the hypertensive patient. The warm-up and cooldown during pre- and post-workouts ensure abrupt heart-rate increases and decreases do not induce injury. Unfortunately, studies have not shown that resistance training produces a decrease in blood pressure for hypertensive individuals. Therefore, the ACSM recommends circuit training with light weights and high repetitions to produce muscle hypertrophy or preservation; isometric weight training should be avoided (ACSM, 1995). Furthermore, strength training should not be the only mode of exercise that is prescribed for clients suffering from hypertension or CV disease.

Arthritis

Association of Exercise and Arthritis

Osteoarthritis and rheumatoid arthritis are two diseases causing pain, stiffness and complaints of loss of motion in obese individuals (Oddis, 1996). Clients with arthritis may have pain or discomfort in the hip, knee, ankle, shoulder, elbow and lower back and, unfortunately, tend to be deconditioned (Oddis, 1996). Vigorous bouts of exercise and competitive athletics have often been associated with orthopedic problems (U.S. Department of Health and Human Services, 1996; Lane, 1995; ACSM, 1995). However, while excessive intensities and durations of exercise programs have worsened arthritic conditions for exercisers, moderate levels of aerobic and resistance exercise of a therapeutic nature have been shown to produce improvements in disability, physical performance and pain (Ettinger et al., 1997). Weight loss should be one of the main goals for the development of an exercise program for the arthritic individual.

Establishing Appropriate Mode of Exercise

Flexibility should be a priority in the development of an exercise program. Stretching exercises prevent injury and improve range of motion for aerobic and strength exercises. Obese individuals carry a great deal of excess weight that further complicates symptoms of arthritis. It is important to find the appropriate mode of exercise for these individuals, and swimming is often cited as the best mode of therapeutic exercise for clients with joint diseases (Oddis, 1996). The water makes the body buoyant, which allows for activity without pounding damaged joints. However, it may be appropriate to have your client engage in swimming that is less intense (i.e., breaststroke, sidestroke, elementary backstroke). While swimming should be suggested as the most effective exercise for the arthritic patient, pool activities, walking and stationary biking can be recommended for those clients preferring other modes of exercise. Pool walking offers the benefits of activity for those who don't enjoy or cannot swim, and low-intensity pool aerobics may be similar to activities they may have performed in the past.

If there isn't a pool where you train your client, encourage them to choose beneficial low-impact land activities. Interview your client to determine areas that have surfaces that are more joint-friendly. If your client has access to indoor facilities and no concurrent injuries exist, treadmill walking or stationary biking could be beneficial. Hard surfaces such as macadam and concrete are widely available, but are also least favorable for the protection of joints. Try to find activities that enable walking on grass, wood chip paths or rubberized tracks. As with all exercise conditions for the obese individual, proper footwear is essential for preventing the onset of injury for non-water-related activities. Ascertain the mileage and usage of the client's sneakers, which provide proper support for approximately 500 to 600 miles of activity, depending on the make and model. It then is advisable to invest in a new pair. The proper exercise program for your arthritic client should improve conditions and not lead to greater complications or pain associated with disease. If in any doubt, refer your client to a physician or request their opinion on providing an effective exercise program. Arthritis is discussed in more detail in Chapter 15.

Respiratory Disorders and Sleep Apnea

Obesity, particularly upper-body obesity, is known to be associated with respiratory problems and with obstructive sleep apnea. Obstructive sleep apnea is defined as an absence of breathing for at least 10 seconds during sleep. The major consequences of severe sleep apnea include arterial hypoxemia, recurrent arousals from sleep, pulmonary and systemic hypertension and cardiac arrhythmias. Sleep apnea is typically associated with increased daytime sleepiness and altered cardiopulmonary function. Weight reduction has been associated with a reduction in the severity of sleep apnea (Schwartz, Gold, Schubert, et al., 1991).

As part of your assessment, determine whether your overweight clients report any daytime sleepiness, or if their sleeping partners report that they snore excessively or are restless sleepers. If you suspect sleep apnea is a problem, your client should be sent to a pulmonary specialist or, preferably, to a sleep disorder specialist in your area.

Case Studies

Three case studies serve as examples of clients that you might encounter. Initial physiological data and demographics are presented for each case-study client. When you work with an obese client, it is important to realize both the physiological and intrapersonal limitations of your client before providing an exercise program and beginning supervised training. Ultimately, you should attempt to optimize the fitness-related components of physical fitness (body composition, muscular strength and endurance, cardiorespiratory fitness and flexibility).

Case Study 1

Tim
Height: 6'5"
Weight: 330 lbs.
Body Mass Index: 39.5 kg/m^2
Age: 45
Body Fat Percentage: 30 percent
Resting Heart Rate: 68
Resting Blood Pressure: 158/110
Nonsmoker
Cholesterol: 225 mg/dl

Past History

Formerly, Tim was a very active person participating in division I football in college. He went on to play professional football for two years and engaged in weight training designed to promote strength. In recent years, he has worked at a desk job and he plays in a rugby club that competes in various weekend tournaments. He has participated in little exercise except an occasional rugby tournament. Most recently, a knee injury has rendered his left leg considerably weaker than his right leg. Tim has tried only sparingly to strengthen the quadriceps of his left leg since he discontinued physical therapy. With the decreased activity that is associated with his knee injury and a rather sedentary job, he now seeks to begin exercising.

Physician Clearance/Recommendations

Tim is recovering from surgery performed one year ago to repair tendons in his left knee. His left quadriceps is considerably weaker and smaller than his right. Some rehabilitation has been done to strengthen his knee at the request of his physician and physical therapist; however, his flexibility and strength have not returned to normal. Tim's physician has prescribed blood pressure medications and has recommended supervised exercise after determining that there were no abnormalities with his EKG.

Client Goals

Tim hopes to reduce his body weight to a figure similar to what he weighed in college, and he has set a weight-loss goal of 60 pounds. He would like to attempt jogging and feels that walking is not competitive enough for him. Tim wants to become fitter and stronger, and again participate in strength training.

Recommendations

Special feedback and encouragement will help Tim in his pursuit to develop an exercise routine and ulti-mately return to a comfortable weight. Tim has previously been successful and fit, and his motivation and previous experience with lifting heavy weights could be potentially dangerous. Tim has had success with athletics in the past, but now he may hurt himself if he doesn't take the proper approach to beginning an exercise program to reduce his weight. A client who is successful with athletics prior to gaining weight may be at greater risk for injury when attempting an ambitious return to the original workouts or trying to return to a previous weight. Safety is a concern. Focus on having Tim realize the importance of health-related components of fitness at this stage in his life (i.e., body composition, muscular strength and endurance, cardiovascular endurance and flexibility) rather than activity geared toward performance components of fitness (speed, power, etc.).

Seek Tim's involvement in the decision-making process of exercise-program design and implementation. Tailor the exercise program and allow for adequate input. Take caution to lead Tim toward trying exercises that are safe and effective, rather than the power lifting of the past. Preparing Tim to expect that he has a say in developing his exercise selection assures him that he is an active participant in the design of a program that meets his interests.

Time Restraints

Tim is willing to devote 90 minutes three to five days during the week.

Flexibility

It is essential to reiterate the importance of flexibility to Tim and to map out stretches that are specific to his previous injury and the activities that you will be prescribing.

Table 12.4

Exercise	Muscles Group(s)	Repetitions	Sets
leg press	quadriceps, gluteals, hamstrings	8 - 12	1 - 2
leg extension	quadriceps	8 - 12	1 - 2
leg curl	hamstrings	8 - 12	1 - 2
chest press	pectorals, deltoids, triceps	8 - 12	1 - 2
chest flies	pectorals	8 - 12	1 - 2
lat pull-downs	latisimus dorsi, biceps	8 - 12	1 - 2
seated row	latisimus dorsi, rhomboids, posterior deltoids, biceps	8 - 12	1 - 2
lateral arm raises	deltoids	8 - 12	1 - 2
tricep push-downs	triceps	8 - 12	1 - 2
arm curls	biceps	8 - 12	1 - 2
modified sit-ups	abdominals	10 - 20	2 - 3

Muscle Strength and Endurance Training

Strength training should focus primarily on multiple-joint exercise with major single-joint exercises using isotonic plate-loaded machines at the fitness center. Stress the leg press, leg extension and leg curl to develop the muscles supporting the knee joint. However, take care that initial intensities are set at a comfortable weight to ensure safety and skill acquisition for each exercise. Closely supervise and advise Tim on form due to his previous experiences with strength training. Because strength training is enjoyable and important to Tim, work toward two sets for each exercise and possibly three in the future if Tim's interest is sustained. Strength training is part of the recommendations for healthy individuals and can be performed during a weight-reduction exercise program to stimulate muscle growth with the goal of preserving lean body mass (ACSM, 1995). (Table 12.4.)

Physical Activity

Tim must become active. Your goal is to increase overall energy expenditure whenever possible in a safe and conservative fashion, and to have your client exercise at an intensity that derives fitness benefits. In Tim's case, walking on a treadmill or stationary biking are low-impact activities that he may enjoy and possibly may progress into brisk walking or jogging. Proper progression allows Tim to integrate exercise activities of the past (i.e., jogging after some weight loss occurs and he feels comfortable with brisk walking).

Tim performs a five-minute warm-up and cool-down before and after the activity, consisting of very-low-intensity walking or cycling. Five to 10 minutes of treadmill walking or stationary biking enables Tim to introduce the aerobic exercise component to his exercise routine and to gradually partake in activity in a safe and effective way. The focus of exercise is light-to-moderate intensity at 50 percent to 65 percent of heart-rate reserve (121 to 138 beats per minute). Explain the necessity of introducing a small amount of light- to moderate-intensity low-impact activity, such as walking, and increasing the duration and intensity as overall fitness improves. Weekly goals focusing on an increase in exercise duration should be set, along with a long-term duration goal of 45 minutes.

Urge Tim to become more active throughout the day by walking at lunch and performing small bouts of physical activity whenever possible to accumulate energy expenditure.

Case Study 2

Mary
Height: 5'3"
Weight: 205 lbs.
Body Mass Index: 36.4 kg/m²
Age: 51
Resting Blood Pressure: 130/88
Resting Pulse: 78
Body Fat Percentage: 34 percent
Nonsmoker
Cholesterol: 203 mg/dl

Past History

Mary is a nurse and is knowledgeable about fitness techniques, such as performing aerobic exercise to increase fitness. Time restraints and difficulty with exercise cause her to continually look for better ways to exercise. Mary feels like a "klutz" and strays from going to fitness centers. She participates in little or no leisure-time physical activity. She dislikes exercise because she doesn't like to sweat, and she doesn't enjoy group exercise because she can't keep up with the instructor in a "beginner's" aerobics class. Mary feels she needs to do something beneficial for her health and seeks your advice.

Physician Clearance/Recommendations

Mary sees her physician annually, and no medical problems are ever reported. However, when Mary questions her physician about the soreness in her knees and ankles after a long day at work, the physician finds no orthopedic problems and comments that the excess weight that Mary carries is solely responsible for the soreness. The physician always mentions that Mary should exercise and maintain a proper diet for weight loss, but hasn't given her any specific suggestions.

Client Goals

Mary's goal is to reduce her body weight by 50 pounds. She realizes that cardiovascular exercise is important for her health, and she tries to perform exercise that expends the maximum amount of calories (i.e., vigorous exercise on the cross-country ski machine), but she has trouble sticking with a program for more than a couple of weeks. Mary is eager to learn how to properly begin a strength-training routine to tone her muscles.

Recommendations

A home setting may be an excellent chance for you to get Mary to try alternative exercises. It is important to teach Mary that the optimum exercise is one that is safe, effective and holds her interest. Considering her lack of skill or coordination, she is a prime candidate for individual exercise. Moderate-intensity walking probably is the activity of choice, as she does not own exercise equipment and has limited options. The limited availability of fitness equipment may actually get her to focus on the most important part of exercise: movement. Suggest that she purchase an inexpensive piece of indoor exercise equipment that she can use on days when the weather is inclement. Trying to get Mary to learn to use cross-country skiers or engage in aerobics classes may turn her off more to exercise. Therefore, stationary cycling may be a more appropriate form of indoor exercise. In addition, Mary lives in a safe neighborhood that is close to a park that offers a variety of trails.

Time Restraints

Mary has one hour to devote to exercise on three to four days a week. However, she works a mixture of night and day shifts at the hospital which doesn't allow her to perform her exercise at the same time each day.

Flexibility

Teach Mary to recognize the feeling of "mild discomfort" during controlled static stretching. Have her hold each stretch for 15 to 30 seconds, and explain the importance of stretching after a bout of walking.

Physical Activity

Encourage Mary to embark on a walking program that allows her to become active without struggling with the coordination necessary to use certain pieces of exercise equipment. Her program should focus on walking outdoors or using a stationary bike indoors; listen to Mary's ideas about which activity she wants to engage in on a particular day. Have her wear quality footwear whenever exercising and look for soft walking surfaces in the nearby park. A rating of perceived exertion of 9 to 13 on the Borg scale should be the intensity goal (fairly light to somewhat hard). If appropriate, increase the initial duration of 10 minutes weekly (as fitness increases, overload duration). These small weekly goals that focus on achieving a set goal time allow Mary to safely expend calories and reap the conditioning benefits of light- to moderate-intensity exercise. Motivation and support are essential to training this client. Convey that the ultimate objective is not to find the exercise that burns the most calories, but to find the one she enjoys and can sustain for a lifetime.

In the future, modify and keep Mary's exercise fresh by introducing strength training using dumbbells at home. Weight reduction is associated with a loss of fat-free mass, and dumbbell strength training may stimulate muscle development for preservation of this tissue. For those who do not enjoy exercise, dumbbells in a home setting may provide an easy and effective strength-training component to a weight-loss program.

Case Study 3

Beth
Height: 5'5"
Weight: 190 lbs.
Body Mass Index: 31.7 kg/m^2

Table 12.5

Exercise	Muscle Group(s)	Repetitions	Sets
leg press	quadriceps, gluteals, hamstrings	8 - 12	1
leg extension	quadriceps	8 - 12	1
leg curl	hamstrings	8 - 12	1
chest press	pectorals, deltoids, triceps	8 - 12	1
lat pull-downs	latisimus dorsi, rhomboids, biceps	8 - 12	1
seated row	latisimus dorsi, rhomboids, posterior deltoids, biceps	8 - 12	1
upright row (pulley machine)	deltoids, trapezius, biceps	8 - 12	1
tricep push-down (pulley machine)	triceps	8 - 12	1
bicep curls (with dumbbells)	biceps	8 - 12	1
abdominal crunches	abdominals	10 - 20	2

Age: 25
Resting Blood Pressure: 110/84
Resting Pulse: 64
Body Composition: 28 percent
Nonsmoker
Cholesterol: 185 mg/dl

Past History

Beth works as an elementary school teacher, and is on her feet all day. She goes to the fitness center three times a week, and currently participates in vigorous aerobic exercise three days a week and strength training on isotonic machines (eight machines in a circuit) two to three days per week. Although she is performing this type of exercise regularly, she still is unable to reach her ideal weight. She strives to fit physical activity into the weekends because she likes to stay active even when she isn't teaching. Beth has noticed that she experiences some difficulty when jogging at this weight. She mentions that she continues to eat the same way as in college when she was 22, and that her activity levels are not as intense. It is frustrating for Beth to continue to exercise when she sees slight improvements in her stamina, yet small amounts of weight loss. She feels that exercise would be much easier at a lighter weight and that she would feel better about herself if she loses a few pounds.

Physician Clearance/Recommendations

Beth's physician recommends exercise. She has no medical concerns.

Client Goals

Beth would like to decrease her body weight by 50 to 60 pounds. She believes she is being realistic by striving for a weight of 130 pounds. Eventually, she would like to join a summer volleyball and softball league and run a 5K race, but feels uncomfortable competing at her current weight.

Recommendations

Beth's exercise program is in need of refinement, and she could benefit from referral to a registered dietitian (R.D.). Many individuals have difficulty losing or maintaining weight due to their inability to monitor portion control and develop proper eating behaviors in conjunction with exercise. An R.D. has experience in sports nutrition, and is better suited to deal with issues of proper and safe restriction of caloric intake and percentage of dietary intake coming from fats, proteins and carbohydrates that meet the daily activity and exercise needs.

Time Restraints

Beth would like to exercise five days a week. She mentions that outdoor exercise is a problem in the fall and winter because she only exercises in the evenings after school and it is usually dark out. She has no problem finding time to exercise in the summer when she is not teaching. She does, however, go to the fitness center religiously after school each day.

Flexibility

Evaluate the stretching exercises Beth is currently performing. Commend her on her commitment to include flexibility exercises in her routine, and have her perform sport-specific stretching if she is not doing so already. Encourage good form and static stretching of 15 to 30 seconds for each of the lower- and upper-body stretches.

Muscular Strength and Endurance

Beth is already strength training, so evaluate her form and specificity of training. Include upper- and lower-body exercises, and a mixture of dumbbell and pulley-machine exercises also may keep her strength-training program fresh. Gradually incorporate these machines into her workout and look to overload when possible. Initially, prescribe a low volume (one set, except for abdominals) of strength training and modify if her goals or needs change. As Beth achieves success, increase the weight by 5 percent and stress to her that strength training preserves lean-body mass while she is restricting calories. Explain the importance of lean-body mass to Beth, and allow her to choose activities that she enjoys and are safe.

Physical Activity

Assessing the effectiveness of her current exercise regimen may provide Beth with a challenging aerobic exercise program. Beth's current program can benefit from modified changes and from your input and supervision. Investigate the quality and safety of her workout, and commend Beth on her commitment to exercise; clients usually insufficiently emphasize their exercise habits in comparison to dietary habits. To achieve fitness benefits, increase the frequency of the cardiovascular workouts and the intensity of the strength-training exercises. Beth suffers from being overweight, but she could benefit from an increase in exercise volume since there are no medical problems associated with her weight (e.g., osteoarthritis, diabetes, etc.) Thirty to 45 minutes of moderate-intensity exercise five days a week should be a goal for Beth. Suggest swimming as an excellent cardiovascular activity that would be easy on the joints and different from her routine of simply walking on the treadmill. She also may cross-train by engaging in various exercises. Stationary biking, swimming, outdoor walking and low-impact aerobics may add variety to a stale routine.

Convey the importance of not only participating in cardiovascular exercise, but of increasing overall energy expenditure by choosing to engage in physical activity throughout the day and using fewer labor-saving devices.

References

Anonymous. (1993). Fifth Report of the Joint Committee on Detection, Evaluation, and Treatment of High Blood Pressure (JNCV). *Archives of Internal Medicine,* 153, 154-183.

American College of Sports Medicine. (1995). *ACSM's Guidelines for Exercise Testing and Prescription* (5th ed.) Baltimore, Md.: Williams & Wilkins.

American Diabetes Association. (1995). Diabetes and exercise: The risk-benefit profile. In J. T. Devlin & N. Ruderman (Eds.) *The Health Professional's Guide to Diabetes and Exercise* (pp. 3-4). Alexandria, Va.: American Diabetes Association.

American Diabetes Association. (1998). Position statement: Diabetes mellitus and exercise. *Diabetes Care,* 21 (Supplement 1), S40-S44.

Andersen, R.E. (1995). Is exercise or increased activity necessary for weight loss and weight management? *Medicine Exercise Nutrition and Health,* 4, 57-59.

Andersen, R.E. & Bartlett, S.J. (1997 April/May). Body composition assessment: The numbers don't always add up. *ACE Certified News,* 3, 8-9.

Andersen, R.E., Brownell, K.D. & Haskell, W.L. (1992). *The Health & Fitness Club Leader's Guide: Administering A Weight Management Program.* Dallas, Texas: American Health Publishing Co.

Andersen, R.E., Crespo, C.J., Bartlett, S.J., Cheskin, L.J. & Pratt, M. (1998). Relationship of physical activity and television watching habits among U.S. children with body weight and level of fatness: Results from the Third National Health and Nutrition Examination Survey. *Journal of the American Medical Association,* 279, 938-942.

Atkinson, R.L. (1993). Proposed standards for judging the success of the treatment of obesity. *Annals of Internal Medicine,* 119 (part 2), 677-680.

Bakris, G.L., Weir, M.R. & Sowers, J.R. (1996). Therapeutic challenges in the obese diabetic patient with hypertension. *American Journal of Medicine,* 101 (suppl. 3A), 33S-46S.

Blackburn, G.L. & Rosofsky, W. (1992). Making the connection between weight loss, dieting, and health: The 10% solution. *Weight Control Digest,* 2, 1, 101-110.

Brownell, K.D. & Wadden, T.A. (1992). Etiology and treatment of obesity: Understanding a serious, prevalent, and refractory disorder. *Journal of Consulting and Clinical Psychology,* 60, 4, 505-517.

Brownell, K.D. (1995). Exercise in the treatment of obesity. In K. D. Brownell & C.G. Fairburn (Eds.) *Eating Disorders and Obesity: A Comprehensive Handbook* (pp. 473-478). New York: The Guilford Press.

Colditz, G.A. (1992). Economic costs of obesity. *American Journal of Clinical Nutrition,* 55, 503S-507S.

Crespo, C.J. & Wright, J.D. (1995). Prevalence of overweight among active and inactive U.S. adults from the Third National Health and Nutrition Examination Survey. *Medicine and Science in Sports and Exercise,* 27, S73.

Crespo, C.J., Andersen, R.E., Pratt, M., Snelling, A. M. & Franckowiak, S. (1998). Obesity and its relation to physical activity and television watching among U.S. children. *Medicine and Science in Sports and Exercise,* 30, S80.

DeBusk, R.F., Stenestrand, U., Sheehan, M. & Haskell, W.L. (1990). Training effects of long versus short bouts of exercise in healthy subjects. *American Journal of Cardiology,* 65, 1010-1013.

Donnelly, J.E., Jacobsen, D.J., Jakicic, J.M. & Whatley, J.E. (1994). Very low calorie diet with concurrent versus delayed and sequential exercise. International Journal of Obesity, 18, 469-475.

Eckel, R.H. & Krauss, R.M. (1998). American Heart Association call to action: Obesity as a major risk factor for coronary heart disease. *Circulation,* 97, 2099-2100.

Ettinger, W.H.J., Burns, R., Messier, S.P., Applegate, W., Rejeski, W.J., Morgan, T., Shumaker, S., Berry, M.J., O'Toole, M., Monu, J. & Craven, T. (1997). A randomized trial comparing aerobic exercise and resistance exercise with a health education program in older adults with knee osteoarthritis. The Fitness Arthritis and Seniors Trial (FAST). *Journal of the American Medical Association,* 277, 1, 25-31.

Institute of Medicine. (1995). *Weighing the Options: Criteria for Evaluating Weight-Management Programs.* Washington, D.C.: National Academy Press.

Kayman, S., Bruvold, W. & Stern, J.S. (1990). Maintenance and relapse after weight loss in women: Behavioral aspects. *American Journal of Clinical Nutrition,* 52, 800-807.

Klem, M.L., Wing, R.R., McGuire, M.T., Seagle, H.M. & Hill, J.O. (1997). A descriptive study of individuals successful at long-term maintenance of substantial weight loss. *American Journal of Clinical Nutrition,* 66, 239-246.

Kuczmarski, R.J., Carrol, M.D., Flegal, K.M. & Troiano, R.P. (1997). Varying body mass index cutoff points to describe overweight prevalence among U.S. adults: NHANES III (1988 to 1994). *Obesity Research,* 5, 6, 542-548.

Lane, N.E. (1995). Exercise: A cause of arthritis. *Journal of Rheumatology,* 22 (suppl. 43), 3-6.

National Institutes of Health. Consensus conference on physical activity and cardiovascular health. Vol. 276.

National Task Force on the Prevention and Treatment of Obesity. (1994). Weight Cycling. *Journal of the American Medical Association,* 272 (15), 1196-1202.

Oddis, C.V. (1996). New perspectives on osteoarthritis. *American Journal of Medicine,* 100 (suppl 2A), 10S-15S.

Pate, R.R., Pratt, M., Blair, S.N., Haskell, W.L., Macera, C.A., Bouchard, C., Buchner, D., Ettinger, W., Heath, G.W., King, A.C., Kriska, A., Leon, A.S., Marcus, B.H., Morris, J., Paffenbarger, R.S. Jr., Patrick, K., Pollock, M.L., Rippe, J.M., Sallis, J. & Wilmore, J.H. (1995). Physical activity and public health: A recommendation from the Centers for Disease Control and Prevention and the American College of Sports Medicine. *Journal of the American Medical Association,* 273, 402-407.

Prentice, A.M. & Jebb, S.A. (1995). Obesity in Britain: Gluttony or sloth? *British Medical Journal,* 311, 437-439.

Sallis, J.F., Haskell, W. L. & Fortmann, S.P. (1986). Predictors of adoption and maintenance of physical activity in a community sample. *Preventive Medicine,* 15, 331-341.

Schwartz, A.R., Gold, A.R., Schubert, N., Stryzak, A., Wise, R.A., Permutt, S. & Smith, P.L. (1991) Effect of weight loss on upper airway collapsibility in obstructive sleep apnea. *American Review of Respiratory Disease,* 144, 494-498.

U.S. Department of Health and Human Services. (1996). *Physical Activity and Health: A Report of the Surgeon General.* Atlanta: U.S. Department of Health and Human Services, Centers for Disease Control and Prevention, National Center for Chronic Disease Prevention and Health Promotion.

Wadden, T. A., Foster, G. D., Letizia, K. A., & Mullen, J. L. (1990). Long-term effects of dieting on resting metabolic rate in obese outpatients. *Journal of the American Medical Association,* 264, 6, 707-711.

Wolf, A. M. (1998a). What is the economic case for treating obesity? *Obesity Research,* 6, 2S-7S.

Wolf, A. M. & Colditz, G.A. (1998b). Current estimates of the economic cost of obesity in the United States. *Obesity Research,* 6, 97-106.

Acknowledgment

Dr. Andersen's work is supported by the John A. Hartford Foundation grant 97214-G.

CHAPTER 13

Blood Lipid Disorders

RALPH LA FORGE

Ralph La Forge, M.S., is a clinical exercise physiologist and managing director of the Duke University Lipid Clinic and Disease Management Preceptorship Program at the Duke University Medical Center's Division of Endocrinology, Metabolism and Nutrition. He also is program director of the Lipid Clinic Preceptorship Program at San Diego Cardiac Center Medical Group. La Forge has worked for 20 years in clinical cardiology and has also served as an instructor of exercise physiology and health promotion at the University of California San Diego and the California School of Professional Psychology. He is the past program director of two large hospital-based preventive medicine and cardiac rehabilitation programs, and is the current exercise science research editor for IDEA Source.

Lipid Response
LDL & Total Cholesterol
Overall Lipid Management

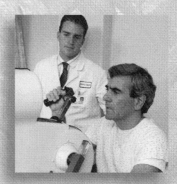

In the United States, cardiovascular disease accounts for 945,000 annual deaths and contributes to substantial morbidity, including 6 million hospital admissions annually. A large body of data has established that serum cholesterol and associated lipoproteins are a crucial risk factor for atherosclerosis. Blood lipid disorders (also called dyslipidemia) represent an important modifiable risk factor for the development and progression of coronary heart disease (CHD). The *1998 Heart and Stroke Statistical Update*, published by the American Heart Association, estimates that 37.7 percent of Americans have lipid abnormalities or dangerously high cholesterol levels.

New landmark primary and secondary prevention trials involving aggressive cholesterol lowering have demonstrated measurable atherosclerotic plaque regression, diminished atherosclerosis progression, improved arterial endothelial function, decreased mortality and/or improved clinical outcomes (Sacks, 1996; Pederson, 1994; Shepard, 1995; Gotto, 1997; Downs, 1998). In a well-controlled trial Pitt et al. demonstrated that early aggressive lipid management significantly reduces clinical events such as heart attack, the need for coronary artery bypass surgery and angioplasty after fewer than six months of therapy (Pitt, 1994). Even in those who were clinically free of coronary heart disease (and had average total cholesterol and LDL), systematic reduction of lipids and lipoproteins has been shown to significantly reduce the incidence of first heart attacks and revascularization procedures (Downs, 1998). Recent evidence also indicates that women benefit from lipid lowering similar to men (Pederson, 1994; Sacks, 1996). Furthermore, adverse changes in plasma lipids and lipoproteins that occur with age in sedentary women are not observed in women who regularly exercise (Stephenson, 1995, 1997; Owens, 1992).

Lipids, Lipoproteins and Atherosclerosis

Cholesterol is a fatty substance that travels in the blood in distinct particles that contain both lipids and proteins. These particles are called lipoproteins. The cholesterol level in the blood is determined partly by genetics and partly by lifestyle factors such as diet, body fat, exercise and even psychological stress. There are three major classes of lipoproteins found in the blood of a fasting individual: low-density lipoproteins (LDL), high-density lipoproteins (HDL) and very-low-density lipoproteins (VLDL).

VLDL is a major carrier of triglycerides in the plasma. Synthesized in the liver, triglyceride-rich VLDL carries endogenously (produced by the body) synthesized triglycerides and choles-

terol to their sites of utilization. VLDL also contains 10 percent to 15 percent of the body's total serum cholesterol. Increased concentrations of VLDL are associated with a number of lipoprotein disorders, such as familial hypertriglyceridemia, obesity, diabetes and nephrotic syndrome. Triglycerides, once thought not to be very important, have been shown to be a major risk factor for atherosclerosis (Austin, 1991).

LDL cholesterol is the major carrier of cholesterol in the circulation. It contains 60 percent to 70 percent of the body's total serum cholesterol and is directly correlated with the risk for coronary heart disease. LDL cholesterol plays a pivotal role in atherogenesis, the early stages of atherosclerosis. This role is illustrated in Figure 13.1, which describes the steps of LDL entry into the arterial endothelium and cholesterol plaque formation. Although all blood lipids play a role in the development of atherosclerosis, epidemiologic studies suggest that LDL cholesterol is the most important blood lipid. Without a threshold level of LDL, atherosclerosis is rare, despite the presence of other risk factors. LDL cholesterol also is the primary focus of most blood-lipid-lowering therapies. Plasma LDL concentrations are regulated by specialized LDL receptors on the arterial endothelium. When there is a defect in the gene for the synthesis of the LDL receptor, plasma LDL concentrations increase, as seen in patients with familial hypercholesterolemia. Table 13.1 depicts various LDL-cholesterol-lowering strategies and their respective efficacy.

HDL cholesterol is formed in the intestine and liver. HDL normally contains 20 percent to 30 percent of the body's total cholesterol, and HDL levels are inversely correlated with coronary heart disease risk. HDL plays an important role in reverse cholesterol transport (i.e., removal of cholesterol from cells and transporting it back to the liver). By removing excess cholesterol from the circulation, HDL may provide a protective mechanism against the development of atherosclerosis. Research has shown that each mg/dl increase in plasma HDL cholesterol concentration is associated with a 3 percent reduction in CHD risk (Gordon, 1989).

There are other lipid fractions such as lipoprotein (a) and various sub-species of HDL and LDL cholesterol, e.g., large- and small-dense LDL cholesterol (LDL phenotype A and B, respectively).

Table 13.1
Comparative LDL Reduction Therapies

Therapy	Percent reduction in LDL
American Heart Association Step I diet	5-10%
American Heart Association Step II diet	10-18%
Very low fat diets, e.g., Ornish (<10-15% fat)	25-35%
Exercise training	5-15+%

Therapy	Percent reduction in LDL
Estrogen therapy	5-15%
Relaxation & stress reduction therapy	5-10%
Pharmacotherapy, statins,	15-60%
Pharmacotherapy, niacin	10-25+%

INFILTRATION AND ENTRAPMENT OF LDL

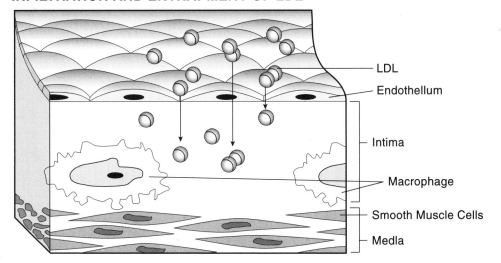

— LDL

— Endothellum

— Intima

— Macrophage

— Smooth Muscle Cells

— Medla

Figure 13.1

*Role of LDL-
cholesterol in
atherosclerosis*

FATTY STREAK

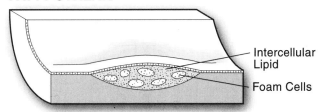

Intercellular
Lipid

Foam Cells

FIBROUS PLAQUE

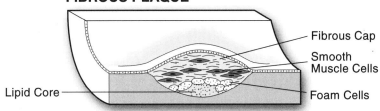

Fibrous Cap

Smooth
Muscle Cells

Lipid Core —

Foam Cells

COMPLICATED LESION

Thrombosis

Ulceration

Hemorrhage

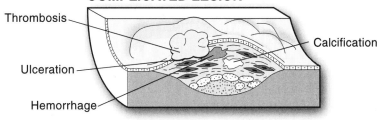

Calcification

Steps in Atherosclerosis:
a) Infiltration of LDL into arterial wall
b) Entrapment of LDL in arterial wall
c) Modification (e.g., oxidation) of LDL
d) Uptake of oxidized LDL by macrophages
 - formation of foam cells
 - formation of fatty streaks
e) Conversion of fatty streaks to fibrous cholesterol plaques

Modified from: Grundy, S.M. (1990). *Lipid Disorders: Cholesterol, Atherosclerosis and Coronary Heart Disease.* New York: Lippincot Co.

Because accurate and reliable measurement for these various lipid fractions is not widely available, and because we lack definitive clinical trial data showing that their modification reduces risk of CHD, they are not relevant to our discussion on exercise therapy.

National Cholesterol Education Program (NCEP) Guidelines

In June of 1993 the Second Report of the Expert Panel on Detection, Evaluation and Treatment of High Blood Cholesterol in Adults advocated more definitive and aggressive management of LDL and HDL cholesterol levels, especially in those with known coronary disease (NCEP, 1993). This second report mirrored the 1988 report in its emphasis on the primary prevention of coronary heart disease. LDL cholesterol remains the primary target of cholesterol-lowering therapy, although the level of HDL cholesterol is now considered an important factor in the assessment of overall risk and choice of drug therapy. The report also states that dietary modification, weight control and increased physical activity are the essential first steps in treatment of high blood cholesterol. These new guidelines also make clear that the intensity of the treatment is determined by the patient's risk of developing CHD. The patient's risk of CHD is, in turn, predicted by the presence of the following risk factors *other than LDL cholesterol* (which is quantified in Table 13.2):

Positive Risk Factors Other Than LDL Cholesterol:
- Men > 45 years
- Women > 55 years

- Family history of premature CVD — defined as sudden death or definite myocardial infarction before the age of 55 in father or other first-degree male relative, or before the age of 65 in mother or other female first-degree relative
- Current cigarette smoking
- Hypertension
- HDL-cholesterol < 35 mg/dl
- Diabetes

Negative Risk Factor:
- HDL cholesterol > 60 mg/dl

Table 13.2 depicts the composition of a typical *lipid profile*. This table also reflects the 1993 NCEP guidelines for total cholesterol and lipoprotein goals and standards. Note that the LDL cholesterol goal for those with documented coronary heart disease (or other clinical atherosclerotic disease, such as carotid artery disease) is 100 mg/dl versus 130mg/dl. These patients are at particularly high risk of myocardial infarction and death, and LDL cholesterol of 100 mg/dl is optimal. The lipid profile requires a 12-hour fast and is the most commonly ordered laboratory blood lipid assessment. It also is the most likely form of blood cholesterol information you will receive from your client's physician.

Lipid-lowering Medications

As indicated in the most recent NCEP guidelines, drug therapy should be considered only after patients have received at least six months of nonpharmacologic therapy, specifically intensive dietary and exercise therapy. Exceptions may include those with overt coronary heart disease, including post-myocardial infarction patients who have lipid

Table 13.2
The Lipid Profile and NCEP Standards

	Desirable Level	Borderline-high	High
Total Cholesterol	≤ 200	200-239	> 240
LDL Cholesterol	≤ 130	130-159	≥ 160
CHD	≤ 100		
HDL Cholesterol	≥ 36*	25-35	< 25
Triglycerides	≤ 200	200-500	> 500
LDL/HDL Ratio	≤ 2.7		

All values are expressed in milligrams per deciliter * HDL >45mg/dl ideal
Source: NCEP, 1993.

disorders. It is important for you to recognize these drugs and understand their effects on blood lipids and lipoproteins. The drug classes and drugs most commonly prescribed for patients with lipid disorders include:

Bile Acid Sequestrants (e.g., Cholestyramine, Colestipol). These agents bind bile acids in the small intestine and cause decreased bile acid absorption, in turn, lowering total and LDL cholesterol. The agents are available as dry powders in bulk or individual packets, and are usually consumed within one hour of eating and/or are taken with the evening meal. The bile acid sequestrants are quite effective for patients younger than age 55 who have LDL cholesterol between 160 and 220 mg/dl. Side effects are primarily gastrointestinal, with constipation being the most common.

Nicotinic Acid (Niacin). Niacin is a water-soluble B vitamin that is very effective in lowering LDL cholesterol and triglycerides, and increasing HDL cholesterol when used in relatively high doses (> 1,500 mg/day). Niacin is relatively inexpensive, making it an attractive choice as either single therapy or in combination with other drugs, such as statins. Its chief side effects include significant cutaneous flushing and vasodilatation. Niacin must be used with extreme caution in patients with liver disease, diabetes or gout and those at risk for peptic ulcer disease.

HMG CoA Reductase Inhibitors, (also known as statins, which includes: Lovastatin, Pravastatin, Simvastatin, Fluvastatin, Atorvastatin and Cerivastatin). These drugs effectively lower LDL cholesterol by interfering with cholesterol synthesis. They are competitive inhibitors of HMG-CoA reductase, the enzyme responsible for the rate-limiting step in the cholesterol biosynthetic pathway. They also block the for-

mation of mevalonic acid and decrease intracellular cholesterol synthesis. These drugs are the most effective and expensive class of medications available for lowering LDL cholesterol. Several of the statins have substantial clinical trial support for reducing cardiovascular morbidity and mortality, as well as clinical events and the need for cardiovascular intervention procedures.

Fibrates (Gemfibrozil, Fenofibrate). Gemfibrozil and Fenofibrate primarily lower triglycerides and, to a lesser extent, increase HDL cholesterol by reducing VLDL (triglyceride) synthesis and increasing VLDL clearance by increasing lipoprotein lipase activity.

Probucol (Lorelco). Probucol is a drug that is normally restricted to patients who have not tolerated or responded to their cholesterol-lowering medications. It has antioxidant properties and moderately lowers LDL cholesterol.

Estrogen Replacement Therapy. Although there are still many issues regarding estrogen replacement therapy, it can be considered as an alternative to drugs and, in many cases, may render drug therapy unnecessary. Estrogen has been shown to moderately lower LDL cholesterol (by approximately 15 percent) and can increase HDL by as much as 15 percent. Estrogens, however, may cause significant increases in serum triglycerides, particularly in women who already have high triglycerides (NCEP, 1993).

Other Agents (non-FDA-approved). Over the next few years, a variety of other nutritive and herbal agents are slated to be marketed and sold to consumers throughout the world. Many of these agents will be accompanied by ad campaigns claiming power to lower blood lipids. For example, the yeast-based supplement Cholestin, produced by Pharmanex, Inc., claims on a

Table 13.3

Client Information to Obtain from Medical Professionals

1) Are there any relevant co-morbidities, such as diabetes or coronary heart disease?

2) Is there any reason that this patient should not exercise? If so, what and with what limitations?

3) What medications is this patient taking?

4) What were the patient's laboratory lipid results over the last two years?

5) Does this patient need an exercise ECG prior to engaging in exercise?

6) What additional relevant concerns do you have with this patient?

promotional insert that it can lower LDL cholesterol 13 percent to 16 percent. Until adequately controlled and statistically based research is conducted and published, these supplements should not be considered primary modes of therapy in lipid management.

Overview of Cholesterol and Exercise

Exercise is not generally considered primary therapy for lipid disorders, especially in the current era of lipid-lowering drug therapy. This is unfortunate because exercise of appropriate volume can induce significant favorable changes in the lipid profile, as well as many other health-related benefits. Barnard recently demonstrated a 19 percent additional reduction in total cholesterol when diet and exercise complemented drug therapy in 93 men and women with dyslipidemia (Barnard, 1997). Dietary reduction of fat, exercise and weight loss are still the cornerstones of therapy for those who have elevated blood lipids, despite the overwhelming number of recent statin drug trials and lipid-lowering drug promotional campaigns extolling the benefits of

statin therapy. With the exception of those who have existing CHD, the essential first steps of therapy should be diet and exercise. This recommendation is clearly emphasized in the 1993 NCEP guidelines.

One of the hallmark findings of lipid-lowering drug therapy is improved arterial endothelial function, primarily through enhanced nitric oxide formation and function (nitric oxide is the most potent endogenous arterial vasodilator). Improved endothelial function is thought by many to be one of the primary mechanisms responsible for reduced CVD morbidity and mortality (Gotto, 1997; Kinlay, 1996). Research also has demonstrated similar improvements in endothelial function with sufficient exercise training (Ultriainen, 1996; Bode-Bloger, 1994).

The Lipid Response to Exercise Training

Exercise training of sufficient volume generally increases HDL cholesterol and lowers LDL cholesterol and triglycerides via a number of mechanisms, including reduced body fat stores and increased lipoprotein lipase activity. Most studies demonstrating exercise-improved lipid profiles have involved subjects

Table 13.4

Typical Activity Guidelines

- In general, a relatively high volume of exercise (e.g., 1,500 kcal per week) is recommended to reduce LDL cholesterol levels by 10 percent to 15 percent. Associated visceral abdominal weight loss is a good predictor of LDL-cholesterol reduction.

- Gradually increase the client's weekly exercise volume from 300 to 1,500 kcals. Use 300-kcal increments (i.e., 300 kcals, 600 kcals, 900 kcals, 1,200 kcals, 1,500 kcals). The client's time investment will range from one to eight hours depending on their initial fitness level and lipid goals.

- The exercise-lipid response generally is independent of exercise mode and intensity. Therefore, exercise intensity is not a major factor and generally can be set between 40 percent and 70 percent of peak work rate.

- Even though a client may not be able to generate an exercise volume of 1,500

kcals per week, a formerly sedentary client who transitions from zero to 600 or 800 kcals per week accrues the greatest relative reduction in cardiovascular risk.

- Provide written exercise guidelines for the client and include mode, frequency, duration, progression and relative intensity.

- Anthropometric measures and changes (e.g., waist circumference, body fat percentage) aid in predicting exercise-associated lipid responses.

- Use caution when training clients with existing exercise ischemic thresholds (relatively low exercise tolerance with s-t segment changes or angina) demonstrated by recent exercise ECG test. Clients with existing cardiovascular disease or diabetes also should follow special guidelines.

- Frequently and aggressively ensure program compliance.

with relatively normal blood lipids. There are very few randomized controlled studies appraising the lipid response to exercise training in patients with lipid disorders. It is very possible that those with lipid disorders may respond differently to a given dose of exercise, depending on the lipid disorder (e.g., those with lipoprotein lipase deficiency). There is some support for higher energy expenditure thresholds (e.g., > 1,000+ kcal/week) for those with elevated total and LDL cholesterol (Crouse, 1997).

Table 13.5 illustrates the variety of factors that play a role in determining serum lipids and the exercise/blood-lipid response. This large number of factors is the reason the exercise/blood-lipid response is complex and very individualized. Most studies indicate that the most important factors determining the exercise lipid response are: total caloric expenditure (exercise volume), co-existing body fat loss and initial lipid values. As a general rule, fat weight reduction is required for the most favorable blood lipid response in those who have elevated total and LDL cholesterol. This volume of exercise (between 1,000 and 2,000 kcal per week) is similar to that recommended for fat weight loss (ACSM, 1995). It is important for you to understand that this weekly energy expenditure is generally higher than that required to favorably alter blood pressure, enhance immune function, reduce platelet aggregation, improve bone mineral density and improve psychological

---

Table 13.5
Primary Factors Influencing Blood Lipids and Exercise Lipid Responses

---

1. Frequency, duration and intensity of exercise (as these increase, total caloric expenditure increases)
2. Total calories expended
3. Length of training period (e.g., one month, six months, 18 months)
4. Coexisting body fat loss
5. Corresponding dietary changes
6. Concomitant alcohol intake
7. Baseline lipid values
8. Plasma volume changes
9. Menopausal status
10. Genetics
11. Biologic variation (seasonal & diurnal changes)

---

well-being (Haskell, 1994). If exercise is of sufficient volume, exercise intensity is not of primary importance in improving the lipid profile, although most research supports a minimum intensity of at least 40 percent of peak work capacity (Durstine, 1997).

Decreased body fat tends to correlate reasonably well with reduced LDL cholesterol and increased HDL cholesterol, which is why it is important to periodically evaluate body-fat composition in dyslipidemic patients. Most exercise trials support between 700 and nearly 2,000 kcal of exercise per week to significantly alter HDL cholesterol and, to a lesser extent, LDL cholesterol (Durstine, 1994; Superko,1991; Taylor, 1993; Williams, 1994; Kokkinos, 1995; King, 1995).

Prospective Exercise Training Lipid Response by Lipid/Lipoprotein

Triglycerides

Compared to other lipids, such as LDL cholesterol, elevated blood triglycerides (TG) are generally easier to reduce with exercise training. Triglyceride mobilization and utilization appears to be in direct proportion to exercise energy expenditure. Blood triglycerides frequently decrease with exercise training, depending on baseline values and volume of exercise. Unlike total and LDL cholesterol, triglycerides generally decrease immediately after a session of high-volume endurance exercise (e.g., greater than 45 to 50 minutes of sustained effort), and remain lower for several days after the session.

The exercise prescription should follow the optimal mode, intensity, duration and frequency for fat weight reduction (e.g., 40 percent to 70 percent of aerobic capacity for 40 to 60+ minutes, four to six days per week). Four days a week of endurance exercise (e.g., four miles/day of jogging or 400+ kcal of energy expenditure) has been shown in a number of research trials to reduce TG significantly, especially in those with elevated baseline triglycerides (Durstine, 1994). Overall, a threshold of fat weight loss may be required for sustained TG reduction. Additionally, a reduction in TG is generally associated with an increase in

HDL cholesterol, especially in hypertriglyceri-
demic subjects.

LDL and Total Cholesterol

Most studies evaluating the total cholesterol
and/or LDL cholesterol response to exercise training have found zero to only moderate decreases in
these lipids. Many studies used inadequate exercise volumes and/or energy expenditure or failed
to control for confounding variables such as training-induced changes in plasma volume, dietary
habits or seasonal variation in cholesterol and
lipoproteins (Durstine, 1994).

The total and LDL cholesterol response to
exercise training is quite variable, but tends to
respond best to associated fat weight loss. LDL
reduction appears to be slightly more responsive to endurance exercise training than
total cholesterol. When LDL concentrations are
lower (e.g., <130mg/dl) the reduction has been
inversely related to the distance run each week
(Wood, 1983). Most studies have provided
mixed findings for plasma cholesterol concentrations for male runners, female runners,
cross-country skiers and other endurance-
trained athletes compared with inactive controls (Superko, 1991; Durstine, 1994). Results
from endurance-training studies have been no
more encouraging. Exercise training that results in weight loss and plasma volume expansion is more likely to result in lower LDL and
total cholesterol. Most research indicates minimal thresholds of a net 800 kcal of exercise per
week (e.g., 10 to 12+ miles of walking/wk).
Ideally, 1,200-1,500 kcal or more per week for
four to six months is required for significant
reductions in LDL cholesterol.

HDL Cholesterol

HDL cholesterol exercise training responsiveness appears to be dependent on the following
factors:
- length of the training period
- the volume of training completed
- frequency of training
- changes in body composition
- dietary intake
- weight loss
- pre-training HDL concentrations

There have been mixed findings among studies investigating the relationship of exercise

intensity and increases in HDL, with some studies reporting the necessity for more vigorous
exercise intensities. Inactive subjects may not increase HDL through energy expenditure as easily as physically active subjects (Durstine, 1997).
It has been my experience at the San Diego
Cardiac Center Medical Group Lipid Clinic that
those with very low HDL cholesterol (<25 mg/dl)
frequently do not respond to exercise training as
well as those with more normal HDL cholesterol.
Increased physical activity can also reduce the
tendency for HDL to decrease and triglycerides
to increase in patients who increase dietary carbohydrate (Thompson, 1988).

Recent research suggests that HDL cholesterol
may transiently increase after a single bout of
endurance exercise in men (Pronk, 1993; Visich
1996). The HDL subspecies HDL-2 and HDL-3
also tend to increase secondary to exercise-generated weight loss. Chronic increases in HDL cholesterol and HDL-2 appear to require a relatively
high exercise threshold (total energy expenditure). This threshold ranges from running seven
miles per week, or approximately 700 kcal
(Kokkinos, 1996), to running 15 miles per week,
or approximately 1,500 kcal (Williams, 1996).
Hartung reported that for each six miles run per
week, the HDL was approx. 3 mg/dl higher in
both men and women (Hartung, 1995). For inactive populations in general, 1,000 kcal per week
or more of exercise may be necessary for significant increases in HDL cholesterol.

There is some evidence that premenopausal
women require greater weekly exercise volumes (e.g., 2,000+ kcal) to significantly increase HDL cholesterol (Taylor, 1993). It is
recommended that one engage in a minimum of
four months of training at four to five sessions
per week to significantly increase HDL cholesterol. There is evidence that HDL may be more
responsive to a higher daily frequency of exercise (e.g., three 15-minute sessions vs. one 40-
minute session). Baseline HDL-cholesterol and
genetic factors have a significant impact on
capacity to increase HDL via exercise. Recent
research also indicates that exercise-induced
HDL increases are independent of exercise
intensity, especially in men and women older
than 45 to 50 years of age (King 1995; Crouse
1997). Studies also demonstrate that older
adults may take longer to increase HDL choles-

terol via exercise, perhaps as long as two years (King, 1995).

Exercise Volume Programming for Overall Lipid Management

Although there will be significant individual variation, it appears that to improve overall lipoprotein status (LDL, HDL, LDL/HDL ratio and triglycerides), an exercise volume of approximately 1,500+ kcal per week (e.g., running 15 miles or walking 20+ miles per week) may be necessary based on available research. Table 13.6 depicts sample exercise protocols with approximate weekly energy expenditures ranging from 500 to 2,000+ kcal per week. The duration of

Table 13.6
Sample Graduated Weekly Exercise Energy Expenditures (assumes 160- to 180-pound body weight)

Protocol A (400-600 kcal/wk)

Monday, Wednesday, Friday: *

Walk 2 miles/day = 400 kcal

Sunday:

20 min of low-level stationary cycling = 100 kcal

Protocol B (800-1,000 kcal/wk net)

Monday, Wednesday, Friday:

Walk 2 miles/day = 400 kcal

Tuesday & Saturday:

Walk 3 miles/day = 400 kcal

Sunday:

Nine holes of golf or 30 minutes

of singles tennis = 200 kcal

Protocol C (1,500+ kcal/wk)

Monday, Wednesday, Friday:

Walk 4 miles/day = 800 kcal

Tuesday & Thursday:

30 min of cycling (60% max VO$_2$) = 350 kcal

Sunday:

60 min of singles tennis plus 3-mile walk = 500 kcal

Protocol D (2,000+ kcal/wk)

5 days per week average 300 kcal workout (e.g., 40- to 45-minute aerobic session) = 1500 kcal

1 day/ week perform long slow-distance workout (e.g., 120-minute variable-terrain walk) = 600+ kcal

* walking at moderate pace (2.5-4mph)

weekly exercise equivalent to 1,500 kcal that is required for overall lipid changes can range from two-and-a-half to seven hours, depending on initial fitness level. For example:

very low fit individuals: 7+ hours of moderate exercise per week

moderately fit individuals: 4 to 6 hours per week

fit individuals: 2.5 to 3 hours per week

Middle-aged and post-menopausal women may require as much as 2,000 kcal or more of exercise per week (Taylor, 1993). Older adults may require more time (e.g., two years) to increase HDL cholesterol (King, 1995).

Resistance Training and Lipid Disorders

As with hypertension management, resistance training is not recommended as the primary form of exercise therapy for those with blood lipid disorders. Resistance training may be recommended as a component of a complete exercise program. Research has shown that the blood lipid response to strength training is negligible, with some studies reporting slight-to-moderate reductions in total and LDL cholesterol and others reporting no change (Tucker, 1997; Boyden, 1993; Kokkinos, 1988). It is likely that the blood lipid response to strength training is related to total net energy expenditure of the session (kcal per workout), as it is with endurance exercise. One example of a relatively high energy expenditure resistance-training session is low-resistance, high- repetition circuit weight training performed for extended periods and approaching 300 kcal or more per session.

Practical Exercise-programming Considerations
Essential Steps in Exercise Programming for Patients with Blood Lipid Disorders
1. **Evaluate health and lifestyle history.**
   - determine any relevant co-morbidities
   - blood lipid history and current blood lipid profile
   - exercise treadmill test history

- medications
- diet and exercise history

Patients with documented or suspected lipid disorders frequently have other related clinical conditions (co-morbidities) that also may influence exercise programming. Prolonged elevations in LDL cholesterol, for example, can increase the likelihood of coronary heart disease. Other conditions, such as diabetes, especially non-insulin-dependent diabetes, and obesity, often co-exist with lipid disorders and can influence the exercise-lipid response. Although many patients who have primary lipid disorders do not have associated co-morbidities, they should be evaluated by a thorough health history for the following conditions or co-morbidities:

- coronary heart disease
- previous myocardial infarction
- angina
- diabetes
- insulin resistance
- hypertension
- obesity
- peripheral vascular disease
- chronic obstructive pulmonary disease

Some of these conditions may necessitate prior thorough examination by a physician and graded exercise tolerance testing with EKG. It is important in these instances that you obtain this medical information and use it to help plan the recommended mode, frequency, duration, intensity and progression of exercise.

2. Determine the necessity for additional tests or evaluations.

Although you may not be in the position to administer or order these tests, you can recommend them to the patient's physician or the lipid clinic that may have referred the patient. Exercise testing with EKG may be required, depending on the patient's risk category and planned level of exercise. If the patient has existing or suspected diabetes or cardiovascular disease, and has not had an exercise EKG in more than two years, it is recommended that this test be administered by the physician or qualified exercise laboratory. Please refer to the current American College of Sports Medicine recommendations for exercise testing (ACSM, 1995).

The following are evaluations that may be appropriate prior to beginning an exercise program for lipid management:

- baseline lipid/lipoprotein profile
- exercise EKG
- physician evaluation
- clinical dietary assessment and diet prescription

3. Anthropometric measures.

Many lipid disorders are sensitive to changes in body fat stores. For this reason, it is essential that you initially and serially assess valid measures of body fat. Body weight, abdominal girth (a measure of central visceral fat stores) and/or total body fat percentage as assessed by skinfold measures should be recorded during the patient's initial visit and at four- to six-week intervals throughout the course of exercise training. Optional measures are hip/waist ratio, bioimpedance body fat evaluation and hydrostatic weighing. It is important to focus on the change in body fat and anthropometric measures rather than their relationship to normative body fat data. Total cholesterol, LDL cholesterol and triglycerides usually decrease with a diminution in body fat, especially abdominal or visceral fat reduction. HDL cholesterol may or may not directly correlate with fat weight changes. Refer to the *ACE Personal Training Manual* (American Council on Exercise, 1997, Chapter 6).

4. Set target lipid goal for exercise therapy.

It is important to emphasize that exercise-lipid responses vary among people and the volume of exercise required for significant changes in blood lipids is generally at a higher weekly energy expenditure threshold than that for reducing blood pressure or improving psychological well-being. For this reason, it may take more time to realize the clinical benefits. Be conservative with short-term lipid reduction goals, especially with total and LDL cholesterol reductions. A 5 percent to 10 percent LDL cholesterol reduction is generally a realistic goal for the first 12 to 16 weeks of exercise training, assuming sufficient weekly exercise energy expenditure. Many patients may take six months or longer to show significant decreases in total and LDL cholesterol. This is not unusual as there are a considerable variety of lipid disorders and blood lipid phenotypes. When possible, employ other co-variants of lipid reduction such as valid measures of overall body fat percentage and/or abdominal-visceral fat.

Laboratory lipid assessment values characteristically vary 8 percent to 12 percent, based on biological and analytic factors. This is important to consider when interpreting serial blood lipid values. Examples of variation in LDL and HDL cholesterol concentration include: *hospitalization, estrogen replacement therapy, pregnancy, Type II diabetes, smoking, acute infection, posture, venous occlusion, and seasonal and circadian biological variation*. The National Heart and Blood Institute published a comprehensive set of recommendations for laboratories and healthcare providers on ensuring valid lipoprotein measurement and interpretation (NHLBI, 1995).

5. Determine exercise plan from prior health history, level of fitness and current lipid profile.

The exercise plan should be written clearly and concisely and include: *exercise mode, frequency, duration, intensity, progression plan and safety precautions*. The patient's health history and initial fitness level are integral to formulating the weekly volume. For example, for patients with stable CHD who have had recent treadmill electrocardiograms, it will be important to review exercise electrocardiographic and hemodynamic data to appropriately set the exercise intensity and duration range. The patient's exercise capacity in METs or measured VO_2 will also be helpful in determining initial exercise work levels.

Overall, it may be easiest to prescribe exercise by energy expenditure or total weekly caloric expenditure. For this approach, it will be necessary for you to be knowledgeable of energy expenditure calculations for a variety of exercise modes (see example below). Initial weekly exercise volumes should be set realistically according to the patient's initial *level of fitness, body composition* and *existing co-morbidities*. Table 13.6 provides a sample set of exercise energy expenditure protocols. Since many patients may be significantly deconditioned and overweight, it may be most appropriate to start the patient on a progressive walking program. In this case, walking distance, speed and terrain should be gradually increased over the course of therapy to generate higher energy expenditures. The following are examples of energy expenditure target goals:

- *Elevated LDL and / or total cholesterol:* Goal 1,500 kcal+ per week
- *Low HDL:* 1,000+ kcal per week

- *Elevated triglycerides:* 1,000+ kcal per week
- *Combined dyslipidemia (elevated LDL & triglycerides with low HDL):* 1,500+ kcal/wk

Calculating Exercise Energy Expenditure

Since overall lipid improvement is responsive to weekly exercise volumes and exercise-generated fat weight loss, it is imperative that you know how to estimate session, daily and weekly exercise energy expenditures in kcal. The following are the approximate energy cost calculations for walking and jogging a given distance (e.g., 1 mile):

Walking. The net caloric cost per mile of walking up to 3.5 mph is 0.77 kcal/kg/mile (e.g., for a 154-pound person this would be 54 net calories per mile). This formula holds true for most walkers.*

Fast walking. The energy cost of walking 3.5 mph to 5 mph (speed walking) is 1.38 kcal/kg/ mile (e.g., for a 154-pound person this would be 97 net calories per mile).

Jogging/running. The net caloric cost per mile is 1.53 kcal/kg/mile (e.g., for a 154-pound person this would be 107 net calories per mile). (McArdle et al., 1997)

*net caloric cost per mile of running is nearly twice that for walking one mile (Howley & Franks, 1997). This is a very important point if you intend to prescribe and quantify walking mileage for fat weight control purposes. The net cost of exercise is the exercise energy expenditure minus resting energy expenditure. The net cost measures the energy used over and above that of just sitting.

6. Keep track of lipid-lowering drugs and other medications, if applicable.

For patients on lipid-lowering drugs, it is wise to know which drug or combination of drugs the patient is taking and any associated dosage changes. The combined use of exercise and lipid-lowering drug therapy can significantly reduce time needed to achieve the lipid goal. As a group, lipid-lowering drugs have little, if any, effect on exercise hemodynamics. Beta-blocking medications, with exception of the few that have intrinsic sympathomimetic activity (acebutolol and pindolol), will have a tendency to increase triglycerides and decrease HDL cholesterol. Patients on significant dosages of niacin therapy (e.g., > 1,500 mg/day) may have a greater tendency to drop their blood pressures after exercise. Niacin can also cause flushing and headaches in early stages of this form of pharmacotherapy. As a final note, many lipid-lowering drugs (e.g., statins and niacin) require periodic liver function tests to assess the possibility of liver toxicity.

Keep track of the patient's musculoskeletal symptom status during the exercise program, much the same as you would for any adult beginning an exercise program. This symptom supervision may be more relevant in those who are on statin drugs. One report suggests lovastatin exacerbated exercise-induced skeletal muscle injury, as measured by elevated creatine kinase levels (an index of skeletal muscle injury), in a group of 59 men who took 40 mg of lovastatin per day while embarking on a five-week vigorous endurance exercise program (Thompson, 1997). Although statins are usually well tolerated, they have occasionally been associated with myopathy (myalgia or muscle weakness) and there is at least a minimal chance that this could be exacerbated with exercise. Myopathy is rapidly reversible if diagnosed early by a physician and treated with discontinuance of drug and hydration. Although the rare occurrence of statin-induced myopathy should not alarm you, it does reinforce the need to keep reasonably close track of musculoskeletal symptoms through at least the early stages of the exercise program.

7. Follow-up.

Encourage follow-up blood lipid profile laboratory evaluations in accordance with the referring physician or lipid clinic's follow-up protocol. Exercise counseling follow-up ideally would be done in conjunction with the routine lipid clinic follow-up visit or at four- to six-week intervals. The exercise plan should be revised, as needed, with documentation of weekly energy expenditures. Anthropometric measures should be assessed at every clinic or at the follow-up visit. Dietary and medication compliance should also be routinely assessed at each follow-up.

8. Be knowledgeable of other nonpharmacologic interventions that can help manage lipid disorders.

For optimal results, it will often be important to use exercise as a complement to other non-pharmacologic (and pharmacologic) measures. For example, exercise stands the best chance of helping the patient reach their NCEP lipid goal if it is combined with dietary therapy (NCEP, 1993). The most recent NCEP guidelines describe in some detail the American Heart Association Step I and Step II dietary fat reduction recommendations.

Supplemental antioxidant vitamin intake (e.g., vitamin E) can be of value in reducing LDL cholesterol oxidation, although these supplements do not directly affect blood lipid levels (Rimm, 1997). Folic acid, vitamin B-6 and vitamin B-12 supplementation may also be of help in reducing serum homocysteine levels. Homocysteine is an amino acid that contributes to build-up of lipids in arteries and increases blood clotting tendency (Wald, 1998).

Stress and anger-management interventions, when applicable, should also be included in a comprehensive lipid-management plan. The rationale for such behavioral programs stems from stress-related catecholamine production and its putative relationship with LDL oxidation, LDL receptor regulation and macrophage activation, all of which are integral in the development of atherosclerosis (Adams, 1994; Williams, 1991).

9. Partner with healthcare professionals.

In many cases, you will be collaborating with a physician-directed lipid clinic team in providing therapy. In this sense, you are part of a medical team and may be required to provide patient progress records to the lipid clinic patient record. I recently published a helpful description of lipid clinic operations and referral affiliations (La Forge, 1996). In other instances, you may act independently through self-referral. In this case, it will be necessary to communicate exercise progress to the patient's physician, and to discuss the relevance of additional tests.

Conclusion

On average, exercise by itself will reduce LDL cholesterol by five percent to 15 percent and increase HDL cholesterol by five percent to 15 percent, depending on exercise volume and the nature of the lipid disorder. Even with a modest five percent to 10 percent reduction in total and LDL cholesterol, there is a significant decrease in coronary risk. Epidemiologic studies have clearly demonstrated that for every one percent reduction in LDL, there is a two percent to three percent reduction in the incidence of CHD (NCEP, 1993). Exercise therapy for the prevention and treatment of coronary heart disease indeed works well beyond its moderate lipid-lowering effects by improving functional capacity, antioxidant defenses, improved arterial endothelial function, fibrinolytic capacity and psychological well-being and by reducing blood pressure and body fat. A recent study of more than 25,000 men clearly demonstrated that attaining a moderate or high level of cardiorespiratory fitness is associated with a marked reduction in cardiovascular disease mortality even when elevated cholesterol is present (Farrell, 1998).

Lipid management in the new millennium represents an important opportunity for you given the growth of supportive clinical trials justifying aggressive lipid therapy in dyslipidemic patients and the burgeoning growth of physician-directed lipid clinics. Currently, the vast majority of lipid clinics do not recognize or adequately address exercise in any systematic manner. If you are interested in lipid disorders you should find this a welcome challenge and seek to forge strong alliances with outpatient lipid clinic teams.

Lastly, you should be prepared for the next NCEP Adult Treatment Panel report. This report (due to be released in the next two years) further clarifies pharmacologic and nonpharmacologic treatment recommendations.

Case Studies

Case Study 1

A 44-year-old female nurse administrator with a family history of cardiovascular disease (mother had myocardial infarction at age 51), a 12-year history of obesity, elevated LDL cholesterol (ranging from 158 mg/dl to 185 mg/dl), HDL ranging from 42 to 52 mg/dl and triglycerides ranging from 155 to 160. Patient is 5' 6" tall, 175 pounds, and has 34 percent body fat.

Goal: <130 mg/dl LDL cholesterol and <30 percent body fat.

She was put on 40 mg/day (20mg bid) of lovastatin, but over the last two years refused to consistently take the complete daily dose. Client was also prescribed an AHA Step II fat reduction diet. Subsequently, patient decreased her LDL to the 140 to 145 mg/dl range with her body weight still at 170 to 175 pounds and body fat at 33 percent to 35 percent (Jackson-Pollock skinfold assessment). Six months ago, the client was represcribed 20 mg of lovastatin once a day and the following exercise program (approximately 1,700+ kcal/wk):

Exercise Plan: 1,700+ kcal/week. Variable-terrain walking four times per week at approximately 60 percent of peak heart rate as determined by treadmill EKG; the walking duration began at 20 minutes per session and progressed to 60 minutes per session after four weeks. Client also attended two 50-minute aerobic exercise sessions a week at a local fitness center, where her average exercise intensity was 65 to 70 percent of peak heart rate.

Follow-up: At six months, her initial follow-up (while on the 20mg lovastatin and 1,700 kcal exercise program) resulted in an LDL cholesterol of 111 mg/dl, triglycerides of 128 mg/dl, HDL cholesterol of 48 mg/dl. Her body weight decreased to 164 pounds and her body fat decreased to 29 percent.

Case Study 2

A 56-year-old male traveling corporate attorney with a six-month-old uncomplicated inferior-wall myocardial infarction. His LDL cholesterol is 155mg/dl; HDL, 29mg/dl; triglycerides, 165 mg/dl; body weight, 181 pounds; height, 5' 9"; body fat, 28 percent; waist, 37 inches. The patient was resistant to taking niacin or other lipid-lowering medications, and had borderline hypertension, with an average of 145/85 mmHg blood pressure over the last two clinic visits. His most recent treadmill EKG was negative at a peak heart rate of 168 and he had an 11 MET exercise capacity.

Goal: To decrease LDL cholesterol to below 100 mg/dl, increase HDL to > 35, decrease body fat to at least 25 percent.

Exercise plan: 1,500+ kcal/wk. Client was already walking two to three miles, three times per week, on his own and was advised to increase this to three to four miles of walking five days per week, with one long variable-terrain hike on weekends (two to two-and-a-half hours). Client was also prescribed an American Heart Association Step II diet.

Follow-up: At four months the client decreased his LDL cholesterol to 122 mg/dl, HDL to 35 mg/dl, triglycerides to 148, body weight to 176 pounds, waist to 35 inches, body fat to 25 percent, resting blood pressure to 135/80. The client was resistant to spending more time with exercise and was moderately adherent to his reduced fat AHA Step II diet plan: Client agreed to take niacin, and over four weeks he increased the dose to 1,500 mg of immediate-release niacin per day, and maintained his existing exercise program. At six and a half months, the patient had tolerated niacin therapy nicely and reduced his LDL to 105 mg/dl, increased his HDL to 39 mg/dl, and further reduced his body fat to 22.5 percent, body weight to 172 pounds and his waist circumference to 34 inches. He plans to continue niacin therapy and 1,500 kcal/week exercise program and add two to three 15-minute resistance exercise sessions a week (at home or on the road).

References

American College of Sports Medicine. (1995). *ACSM's Guidelines for Exercise Testing and Prescription.* (5th ed.). Baltimore: Williams & Wilkins.

Adams, D.O. (1994). Molecular biology of macrophage activation: A pathway whereby psychosocial factors can potentially affect health. *Psychosomatic Medicine,* 56, 316-327.

American Council on Exercise. (1997). *Ace Personal Trainer Manual.* San Diego, Calif.: American Council on Exercise.

Austin, M.A. (1991). Plasma triglyceride and coronary heart disease. *Arterioscleroptic Thrombosis,* 11, 2-14.

Barnard, R.J., DiLauro, S.C. & Inkeles, S.B. (1997). Effects of intensive diet and exercise intervention in patients taking cholesterol-lowering drugs. *American Journal of Cardiology,* 79, 1112-1114.

Bode-Bioger, S.M., Bioger, R.H., Schrloder, E.P. & Frololich, J.C. (1994). Exercise increases systemic nitric oxide production in men. *Journal of Cardiovascular Risk,* 1, 173.

Boyden, T.W., Pamenter, R.W., Going, S.B. et al. (1993). Resistance exercise training is associated with decreases in serum low-density lipoprotein cholesterol levels in premenopausal women. *Archives of Internal Medicine,* 153, 97-100.

Crouse, S.F., O'Brien, B.C., Grandjean, P.W. et al. (1997). Training intensity, blood lipids and apolipoproteins in men with high cholesterol. *Journal of Applied Physiology,* 82, 270-277.

Downs, J.R., Clearfield. M., Weis, S. et al. (1998). Primary prevention of acute coronary events with lovastatin in men and women with average cholesterol levels. *Journal of the American Medical Association,* 279, 1615-1622.

Durstine, J.L., & Moore, G.E. (1997). Hyperlipidemia. In: Durstine (Ed.) *ACSM's Exercise Management for Persons with Chronic Diseases and Disabilities.* Champaign, Ill.: Human Kinetics.

Durstine, J.L. & Haskell, W. (1994). Effects of Exercise Training on Plasma Lipids and Lipoproteins. In *Exercise and Sports Sciences Reviews,* 22, 477-522. Baltimore: Williams & Wilkins.

Farrell, S.W., Kampert ,J.B., Kohl, H.W. et al. (1998). Influences of cardiorespiratory fitness levels and other predictors on cardiovascular disease mortality in men. *Medicine & Science in Sports & Exercise,* 30, 899-905.

Gordon, D.J., Probstfield, J.L. & Garrison, R.F. (1989). High density lipoprotein cholesterol and cardiovascular disease: Four prospective studies. *Circulation,* 79, 8-15.

Hartung, G.H. (1995). Physical activity and high-density lipoprotein cholesterol. *Journal of Sports Medicine and Physical Fitness,* 35, 1-5.

Haskell, W. (1994). Health Consequences of Physical Activity: Understanding and Challenges Regarding Dose-Response. *Medicine & Science in Sports & Exercise,* 26, 649-660.

Howley, E.T. & Franks B.D. (1997). *Health and Fitness Instructor's Handbook.* (3rd ed.). Champaign, Ill.: Human Kinetics.

King, A. Haskell, W.L., Young, D.R. et al. (1995). Long-term effects of varying intensities and formats of physical activity on participation rates, fitness and lipoproteins in men and women aged 50 to 65 years. *Circulation,* 91, 2595-2604.

Kinlay, S., Selwyn, A.P., Delagrange. D. et al. (1996). Biological mechanisms for the clinical success of lipid-lowering in coronary artery disease and the use of surrogate end-points. *Current Opinion in Cardiology,* 7, 389-397.

Kokkinos, P.F., Hurley, B.F., Vaccaro, P. et al. (1988). Effects of low and high-repetition resistive training on lipoprotein lipid levels. *Medicine & Science in Sports & Exercise.* 20, 50-54.

Kokkinos, P., Holland, J.C., Harayan. P. et al. (1995). Miles run per week and high-density lipoprotein cholesterol levels in healthy, middle-aged men. *Archives of Internal Medicine,* 155, 415-420.

La Forge, R. & Thomas T. (1996). Design and Operation of A Comprehensive Outpatient Lipid Clinic. *Journal of Cardiovascular Nursing,* 11, 39-53.

NCEP. (1993). Expert Panel on Detection, Evaluation and Treatment of High Blood Cholesterol in Adults. Summary of the 2nd Report of NCEP Expert Panel on Detection, Evaluation and Treatment of High Blood Cholesterol in Adults (Adult Treatment Panel II). *Journal of American Medical Association,* 269, 3015-3023.

National Heart Lung and Blood Institute, National Institutes of Health. (1995). *Recommendations on Lipoprotein Measurement.* NIH Publication # 95-3044 (single copies are free from NIH, call (301)251-1222).

Owens, J. Matthews, K., Wing, R. & Kuller, L. (1992). Can physical activity mitigate the effects of aging in middle aged women? *Circulation,* 85, 265-1270.

Pederson, T.R. & the Scandinavian Simvastatin Survival Study Group (1994). Randomized trial of cholesterol lowering in 4,444 patients with coronary heart disease. *Lancet,* 344, 1383-1389.

Pitt, B., Mancini. G.B. & Ellis, S.G. (1995). Pravastatin limitation of atherosclerosis in the coronary arteries (PLAC I). *JACC,* 26, 133-139.

Pronk, N.P. (1993). Short-term effects of exercise on plasma lipids and lipoproteins in humans. *Sports Medicine,* 16, 431-448.

Rimm, E.B. & Stampfer, M.J. (1997). The role of antioxidants in preventive cardiology. *Current Opinion in Cardiology,* 12, 188-194.

Sacks, F.M., Pfeffer, M.A., Moye, L.A. et al. (1996). The effect of pravastatin on coronary events after myocardial infarction in patients with average cholesterol levels. *New England Journal of Medicine,* 225,1001-1009.

Shepard. J., Cobbe, S.M., Ford, I. et al. (1995). Prevention of coronary heart disease with Pravastatin in men with hypercholesterolemia. (West of Scotland Coronary Prevention Study). *New England Journal of Medicine,* 333, 1301-1307.

Stevenson, E.T., DeSouza, C.A., Jones, P.P. et al. (1997). Physically active women demonstrate less adverse age-related changes in plasma lipids and lipoproteins. *American Journal of Cardiology,* 80, 1360-1364

Stevenson, E.T., Davy, K.P., Seals, D.R. et al. (1995). Physical activity is associated with favorable hemostatic and metabolic risk factors for coronary heart disease in healthy non-obese postmenopausal women. *Arteriosclerosis Thrombosis Vascular Biology,* 15, 669-677.

Superko, R. (1991). Exercise Training, Serum Lipids and Lipoprotein Particles: Is There A Change Threshold? *Medicine & Science in Sports & Exercise,* 23, 677.

Taylor, P. & Ward, A. (1993). Women, high-density lipoprotein cholesterol and exercise. *Archives of Internal Medicine,*153, 1178-1184.

Thompson, P.D. (1988). The benefits and risks of exercise training in patients with chronic coronary disease. Journal of the *American Medical Association,* 259, 1537-1540.

Thompson P.D, Zmuda, J.M., Domalik, L.J. et al. (1997). Lovastatin increases exercise-induced skeletal muscle injury. *Metabolism,* 46, 1206-1210.

Tucker, L.A., Martin, J.R. & Harris K. (1997). Effects of a strength-training program on the blood lipid levels of sedentary adult women. *American Journal of Health Behavior,* 21, 323-332.

Visich, P.S., Goss, F.L., Gordon, P.M. et al. (1996). Effects of exercise with varying energy expenditure on high-density lipoprotein cholesterol. *European Journal of Applied Physiology,* 72, 242-248.

Wald, N., Watt, H.C., Malcolm, R. et al (1998). Homocysteine and ischemic heart disease. *Archives of Internal Medicine,* 158, 862-867

Williams, P. (1997). Relationship of distance run per week to coronary heart disease risk factors in 8,283 male runners. *Archives of Internal Medicine,* 157, 191-198.

Williams, R.B., Suarez, E.C., Kuhn, C.M. et al. (1991) Biobehavioral basis of coronary-prone behavior in middle-aged men. Part I: Evidence for chronic SNS activation in type A's. *Psychosomatic Medicine,* 53, 517-527.

Wood, P.D., Haskell, W.L., Blair, S.N. et al. (1983). Increased exercise level and plasma lipoprotein concentrations: A one-year randomized, controlled study in sedentary middle-aged men. *Metabolism,* 32, 31-39.

Utriainen, T., Miakimattila, S., Virkamlaki, A. et al. (1996). Physical fitness and endothelial function (nitric oxide synthesis) are independent determinants of insulin-stimulated blood flow in normal subjects. *Journal of Clinical Endocrinology Metabolism,* 81, 4258-4263.

Suggested Reading

Durstine, J.L. & Haskell, W. (1994). Effects of Exercise Training on Plasma Lipids and Lipoproteins. *In Exercise and Sports Sciences Reviews,* 22, 477-522. Baltimore: Williams & Wilkins.
Perhaps the most thorough scientific review of the literature on the effects of exercise on lipids and lipoproteins (with more than 200 references).

Miller, N.H., Stoy, D.B. & Thomas T. (1994). *A Nurse's Guide to the Management of Cholesterol and Coronary Disease.* A Bristol-Myers Squibb Company educational monograph available through BMS representatives. *Although it was written primarily for nurse specialists, you will find that this is a user-friendly, 41-page overview of lipid disorders, the effects of lipid-lowering drugs and dietary therapy, including case studies.*

National Cholesterol Education Program (1993). Expert Panel on Detection, Evaluation and Treatment of High Blood Cholesterol in Adults. Summary of the 2nd Report of the NCEP Expert Panel on Detection, Evaluation and Treatment of High Blood Cholesterol in Adults (Adult Treatment Panel II). *Journal of the American Medical Association,* 269, 3015-3023.
This is essential reading for those who plan to work with those who have lipid disorders. It is written in a nontechnical but professional format, and available at no cost or at minimal cost through the NIH printing office.

Section Five

Immunological/ Hematological Disorders

CHAPTER 14

Cancer

DAVID C. NIEMAN

David C. Nieman, Dr. P.H., F.A.C.S.M,
is a professor of health and exercise
science at Appalachian State
University in Boone, N.C. He has
taught at the college and university
level since 1972, and is the author of
five textbooks and more than 120
research articles in the areas of
sports medicine, exercise and health,
exercise immunology, sports
nutrition and obesity.

Risk Factors
Client Assessment
Exercise Training Benefits

There are many types of cancers, but they can all be characterized by uncontrolled growth and spread of abnormal cells (American Cancer Society, 1997; Parker et al., 1997). If the spread is not controlled, it can result in death as vital passageways are blocked and the body's oxygen and nutrient supply is diverted to support the rapidly growing cancer.

The term cancer is used to indicate any of the more than 100 types of malignant tumors or neoplasms (American Cancer Society, 1997). A neoplasm is defined as an abnormal tissue that grows by cellular proliferation more rapidly than normal, and continues to grow after the stimuli that initiated the new growth cease.

Neoplasms show a lack of structural organization and coordination with the surrounding normal tissue, and usually form a distinct mass of tissue which may be either benign (benign tumor) or malignant (cancerous tumor). A malignant cancer is one that invades surrounding tissues and is usually capable of producing metastases (the spread of **cancer** cells from one part of the body to another). Often the malignant cancer may recur after attempted removal, and is likely to cause death unless adequately treated through **radiation, chemotherapy** and surgery.

Two common classifications of cancerous tumors are **carcinoma** and **sarcoma**. A carcinoma is any of the various types of malignant neoplasms derived from epithelial tissue (the lining or covering cells of tissues). Carcinomas occur more frequently in the skin and large intestine in both sexes, and in the lung and prostate gland in men, and the lung and breast in women. A sarcoma is a connective tissue neoplasm, and is usually highly malignant.

Cancer Statistics

Although heart disease during the last half century has been the leading cause of death in the United States, cancer will probably replace heart disease as the top killer soon after the year 2000 (National Center for Health Statistics, 1997) (Tables 14.1 and 14.2). Since the 1950s, death rates for heart disease have fallen steeply (55 percent). Meanwhile, the war against cancer has been largely unsuccessful. Between 1950 and 1990, age-adjusted death rates for cancer rose 7.7 percent, due primarily to the sharp increase in lung cancer. From 1991 to 1995, total cancer deaths fell 3.1 percent, marking the first decline since cancer statistics were first documented in the 1930s (Cole & Rodu, 1996). The decline is expected to continue at about 2 percent per year, and has been attributed to reduced cigarette smoking (and a

concomitant decrease in male lung cancer death rates) and improved screening and treatment.

The American Cancer Society has estimated that the lifetime risk of developing cancer is a staggering 48 percent for men and 38 percent for women (Table 14.2). About 1.4 million Americans are diagnosed with cancer each year (not including the more than 900,000 cases of skin cancer) (Parker et al., 1997). Each year, more than one-half million Americans die of cancer, about 1,500 each day. Just fewer than one in four deaths each year in the U.S. is the result of cancer. The leading cancer killer for both men and women is lung cancer, followed by prostate or breast cancer, and colorectal cancer (American Cancer Society, 1997). (Figure 14.1).

Cancer Prognosis

In the early 1900s, few cancer patients had much hope of long-term survival. In the 1930s, fewer than one in five was alive five years after treatment. Now, four of 10 patients who get cancer live five or more years after diagnosis (Parker et al., 1997). With regular screening and self-exams, cancer can often be detected early, greatly enhancing the success of treatment. Table 14.3 summarizes the American Cancer Society recommendations for the early detection of cancer in the general population. Table 14.4 outlines signs and symptoms for five major cancers. Screening examinations, conducted regularly by a healthcare professional, can result in the detection of cancers at earlier stages when treatment is more likely to be successful. More

Table 14.1
Ten Leading Causes of Death, United States, 1995

Rank	Cause of Death	Crude Death Rate per 100,000 Population	Percent of Total Deaths
1	Heart Diseases	280.7	31.9
2	Cancer	204.9	23.3
3	Cerebrovascular Diseases	60.1	6.8
4	Chronic Obstructive Pulmonary Diseases	39.2	4.5
5	Accidents	35.5	4.0
6	Pneumonia & Influenza	31.6	3.6
7	Diabetes Mellitus	22.6	2.6
8	HIV Infection	16.4	1.9
9	Suicide	11.9	1.4
10	Cirrhosis of Liver	9.6	1.1

Source: National Center for Health Statistic (1997). *Monthly Vital Statistics Report*, 45, 11, 2.

Table 14.2
Basic Cancer Facts and Figures, United States

New cancer cases per year . . . . .1,400,000 (plus 900,000 skin cancers)
Cancer deaths per year . . . . .560,000 (1,500 per day)
Rank as cause of death . . . . .Second (behind heart disease)
Percent of total U.S. deaths 23.3%
Cancer death trends . . . . .Steady, slight rise from 1950 to 1990;
                                            small decrease since 1990
Lifetime risk of developing cancer . . . . .48% for males, 38% for females
Survival rate for all cancers, five years 40%
Americans alive with a history of cancer . . . . .7.4 million
Cost of cancer . . . .$104 billion per year
Cancer causes . . . . .33% poor nutrition
                                            30% tobacco use

than half of all new cancer cases occur in nine screening-accessible cancer sites (breast, colon, rectum, prostate, tongue, mouth, cervix, testis and skin). The relative survival rate for these cancers is 80 percent, but could rise to 95 percent if all Americans participated in regular cancer screenings (American Cancer Society, 1997). As shown in Figure 14.2, five-year relative survival rates for cancer are much improved when the cancer is diagnosed prior to regional and distant body spread (American Cancer Society, 1997; Parker et al., 1997).

Risk Factors for Cancer Causation

Table 14.4 lists the important risk factors for the leading cancer sites (American Cancer Society, 1997). Dietary factors (33 percent of all cancers) and cigarette smoking (30 percent of all cancers) account for nearly two-thirds of all cancers. Other important risk factors include reproductive factors (especially for breast cancer), environmental factors (especially radiation and radon exposure, and air pollution), family history, and physical inactivity and obesity.

The American Cancer Society has urged that to reduce cancer risk, people should avoid all tobacco use, consume low-fat, high-fiber diets containing plenty of whole grains, fruits and vegetables, be physically active and maintain a healthy weight, limit consumption of alcoholic beverages, and limit exposure to ultraviolet radiation (American Cancer Society, 1996; 1997)

Table 14.3
Summary of American Cancer Society Recommendations for the Early Detection of Cancer in Asymptomatic People

Test	Population Sex	Population Age	Frequency
Sigmoidoscopy, preferably flexible	M & F	50 and over	Every 3-5 years
Fecal Occult Blood Test	M & F	50 and over	Every year
Digital Rectal Exam	M & F	40 and over	Every year
Prostate Exam*	M	50 and over	Every year
Pap Test	F	All women who are, or who have been, sexually active, or have reached age 18, should have an annual Pap test and pelvic examination. After a woman has had three or more consecutive satisfactory normal annual examinations, the Pap test may be performed less frequently at the discretion of her physician.	
Breast Self-examination	F	20 and over	Every month
Breast clinical examination	F	20-40 / Over 40	Every 3 years / Every year
Mammography**	F	40 and over	Every year

*Annual digital rectal examination and prostate-specific antigen should be performed on men 50 years and older. If either result is abnormal, further evaluation should be considered.**Screening mammography should begin by age 40.
Source: American Cancer Society

Table 14.4
Major Risk Factors and Signs & Symptoms For Major Cancer Sites

Lung Cancer

Risk Factors:	cigarette smoke; exposure to certain industrial substances (e.g., arsenic, asbestos); radiation exposure; residential radon exposure; air pollution; tuberculosis; exposure to environmental tobacco smoke in nonsmokers
Signs & Symptoms:	persistent cough; sputum streaked with blood; chest pain; recurring pneumonia or bronchitis

Colon and Rectum Cancer

Risk Factors:	personal/family history of colorectal cancer or polyps; inflammatory bowel disease; physical inactivity; high fat and/or low fiber diet; inadequate intake of fruits and vegetables
Signs & Symptoms:	rectal bleeding or blood in the stool; change in bowel habits

Breast Cancer

Risk Factors:	increasing age; personal or family history of breast cancer; never had children; some forms of benign breast disease; first childbirth after age 30; BRCA1 and BRCA2 gene mutations; early menarche; late menopause; higher education; lengthy exposure to postmenopausal estrogen; alcohol consumption; higher socioeconomic status; physical inactivity; high dietary fat intake (international contrast); obesity
Signs & Symptoms:	abnormality that shows up on a mammogram before it can be felt; breast changes that persist (lump; thickening; swelling; dimpling; skin irritation; distortion; retraction; scaliness; pain; nipple tenderness)

Prostate Cancer

Risk Factors:	age (more than 80 percent are diagnosed after age 65); African-American race has highest incidence rate in the world; high dietary fat intake (international contrast); family history (may be genetic or environmental); live in North America or northwestern Europe
Signs & Symptoms:	weak or interrupted urine flow; itchiness, tenderness or pain

Source: American Cancer Society. *Cancer Facts & Figures,* 1997. Atlanta: Author.

(Table 14.5). (Visit the American Cancer Society's WWW home page at: http://www.cancer.org).

Exercise Benefits in the Treatment and Rehabilitation of Cancer

The relationship between physical activity and cancer (both prevention and treatment) has not received sufficient attention from researchers until recently. In the area of cancer prevention, regular physical activity was finally added in 1996 to the list of measures advocated by the American Cancer Society (Table 14.5).

Physical Activity and Prevention of Cancer

Evidence is mounting in animal and human studies that regular physical activity does contribute to the prevention of cancer. Investigators have injected animals with cancer-causing chemicals, divided them into exercise and nonexercise groups, and then measured the size and time of cancer appearance. Results show that exercise retards cancer growth at several different sites (MacNeil & Hoffman-Goetz, 1993; Roebuck et al., 1990; Thompson, 1994; Thompson et al., 1995; Woods & Davis, 1994). Exercise appears to enhance the activity of certain cells in the immune system, especially **natural killer cells,** cytotoxic T cells and macrophages, which improves cancer-fighting proficiency (MacNeil & Hoffman-Goetz, 1993; Woods & Davis, 1994).

Large groups of people have been followed for extended periods to see if those who exercise regularly have less incidence of cancer than those who lead an inactive lifestyle. The most impressive results have shown a protective effect of exercise against three common cancer killers: colon, breast and prostate cancer (Lee, 1994, 1995; Martinez et al., 1997; Shephard, 1993, 1995; Thune et al., 1997; U.S. Department of Health and Human Services, 1996). In 1997, an international panel of cancer experts concluded that as many as 30 percent to 40 percent of all cancer cases worldwide could be avoided if people ate a healthy diet, avoided obesity and participated in an adequate amount of exercise (American Institute for Cancer Research, 1997). The panel proposed a rigorous exercise goal: Take a brisk walk for about an hour daily (or the equivalent) and exercise vigorously at least one hour per week if one's occupation is sedentary.

Although the link between physical activity and prevention of cancer is now well established, more research is needed to determine whether exercise can play a role in treatment after cancer development.

Physical Activity and Rehabilitation of the Cancer Patient

Fred Lebow, founder of the New York City Marathon and an active marathoner, was diag- nosed with brain cancer in 1990. Even as he underwent chemotherapy, he continued to run, first on the roof of the hospital and then on the roads and paths of New York's Central Park. In 1992, he and an old friend, nine-time New York City Marathon winner Grete Waitz of Norway, ran the entire 26.2-mile course. Just before the 1994 New York City Marathon, runners throughout the world were saddened to hear that Fred Lebow had died at age 62 after a second bout with brain cancer.

Lebow's fight against cancer is well known, and has raised the question of whether he should have curtailed his training after being diagnosed with cancer. Specifically, the questions asked were: Can too much exercise be harmful to the cancer patient? And, on the other hand, can moderate amounts be beneficial?

Although the link between physical activity and cancer prevention is finally being acknowl-

---

Table 14.5
Cancer Prevention Guidelines from the American Cancer Society

---

Practice Good Nutrition and Exercise Habits

---

1. **Choose most of the foods you eat from plant sources.**
   Eat five or more servings of fruits and vegetables each day; eat other foods from plant sources, such as breads, cereals, grain products, rice, pasta or beans several times each day.

2. **Limit your intake of high-fat foods, particularly from animal sources.**
   Choose foods low in fat; limit consumption of meats, especially high-fat meats.

3. **Be physically active; achieve and maintain a healthy weight.**
   Physical activity can help protect against some cancers, either by balancing caloric intake with energy expenditure or by other mechanisms.

4. **Limit consumption of alcoholic beverages, if you drink at all.**
   Alcoholic beverages, along with cigarette smoking and use of snuff and chewing tobacco, cause cancers of the oral cavity, esophagus and larynx. Studies have also noted an association between alcohol consumption and an increased risk of breast cancer.

Avoid All Tobacco

Lung cancer mortality rates are 23 times higher for male smokers and 11 times higher for female smokers. In addition to being responsible for 87 percent of lung cancers, smoking is also associated with cancers of the mouth, pharynx, larynx, esophagus, pancreas, uterine cervix, kidney and bladder. Smoking accounts for 29 percent of all cancer deaths. Oral cancer occurs several times more frequently among snuff dippers compared with non-tobacco users. The excess risk of cancer of the cheek and gum may reach nearly 50-fold among long-term snuff users. Cigar smokers have four to 10 times the risk of nonsmokers of dying from laryngeal, oral or esophageal cancers. Each year, about 3,000 nonsmoking adults die of lung cancer as a result of breathing the smoke of others' cigarettes. Secondhand smoke contains at least 14 known or probable human carcinogenic chemicals.

Environmental Cancer Risks

---

1. **Chemicals:** Some show definite evidence of human carcinogenicity (e.g., benzene, asbestos, vinyl chloride, arsenic, aflatoxin).

2. **Radiation:** Only high-frequency radiation, ionizing radiation (e.g., radon and x-rays) and ultraviolet radiation have been proven to cause human cancer.

3. **Unproven risks:** Pesticides, non-ionizing radiation (e.g., radiowaves, microwaves, radar, and electric and magnetic fields associated with electric currents), toxic wastes and nuclear power plants.

Source: American Cancer Society. *Cancer Facts & Figures,* 1997. Atlanta: Author.

---

edged, little attention has been directed toward exercise and rehabilitation from cancer (Gerhardsson, 1997). Of the studies currently available, numerous methodological limitations exist, and results must be considered preliminary (Friendenreich & Courneya, 1996). Despite limited research data, some experts still feel that moderate exercise may have important benefits for the cancer patient. According to Dr. Roy Shephard of the University of Toronto in Canada, "Exercise has an immediate mood-elevating effect, and thus can be of particular help to the cancer victim. It also stimulates appetite, and encourages the retention of muscle tissue. These effects should slow the clinical course of the disease, setting back the age at death, while also increasing the quality of the remaining years of life" (Shephard, 1993).

Of the 1.4 million Americans diagnosed with cancer each year, about 40 percent will be alive five years after treatment (American Cancer Society, 1997). Most cancer patients will receive adjuvant chemotherapy, radiation or both after surgery in an effort to prevent disease recurrence. Side effects of chemotherapy include nausea, vomiting, fatigue, alopecia,

mucositis, **cytopenia** and weight change (Demark-Wahnefried et al., 1997). Breast cancer patients often gain weight, decrease physical activity and lose physical fitness. Due to the large number of cancer survivors and the important role physical exercise may have in countering treatment-related symptoms, fitness assessment and programming should receive growing attention during the next decade.

Client Assessment of Physical Fitness

According to the American College of Sports Medicine (1997), formal exercise testing is appropriate for patients whose cancer is in remission. Patients undergoing treatment with chemotherapy or radiation therapy do not need exercise testing, but may benefit from bedside assessment to develop an exercise program individualized to their condition.

ACSM has listed two primary objectives of exercise testing of cancer patients:

➤ Assess aerobic capacity, submaximal endurance, strength and functional performance.

➤ Reveal other co-morbidity, such as coronary heart disease, diabetes, etc.

Exercise testing must be individualized to the condition of the cancer patient, but usually can be performed using standard protocols. ACSM recommends that patients who have received chest irradiation or chemotherapy that is toxic to the heart or lungs must be monitored during exercise testing. Frequently assess heart rate and blood pressure, as well as arterial oximetry, to guard against cardiopulmonary decompensation.

Aerobic power can be assessed in frail cancer patients using the six-minute walk test (distance covered in six minutes) (Nieman et al., 1995). If the cancer survivor has no contraindications to exercise, treadmill-and-cycle ergometer graded exercise testing can be used to assess aerobic power. Patients who are recovering from high dose chemotherapy often experience mucositis and therefore cannot tolerate a mouthpiece for direct assessment of VO_2max (Dimeo et al., 1997b). Strength can be measured with one repetition maximum (1-RM) weight lifts, depending on the cancer patient or survivor. Most importantly, progress should be monitored over time, and the testing

Figure 14.1

Sixty percent of all cancer deaths for each sex are caused by four different cancers.

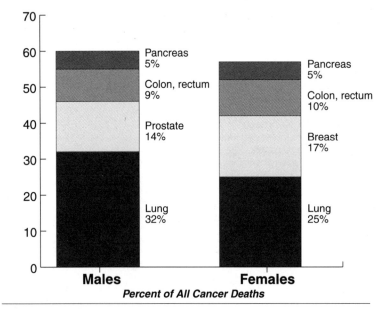

Pancreas 5%
Colon, rectum 9%
Prostate 14%
Lung 32%

Pancreas 5%
Colon, rectum 10%
Breast 17%
Lung 25%

Males   **Females**
Percent of All Cancer Deaths

Source: American Cancer Society, 1997

program should be individualized to the cancer patient.

Exercise Programming and Leadership for Cancer Patients

The development of an individualized exercise plan for patients with cancer involves screening, assessment, prescription, goal setting, evaluation and communication (Smith, 1996). Physical activity has the potential to influence all dimensions of life for the cancer patient, but the Advanced Personal Trainer must use sound clinical judgment and creativity, as well as collaborate with other healthcare professionals, when prescribing exercise.

Fatigue, loss of fitness, impaired exercise tolerance, anxiety and difficulty sleeping are commonly reported symptoms in cancer patients during treatment (Pihkala et al., 1995; Monga et al., 1997; Mock et al., 1997). Most cancer patients reduce levels of physical activity and energy expenditure during treatment, which has been linked to a lowered quality of life (Demark-Wahnefried et al., 1997; Courneya & Friedenreich, 1997). Following treatment, surviving cancer patients often report diminished strength and muscle mass, weakness and low cardiorespiratory fitness (Hovi et al., 1993). Almost 30 percent of cancer survivors experience a loss of energy for years after treatment cessation, and loss of physical fitness has been postulated to be a major cause (Dimeo et al., 1997b). Often a vicious cycle sets in with cancer survivors: Cancer treatment-related fatigue leads to a decrease in physical activity which further lowers fitness and muscle mass, causing even greater fatigue. Cancer patients report other important barriers to exercise training including lack of time and inertia (Leddy, 1997).

With the improving cure rate in childhood and adult cancers, increasing interest has been focused on the long-term survivors and their quality of life. In some studies of survivors of childhood cancer, disabilities have been detected in as many as 40 percent (Hovi et al., 1993). Growth, endocrinologic systems and neuropsychological performance are often affected. During treatment of **leukemia**, physical fitness can be impaired by infections and nutritional disturbances. Radiation therapy and chemotherapy may have long-term effects on muscle and nerve tissue in survivors of childhood cancer. Some chemotherapeutic agents, especially vincristine, can cause acute or prolonged peripheral nerve damage that may be clinically detectable for years after therapy (Hovi et al., 1993).

There are many types of cancers, and individuals vary widely in physical fitness changes following therapy. With this in mind, the ACSM (1997) has made several recommendations regarding exercise testing and training for cancer patients:

➤ Exercise testing and training should be individualized to the patient.

➤ For persons who are undergoing therapy for cancer, exercise training should have the objective of maintaining endurance, strength and level of function. Cancer therapy exhausts physical and emotional reserves, so a good use of exercise training is an attempt to maintain these resources.

➤ For survivors of cancer (in remission or after cure), exercise training should have the objective of returning them to their former level of physical and psychological function.

Exercise programming for the cancer patient should include all components of physical fitness, and strive to improve quality of life,

Table 14.6

Client Information to Obtain from Medical Professionals

1) Are there any signs or symptoms that I should be aware of that would indicate a problem or need for immediate referral back to the physician?

2) What exercises are contraindicated? Is this patient at any increased risk for fractures, anemia, bleeding, etc.?

3) What are the long-term goals for the patient?

4) What is the long-term prognosis for the patient? What type of progress can I expect from the patient?

5) Is the patient on any medications that will affect his/her exercise performance?

enhance ability to accomplish daily activities of living and allow the individual to return to work (ACSM, 1997):

> ➤ *Cardiorespiratory endurance:* Increase peak VO₂max and endurance.
> ➤ *Muscular strength and endurance:* Increase muscle strength, endurance and mass.
> ➤ *Flexibility:* Increase range of motion of major joints, especially those affected by the disease process.
> ➤ *Neuromuscular:* Improve balance, hand-eye and foot-eye coordination, and walking gait.

In the early 1980s, Dr. Meryl Winningham developed aerobic testing and training programs for cancer patients (Winningham et al., 1986). Her Winningham Aerobic Interval Training (WAIT) scale was created to engage patients in moderate aerobic training in a work-rest interval program, providing a progressive increase in overall aerobic fitness levels.

In 1994, an exercise and wellness program for cancer patients was started at the Santa Barbara Athletic Club (SBAC) (Durak & Lilly, 1997). The SBAC program is provided as a

community service for cancer patients who are referred from a local cancer treatment center. The program focuses on three components: aerobic, strength and stretching/relaxation. The aerobics component includes ergometer and treadmill exercise, and group walks. The strength component builds upper- and lower-body strength with machine weights. Those with special needs use resistance exercise bands or manual resistance from trainers. A typical program is as follows:

Cardiorespiratory endurance:
• Warm-up (5 minutes)
• Treadmill, stationary cycle or group walking (10-25 minutes)

Muscular strength and endurance:
• Bench press, lat pulls (2-4 sets, 6-10 reps)
• Shoulder press, T-rows (1-2 sets, 10 reps)
• Biceps, triceps, abdominals (1-2 sets, 10 reps)
• Leg press, leg extensions (2-3 sets, 6-10 reps)
• Leg curls, toe extensions (1-2 sets, 10 reps)
• Elastic band exercises, personal trainer exercises for specific cancer types (as needed)

Relaxation/flexibility:
• Stretching exercises (5-10 minutes, all major joints)
• Breathing, visualization, yoga (5-10 minutes)

Dimeo et al. (1997b) used a progressive, interval training treadmill walking program in their randomized six-week study of 32 cancer patients who had completed a regimen of high dose chemotherapy. Patients exercised at 80 percent of maximal heart rate, five times per week. The duration of each exercise session progressively increased according to the following regimen:

> *Week 1:* five three-minute sessions (three minutes walking at half-speed between intervals)
> *Week 2:* four five-minute sessions
> *Week 3:* three eight-minute sessions
> *Week 4:* three 10-minute sessions
> *Week 5:* two 15-minute sessions
> *Week 6:* one 30-minute session

Dimeo et al. (1997b) suggest that intensive aerobic exercise may be contraindicated, especially in patients with infections, fever, malnourishment or bony metastases. These inves-

Figure 14.2

Five-year survival rates for cancer are much improved if cancer is detected early before spreading to distant sites.

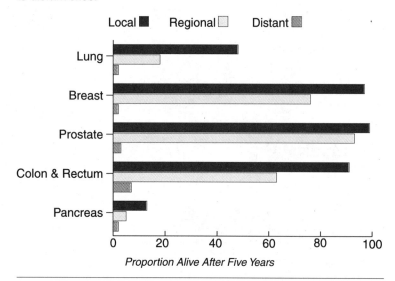

Source: American Cancer Society, 1997

tigators feel that assessment of hematopoietic function is indispensable before starting an aerobic training program. To diminish the risk of hemorrhages and infections, patients should not start training until their platelet counts surpass 20 x 109/L, and their leukocyte counts 1.5 x 109/L. Although anemia is sometimes used as a contraindication to aerobic exercise training, Dimeo et al. (1997b) feel that this would exclude nearly all cancer patients who have undergone high dose chemotherapy. Because in their study exercise was linked to an improvement in iron status, they recommend that cancer patients with anemia be allowed to exercise aerobically (using gradual progression as summarized above).

There is some concern that intensive exercise engaged in for extended periods may be detrimental (Kent, 1996). Several studies suggest that in animals, intense, forced, high-volume exercise enhances the spread of certain types of cancer (Cohen et al., 1988; Hoffman-Goetz & Husted, 1994). Data in humans is lacking, and as a result, most health professionals err on the side of caution when advising patients about exercise intensity, duration and frequency (Kent, 1996; Dimeo et al., 1997b). Until more is known, it would be prudent to urge cancer patients undergoing treatment to exercise moderately each day, and to avoid unusually prolonged and intensive exercise.

Exercise Training Benefits for the Cancer Patient

Several reports from the literature indicate that cancer patients benefit physiologically and psychologically from regular exercise during and after treatment (Friendenreich & Cour-

neya, 1996). For the cancer patient undergoing treatment (e.g., chemotherapy), exercise can help counter feelings of fatigue and anxiety, and loss of muscular and cardiorespiratory fitness. For cancer survivors, a fitness program can help them regain their former state of health and function (and more, depending on their initial status).

Researchers from Germany have studied the feasibility and effects of aerobic training in the rehabilitation of cancer patients after completing high dose chemotherapy (Dimeo et al., 1997a,b). In two studies, Dimeo et al. (1997a,b) have shown that daily, moderate aerobic activity (30 minutes of biking on an ergometer in the supine position, or treadmill walking) can be safely performed immediately after high dose chemotherapy, and helps prevent loss of cardiorespiratory fitness. According to these researchers, "to reduce fatigue, this group of patients should be counseled to increase physical activity rather than rest after treatment."

Researchers from Ohio State University and Johns Hopkins Hospital have also demonstrated that breast cancer patients undergoing chemotherapy can improve aerobic power and reduce symptoms of fatigue and anxiety by exercising regularly (cycle ergometry exercise and walking) (MacVicar et al., 1989; Mock et al., 1997).

The Santa Barbara Athletic Club (mentioned previously) provides an exercise training program for cancer patients who are referred from a local cancer treatment center (Durak & Lilly, 1997). The program focuses on three components — aerobic, strength and stretching/ relaxation. Results show that cancer patients can experience strong gains in aerobic fitness and upper- and lower-body strength. Patients also

---

Table 14.7

Typical Activity Guidelines

- ■ Try to maintain some kind of exercise through the treatment process. This will help to preserve muscle mass and can provide a psychological boost.

- ■ Be careful not to push too hard. If you feel fatigued more than an hour past your exercise session, you probably pushed too hard.

- ■ Once you have recovered from the cancer and/or the treatment, you can gradually increase your activity up to your desired intensity and duration.

- ■ Find out if your doctor has any concerns about any of your exercise or physical activity plans.

reported improvement in ability to engage in household tasks and recreational activities.

In a study performed in Sweden, researchers assigned 200 cancer patients either to the "Starting Again" program or to the control condition (Berglund et al., 1994). The program emphasized physical training, information and coping skills. According to the researchers from the Karolinska Hospital in Stockholm, the patients in the program experienced greater physical strength and an improved mood state than those in the control condition.

Researchers at Wake Forest University in North Carolina randomized 16 breast cancer survivors to exercise and nonexercise groups (Nieman et al., 1995). Exercise training consisted of 60 minutes of supervised weight training and aerobic activity, three times a week for eight weeks. Improvements in various measures of aerobic and strength tests were reported, demonstrating that breast cancer survivors are capable of engaging in exercise programs normally prescribed to individuals without cancer.

Can exercise training improve long-term survival in cancer patients? Few studies have been conducted in this area. In one study, researchers followed 451 breast cancer patients for an average of five to six years. During that time, patients reported their weekly levels of light, moderate and vigorous physical activity (Rohan et al., 1995). No link between exercise habits and survival from breast cancer could be measured. Animal research has determined that breast cancer risk is decreased by exercise during the earliest stages of cancer formation, but not after the cancer has become established (Hoffman-Goetz & Husted, 1994).

There are several potential mechanisms whereby exercise training might have a favorable influence on the prognosis of breast cancer patients. Higher body mass has been linked to an adverse effect on life expectancy in women with breast carcinoma (Stoll, 1996). Physical exercise is an important component in the management of obesity (Shephard, 1993, 1995). Regular physical exercise also reduces insulin and estrogen levels, helping to counter the effect these hormones have in supporting breast carcinoma growth (Stoll, 1996). Clinical trials are currently underway to more fully measure the role of physical exercise and weight management on the prognosis of breast cancer patients.

Medications and Disease-specific Limitations

Cancer therapy has major physiological and psychological effects on the patient. Cancer patients and survivors may have disease- or treatment-specific obstacles to exercise training, according to ACSM (1997). Some side effects of anti-cancer treatment are acute (e.g., inflammatory lung tissue responses and impaired oxygen transfer to radiation), while others are delayed (e.g., radiation-induced lung scarring or daunorubicin-induced cardiomyopathy months after treatment). Further research with cancer patients is needed to determine the effect some of these drugs have on the ability to exercise. Dimeo et al. (1997b) have demonstrated that cancer patients with no signs of impaired cardiac function after high dose chemotherapy and autologous peripheral blood stem cell transplantation can participate in an aerobic training program without fear of cardiac complications, despite their recent exposure to potentially cardiotoxic agents.

➤ Surgery can cause pain, loss of flexibility, amputation, and motor and sensory nerve damage.

➤ Radiation can cause loss of flexibility in irradiated joints and cardiac or lung scarring, or both.

➤ Chemotherapy uses several drugs that have characteristic side effects:
- *Vinca alkaloids*—Vincristine, Velban (effects include peripheral nerve damage)
- *Daunorubicin*—Cerubidine (effects include cardiomyopathy)
- *Doxorubicin*—Adriamycin (effects include cardiomyopathy)
- *Mitoxantrone*—Novantrone (effects include cardiomyopathy)
- *Bleomycin*—Blenoxane (effects include pulmonary fibrosis)
- *Corticosteroids*—Decadron, prednisone (effects include myopathy)
- *Most chemotherapy drugs*—(effects include anemia)

Case Study 1

Data from Medical/Health Questionnaire

Age: 45 years; *Height:* 64 inches; *Weight:* 165 pounds; *Sex:* Female; *Desired weight:* 130 pounds

Smoking status: quit 9 years ago

Exercise habits: sedentary both at work and during leisure for all of adult life.

Family history of disease: mother developed breast cancer at age 52 years; father developed heart disease at age 55 years.

Personal history of disease: developed breast cancer at age 43. The left breast was removed, and chemotherapy and radiation treatment were successful in removing the cancer. During the two years of treatment, the patient gained 20 pounds of body weight, and experienced significant loss of aerobic and muscular fitness.

Signs or symptoms suggestive of cardiopulmonary or metabolic disease: negative

Dietary habits: fruits/vegetables, 2 serving/day (low); cereals/grains, 5/day (low and refined)

Personal goals: gain back original energy levels, lose weight, improve appearance and muscle tone, decrease risk of heart disease

Preferred modes of aerobic exercise: brisk walking, stationary bicycling

Data from Physical Fitness Testing Session (Physician's Office and Fitness Center)

Resting heart rate: 81 bpm (poor)

Resting blood pressure: 150/98 mm Hg (mild hypertension) (from 2 measurements on 2 days)

Serum cholesterol: 260 mg/dl (high risk)

HDL-cholesterol: 33 mg/dl (low)

Cholesterol/HDL-cholesterol ratio: 7.9 (high risk)

Percent body fat: 37 percent (obese)

VO_2max: estimated from Bruce treadmill test with EKG—24 ml•kg•min (low); EKG, negative

Sit-and-reach flexibility test: -2 inches from footline (fair)

Hand grip dynamometer (sum of right and left hands): 55 kg (below average)

Comments

Using the medical/health questionnaire and laboratory data from recent testing, this breast cancer client was also classified as an "individual at increased risk" for heart disease using ACSM criteria.

This classification was given because she has two or more major coronary risk factors (family history, hypertension, hypercholesterolemia, sedentary lifestyle). Due to the number of risk factors and family history of coronary heart disease, and the client's desire to engage in moderate-to-vigorous exercise, a medical exam and diagnostic exercise test were recommended. The treadmill-EKG test was negative (no evidence of ischemia or arrhythmias), and physician clearance was given for the client to begin a moderate exercise program with gradual progression. Additional physical fitness tests were conducted at a fitness center to determine body composition and musculoskeletal fitness.

Recommended Exercise Program

The cancer rehabilitation program initiated by the Santa Barbara Athletic Club is recommended for this breast cancer patient (Durak & Lilly, 1997).

Cardiorespiratory endurance:

- Warm-up (5 minutes)
- Treadmill, stationary cycle or group walking (10-25 minutes)

Muscular strength and endurance:

- Bench press, lat pulls (2-4 sets, 6-10 reps)
- Shoulder press, T-rows (1-2 sets, 10 reps)
- Biceps, triceps, abdominals (1-2 sets, 10 reps)
- Leg press, leg extensions (2-3 sets, 6-10 reps)
- Leg curls, toe extensions (1-2 sets, 10 reps)
- Elastic band exercises, personal trainer exercises for specific cancer types (as needed)

Relaxation/flexibility:

- Stretching exercises (5-10 minutes, all major joints)
- Breathing, visualization, yoga (5-10 minutes)

During the first month, have the client warm up with range-of-motion calisthenics and walking for five minutes, followed by 15 minutes of brisk walking and/or stationary cycling at 50 percent to 60 percent heart rate reserve, three days per week. After warming down, the client should engage in resistance exercise for 20 to 30 minutes, starting with one set. Give special attention to the left chest area, using elastic band butterfly movements. End with static stretching activities for five to 10 minutes, followed by 10 minutes of yoga.

After the first month, gradually increase the duration of brisk walking and/or cycling to 25 minutes per session, and the frequency to five days per week. The intensity of exercise can also be gradually increased to 70 percent of heart rate reserve. These increases, along with careful control of dietary habits, will help ensure a steady weight loss of about 1 pound per week. Since the client has 35 pounds of body fat to lose, ideal body weight should be attained after approximately one-half year of training. This degree of weight loss combined with improvements in physical fitness should help improve muscle tone and aerobic fitness, and bring both hypertension and hypercholesterolemia under control if improvements in dietary quality are made (i.e., less saturated fat and cholesterol, more fruits, vegetables and whole grains, less sodium and alcohol). The client has a high risk of coronary heart disease, and it is imperative that the risk factors be brought under control through weight loss and dietary and exercise lifestyle changes. Enlist the services of a dietitian to ensure adherence to an anti-atherogenic diet.

Retest every three months to help ensure motivation and attainment of goals. Long-term compliance can be enhanced by encouraging family support, goal setting and contracting, establishing rewards for attainment of goals, and combating time obstacles.

Case Study 2

Data from Medical/Health Questionnaire

Age: 25 years; *Height:* 70 inches; *Weight:* 165 pounds; *Sex:* Male; *Desired weight:* 165 pounds
Smoking status: never smoked
Exercise habits: prior to the cancer, running 90 miles per week. Competed successfully at the regional level in 10km and 15km road races (personal best time of 29:30 in the 10km).
Family history of disease: none in parents or siblings.
Personal history of disease: Testicular cancer was diagnosed two months ago. The left testicle and 35 lymph nodes from the groin to the lungs were removed through surgery. Biopsies revealed some spread of cancer cells, and a 12-week chemotherapy regimen was initiated to kill the cancer but prevent scarring of the lungs (to preserve his running career). The chemotherapy has been successful thus far, and the levels of proteins in the blood that are produced by the cancer have dropped to nearly undetectable levels. Doctors put his chances of full recovery at 85 percent. Between chemotherapy sessions (every two weeks), the patient has attempted to put in 30 to 45 minutes a day of moderate running. Nonetheless,

the patient complains of a lack of strength and energy, and has lost 10 pounds of fat free mass (nausea has diminished appetite).

Personal goals: gain back original energy levels and muscle weight; slowly build back to original aerobic fitness and competitive running level.

Data from Physical Fitness Testing Session (Physician's Office and Fitness Center)

Resting heart rate: 40 bpm (excellent)
Resting blood pressure: 110/65 mm Hg (excellent)
Serum cholesterol: 160 mg/dl (excellent)
HDL-cholesterol: 60 mg/dl (excellent)
Percent body fat: 6 percent (very lean)
VO_2max: Series of treadmill-graded exercise tests prior to development of the cancer indicated a VO_2max of 70 ml.kg.-1min-1.
1-RM bench press test: 0.75 of body weight (fair)

Comments

The decision is made to build back muscle mass through a progressive, weight training program (eight different exercises, 10 to 12 reps, one set for the first two weeks, building up to two to three sets over the next month). The patient agrees to report to the health/fitness club every three days for these weight-training sessions under the guidance of an advanced personal trainer. Emphasis is placed on a total body regimen. The patient also agrees to see a dietitian to adopt a diet compatible with cancer treatment.

A progressive running program is established (between chemotherapy sessions), and the patient agrees to avoid intensive running sessions until chemotherapy has been completed. Following successful treatment, the patient will allow four to six months of progressive training (and retesting) until resuming intensive training, and then finally competitive racing.

References

American Cancer Society. (1997). *Cancer Facts & Figures - 1997.* Atlanta: Author.

American Cancer Society. (1996). Guidelines on diet, nutrition, and cancer prevention: Reducing the risk of cancer with healthy food choices and physical activity. *CA: A Cancer Journal for Clinicians, 46,* 325-341.

American College of Sports Medicine. (1997). *ACSM's Exercise Management for Persons with Chronic Diseases and Disabilities.* Champaign, Ill.: Human Kinetics.

American Institute for Cancer Research. (1997). Prevention of cancer: A global priority. *Vegetarian Nutrition: An International Journal,* 1, 112.

Berglund, G., Bolund, C., Gustafsson, U.L. & Sjoden, P.O. (1994). One-year follow-up of the 'Starting Again' group rehabilitation program for cancer patients. *European Journal of Cancer,* 30A, 1744-1751.

Cohen, L.A., Choi, K. & Wang, C.X. (1988). Influence of dietary fat, caloric restriction, and voluntary exercise in N-nitrosomethylurea induced mammary tumorigenesis in rats. *Cancer Research,* 48, 4276, 4283.

Cole, P. & Rodu, B. (1996). Declining cancer mortality in the United States. *Cancer,* 78, 2045-2048.

Courneya, K.S. & Friedenreich, C.M. (1997). Relationship between exercise pattern across the cancer experience and current quality of life in colorectal cancer survivors. *Journal of Alternative and Complementary Medicine,* 3, 215-226.

Demark-Wahnefried, W., Hars, V., Conaway, M.R., Havlin, K., Rimer B.K., McElveen, G. & Winer, E.P. (1997). Reduced rates of metabolism and decreased physical activity in breast cancer patients receiving adjuvant chemotherapy. *American Journal of Clinical Nutrition,* 65, 1495-14501.

Dimeo, F., Fetscher, S., Lange, W., Mertelsmann, R. & Keul, J. (1997a). Effects of aerobic exercise on the physical performance and incidence of treatment-related complications after high-dose chemotherapy. *Blood,* 90, 3390-3394.

Dimeo, F.C., Tilmann, M.H., Bertz, H., Kanz, L., Mertelsmann, R. & Keul, J. (1997b). Aerobic exercise in the rehabilitation of cancer patients after high dose chemotherapy and autologous peripheral stem cell transplantation. *Cancer,* 79, 1717-1722.

Friendenreich, C.M. & Courneya, K.S. (1996). Exercise as rehabilitation for cancer patients. *Clinical Journal of Sports Medicine,* 6, 237-244.

Gerhardsson, D.V.M. (1997). Physical activity in the prevention and management of cancer. *World Review of Nutrition and Diet,* 82, 240-249.

Hoffman-Goetz, L. & Husted, J. (1994). Exercise and breast cancer: Review and critical analysis of the literature. *Canadian Journal of Applied Physiology,* 19, 237-252.

Hovi, L., Era, P., Rautonen, J. & Siimes, M.A. (1993). Impaired muscle strength in female adolescents and young adults surviving leukemia in childhood. *Cancer,* 72, 276-281.

Kent, H. (1996). Breast-cancer survivors begin to challenge exercise taboos. *CMAJ,* 155, 969-971.

Leddy, S.K. (1997). Incentives and barriers to exercise in women with a history of breast cancer. *Oncology Nursing Forum,* 24, 885-890.

Lee, I.-M. (1995). Exercise and physical health: Cancer and immune function. *Research Quarterly of Exercise and Sport,* 66, 286-291.

Lee, I.-M. (1994). Physical activity, fitness and cancer. Bouchard, C., Shephard, R.J. & Stephens, T. (eds.) *Physical Activity, Fitness, and Health: International Proceedings and Consensus Statement.* Champaign, Ill.: Human Kinetics.

MacNeil, B. & Hoffman Goetz, L. (1993). Chronic exercise enhances in vivo and in vitro cytotoxic mechanisms of natural immunity in mice. *Journal of Applied Physiology,* 74, 388, 395.

MacVicar, M.G., Winningham, M.L. & Nickel, J.L. (1989). Effects of aerobic interval training on cancer patients' functional capacity. *Nursing Research,* 38, 348-351.

Martinez, M.E., Giovannucci, E., Spiegelman, D., Hunter, D.J., Willett, W.C. & Colditz, G.A. (1997). Leisure-time physical activity, body size, and colon cancer in women. *Journal of the National Cancer Institute,* 89, 948-955.

Mock, V., Dow, K.H., Meares, C.J., Grimm, P.M., Dienemann, J.A., Haisfield-Wolfe, M.E., Quitasol, W., Mitchell, S., Chakravarthy, A. & Gage, I. (1997). Effects of exercise on fatigue, physical functioning, and emotional distress during radiation therapy for breast cancer. *Oncology Nursing Forum,* 24, 991-1000.

Monga, U., Jaweed, M., Kerrigan, A.J., Lawhon, L., Johnson, J., Valibona, C. & Monga, T.N. (1997). Neuromuscular fatigue in prostate cancer patients undergoing radiation therapy. *Archives of Physical Medicine and Rehabilitation,* 78, 961-966.

National Center for Health Statistics. (1997). *Health, United States,* 1996-97 and *Injury Chartbook.* Hyattsville: Author.

Nieman, D.C., Cook, V.D., Henson, D.A., Suttles, J., Rejeski, W.J., Ribisl, P.M., Fagoaga, O.R. & Nehslen-Cannarella, S.L. (1995). Moderate exercise training and natural killer cell cytotoxic activity in breast cancer patients. *International Journal of Sports Medicine,* 16, 334-337.

Parker, S.L., Tong, T., Bolden, S. & Wingo, P.A. (1997). Cancer statistics, 1997. *CA: A Cancer Journal for Clinicians,* 47, 5-27, 1997.

Pihkala, J., Happonen, J.M., Virtanen, K., Sovijarvi, A., Siimes, M.A., Pesonen, E. & Saarinen, U.M. (1995). Cardiopulmonary evaluation of exercise tolerance after chest irradiation and anticancer chemotherapy in children and adolescents. *Pediatrics,* 95, 722-726.

Roebuck, B.D., McCaffrey, J. & Baumgartner, K.J. (1990). Protective effects of voluntary exercise during the postinitiation phase of pancreatic carcinogenesis in the rat. *Cancer Research,* 50, 6811, 6816.

Rohan, T.E., Fu, W. & Hiller, J.E. (1995). Physical activity and survival from breast cancer. *European Journal of Cancer Prevention,* 4, 419-424.

Shephard, R.J. (1995). Exercise and cancer: Linkages with obesity? *International Journal of Obesity,* 19(suppl. 4), S62-S68.

Shephard, R.J. (1993). Exercise in the prevention and treatment of cancer. An Update. *Sports Medicine,* 15, 258, 280.

Smith, S.L. (1996). Physical exercise as an oncology nursing intervention to enhance quality of life. *Oncology Nursing Forum,* 23, 771-778.

Stoll, B.A. (1996). Diet and exercise regimens to improve breast carcinoma prognosis. *Cancer,* 78, 2465-2470.

Thompson, H.J., Westerlind, K.C., Snedden, J.R., Briggs, S. & Singh, M. (1995). Inhibition of mammary carcinogenesis by treadmill exercise. *Journal of the National Cancer Institute,* 87, 453-455.

Thompson, H.J. (1994). Effect of exercise intensity and duration on the induction of mammary carcinogenesis. *Cancer Research,* 54 (7 suppl.), 1960S-1963S.

Thune, I., Brenn, T., Lund, E. & Gaard, M. (1997). Physical activity and the risk of breast cancer. *New England Journal of Medicine,* 336, 1269-1275.

Winningham, M.L., MacVicar, M.G. & Burke, C.A. (1986). Exercise for cancer patients: Guidelines and precautions. *The Physician and Sportsmedicine,* 14, 10, 152-157.

U.S. Department of Health and Human Services. (1996). *Physical Activity and Health: A Report of the Surgeon General.* Atlanta, GA: U.S. Department of Health and Human Services, Centers for Disease Control and Prevention, National Center for Chronic Disease Prevention and Health Promotion.

Woods, J.A. & Davis, J.M. (1994). Exercise, monocyte/macrophage function, and cancer. *Medicine and Science in Sports and Exercise,* 26, 147-156.

Suggested Reading

American College of Sports Medicine. (1997). *ACSM's Exercise Management for Persons with Chronic Diseases and Disabilities.* Champaign, Ill.: Human Kinetics.

Hamann, B.P. (1994). *Disease: Identification, Prevention, and Control.* St. Louis, Mo.: Mosby.

Nieman, D.C. (1999). *Exercise Testing and Prescription: A Health-Related Approach* (4th ed.). Mountain View: Mayfield Publishing Company.

Rothstein, J.M., Roy, S.H. & Wolf, S.L. (1998). *The Rehabilitation Specialist's Handbook* (2nd ed.). Philadelphia, Pa.: E.A. Davis Company.

Torg, J.S. & Shephard, R.J. (1995). *Current Therapy in Sports Medicine* (3rd ed.). St. Louis, Mo.: Mosby.

CHAPTER 15

Arthritis

DAVID C. NIEMAN

David C. Nieman, Dr. P.H., F.A.C.S.M., is a professor of health and exercise science at Appalachian State University in Boone, N.C. He has taught at the college and university level since 1972, and is the author of five textbooks and more than 120 research articles in the areas of sports medicine, exercise and health, exercise immunology, sports nutrition and obesity.

Osteoarthritis
Complications in Exercise
Rheumatoid Arthritis

Arthritis and other rheumatic conditions are among the most prevalent chronic conditions in the United States, affecting an estimated 40 million persons in 1995 (one in seven) and a projected 60 million by 2020, according to the Centers for Disease Control and Prevention (CDC) (CDC, 1996 a,b; Strange, 1996). Women are affected by arthritis more than men — nearly two-thirds of people with arthritis are women. Arthritis is the No. 1 cause of disability in America, and limits everyday activities such as dressing, climbing stairs, getting in and out of bed, or walking for about 7 million Americans.

Arthritis means joint inflammation, a general term that includes more than 100 kinds of rheumatic diseases (Arthritis Foundation, 1996; Harris, 1993). Rheumatic diseases are those affecting joints, muscles and connective tissue, which make up or support various structures of the body. Arthritis is usually chronic and lasts a lifetime. The early warning signs of arthritis include pain, swelling and limited movement that lasts for more than two weeks.

The most common type of arthritis is osteoarthritis, affecting more than 16 million Americans, about half of whom are age 65 or older (CDC, 1996 a,b; Arthritis Foundation, 1996) (Table 15.1). Although this degenerative joint disease is common among the elderly, it may appear decades earlier. **Osteoarthritis** begins when joint cartilage breaks down, sometimes eroding entirely to leave a bone-on-bone joint. The joint then loses shape, bone ends thicken, and spurs (bony growths) develop. Any joint can be affected, but the feet, knees, hips and fingers are most common.

Osteoarthritis is not fatal, but it is incurable, with few effective treatments. Symptoms of pain and stiffness can persist for long periods, leading to difficulty in walking, stair climbing, rising from a chair, transferring in and out of a car, and lifting and carrying.

The second most common form of **arthritis** is **rheumatoid arthritis,** an autoimmune disease that affects 2.5 million Americans, three times more women than men (CDC, 1996 a,b; Arthritis Foundation, 1996; Semble, 1995). It can strike at any age, but usually appears between ages 20 and 50. Rheumatoid arthritis starts slowly over several weeks to months. The small joints of the hands and the knee joint are most commonly affected, but it can affect most joints of the body. In general, rheumatoid arthritis is frequently related to severe complications and decline in ability to function, with most patients dying 10 to 15 years earlier than those who are non-afflicted.

Many joints of the body have a tough capsule lined with a synovial membrane that seals the joint and provides a lubricating fluid. In rheumatoid arthritis, inflammation begins in the synovial lining of the joint and can spread to the entire joint. The inflamed joint lining leads to damage of the bone and cartilage. The space between joints diminishes, and the joint loses shape and alignment. Highly variable (some sufferers become bedridden, others can run marathons) and difficult to control, the disease can severely deform joints. Depending on functional capacity,

rheumatoid arthritis can be divided into four classes (Hochberg, 1992):

➤ **Class I** — Completely able to perform usual activities of daily living (self-care, vocational and avocational).

➤ **Class II** — Able to perform usual self-care and vocational activities, but limited in avocational activities.

➤ **Class III** — Able to perform usual self-care activities, but limited in vocational and avocational activities.

➤ **Class IV** — Limited in ability to perform usual self-care, vocational and avocational activities.

Other common types of arthritis include **gout** (a metabolic disorder leading to high uric acid and crystal formation in joints), **ankylosing spondylitis** (inflammatory disease of the spine that can result in fused vertebrae and rigid spine), **juvenile arthritis** (involving 200,000 American children), **psoriatic arthritis** (affecting about 5 percent of people with psoriasis, a chronic skin disease), and systemic **lupus** erythematosus (symptoms usually appear in women of childbearing age) (Arthritis Foundation, 1996).

Treatment of Arthritis

The key to treatment of arthritis is early diagnosis and a plan that is individualized to the needs of each patient (Arthritis Foundation, 1996; Semble, 1995). Therapy of arthritis has four major goals:

➤ ease of pain
➤ decrease of pain inflammation
➤ improvement in function
➤ lessening of joint damage

Most treatment programs include a combination of patient education, medication, exercise, rest, use of heat and cold, joint protection tech-

Table 15.1
Common Forms of Arthritis and Prevalence*

Arthritis Type	# of Cases, U.S.	Commonly Affected Joints
Osteoarthritis	16 million	Hands, spine, hips, knees
Rheumatoid arthritis	2.5 million	Wrist, hands, knees, feet, cervical spine
Gout	1 million	Great toe, ankles, knees, wrists
Ankylosing spondylitis	318,000	Spine, hip, shoulder girdle, knees
Juvenile arthritis	200,000	Wrist, hands, knees, feet, cervical spine
Psoriatic arthritis	160,000	Spine, hip, shoulder girdle, knees
Lupus	131,000	Hands, knees, elbows, feet

Coping with arthritis in its many forms. *FDA Consumer: The Official Magazine of the Food and Drug Administration*, 3, 17-21 (1996).

* See text for a description

niques and sometimes surgery (for example, total hip replacement surgery). Total hip arthroplasty (THA) is commonly used to treat severe osteoarthritis of the hip, with more than 120,000 such operations performed each year in the U.S. (Chang et al., 1996).

The Arthritis Foundation (1996) guidelines advise that treatment include:

➤ **Lifestyle changes.** Exercise to strengthen muscles, weight loss to reduce stress on joints, and assistive devices such as canes and wall bars when needed.

➤ **Pain management.** Physical therapy, acetaminophen as first-line therapy; prescription drugs or surgery for more severe pain.

➤ **Patient education.** To inform patients about the disease, provide tools to help overcome pain and help them adjust to their situation.

Arthritis symptoms come and go. A worsening or reappearance of the disease is called a **flare.** This can be followed by a remission period that brings welcomed relief. During a flare-up, physical activity is painful and difficult. The normal up-and-down nature of this painful, incurable disease has led to widespread fraud and quackery (Arthritis Foundation, 1996). People with arthritis spend nearly $1 billion per year on unproven remedies, diets and supplements. Arthritis patients have been lured by an astounding array of quack devices, including copper or magnetic bracelets, electronic mechanisms, vibrating chairs, pressurized edema devices, snake venom and countless nutritional supplements including cod liver oil, alfalfa, pokeberries, vinegar, iodine and kelp. While some of these remedies seem harmless, they can become dangerous if they cause people to abandon conventional therapy.

The FDA also cautions that diet has little to do with arthritis (Strange, 1996). Gout is the only **rheumatic disease** known to be helped by avoiding certain foods. Regarding diet, the American College of Rheumatology advises that until more data is available, patients should continue to follow balanced and healthful diets, be skeptical of miraculous claims and avoid elimination diets and fad nutritional practices.

Overweight persons are at high risk of osteoarthritis in the knee, hips and hands (Felson, 1996). For example, the heaviest Americans (those in the upper 20 percent of body weight) have seven to 10 times the risk of developing osteoarthritis of the knee than those of normal weight. Weight control is an important concern for people with arthritis to help decrease the pressure on the knees and hips.

Medications for Arthritis Treatment

There are many different kinds of drugs used to treat arthritis (Strange, 1996; Arthritis Foundation, 1996; O'Dell et al., 1996). Anti-inflammatory agents generally work by slowing the body's production of prostaglandins, substances that play a role in inflammation. The most familiar anti-inflammatory agent is aspirin, often a good arthritis treatment. Acetaminophen is recommended as a first-line therapy, at doses up to 4,000 milligrams a day. More than a dozen nonsteroidal anti-inflammatory drugs (NSAIDS) are available (most by prescription only) to fight pain and inflammation. The FDA has approved three NSAIDS for over-the-counter marketing: ibuprofen (marketed as Advil, Nuprin, Motrin and others), naproxen sodium (sold as Aleve) and ketoprofen (marketed as Actron and Orudis). The most potent anti-inflammatories are corticosteroids.

Disease-modifying drugs are also prescribed by doctors to slow rheumatoid arthritis (Strange, 1996). These drugs are now used early in the course of the illness to slow disease advancement. Gold salts, penicillamine, methotrexate, hydroxychloroquine, sulfasalazine and other powerful drugs often used in combination, are prescribed to help suppress the immune system.

Role of Exercise in Treatment of Arthritis

In the past, doctors often advised arthritis patients to rest and avoid exercise (Hoffman, 1993; DiNubile, 1997; Ytterberg et al., 1994; Panush, 1994). Rest remains important, especially during flares. But inactivity can lead to weak muscles, stiff joints, reduced joint range of motion, and decreased energy and vitality. Rheumatologists today routinely advise a balance of physical activity and rest, individualized to meet special patient needs.

Arthritis

As a clinical exercise specialist, you should work within a multidisciplinary setting that offers preventive, medical and rehabilitative care. Patient safety, health and physical fitness development can best be achieved by ongoing consultation with healthcare providers experienced in rheumatologic care and rehabilitation.

Client Assessment of Physical Fitness

Studies have consistently shown that people with arthritis have weaker muscles, less joint flexibility and range of motion, and lower aerobic capacity compared to those without arthritis (Hoffman, 1993). In addition, individuals with arthritis have been found to be at higher risk for several other chronic diseases including coronary heart disease, diabetes mellitus and osteoporosis. Thus, it makes sense that a well-rounded physical fitness program may be of benefit to those suffering from arthritis. Prior to initiating an exercise program, however, each patient should have an extensive evaluation to assess the severity and extent of joint involvement, presence of systemic involvement, overall functional capacity, and presence of other medical conditions that may interfere with exercise (DiNubile, 1997).

The ACSM (1997) recommends the following exercise testing program for patients with arthritis:

➤ **Muscular strength and endurance:** Use isokinetic machines at 90-120E/second to measure the strength and endurance of major muscle groups.
➤ **Aerobic endurance:** Various walking tests including the six-minute walk or the one-mile walk test.
➤ **Joint flexibility and range of motion:** Use a goniometer to measure joint range of motion. Assess asymmetry.
➤ **Neuromuscular fitness:** Gait analysis may be necessary for people who have severe disease, altered biomechanics and a need for orthotics. Also assess balance.
➤ **Functional capacity:** Assess capacity to accomplish activities of daily living by observing ability to walk with balance and symmetry, ability to sit and then stand up several times, and ability to stand in one place without difficulty.

Exercise Programming and Leadership for Patients with Arthritis

Individuals with arthritis will often respond to their pain by limiting physical activity (CDC, 1997). Over time, this leads to loss of muscle strength and endurance, further weakening the joints and leading to a vicious cycle that accelerates arthritis. Thus, one of the chief goals of exercise training for the patient with arthritis is to counter the effects of inactivity (ACSM, 1997). There are three objectives of exercise for patients with arthritis (Ytterberg et al., 1994):

➤ Preserve or restore range of motion and flexibility around each affected joint.
➤ Increase muscle strength and endurance to enhance joint stability.
➤ Increase aerobic conditioning to improve psychological mood state and decrease risk of disease.

As depicted in Figure 15.1, the exercise program should be organized according to the exercise pyramid, with exercises that develop joint range of motion and flexibility providing the foundation (Hoffman, 1993).

➤ **Range-of-motion and stretching exercises:** Maintaining joint mobility is very important for all patients with arthritis. Loss of joint range of motion results in a tightening of surrounding tendons, muscles and other tissues. Acutely inflamed joints should be put through gentle range-of-motion exercises several times a day with the assistance of a therapist or trained family member. Overzealous stretching or improper technique can cause harmful effects on a joint, especially if it is inflamed or unstable. Utilizing a trained therapist to initially monitor and teach the patient proper technique is recommended. Once the joints become less inflamed, the patient can gradually work up to several sets of 10 repetitions daily of stretching and range-of-motion exercises.
➤ **Muscle strengthening:** Both isometric and isotonic strengthening exercises are recommended. Isometric exercises can build muscle strength without adverse effects on an acutely inflamed joint. Isotonic exercises (e.g., weight lifting, calisthenics) allow the joints to move through a

limited or full range of motion while the muscles are contracting. This type of exercise is recommended when pain and joint inflammation have been controlled and sufficient strength has been achieved through isometric exercise. The ACSM (1997) recommends that patients build up to two to three sessions per week. High-repetition, high-resistance and high-impact muscle strengthening exercises are not recommended.

➤ **Aerobic exercise:** In the past, the treatment of arthritis has often excluded aerobic exercise for fear of increasing joint inflammation and accelerating the disease process. Aerobic exercise, however, has been demonstrated to be a safe and effective treatment for patients who are not in acute flares. Low-impact activities such as swimming, water aerobics, walking, bicycling, low-impact dance aerobics and rowing can improve aerobic fitness without negatively affecting arthritis. Patients should start with 10 to 15 minutes of aerobic activity every other day, gradually progressing toward near daily activity of 30 to 45 minutes duration at a moderate to somewhat-hard intensity. For some patients, exercise can be accumulated throughout the day in several short sessions. Discontinuous exercise (mixture of exercise and rest intervals) should be considered for some patients. Each aerobic session should begin and end with range-of-motion exercises. Stair climbing, running and other high-impact activities should be avoided in patients with arthritic knees or hips. Shoes and insoles should be selected that provide maximum shock attenuation during exercise. Rigid or semi-rigid orthotics should be considered for biomechanical correction at the ankles and knees (ACSM, 1997).

➤ **Recreational exercise:** Golfing, gardening, hiking on gentle terrain and other hobbies requiring physical activity are a few activities patients with arthritis commonly find enjoyable. Many organizations, including the Arthritis Foundation and PACE (People with Arthritis Can Exercise), offer aquatic exercise classes or other group activities. Patients may experience improvements in both fitness and psychological mood state as they engage in group recreational activities.

Complications in Exercise Programming for the Patient with Arthritis

The ACSM has described several potential complications of exercise training for patients with arthritis:

➤ Pain, stiffness, biomechanical inefficiency and gait abnormalities can increase the metabolic cost of physical activity by as much as 50 percent. Patients with arthritis tend to be less physically fit than others and, as a result, gradual progression in exercise training is recommended.

➤ Joint range of motion may be restricted by stiffness, swelling, pain, bone changes, fibrosis and **ankylosis**. It is critical that you adapt the exercise program to ensure joint protection and safety. The site and severity of joint involvement determines the activity mode for both exercise testing and prescription. Deconditioned and poorly supported joints are at high risk for injury from high-impact or poorly controlled movements.

➤ Many patients with arthritis are unable to perform rapid, repetitive movements. Exercise modes should be adapted to the individual patient to protect the involved joints.

➤ Depending on the type of arthritis, consideration should be given to the following complications:

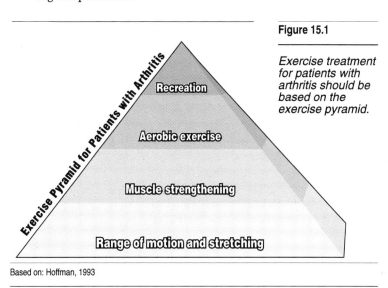

Figure 15.1

Exercise treatment for patients with arthritis should be based on the exercise pyramid.

Based on: Hoffman, 1993

Osteoarthritis: Spinal stenosis, **spondylosis** (causing localized and radiating back pain)
Rheumatoid arthritis: Cervical spine **subluxation** (cervical instability, spinal cord decompression, numbness, tingling, weakness); foot disease (foot pain and instability); wrist and hand disease (pain, instability, loss of grip strength)
Lupus: **Necrosis** of femoral head (hip pain, often associated with long-term corticosteroid use)

Osteoarthritis and Potential Exercise Precautions

Some clinicians have defined osteoarthritis as a wear-and-tear disease, and fear that high amounts of weight-bearing exercise may increase the risk for osteoarthritis (Hannan et al., 1993; Lane et al., 1993 a,b; Rangger et al., 1997). Several important risk factors for osteoarthritis include (Hoffman, 1993):

➤ Increasing age: By age 75, 85 percent of people have evidence of osteoarthritis.

➤ Joint malalignment: If the joint is not aligned correctly, a smaller contact area may create stresses that exceed the shock-absorbing capabilities of the joint.

➤ Obesity: Several studies have suggested that obesity increases the risk of osteoarthritis.

➤ Repetitive impact to the joint.

Together, these risk factors and animal studies appear to suggest that osteoarthritis is a wear-and-tear disease. Some animal studies have suggested that animals trained intensely for long periods have more osteoarthritis (Hoffman, 1993). For example, the Husky breed of dogs has increased hip and shoulder arthritis from pulling sleds, while racehorses and workhorses can develop arthritis in their forelegs and hind legs, respectively. Good evidence to confirm these findings in humans is lacking. Earlier studies had suggested that repetitive trauma to joints during work may lead to arthritis. For example, some studies reported increased osteoarthritis in the elbows and knees of miners, the shoulders and elbows of pneumatic drill operators, the hands of cotton workers and diamond cutters, and the spines of dock workers. However, not all these studies were carried out to contemporary standards, nor have they been confirmed.

Many athletic endeavors place tremendous stress on joints. Baseball, football, basketball, gymnastics, soccer, wrestling and ballet dancing have each been studied for their effect on osteoarthritis (Hannan et al., 1993; Lane et al., 1993 a,b; Rangger et al., 1997). There are many anecdotal reports of famous athletes developing arthritis. Los Angeles Dodger Sandy Koufax, for example, was forced to retire from pitching in 1966 because of an arthritic elbow. However, most experts now feel that participation in vigorous exercise and sports does not increase the risk of osteoarthritis unless the involved joint has some sort of abnormality or previous major injury (Rangger et al., 1997). Normal joints are well designed to withstand the repetitive stress that comes with physical activity. But an injury to the joint alters its ability to handle exercise stress. Several studies of athletes with major knee injuries, for example, have shown that they are at increased risk of premature osteoarthritis (Rangger et al., 1997).

Long-distance runners have been studied more than any other type of athlete because of the long-term and repetitive stress their leg

Table 15.2

Client Information to Obtain from Medical Professionals

1) What type of arthritis does this patient have?

2) What symptoms are experienced by this patient? Are there limitations to certain forms of physical activity?

3) What medications are used by this patient? What are the side effects?

4) Does this patient have other medical conditions that may limit physical activity?

5) What specific joints are most painful and unstable?

6) Can this patient engage in a total fitness program emphasizing range-of-motion exercise, resistance training and aerobic conditioning?

joints are subjected to. During running, two-and-one-half to three times the body weight is transmitted to the lower limbs at heel strike. The stresses that the feet and ankles do not absorb are shifted to the knees, hips and spine. Despite the repetitive stress to their feet and legs, long-distance runners who train for many years do not appear to be at increased risk of osteoarthritis unless they have abnormal bio-mechanical problems or prior injuries in the hips, knees or ankles (Lane et al., 1993 a,b).

The injury rate among participants in many sports is quite high. Fortunately, most injuries appear to be limited, with no long-term consequences. If the injury leads to long-term joint instability, however, the risk for osteoarthritis climbs sharply (Rangger et al., 1997).

Exercise Training Benefits for the Patient with Arthritis

There are many potential benefits of exercise for the individual with arthritis (Hoffman, 1993; DiNubile, 1997; Ytterberg et al., 1994; Panush, 1994):

➤ improved joint function and range of motion

➤ increased muscular strength and aerobic fitness to enhance activities of daily living

➤ elevated psychological mood state

➤ decreased loss of bone mass

➤ decreased risk of heart disease, diabetes, hypertension and other chronic diseases

Can regular exercise improve, retard the progression, or even cure arthritis? Most researchers who have studied this question now answer, No. (Coleman et al., 1996; Ettinger et al., 1994, 1997; Hochberg et al., 1995; Kovar et al., 1992; Häkkinen et al., 1992; Hanson et al., 1993; Lyngberg et al., 1994; Noreau et al., 1997; Rall et al., 1996; Rintala et al., 1996). While exercise for people with arthritis is important for all the reasons listed above, investigators have typically found that exercise training does not improve arthritis and does not worsen the disease process either. In other words, exercise does not affect the underlying disease state in people with arthritis one way or the other, but does improve many other areas that pertain to life quality.

In one study, researchers randomly divided 102 patients with osteoarthritis of the knee into walking and control groups (Kovar et al., 1992).

Those in the walking group walked up to 30 minutes, three times a week, for eight weeks. As shown in Figure 15.2, the walkers experienced a strong increase in their performance during a six-minute walking test, an effect that was achieved without exacerbating pain or triggering flares. Therefore, those with osteoarthritis became fitter with the exercise program, but their disease was not reversed.

In another study, elderly subjects with a history of mild-to-moderate arthritis were divided into four groups: strength training (two sets and 10 reps of eight different weight machine exercises, three days a week), stationary cycle training (35 minutes at 60 percent to 75 percent intensity, three days a week), both strength and cycle training, and controls (Coleman et al., 1996). After six months of training, strength improved significantly in all exercise groups, but especially in those who exercised on the weight machines. Joint pain symptoms did not improve or worsen in any group.

In the 18-month FAST study (The Fitness Arthritis and Seniors Trial), 439 adults aged 60 years or older with osteoarthritis were randomly divided into one of three groups: health education (no exercise), aerobic exercise (three 40-minute sessions per week), or resistance exercise (three 40-minutes sessions per week, with two sets of 12 repetitions of nine exercises) (Ettinger

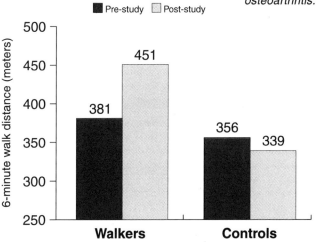

Supervised Fitness Walking in Patients with Osteoarthritis of the Knee
47 Walkers Compared to 45 Controls After 8 Weeks of Training (3/wk, 90 min/session)

Source: Kovar et al., 1992

Figure 15.2

Exercise training improves walking performance in patients with knee osteoarthritis.

et al., 1997). As shown in Figure 15.3, the mean score on the physical disability questionnaire was significantly improved for both exercise groups. Other tests revealed lower pain scores, and improved measures of performance with exercise. The researchers concluded that older disabled persons with osteoarthritis of the knee can experience modest improvements in measures of disability, physical performance and pain from participating in a regular exercise program.

Other researchers have come to the same conclusion: Patients with arthritis are trainable (i.e., they can get stronger and more aerobically fit), and the exercise can be done safely without detrimental effects on the joints (Panush, 1994). However, the results show no effect of training on the disease activity or on the progression of the disease.

Case Study 1

Data from Medical/Health Questionnaire

Age: 62 years; *Height:* 68 inches; *Weight:* 250 pounds; *Sex:* Male; *Desired weight:* 170 pounds

Osteoarthritis: diagnosed in knees two years ago; controls pain with NSAIDS

Figure 15.3

Physical disability symptoms are reduced in adults with knee osteoporosis who exercise regularly.

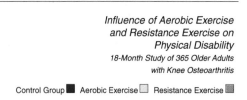

Influence of Aerobic Exercise and Resistance Exercise on Physical Disability

18-Month Study of 365 Older Adults with Knee Osteoarthritis

Control Group ■ Aerobic Exercise □ Resistance Exercise ▨

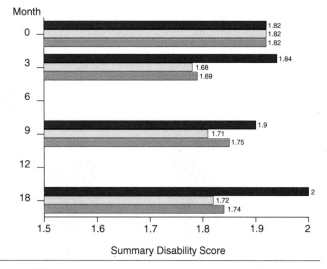

Summary Disability Score

Source: Ettinger et al., 1997

Smoking status: quit 20 years ago

Exercise habits: walks occasionally for a short distance after supper with wife, but no other formal exercise

Family history of disease: negative

Personal history of disease: Type 2 diabetic, diagnosed five years ago

Signs or symptoms suggestive of cardiopulmonary or metabolic disease: negative, but has low energy and feels tired much of the day; feels out of breath after climbing stairs; feels weak

Dietary habits: low in fruits and vegetables (2 servings/day); low in whole grains and cereals (3 servings/day); uses whole milk and cheese; likes red meat (2 servings/day)

Personal goals: lose weight to help control diabetes and lessen strain on joints; improve aerobic fitness and increase energy level; increase muscle strength moderately

Preferred modes of aerobic exercise: walking outside on good weather days; use of a treadmill on bad weather days

Data from Physical Fitness Testing Session (Physician's Office and Testing at Home)

Resting heart rate: 88 bpm (poor)

Resting blood pressure: 155/97 mmHg (mild hypertension) (from 2 measurements on 2 days)

Serum cholesterol: 256 mg/dl (high risk)

HDL-cholesterol: 30 mg/dl (low)

Cholesterol/HDL-cholesterol ratio: 8.5 (high risk)

Percent body fat: 38 percent (obese)

VO_2max: estimated from timed, modified Bruce treadmill-EKG test — 20 ml·kg^{-1}·min^{-1} (low); EKG (negative)

Sit-and-reach flexibility test: -3.5 inches from footline (poor)

Hand grip dynamometer (sum of right and left hands): 75 kg (poor)

Comments

Using the medical/health questionnaire and laboratory data from recent testing at the doctor's office, this client was classified as an "individual with disease," using ACSM criteria. This is because he is a diagnosed Type 2 diabetic, a condition that can often be controlled through weight loss, exercise and improvements in the diet (especially more dietary fiber and carbohydrate). After consulting with the client's physician (who determined that the EKG results were negative), you have been given approval to put the client on a moderate-intensity exercise program. The doctor urges gradual progression to avoid aggravating the osteoarthritis in the knees, and to avoid an exercise-induced heart attack (the client is considered to be at high risk for heart disease because of the presence of multiple risk factors including age, diabetes, hypercholesterolemia and sedentary lifestyle). The physician has advised that retesting be conducted every three months to monitor progress. Additionally, the services of a dietitian have been advised to help the client improve dietary intake.

Recommended Exercise Program

A home-based program, using walking, supported with a basic weight-training program and calisthenics for general muscle toning, is recommended. During the first month, have the client warm up with range-of-motion calisthenics and treadmill walking for five to 10 minutes, followed by 15 minutes of treadmill walking at 40 percent to 50 percent of heart-rate reserve, three days per week. After warming down, the client should engage in range-of-motion stretching activities for five to 10 minutes, followed by toning calisthenics and weight training (one set, 10 reps, eight different exercises) for 20 minutes.

After the first month has passed, gradually increase the duration of treadmill walking to 30 minutes per session, and the frequency to five days per week. Urge that stationary cycling be included in the exercise regimen twice per week to minimize strain on the knees. The intensity of exercise can also be gradually increased to 60 percent of heart-rate reserve. Flexibility and strength exercises should be included with each exercise session. These increases, along with careful control of dietary habits, will help ensure a steady weight loss of about 0.5 to 1 pound per week. The client has 80 pounds of body mass to lose, which is considered critical in treating both osteoarthritis and Type 2 diabetes. At the same time, this degree of weight loss combined with improvements in physical fitness should help bring hypertension and hypercholesterolemia under control if improvements in dietary quality are made. Patients with osteoarthritis and diabetes tend to be at high risk for coronary heart dis-

ease, and attainment of normal blood pressure, serum cholesterol and HDL-cholesterol is an important goal.

To ensure long-term success, seek family support of all lifestyle changes. If various goals are met during retesting sessions, organize an incentive system to improve client motivation and interest. During the entire exercise program, close communication and cooperation with the physician and dietitian are crucial.

Case Study 2

Data from Medical/Health Questionnaire

Age: 45 years; *Height:* 64 inches; *Weight:* 175 pounds; *Sex:* Female; *Desired weight:* 135 pounds

Arthritis status: diagnosed with rheumatoid arthritis five years ago; has progressed to class II (able to perform usual self-care and vocational activities, but limited in avocational activities); small joints of the hands and the knee joint are now affected.

Smoking status: quit five years ago

Exercise habits: sedentary both at work and during leisure for all of adult life

Family history of disease: father died of coronary artery disease at age 52 years

Personal history of disease other than arthritis: negative

Signs or symptoms suggestive of cardiopulmonary or metabolic disease: negative

Dietary habits: low in fruit/vegetables (2 servings/day); low and refined in cereals/grains, (5 servings/day)

Personal goals: lose weight, improve ability to use hands and knee joints, improve appearance and muscle tone, decrease risk of heart disease

Preferred modes of aerobic exercise: brisk walking

Data from Physical Fitness Testing Session (Physician's Office)

Resting heart rate: 82 bpm (poor)

Resting blood pressure: 153/96 mmHg (mild hypertension) (from 2 measurements on 2 days)

Table 15.3

Typical Activity Guidelines

■ Preserve or restore joint range of motion and flexibility.

■ Increase muscle strength and endurance to enhance joint stability.

■ Increase aerobic conditioning to improve

psychological mood state and decrease risk of disease.

■ Encourage recreational activity to promote long-term compliance.

■ Do not harm inflamed or unstable joints.

Serum cholesterol: 267 mg/dl (high risk)

HDL-cholesterol: 29 mg/dl (low)

Cholesterol/HDL-cholesterol ratio: 9.2 (high risk)

Percent body fat: 39 percent (obese)

VO_2max: estimated from modified Bruce treadmill-EKG test — 23 ml•kg^{-1}•min^{-1} (low); EKG, (negative)

Sit-and-reach flexibility test: -2 inches from footline (fair)

Hand grip dynamometer (sum of right and left hands): 35 kg (poor)

Comments

Using the medical/health questionnaire and laboratory data from recent testing, this client was classified as an "individual at increased risk," using ACSM criteria. This classification was given because she has two or more major coronary risk factors (family history, hypertension, hypercholesterolemia, sedentary lifestyle). Due to the number of risk factors and family history of coronary heart disease, and the client's desire to engage in moderate-to-vigorous exercise, a medical exam and diagnostic exercise test were recommended. The treadmill-EKG test was negative (no evidence of ischemia or arrhythmias), and physician clearance was given for the client to begin a moderate exercise program with gradual progression. Additional physical fitness tests were conducted at a fitness center to determine body composition and musculoskeletal fitness.

Recommended Exercise Program

The pain and inflammation of the small joints of the hand and the knee joints are being controlled with medication. The physician has asked you to help his patient lose weight, strengthen all of the major muscle groups of her body, increase range of motion in all her major joints, and improve cardiorespiratory endurance. A home-based program, using treadmill walking and indoor stationary bicycling, supported with range-of-motion exercises, calisthenics and weightlifting for general muscle toning, is recommended.

During the first month, have the client warm up with range-of-motion calisthenics and treadmill walking for 10 to 15 minutes. Follow this with 12 minutes of brisk treadmill walking and/or stationary cycling at 50 percent to 60 percent heart-rate reserve, three days per week. To protect her knee joints, use a discontinuous exercise protocol (three minutes walking, one minute rest, three minutes cycling, one minute rest, two complete cycles). After warming down, the client should engage in static stretching activities for five to 10 minutes, followed by toning calisthenics and weightlifting for 20 to 30 minutes (one set,

eight exercises, 10 repetitions). Develop specific muscle strengthening and range-of-motion exercises for the hands, with special care given to protection of the joints.

After the first month has passed, gradually increase the duration of treadmill walking and cycling to 30 to 45 minutes per session, and the frequency to five to six days per week. Continue the discontinuous exercise protocol until fitness is improved sufficiently to allow 30 to 45 minutes of continuous walking/cycling. The intensity of exercise can also be gradually increased to 70 percent of heart-rate reserve. These increases, along with careful control of dietary habits, will help ensure a steady weight loss of about one pound per week. Since the client has 40 pounds of body fat to lose, ideal body weight should be attained after 30 to 40 weeks of training. This degree of weight loss, combined with improvements in physical fitness, should help to improve joint strength and range of motion, and cardiorespiratory fitness, and bring heart disease risk factors under control if improvements in dietary quality are made (i.e., less saturated fat and cholesterol; more fruits, vegetables and whole grains; less sodium and alcohol). The client has a high risk of coronary artery disease, and it is imperative that the risk factors be brought under control through weight loss and dietary and exercise lifestyle changes. Enlist the services of a dietitian to ensure adherence to an anti-atherogenic diet.

Retest every three months to help ensure motivation and attainment of goals. Long-term compliance can be enhanced by encouraging family support, goal setting and contracting, establishing rewards for attainment of goals, and combating time obstacles. After a sufficient fitness level has been increased, encourage the client to join an aquatic exercise class or group activity program (e.g., PACE).

References

American College of Sports Medicine. (1997). *ACSM's Exercise Management for Persons with Chronic Diseases and Disabilities.* Champaign, Ill.: Human Kinetics.

Arthritis Foundation. (1996). *Arthritis Fact Sheet.* http://www.arthritis.org.

CDC. (1996a). Factors associated with prevalent self-reported arthritis and other rheumatic conditions—United States, 1989-1991.

Morbidity and Mortality Weekly Report, 45, 487-491.

CDC. (1996b). Prevalence and impact of arthritis by race and ethnicity—United States, 1989-1991.

Morbidity and Mortality Weekly Report, 45, 373-367.

CDC. (1997). Prevalence of leisure-time physical activity among persons with arthritis and other rheumatic conditions—United States, 1990-1991.

Morbidity and Mortality Weekly Report, 46, 389-393.

Chang, R.W., Pellissier, J.M. & Hazen, G.B. (1996). A cost-effectiveness analysis of total hip arthroplasty for osteoarthritis of the hip. *Journal of the American Medical Association, 275*, 858-865.

Coleman, E.A., Buchner, D.M., Cress, M.E., Chan, B.K.S. & De Lateur, B.J. (1996). The relationship of joint symptoms with exercise performance in older adults. *Journal of the American Geriatric Society, 44*, 14-21.

DiNubile, N.A. (1997). Osteoarthritis: How to make exercise part of your treatment plan. *Physician and Sportsmedicine, 25*, 7, 47-56.

Ettinger, W.H. & Afable, R.F. (1994). Physical disability from knee osteoarthritis: the role of exercise as an intervention. *Medicine: Science in Sports & Exercise, 26*, 1435-1440.

Ettinger, W.H. Burns, R. & Messier, S.P. (1997). A randomized trial comparing aerobic exercise and resistance exercise with a health education program in older adults with knee osteoarthritis. The Fitness Arthritis and Seniors Trial (FAST). *Journal of the American Medical Association, 277*, 25-31.

Felson, D.T. (1996). Weight and osteoarthritis. *American Journal of Clinical Nutrition, 63* (suppl), 430S-432S.

Häkkinen, A., Häkkinen, K. & Hannonen, P. (1994). Effects of strength training on neuromuscular function and disease activity in patients with recent-onset inflammatory arthritis. *Scandinavian Journal of Rheumatology, 23*, 237-242.

Hannan, M.T., Felson, D.T., Anderson, J.J. & Naimark, A. (1993). Habitual physical activity is not associated with knee osteoarthritis: The Framingham Study. *Journal of Rheumatology, 20*, 704-709.

Hanson, T.M., Hansen, G., Langgaard, A.M. & Rasmussen, J.O. (1993). Long-term physical training in rheumatoid arthritis. A randomized trial with different training programs and blinded observers. *Scandinavian Journal of Rheumatology, 22*, 107-112.

Harris, C. (1993). Osteoarthritis: How to diagnose and treat the painful joint. *Geriatrics, 48*, 39-46.

Hochberg, M.D. (1992). The American College of Rheumatology 1991 revised criteria for the classification of global functional status in rheumatoid arthritis. *Arthritis & Rheumatology, 35*, 498.

Hochberg, M.C., Altman, R.D. & Brandt, K.D. (1995). Guidelines for the medical management of knee osteoarthritis. *Arthritis Rheumatology, 38*, 1541-1546.

Hoffman, D.F. (1993). Arthritis and exercise. *Primary Care, 20*, 895-910.

Kovar, P.A., Allegrante, J.P., MacKenzie, R., Peterson, M.G.E., Gutin, B. & Charlson, M.E. (1992). Supervised fitness walking in patients with osteo-arthritis of the knee. *Annals of Internal Medicine, 116*, 529-534.

Lane, N.E. & Buckwalter, J.A. (1993). Exercise: A cause of osteoarthritis? *Rheumatic Diseases, Clinics of North America, 19*, 617-633.

Lane, N.E., Michel, B., Bjorkengren, A., Oehlert, J., Shi, H., Bloch, D.A. & Fries, J.F. (1993a). The risk of osteoarthritis with running and aging: A 5-year longitudinal study. *Journal of Rheumatology, 20*, 461-468.

Lyngberg, K.K., Harreby, M., Bentzen, H., Frost, B. & Danneskiold-Samsøe, B. (1994). Elderly rheumatoid arthritis patients on steroid treatment tolerate physical training without an increase in disease activity. *Archives of Physical Medicine and Rehabilitation, 75*,1189-1195.

Noreau, L., Moffet, H., Drolet, M. & Parent, E. (1997). Dance-based exercise program in rheumatoid arthritis. Feasibility in individuals with American College of Rheumatology functional class III disease. *American Journal of Physical Medicine and Rehabilitation, 76*, 109-113.

O'Dell, J.R., Haire, C.E. & Erikson, N. (1996). Treatment of rheumatoid arthritis with methotrexate alone, sulfasalazine and hydroxychloroquine, or a combination of all three medications. *New England Journal of Medicine, 334*,1287-1291.

Panush, R.S. (1994). Physical activity, fitness, and osteoarthritis. Bouchard, C., Shephard, R.J. & Stephens, T. (Eds.). *Physical Activity, Fitness, and Health: International Proceedings and Consensus Statement.* Champaign, Ill.: Human Kinetics.

Rall, L.C., Meydani, S.N., Kehayias, J.J., Dawson-Hughes, B. & Roubenoff, R. (1996). The effect of progressive resistance training in rheumatoid arthritis. Increased strength without changes in energy balance or body composition. *Arthritis Rheumatology, 39*, 415-426.

Rangger, C., Kathrein, A., Klestil, T. & Glotzer, W. (1997). Partial meniscectomy and osteoarthritis. Implications for treatment of athletes. *Sports Medicine, 23*, 61-68.

Rintala, P., Kettunen, H. & McCubbin, J.A. (1996). Effects of a water exercise program for individuals with rheumatoid arthritis. *Sports Medicine, Training, and Rehabilitation, 7*, 31-38.

Semble, E.L. (1995). Rheumatoid arthritis: New approaches for its evaluation and management. *Archives of Physical Medicine and Rehabilitation, 76*, 190-201.

Strange, C.J. (1996). Coping with arthritis in its many forms. *FDA Consumer, 3*, 17-21.

Ytterberg, S.R. Mahowald, M.L. & Krug, H.E. (1994). Exercise for arthritis. *Baillières Clinical Rheumatology, 8*, 161-189

Suggested Reading

American College of Sports Medicine. (1997). *ACSM's Exercise Management for Persons with Chronic Diseases and Disabilities.* Champaign, Ill.: Human Kinetics.

American College of Sports Medicine. (1995). *Guidelines for Exercise Testing and Prescription* (5th ed). Philadelphia, Pa.: Lea & Febiger.

Arthritis Foundation. (1993). *Primer on the Rheumatic Diseases* (10th ed.). Atlanta, Ga.: Arthritis Foundation.

Baechle, T.R. (1994). *Essentials of Strength Training and Conditioning.* Champaign, Ill.: Human Kinetics.

Nieman, D.C. (1999). *Exercise Testing and Prescription: A Health-Related Approach* (4th ed.). Mountain View: Mayfield Publishing Company.

Nieman, D.C. (1998). *The Exercise-Health Connection.* Champaign, Ill.: Human Kinetics.

Rothstein, J.M., Roy, S.H., & Wolf, S.L. (1998). *The Rehabilitation Specialists Handbook* (2nd ed.). Philadelphia, Pa.: E.A. Davis Co.

CHAPTER 16

Acquired Immune Deficiency Syndrome

CONNIE B. SCANGA
MICHAEL YOUSSOUF

Connie B. Scanga, Ph.D., earned her B.A. in psychology at the University of Pennsylvania, which opened the door to an extensive career in counseling and crisis intervention. After completing graduate study in exercise physiology at Temple University, Dr. Scanga went on to become assistant professor at Temple University and Eastern College, both in southeastern Pennsylvania. Currently she is a research fellow at the Malaghan Institute of Medical Research in Wellington, New Zealand, pursuing research into the role played by various components of the immune system in the disease process of atopic asthma.

Michael Youssouf, M.A., is a certified medical exercise specialist and an international fitness educator working with a wide range of populations, training HIV/AIDS individuals since 1984. He holds a bachelor of science degree in kinesiology and dance education from New York State University at Brockport and received a graduate fellowship to obtain a masters of arts degree from Ohio State University. Youssouf is certified as a personal trainer by the American Council on Exercise, the National Academy of Sports Medicine and the American Academy of Fitness Professionals, and a certified instructor for the American Red Cross in Community CPR, First Aid and Sport Safety.

HIV Infection
Exercise Leadership
Case Studies

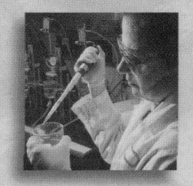

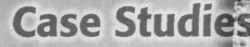

In 1981 the first cases of acquired immun-odeficiency syndrome (AIDS) were reported. Affected individuals were diagnosed with Pneumocystis carinii pneumonia and Kaposi's sarcoma and were immunosuppressed with no apparent cause (Gottlieb et al., 1981; Hymes et al., 1981). Nearly two years later the causative agent of AIDS, the human immunodeficiency virus (HIV), was isolated and identified (Barré-Sinoussi et al., 1983). Although there are still large gaps in our knowledge, much progress has been made since 1981 in understanding HIV/AIDS and in managing the disease process. In this chapter we will review HIV/AIDS and provide guidelines for exercise training of HIV-infected individuals.

The Human Immunodeficiency Virus

Viruses are microscopic **pathogen**s that parasitize host cells, using the cellular organelles for replication and destroying the host cell in the process. **HIV** is a **retrovirus** and like others of its class it is composed of three main parts:

➤ nucleic acid -- specifically, duplicate copies of single-stranded ribonucleic acid (RNA) which code for the virus' structural and regulatory proteins;

➤ the capsid -- this is the protein shell that surrounds and protects the viral RNA;

➤ the (outer) envelope -- a phospholipid bilayer coating which forms as the newly-replicated **virion** (i.e., an intact viral particle) buds through the host cell membrane into the extracellular space (Barré-Sinoussi, 1996; McCullough, Firth & Reade, 1997).

Retroviruses (e.g., HIV) contain the enzyme **reverse transcriptase,** which directs the synthesis of a DNA copy of the viral genome based on the RNA template. This genetic flow of information (RNA ➔ DNA) is the reverse of the typical **transcription** pattern (DNA ➔ RNA), hence the enzyme's name. Viral replication can begin after the virion enters the **cytoplasm** of the host cell and is uncoated. Under the direction of reverse transcriptase the viral genome is translated into a double-stranded DNA provirus. The provirus is inserted into the host cell genome by the viral enzyme integrase, allowing new viral RNA to be replicated along with the host cell genome. New virus particles are subsequently assembled in the cytoplasm of the cell. During viral assembly an HIV-derived protease cleaves a protein precursor molecule to produce the viral capsid proteins. Virions are released from the host cell through a process called budding, destroying the host cell as they leave (Epstein, 1991; Stryer, 1995).

The cell surface **antigen** designated **CD4** is the primary receptor for HIV. The HIV envelope contains a special glycoprotein (called the gp120 protein) which can attach to the CD4 antigen. CD4 is present on the helper subset of T-lymphocytes (Th cells), as well as monocytes, macrophages and **dendritic cells** (i.e., the immune system's antigen-presenting cells), microglial cells of the brain, and gut **epithelial** cells. Thus it is these cells that are potential targets for HIV infection (Dimitrov, 1997; Moore, 1997).

In 1996 exciting discoveries were reported regarding the role of HIV-1 coreceptors, which mediate the entry of HIV into host cells. There are two main types (i.e., CCR5 and CXCR4) and they normally function as chemokine receptors for the host cell. It has now become clear that it is not only the expression of CD4 but also the type and number of chemokine receptors expressed by host cells which make them vulnerable to infection at various stages of the disease (Dimitrov, 1997; Moore, 1997).

Two main strains of the HIV-1 virus are now recognized: M-tropic and T-tropic (Figure 16.1). The M-tropic strain is involved in most transmission of HIV across epithelial membranes. This strain replicates primarily in CD4+ T cells (the Th subset) and monocytes-macrophages, and usually uses CCR5 as its coreceptor. HIV tends to mutate frequently within the host and eventually the T-tropic **phenotype** emerges. The T-tropic strain, which is considered to be the more destructive in terms of Th cell function, tends to use CXCR4 as its coreceptor and becomes the more predominant strain within the host as HIV infection progresses and the virus evolves within its host (Barré-Sinoussi, 1996; Moore, 1997) (Figure 16.2).

HIV Infection

The early weeks of HIV infection have sometimes been described as a viral "incubation" period. During this time the virus replicates and becomes widely disseminated in the host. Within three to six weeks after the primary infection, 50 percent to 70 percent of infected individuals experience an acute mononucleosis-like illness. The illness is associated with high levels of the virus in the blood and coincides with the immune system's production of HIV-specific antibodies. Around the time of the acute illness the host's blood levels of HIV-specific **antibody** rise to detectable levels, signaling **seroconversion** to the HIV+ state.

This initial activation of the immune system is only partially successful in eradicating the virus; plasma viral levels do decline markedly, but it has become clear that viral replication continues.

Early understanding of HIV infection and disease progression was that HIV became latent after the primary infection. However, in the early- to mid-1990s, exciting developments in HIV research led to an enhanced understanding of "latent phase" events. First, it was reported that HIV replication and disease progression is active in lymphoid tissue during this period, even when minimal HIV RNA (i.e., viral load) is detectable in the blood (Embretson et al., 1993; Pantaleo et al., 1993). These groups demonstrated a preferential localization of HIV-infected cells in lymph tissue versus the blood during earlier stages of the disease, specifically reporting that during this period infected CD4+ T cells and macrophages were five to 10 times more prevalent in the lymph nodes than in the blood. In contrast, infected cells were more equally distributed between the lymph nodes and the blood in advanced stages of the disease (Pantaleo et al., 1993). The actual numbers of latently infected CD4+ lymphocytes and macrophages were quite large throughout the course of the disease (Embretson et al., 1993). Subsequently, two different research groups demonstrated that HIV-1 was actually replicating (even during the "latent" phase) at the rate of 109-1010 virions/day (Ho, Neumann, Perelson, Chen, Leonard & Markowitz, 1995; Wei et al, 1995), and that the viral half-life was approximately six hours (Perelson, Neumann, Markowitz, Leonard & Ho, 1996) (Figure 16.3).

The viral replication occurring during the clinically latent stage is associated with progressive damage to lymphoid tissue, which alters lymphocyte trafficking and contributes to progressive compromise of the immune system (Embretson et al., 1993; Pantaleo et al., 1993; Rosenberg, Anderson & Pabst). The high rate of viral production may have a significant impact on CD4+ cell turnover as well. It was calculated that the CD4+ cell death rate without antiretroviral therapy was approximately 2 x 109 cells/day, representing as much as a 78-fold increase above normal (Ho et al, 1995; Wei et al, 1995). This continuous onslaught against the host immune system results in a gradual and progressive immune depletion, which is associated with a gradual reduction in CD4+ T cells. More recently, Ullum et al. (1997) have demonstrated a differential pattern of depletion in naive (i.e., cell populations which have not yet encountered specific antigen challenge) and memory CD4+ T cell subsets. They showed a selective loss of memory T-cells during the early stages of the disease, followed by a depletion of naive cells as the disease progresses and the immune system becomes more comprised. The authors note that the increased depletion of naive CD4+ cells seems to be especially detrimental in advanced stages of the disease, and may be an indication that the immune system's regenerative capacity has been exceeded.

In the early years of the HIV/**AIDS** epidemic, disease progression was monitored in HIV+ individuals by measuring blood CD4+ cell depletion. In 1996, two research groups (Koot, van't Wout, Kootstra, deGoede, Tersmette & Schuitemaker, 1996; Mellors, Rinaldo, Gupta, White, Todd & Kingsley, 1996) reported the correlation between the amount of free HIV in the blood (i.e., viral load), the decline in circulating CD4+ cells and disease progression. Specifically, they demonstrated that as the virus evolved from expressing primarily its M-tropic phenotype to expressing the T-tropic lymphocyte, viral load increased. They found a strong correlation between the level of blood-borne virus and the probability of progression to AIDS, while the predictive value of CD4+ cell counts alone was low. In a study that corroborates these findings, O'Brien et al. reported that taken together, plasma HIV-1 RNA level and the CD4+ lymphocyte count are more reliable predictors of disease progression than other measures tested, and that these two measures can be used to monitor disease status and the efficacy of treatments. Coffin (1996) proposes that neither viral load nor CD4+ cell counts alone provide a complete picture of the disease progression. He suggests that viral load provides a relative measure of the number of cells infected and killed by HIV. The correlation between viral load and disease progression underscores the role of cumulative killing of CD4+ target cells in disease progression. Thus, according to Coffin, CD4+ counts provide a static measure of how far away the disease is from progressing to AIDS, while viral load indicates how fast the disease is progressing in the infected person. Taken together the two pieces of information create a more complete picture than either could provide individually.

Pathogenesis of HIV/AIDS

HIV is a member of the lentivirus family. Like other viruses in this family, HIV produces chronic disease characterized by a long period between primary infection and clinical manifestations and by central nervous system involvement. The dominant feature of HIV infection is the progressive depletion of CD4+ T lymphocytes, the T-helper subset of lymphocytes. The exact mechanisms for CD4+ cell depletion are unclear, but may include direct T-cell killing (due, for example, to membrane degradation during viral budding), immune-mediated killing, or premature triggering of programmed T-cell death (Powderly, Landay & Lederman, 1998).

The helper T-cell plays a central role in immune function. T-helper lymphocytes are activated by antigens displayed by antigen-presenting cells (in the presence of costimulatory **cytokines**). After activation, T-helper cells themselves secrete various cytokines that help regulate cytotoxic T-lymphocytes, B-lymphocytes, natural killer (NK) cells and other components of the immune system. Cytotoxic T-cells and NK-cells provide cell-mediated immunity, while B-lymphocytes are involved in antibody

production. Thus, the progressive depletion of T-helper cells leads eventually to profound **immunosuppression**.

The CD4 molecule is also present on other cells of the immune system, rendering these cells susceptible to HIV infection as well. Other CD4+ cells include antigen-presenting cells (i.e., monocytes-macrophages and dendritic cells), microglial cells of the brain and epithelial cells of the gut. Although the M-tropic virus that infects monocytes-macrophages is considered the less virulent phenotype, it can nonetheless interfere with normal antigen-presenting function and cytokine secretion. The presence in the central nervous system of CD4+ microglial cells which also express the requisite HIV coreceptors is thought to play a role in the **pathogenesis** of HIV-associated dementia (Lavi, Kolson, Ulrich, Fu & González-Scarano, 1998).

Epidemiology

The AIDS epidemic began in the U.S. in 1981, with the first recognized cases of **Kaposi's sarcoma** and **pneumocystis carinii pneumonia** among previously healthy homosexual men living in urban centers on the East and West Coasts. It was later documented in hemophiliacs, transfusion recipients and heterosexual intravenous drug users and their sex partners. It was not until 1983 that the disease and its transmission were linked to the retrovirus HIV (McCullough, Firth & Reade, 1997). In 1986 a second variant of HIV (i.e., HIV type 2 [HIV-2]) was identified in West Africa. Although HIV-2 has spread to the U.S. and Europe, HIV-1 remains the main etiologic agent for AIDS in the U.S. (Clavel et al., 1986).

In the early 1990s, but prior to the introduction of combination antiretroviral therapies, the incidence of AIDS was increasing at a rate of less than 5 percent per year. According to the CDC, as of December 1997 more than 640,000 Americans had been diagnosed with AIDS. Of those, at least 385,000 had died. The benefits of new therapeutic strategies are reflected in more recent data reported by the CDC. Specifically, in 1996 there was a first-time decrease in the estimated incidence of AIDS (6 percent decrease) and in AIDS-related deaths (25 percent decrease). An estimated 242,000 patients were living with AIDS, a 12 percent

Figure 16.1

Life cycle of HIV-1

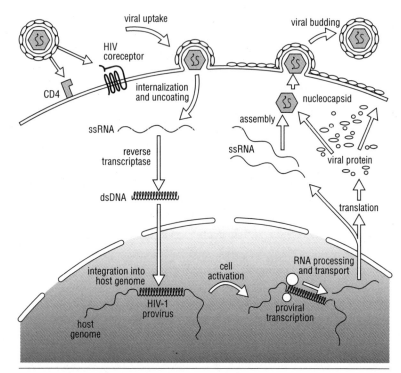

Adapted from Greene, W.C. (1990). *New England Journal of Medicine*, 324, 309.

improvement from the previous year (CDC, 1997). Currently in the U.S., the incidence of HIV infection is increasing most rapidly among women, minorities and young adults and transmission is mainly attributed to heterosexual transmission and intravenous drug use (Graham, 1997).

Clinical Manifestations and Course of the Disease

Screening for HIV Infection

HIV infection can manifest in a variety of ways, ranging from asymptomatic infection early in the disease process to profound immunosuppression with consequent secondary infection or cancers in later stages of the disease. There are two screening tests most often used for HIV, the **enzyme-linked immunosorbent assay (ELISA)** and Western blot. Both procedures are used to detect serum antibodies to HIV. When a repeatedly reactive ELISA is confirmed by **Western blot analysis**, a patient is considered HIV-infected (and infectious). One obvious limitation of these screenings is that it takes some time for the immune system to "gear up" and secrete antibodies in detectable amounts. Thus, there may be a period of weeks to months following primary infection when a screening test returns a false negative response, and the screening tests themselves cannot pinpoint the actual onset of HIV infection.

Case Definition

In 1986, the CDC published guidelines for classifying the stages of HIV/AIDS disease progression (CDC, 1986). These guidelines were subsequently revised to reflect expanded knowledge of the disease (CDC, 1992). A brief description of the stages follows:

Stage 1: Acute infection
- the period of several weeks to several months just after HIV infection
- individuals may experience transient symptoms during this period, including a mononucleosis-like infection around the time of seroconversion

Stage 2: Asymptomatic infection
- infected people are free of signs and symptoms of HIV disease

- this stage can last for as long as 10 to 15 years before clinical manifestations of HIV disease appear

Stage 3: Symptomatic HIV infection
- the number of CD4+ cells is moderately reduced, resulting in the onset of various persistent and nonspecific symptoms, including generalized **lymphadenopathy**, fever, night sweats, anorexia, nausea and diarrhea, **myalgia** and **malaise**
- the constellation of symptoms marking this stage is often referred to as **AIDS-related complex (ARC)**

Stage 4: AIDS--a number of opportunistic infections and cancers were felt to be sufficiently indicative of severe immunosuppression that, in the absence of other identifiable causes, they were included in the CDC's initial case definition of AIDS (1982); these include:
- *opportunistic infections:* Pneumocystis carinii pneumonia, chronic **cryptosporidiosis**, **toxoplasmosis**, extraintestinal **strongyloidiasis** (a parasitic infection), esophageal or lower respiratory tract **candidiasis**, disseminated or CNS **cryptococcosis**, isoporiasis, disseminated atypical mycobacterial infection, **cytomegalovirus** (CMV) infection, chronic mucocutaneous or disseminated **herpes simplex** virus infection, and progressive multifocal **leukoencephalopathy**
- *cancers:* Kaposi's sarcoma, non-Hodgkin's **lymphoma** and primary B-cell lymphoma of the brain

In 1987 the CDC criteria was revised to include additional indicator diseases (e.g., **wasting syndrome**, neurologic disease (e.g., HIV dementia or sensory **neuropathy**) and extrapulmonary **tuberculosis**).

More recently, the case definition was revised (CDC, 1992) to emphasize the clinical importance of the CD4+ T-lymphocyte count in categorizing HIV-related clinical conditions. Included in the expanded case definition are all HIV-infected adults and adolescents over the age of 13 who have either: a) pulmonary tuberculosis, recurrent pneumonia or invasive cervical cancer; b) a CD4+ T-lymphocyte count of less than 200 cells/mL; or c) a CD4+ T-lymphocyte percentage of total lymphocytes of less than 14 percent.

Clinical Manifestations

The HIV disease process is heterogeneous. Infected people may manifest a variety of symptoms and become vulnerable to opportunistic infection and cancers as the disease progresses. Some clinical manifestations are caused by the direct action of the virus on tissues or organs, others develop as secondary infections or disease; still others may be induced by the potent drugs used to treat the primary HIV infection. In addition to the immune and lymphatic system deterioration already described, other common symptoms and infections are described below.

- *Cardiovascular System.* A range of cardiovascular abnormalities can occur with HIV infection. Conditions commonly described in HIV-infected patients are dilated **cardiomyopathy**, **myocarditis**, cardiac lymphoma, cardiac and vascular lesions associated with Kaposi's sarcoma, **endocarditis**, **pericarditis** and noninflammatory myocardial **necrosis**. Symptoms such as **dyspnea**, chest pain or discomfort, fever, cough, generalized weakness or lethargy, and tachycardia may signal underlying cardiovascular disease (Yunis & Stone, 1998).

- *Respiratory System.* Persistent sinusitis, high frequency of upper respiratory tract infections, acute bronchitis, reactive airway disease and pneumonia are not uncommon. Tuberculosis is the leading cause of HIV-related mortality worldwide. Although only about 4 percent of AIDS patients in the U.S. have been diagnosed with tuberculosis, drug-resistant strains of the causative mycobacterium emerged in HIV-infected patients in the 1980s. As a result, tuberculosis is aggressively treated with multiple antibacterial agents today. Kaposi's sarcoma may also exhibit respiratory manifestations. (Allworth & Bowden, 1996; Beiser, 1997; Cavert, 1997; Murray, 1996; Smith & Pigott, 1996)

- *Digestive System.* Virus and fungal infection (e.g., cytomegalovirus and candidiasis, respectively) may cause gastrointestinal inflamma-

tion, **esophagitis** and **oral thrush**. Bacterial infection may also occur. Diarrhea, nausea, vomiting and anorexia are common (Allworth & Bowden, 1996; Cavert, 1997). HIV-associated wasting syndrome may occur. The wasting seems to preferentially catabolize muscle tissue, and may occur even without significant decreases in caloric intake. There is evidence of altered lipid and protein metabolism in advanced HIV infection that may partially account for the disproportionate degree of protein catabolism (Cavert, 1997; Kelly, Lloyd & Kemp, 1996).

- *Nervous System.* HIV infection is frequently associated with disorders of both the central and peripheral nervous systems. HIV is thought to enter the cerebrospinal fluid early in the disease process, probably at the time of seroconversion. Macrophage-lineage cells (e.g., microglial cells of the brain) are targeted by the virus, and more debilitating neural conditions develop as the HIV disease progresses. Common nervous system complications include peripheral neuropathy, encephalitis, cytomegaloviral retinitis (which can progress quickly to blindness if untreated) and **AIDS dementia complex.** The latter is characterized by poor concentration, disturbed cognition and short-term memory deficits, motor coordination deficits and gait unsteadiness, and affective changes (Brew, Wesselingh, Gonzales, Heyes & Price, 1996).

- *Cutaneous Manifestations.* Dry skin, **seborrheic dermatitis** and Kaposi's sarcoma lesions of the skin and mucous membranes are not uncommon (Allworth & Bowden, 1996; Legg & Balano, 1997; Murray, 1996).

Treatment of the Disease

In the early to mid 1990s major advances occurred in antiretroviral therapy. Early antiretroviral agents provided relatively short-lived benefits and were not as successful in limiting viral replication as those currently used (Powderly, Landay & Lederman, 1998). That the CDC could report for 1996 the first decrease in new AIDS cases and deaths (CDC, 1997) can in part be attributed to the introduction of HIV-1 **protease inhibitors** and the use of combination antiretroviral therapies. Recent recommendations from both the NIH ("Guidelines for the Use of Antiretroviral Agents," 1998; "Report of the NIH Panel," 1998) and the International AIDS Society (Carpenter et al., 1998) endorse the early introduction of potent antiretroviral therapy with the goal of improving survival and decreasing morbidity through ongoing maximal suppression of HIV replication. Combination antiretroviral therapy involves the use of three types of agents. A general description of each type follows.

Nucleoside analog reverse transcriptase inhibitors (NRTIs)

- these agents act by incorporating themselves into the HIV DNA and then interfering with the viral transcription process
- NRTIs currently available for use:
- zidovudine (ZDV, AZT) — i.e., Retrovir™
- didanosine (ddl) — i.e., Videx™
- lamivudine (3TC) — i.e., Epivir™
- zalcitabine (ddc) — i.e., HIVID™
- stavudine (d4T) — i.e., Zerit™
- common side effects: headache, fatigue, myalgia, nausea, fever, chills; some types may also cause anemia, diarrhea, and/or pancreatitis; zidovudine has been associated with cardiomyopathy

Non-nucleoside reverse transcriptase inhibitors (NNRTIs)

- these agents act by binding to the viral reverse transcriptase, preventing RNA → DNA transcription
- NNRTIs currently available for use:
- nevirapine — i.e., Viramune™
- delavirdine — .e, Rescriptor™
- common side effects: rash, headache, nausea; may also cause fatigue, anemia, **leukopenia** and/or **hepatitis**

Protease inhibitors (PIs)

- these agents inhibit HIV assembly and release from infected cells
- PIs currently available for use:
- indinavir — i.e., Crixivan™
- ritonavir — i.e, Norvir™
- saquinavir-SGC (soft gel capsule) — i.e., Fortovase™
- nelfinavir — i.e., Varacept™
- common side effects: headache, nausea, elevated values on liver function tests; some types may also cause vomiting, diarrhea, kidney stones, confusion and/or weakness (Carpenter et al., 1998; Henry, Stiffman & Feldman, 1997)

Although combination retroviral therapy is effective in slowing the progress of HIV disease, compliance is sometimes a problem. The therapy is expensive (costing as much as $15,000 annually) and involves taking many pills at varied times of the day. Additionally, the side effects of the medications can be unpleasant at best; this problem is compounded by the many types of drug interactions that can also occur.

A variety of medications are also used to treat the secondary complications of HIV/AIDS. These include antiviral, antifungal and antibacterial agents. Specific medications will vary, based on individual disease manifestations.

Novel or alternative treatments (e.g., megavitamin therapy, hypnotherapy and purported immune-boosting substances) are attractive to some HIV+ individuals. Often these therapies have not been rigorously tested or approved as safe and effective for persons with HIV/AIDS. While alternative therapies cannot be seen as a substitute for standard medical treatment, some physicians may recommend an alternative therapy as an adjunct to conventional medical care. Avoid offering advice about alternative therapies that are beyond your scope of practice.

Exercise and HIV Infection

HIV infection can lead to deconditioning, loss of muscle strength and reduced aerobic capacity. Several controlled studies have reported reduced ventilation, lower lactate and ventilatory thresholds, and reduced VO_2max in asymptomatic HIV+ individuals (Johnson et al., 1990; Pothoff, Wasserman & Ostmann, 1994). Baigis-Smith and her colleagues (1994) found that 65 percent (N=178) of HIV-infected subjects who received clinical nursing care in dedicated inpatient AIDS units, homes, clinic and long-term care facilities had decreased physical endurance. Specifically, 23 percent of their subjects lacked sufficient endurance to complete activities of daily living (ADLs) and 42 percent were unable to perform activities beyond ADLs. Thus, the deconditioning associated with early HIV disease appears to become increasingly problematic as the disease progresses.

An obvious question is to what extent acute and chronic exercise affects immune function in HIV+ individuals. Most studies of exercise and immune function (in seronegative as well as seropositive populations) have attempted to answer this question by enumerating leukocyte subsets in peripheral blood or through in vitro assessment of cell function. In longitudinal studies involving seronegative subjects, several studies have reported no change in absolute numbers of peripheral blood leukocytes and in the total proportion of T-lymphocytes (Soppi, Varjo, Eskola & Laitenen, 1982; Watson, Moriguchi, Jackson, Werner, Wilmore & Freund, 1986). Acute exercise is associated with transient changes in peripheral blood cell number and relative proportion. Immediately following a bout of exercise there is an increase in peripheral blood lymphocyte and granulocyte number. Typically, there is a dramatic increase in the proportion of peripheral blood granulocytes. Although this results in a decreased proportion of total lymphocytes, the CD4+/CD8+ T-cell ratio may be either increased, decreased or unchanged. Post-exercise changes in peripheral blood cell number and function and the period of recovery to baseline levels following a single bout of exercise tend to be transient; the magnitude and duration of changes is related to the duration and relative intensity of the exercise session (Kendall, Hoffman-Goetz, Houston, Mac-Neil & Arumugam, 1990; Lewicki, Tchorzewski, Majewska, Nowak & Baj; Neiman et al., 1994). It appears that, while the total number of T-lymphocytes in peripheral blood of HIV+ people may be suppressed, the pattern of change in T lymphocyte subsets after a bout of acute exercise is similar to that of healthy seronegative controls. However, the increase in circulating neutrophils and NK cells was blunted in HIV+ individuals versus controls, as was the cytotoxic activity of NK cells and lymphokine activated killer cells (Ullum et al., 1994). It has been suggested that the period immediately following an exercise bout may present a "window of vulnerability" during which susceptibility to infection is increased (Lawless, Jackson & Greenleaf, 1995; Nieman, Johanssen, Lee, Cermak & Arabatzis, 1990).

The physical and psychological benefits of exercise training in HIV-infected persons have been documented. Several studies have demonstrated improvements in submaximal and maximal exercise performance in seropositive subjects following 10 and 12 weeks of aerobic training, accompanied by a stable (or nonsignificant increase) in peripheral blood CD4+ numbers following training (LaPerriere, Fletcher, Antoni, Klimas, Ironson & Schneiderman, 1991; LaPerriere et al, 1990; Macarthur, Levine & Birk, 1993; Rigsby, Dishman, Jackson, Maclean & Raven, 1992). Consistently, however, these authors note the problem of noncompliance (i.e., not regularly attending exercise sessions or subject withdrawal from the study) among study participants. Reasons for not completing the study included transportation problems, the difficulty of exercise and acute episodes of poor health. The rate of noncompliance tended to be higher in those with AIDS. Anxiety and depression have been correlated with decrements in immune function (for review, see LaPerriere, Ironson, Antoni, Schneiderman, Klimas & Fletcher, 1994). Significantly, improvements in mood state and quality of life were also reported in exercised-trained HIV+ subjects versus non-exercising HIV+ controls (LaPerriere et al., 1990; Macarthur, Levine & Birk, 1993).

Weight loss and **cachexia** (i.e., preferential loss of lean body mass versus adipose tissue, often in the absence of weight loss per se) are common beginning in the early stages of HIV infection and may in part be attributed to anorexia and loss of appetite, or gastrointestinal discomfort and dysfunction. Several studies have examined the effects in HIV+ individuals of progressive resistance training and report post-training increases in body mass and muscle strength. These authors report no increase in plasma viral load (Evans, Roubenoff & Shevitz, 1998), no exercise-related decline in T lymphocyte (CD4+ and CD8+) proportions (Rigsby, Dishman, Jackson, Maclean & Raven, 1992), and no adverse changes in immune function (Spence, Galantino, Mossberg & Zimmerman, 1990) following chronic resistance exercise training.

Most recently, Stringer and colleagues (1998) investigated the effects of a six-week program of either moderate or heavy aerobic exercise training on immune function in HIV+ individuals versus controls. Subjects were in the asymptomatic phase of disease (CD4+ counts of 100-500 cells/mm3), had been on average seropositive for over three years, were without signs of opportunistic infection and nearly all were receiving antiretroviral therapy. While the lactate threshold increased in both treatment groups, maximal exercise capacity was increased in only the heavy training group. The effects of training on immune function seem to highlight the benefits of training at moderate intensity. There was no change in CD4 counts following treatment in either the exercise or control groups. However, skin reactivity to candida albicans antigen increased significantly in the moderate exercise group, while declining nonsignificantly in the control and heavy exercise group. Additionally, although plasma viral RNA levels decreased in all groups, the most dramatic decrease in viral load occurred in the moderate exercise group.

The Pre-exercise Screening and Assessment

There is a growing body of evidence that exercise training can improve mood state and quality of life for HIV+ individuals, and there is widespread belief among the HIV community that exercise training will make them stronger, improve their endurance and protect them from infection. However, healthcare providers do not always endorse exercise as an adjunct therapy for HIV-infected patients (Baigis-Smith, Coombs & Larson, 1994). Thus, not all of your HIV+ clients will initiate exercise training on their physician's recommendation. Your familiarity with the HIV disease process and treatments will help in building bridges with the medical community and in reassuring your client regarding potential benefits of exercise training.

The Assessment

Prior to the initial screening and fitness assessment, it is prudent to notify the primary-care physician of the client's intent to exercise and request pertinent medical information. This contact can be made by letter and should include a copy of the client's signed consent for the release of information. Specific medical information that will be useful in planning a safe assessment and subsequent exercise program should be obtained.

To ensure client safety during subsequent fitness testing, the client should complete the PAR-Q (Physical Activity Readiness Questionnaire) form prior to the screening session.

As noted previously, combination therapies using several antiretroviral agents are likely. Specific medications prescribed will vary depending on the success of treatment with a particular antiretroviral agent and also on the type and severity of secondary infection present. You should become specifically informed about side effects associated with common antiretroviral agents, and should solicit advice when necessary from the client's physician regarding drug interactions and synergy that could affect the exercise response. The client should be instructed to notify you when medication changes are made.

The initial pre-exercise screening provides the opportunity for you to review the client's medical history and form a positive relationship with the client. During this session it will be helpful to gather information about the physical symptoms the HIV+ client is experiencing (or has recently experienced) and their coping strategies, as well as the client's goals and motivation for exercise training.

Fitness Testing

The complete fitness evaluation may include assessments of body composition, cardiorespiratory endurance, muscular endurance and flexibility. Follow your center's standard procedures in assessing body composition, muscular endurance and flexibility.

Submaximal cycle ergometry tests are recommended for evaluating cardiorespiratory fitness and deriving an estimated VO_2max. HIV+ clients may be severely deconditioned due to prolonged periods of physical inactivity. The test should be limited to eight to 12 minutes (i.e., two to four three-minute stages). If neuromuscular dysfunction is obvious, the exercise test could be administered via recumbent cycle ergometry or upper-body ergometry. Under these circumstances, gait analysis may provide useful information for designing a safe exercise program.

Contraindications to Exercise

If the client's temperature is elevated or if the client is in the acute phase of a secondary infection, exercise is not recommended.

Exercise Programming

When planning an initial exercise program for HIV+ clients, remember the following:

- the primary goal of exercise training for HIV+ clients should be to prevent further deconditioning and progressive physical disability, while maintaining the highest possible degree of immune function;
- initial phases of the exercise program should be more conservative and less intense than programming for a seronegative person of the same age, gender and fitness level;
- help the client develop realistic long-term fitness goals, and be prepared to offer a backup fitness plan if the client's status deteriorates.

Exercise Guidelines

When developing the aerobic portion of the exercise program for an HIV+ client, take into account not only the individual's exercise capacity, but also their clinical status, adjusting the duration and intensity of exercise bouts to correspond to immune decrements. The following guidelines for aerobic training are recommended:

Asymptomatic infection — these clients have likely developed some degree of immunosuppression, but CD4+ cell counts are still fairly robust (CD4+ cells greater than 500-600 cells/mm3)

- *intensity:* initially 55 percent to 65 percent of estimated VO$_2$max, progress incrementally over the first 10 to 15 weeks, should not exceed 85 percent of estimated VO$_2$max
- *duration:* 20 to 30 minutes initially, with increased duration as training progresses
- *frequency:* three to five times per week

Stage 3: Symptomatic HIV infection — these clients may be experiencing a range of nonspecific symptoms (e.g., anorexia, fatigue, lymphadenopathy, chronic diarrhea) related to progressive immunosuppression (CD4+ cell range: 200-500 cells/mm3)

- *intensity:* initially 50 percent to 60 percent of estimated VO$_2$max, progress incrementally over the first 10 to 15 weeks to 55 percent to 75 percent of estimated VO$_2$max

- *duration:* 15 to 20 minutes initially; increase duration up to 40 minutes as training progresses
- *frequency:* three to four times per week

Stage 4: AIDS — these clients may be experiencing secondary infections and cancers indicative of severe immunosuppression (CD4+ cells less than 200 cells/mm3)

- *intensity:* initially 45 percent to 50 percent of estimated VO$_2$max, progress incrementally over the first 10 to 15 weeks, should not exceed 50 percent of estimated VO$_2$max
- *duration:* 15 to 20 minutes initially, progressing to a maximum duration of 20 to 30 minutes
- *frequency:* three times per week (when able)

(Birk, 1996; LaPerriere, Klimas, Major & Perry, 1997)

Aerobic Training Modalities: Walking is excellent in initial stages of programming for deconditioned individuals. After the client becomes more comfortable with exercise training and adept at monitoring exercise intensity, other aerobic options can be introduced. Recommend alternatives such as recumbent bikes, upper body cycling or water activities for those with impaired balance.

Stretching and Flexibility: Clients should be instructed to complete slow, static stretching exercises at the beginning and end of the exercise session. Stretching exercises should focus on the hip/thigh and shoulder girdle. Prescribe one to three repetitions of each stretching exercise, and recommend that each stretch be held for 10 to 30 seconds. Gentle stretching may help relieve muscle discomfort, and can also be performed at home on rest days. Tai chi and yoga could be recommended not only for their strengthening and flexibility benefits, but also for their stress-management value.

Resistance Training: In most HIV+ clients the goal of resistance training should be to maintain or improve muscle mass. Resistance training may incorporate eight to 10 exercises that train major muscle groups. Asymptomatic HIV+ clients should generally complete one set of eight to 12 repetitions, while symptomatic HIV+ clients and those with AIDS should complete one set of 12 to 15 repetitions. The exercise program should include eight to 10 exercises. Resistance training can be performed three days/week on alternate days.

Risk of HIV Transmission in the Exercise Setting

During the earliest years of the AIDS epidemic, it became clear that HIV transmission is restricted to several routes:

- across mucous membranes during sexual contact
- hematological exposure to virally contaminated blood or blood products
- perinatal transmission (i.e., transmission from mother to child before or at the time of birth) (Kaldor & Rubin, 1994; McCullough, Firth & Reade, 1997)

The CDC has published recommendations for blood and body fluid precautions to be used with all patients in healthcare settings to reduce the risk of transmission of bloodborne pathogens. These guidelines (known as "universal precautions") were developed to protect healthcare workers against transmission across mucous membranes (e.g., conjunctiva of the eyes, the lining of the nose or mouth) and through breaks or cuts in the skin. Further, they advise that blood and certain body fluids of all patients should be considered potentially infectious for HIV, hepatitis B and other bloodborne pathogens. The risk of disease transmission is controlled by minimizing the risk of exposure to blood and body fluids. Essentially, the guideline recommendations are as follows (CDC, 1988):

- body fluids to which universal precautions apply: blood and other body fluids containing visible blood, semen and vaginal secretions, tissues and certain specific body fluids (i.e., synovial, cerebrospinal, pleural, pericardial, peritoneal and amniotic)
- body fluids to which universal precautions do not apply: feces, nasal secretions, sputum, sweat, tears, urine, vomit and saliva (unless any of these contain visible blood)
- use protective barriers to prevent exposure to the body fluids to which universal pre-

cautions apply (these will vary, based on the situation)
- immediately and thoroughly wash hands or other skin surfaces that have been contaminated with any of the fluids to which universal precautions apply
- a 1:10 dilution of household bleach will disinfect contaminated equipment surfaces.

Application of universal precautions is prudent for clinical exercise specialists as well as healthcare workers and should be practiced until they are habitual.

Athletics and HIV/AIDS

HIV+ persons in early stages of the disease may enjoy participation in group sporting activities and competitive athletics. There is no evidence for transmission of HIV when seropositive individuals without bleeding wounds or skin lesions participate in sports. And there is very low risk of transmission when an HIV-infected person with a bleeding wound or skin lesion with exudate physically contacts another athlete with a skin lesion. Follow universal precautions (CDC, 1988) with all clients to minimize the risk of transmission of infectious disease.

Consensus statements issued by the World Health Organization (Goldsmith, 1992), the American Academy of Pediatrics (1991) and the National Football League (1994) establish guidelines for dealing with HIV in athletic settings. The following is a summary of these guidelines:

- No evidence exists for a risk of transmission of HIV when infected persons, without bleeding wounds or skin lesions, engage in sports. Thus, athletes infected with HIV should be allowed to participate in all competitive sports.
- There is no medical or public health justification for testing or screening for HIV infection prior to participation in sports activities. HIV testing should remain voluntary.
- There is a very low risk of HIV transmission during combative sports when an infected individual with a bleeding wound or a skin lesion with exudate comes in contact with another athlete with a skin lesion or an exposed mucous membrane. Olympic sports with the greatest risk include boxing, tae kwon do and wrestling, while basketball,

field hockey, judo, soccer and team handball pose only moderate risk.

- It should be the responsibility of any athlete participating in a combative sport who has a wound or other skin lesion to report it immediately to a responsible official and seek medical attention. Athletes who know they are HIV-infected should seek medical counseling about further participation in sports, especially in sports such as wrestling or boxing that pose a high theoretical risk of contagion to other athletes.
- Each coach and athletic trainer should receive training in how to clean skin and athletic equipment surfaces exposed to blood or other body fluids.

Exercise Leadership

Note the following when monitoring exercise in HIV+ clients:

- Planned rest is important and should be incorporated into the exercise program. Encourage the client to avoid inconsistent and variable activity.
- Clients should reduce or discontinue exercise activities when they have acute infections and/or when their temperature is elevated.
- Consider environmental factors (e.g., pollen, automobile exhaust, insects, etc.) that may induce an allergic reaction in the HIV+ client. Allergic reactions can be severe and/or unpredictable. It may be prudent to move workouts indoors to avoid the stress of environmental challenges.
- Conversely, there may an increased risk of exposure to airborne pathogens when exercising indoors during cold or flu season.

Consider scheduling training appointments in fitness facilities at off-peak times to lessen exposure.

- HIV+ clients have an above normal risk of fungal infection. Encourage clients to wear sandals in shower and pool areas to reduce the risk of fungal infection.

Provide written follow-up reports to the client's physician every three months. These reports should summarize the modes of exercise employed, exercise progression since the last report and information regarding the client's response to exercise programming.

Other Considerations:

- If you are experiencing an active illness or infection (e.g., the common cold) that can be socially transmitted via touch, sneezing and coughing, you could transmit this infection to your HIV+ client. It would most likely be in your client's best interest to postpone a training session until your infection has cleared.
- Chronic diarrhea is a common symptom in HIV/AIDS, and it can result in dehydration and electrolyte imbalances. Educate your client about the impact of dehydration on exercise capacity, and also give instruction about maintaining adequate hydration.
- Abnormal lipid metabolism has been reported in advanced HIV infection, and is associated with abnormal elevations in serum triglycerides and abnormally low HDL cholesterol fractions. This may increase the risk of coronary artery disease in advanced stages of HIV infection (Birk, 1996).
- HIV-infected clients can often benefit greatly from professional nutritional

Table 16.1

Client Information to Obtain from Medical Professionals

1) Is the client permitted to exercise? Are there any potential adverse effects of exercise for this individual?

2) What is the status of the client's general health and immune function?

3) What medications is the client taking? Are there any side effects, and will the medication affect the client's ability to exercise?

4) Does the client have any other associated medical conditions?

5) What are your goals for this client?

6) Do you have any recommendations regarding exercise intensity and duration?

7) What was the date of the client's last appointment and physical exam?

counseling, especially in light of the gastrointestinal symptoms (e.g., diarrhea, nausea, suppressed appetite) frequently experienced. Nutritionists are most qualified to review diets and make dietary suggestions.

- Depression, anxiety and pain are common in HIV/AIDS patients. Your client may benefit from progressive relaxation, breathing exercises, meditation, or other types of stress and pain management techniques.

Case Study 1

Case Study of Mitchell Lewis

Mitchell is an attorney in the entertainment industry. He is 55 years old, divorced and travels often for his business. Mitchell has smoked for more than 35 years (two packs/day) and has mild hypertension (138/90). Mitchell was diagnosed as HIV+ approximately four months ago. After diagnosis, his physician's primary and immediate concern was to stabilize Mitchell's CD4+ T-cell count and plasma HIV RNA. His physician also recommended various lifestyle changes, including exercise, diet and smoking cessation. Initially, Mitchell tried to structure his own exercise plan, but was inconsistent in his follow-through and was not sure that his program was safe or effective.

At Mitchell's initial session, we reviewed the medical information that had been sent to our center by his physician. Mitchell is asymptomatic and feels well. His T-cell count is currently 750/mm3 and his plasma HIV RNA is low and stable. He is compliant with his medication regimen, which includes ZDV, ddl (both NRTIs) and indinavir (a protease inhibitor). His blood lipid profile is normal and his physician does not note any contraindications for exercise. I reviewed with Mitchell his responses to the PAR-Q and agreed that there were no immediate contraindications to his involvement in an exercise program.

The initial fitness assessment included a three-stage cycle ergometry test (with resting and exercise blood pressures), modified push-ups, body composition assessment (skinfold measures) and evaluation of flexibility (sit-and-reach test). His estimated VO$_2$max (approximately 31.5 ml/kg^{-1}/min^{-1}) and muscular endurance were low. Happily, his exercise blood pressure response was normal. We estimated approximately 25 percent body fat.

Mitchell's exercise prescription emphasized endurance training. His initial program consisted of 20 minutes aerobic training (cycle ergometry was Mitchell's preference) at an intensity of 55 percent to 60 percent VO$_2$max, with stretching included after a brief warm-up. Mitchell was instructed to exercise three times the first week (on alternate days). We agreed to meet at the end of the first week to review his progress and implement the resistance training portion of his exercise program.

At the first follow-up meeting (and subsequent follow-ups), I monitored Mitchell's blood pressure and discussed his physical status during the past week. After the first week of exercise Mitchell was not experiencing any new symptoms, so the duration of the aerobic phase of exercise was progressed (to 25 minutes). In subsequent weeks, we continued the progression of the aerobic phase of training to 30 minutes per session and Mitchell was encouraged to exercise up to five days per week.

A basic resistance-training program was introduced in the second week of exercise, with goals of improving muscular endurance and muscle tone. Mitchell was instructed to complete one set (10 to 12 repetitions) of each of 10 exercises, three times per week.

In addition to exercise programming, I discussed lifestyle modifications with Mitchell. These included smoking cessation, stress management and nutritional counseling.

Case Study 2

Case Study of Joy Chan

Joy Chan is a 26-year-old woman who has worked as a professional dancer most of her adult life. Approximately two years ago she discovered she was HIV+. Currently, her CD4+ T-cell count is just over 300 cells/mm3 and plasma HIV RNA is low. She experiences various nonspecific symptoms, including fatigue, nausea, loss of appetite and lymphadenopathy. Her current medications are ZDV, ddc (both NRTIs) and ritonavir (a protease inhibitor). In the past few months Joy has not had enough stamina to work regularly. She hopes to regain strength and endurance through formal exercise programming.

The initial fitness assessment included a three-stage cycle ergometry test (with resting and exercise blood pressures), modified push-ups, body composition assessment (skinfold measures) and evaluation of flexibility (sit and reach test). Joy's estimated VO$_2$max (approximately

35.5 ml/kg-1/min-1) and muscular endurance were average and her body fat was approximately 18 percent.

Joy's exercise prescription included both endurance and resistance training, corresponding to her goal of increasing her strength and endurance. Additionally, this program should help Joy maintain or (hopefully) increase her lean body mass. Her initial program consisted of 20 minutes aerobic training (treadmill walking or cycling) at an intensity of 50 percent to 55 percent VO_2max, with stretching at the beginning and end of the exercise session. Resistance training exercises were introduced at Joy's first two exercise sessions (one set, 10 to 12 repetitions, three times per week).

In the initial weeks of training, we gradually increased the duration and intensity of the aerobic phase of Joy's workout (to 30 minutes at 60 percent to 65 percent VO_2max, three days per week). Unfortunately, during the seventh week of programming, Joy experienced a viral infection and could not exercise for three weeks. When Joy returned to the health club, we advised her to gradually resume her previous level of aerobic training beginning with 20 to 30 minutes, 50 percent to 55 percent VO_2max.

References

Allworth, A.M. & Bowden, F.J. (1996). HIV and bacterial infections. *Medical Journal of Australia,* 164, 546-548.

American Academy of Pediatrics, Committee on Sports Medicine and Fitness. (1991). Human immunodeficiency virus [acquired immunodeficiency syndrome (AIDS) virus] in the athletic setting. *Pediatrics,* 88, 640-641.

Baigis-Smith, J., Coombs, V.J. & Larson, E. (1994). HIV infection, exercise and immune function. IMAGE: *Journal of Nursing Scholarship,* 26, 277-281.

Barré-Sinoussi, F. (1996). HIV as the cause of AIDS. *Lancet,* 348, 31-35.

Barré-Sinoussi, F., Chermann, J. C., Rey, F., Nugeyre, M.T., Chamaret, S., Gruest, J., Dauguet, C., Axler-Blin, C., Vezinet-Brun, F., Rouzioux, C., Rozenbaum, W. & Montagnier, L. (1983). Isolation of a T lymphotropic retrovirus from a patient at risk for acquired immunodeficiency syndrome (AIDS). *Science,* 220, 868-871.

Beiser, C. (1997). HIV infection--II. *British Medical Journal,* 314, 579-583.

Birk, T.J. (1996). HIV and exercise. *Exercise Immunology Review,* 2, 84-95.

Brew, B.J., Wesselingh, S.L., Gonzales, M., Heyes, M.P. & Price, R.W. (1996). How HIV leads to neurological disease. *Medical Journal of Australia,* 164, 233-234.

Brown, L.S., Phillips, R.Y., Brown, C.L., Knowlan, D., Castle, L. & Moyer, J. HIV/AIDS policies and sports: The National Football League. *Medicine and Science in Sports and Exercise,* 26, 403-407.

Carpenter, C.C.J., Fischl, M.A., Hammer, S.M., Hirsch, M.S., Jacobsen, D.M., Katzenstein, D.A., Montaner, J.S.G., Richman, D.D., Saag, M.S., Schooley, R.T., Thompson, M.A., Vella, S., Yeni, P.G. & Volberding, P.A. (1998). Antiretroviral therapy for HIV infection in 1998. Updated recommendations of the International AIDS Society--USA Panel. *Journal of the American Medical Association,* 280, 78-86.

Cavert, W. (1997). Preventing and treating major opportunistic infections in AIDS. *Postgraduate Medicine,* 102, 125-140.

CDC. (1982). Update on acquired immune deficiency syndrome (AIDS) -- United States. *Morbidity and Mortality Weekly Report,* 31, 507-508, 513-514.

CDC. (1986). Current trends classification system for human T-lymphotropic virus type III/lymphadeno-pathy-associated virus infections. *Morbidity and Mortality Weekly Report,* 35, 334-339.

CDC. (1987). Revision of the CDC surveillance case definition for acquired immunodeficiency syndrome. *Morbidity and Mortality Weekly Report,* 36(suppl.), 1-15s.

CDC (1988). Perspectives in disease prevention and health promotion update: Universal precautions for prevention of transmission of human immunodeficiency virus, hepatitis B virus and other bloodborne pathogens in health care settings. *Morbidity and Mortality Weekly Report,* 37, 377-388.

CDC. (1992). 1993 revised classification system for HIV infection and expanded surveillance case definition for AIDS among adolescents and adults. *Morbidity and Mortality Weekly Report,* 41(no. RR-17).

CDC. (1997). Update: Trends in AIDS incidence 1996. *Morbidity and Mortality Weekly Report,* 46, 861-867.

Clavel, F., Guetard, D., Brun-Vezinet, F., Chamaret, S., Rey, M. A., Santos-Ferreira, M. O., Laurent, A. G., Dauguet, C., Katlama, C., Rouzioux, C., Klatzman, D., Champalimaud, J. L., & Montagnier, L. (1986). Isolation of a new human retrovirus from West African patients with AIDS. *Science,* 233, 343-346.

Coffin, J.M. (1996). HIV viral dynamics. *AIDS,* 10(suppl 3), S75-S84.

Dimitrov, D.S. (1997). How do viruses enter cells? The HIV coreceptors teach us a lesson of complexity. *Cell,* 91, 721-730.

Embretson, J., Zupancic, M., Ribas, J. L., Burke, A., Racz, P., Tenner-Racz, K. & Haase, A.T. (1993). Massive covert infection of helper T-lymphocytes and macrophages by HIV during the incubation period of AIDS. *Nature,* 362, 359-362.

Epstein, F.H. (1991). The molecular biology of human immunodeficiency virus type 1 infection. *New England Journal of Medicine,* 324, 308-317.

Evans, W.J., Roubenoff, R. & Shevitz, A. (1998). Exercise and the treatment of wasting: Aging and human immunodeficiency virus infection. *Seminars in Oncology,* 25 (suppl 6), 112-122.

Goldsmith, M.F. (1992). World Health Organization consensus statement. Consultation on AIDS and sports. *Journal of the American Medical Association,* 267, 1312-1314.

Gottlieb, M.S., Schroff, R., Schanker, H.M., Weisman, J.D., Fan, P.T., Wolf, R.A. & Saxon, A. (1981). Pneumocystis carinii pneumonia and mucosal candidiasis in previously healthy homosexual men: Evidence of a new acquired cellular immunodeficiency. *New England Journal of Medicine,* 305, 1425-1431.

Graham, N.M.H. (1997). Epidemiology of acquired immunodefieciency syndrome: Advancing to an endemic era. *American Journal of Medicine, 102* (suppl 4A), 2-8.

Guidelines for the use of antiretroviral agents in HIV-infected adults and adolescents. (1998). *Annals of Internal Medicine, 128,* 1079-1100.

Henry, K., Stiffman, M. & Feldman, J. (1997). Anti-retroviral therapy for HIV infection. *Postgraduate Medicine, 102,* 100-120.

Ho, D.D., Neumann, A. ., Perelson, A.S., Chen, W., Leonard, J.M. & Markowitz, M. (1995). Rapid turnover of plasma virions and CD4 lymphocytes in HIV-1 infection. *Nature, 373,* 123-126.

Hymes, K.B., Cheung, T., Greene, J.B., Prose, N.S., Marcus, A., Ballard, H., William, D. C. & Laubenstein, L. J. (1981). Kaposi's sarcoma in homosexual men -- a report of eight cases. *Lancet, 2,* 598-600.

Johnson, J.E., Anders, G.T., Blanton, H.M., Hawkes, C.E., Bush, B.A., McAllister, C.K. & Matthews, J. I. (1990). Exercise dysfunction in patients seropositive for the human immunodeficiency virus. *American Review of Respiratory Disease, 141,* 618-622.

Kaldor, J. & Rubin, G. (1994). Epidemiology of HIV infection. In Albion Street Center (Ed.), *The AIDS Manual* (pp. 1-11). Sydney, Australia: MacLennan & Petty.

Kendall, A., Hoffman-Goetz, L., Houston, M., MacNeil, B. & Arumugam, Y. (1990). Exercise and blood lymphocyte subset responses: Intensity, duration and subject fitness effects. *Journal of Applied Physiology, 69,* 251-260.

Koot, M., van't Wout, A.B., Kootstra, N.A., deGoede, R.E.Y., Tersmette, M. & Schuitemaker, H. (1996). Relation between changes in cellular load, evolution of viral phenotype and the clonal composition of virus populations in the course of human immunodeficiency virus type 1 infection. *Journal of Infectious Diseases, 173,* 349-354.

LaPerriere, A.R., Antoni, M.H., Schneiderman, N., Ironson, G., Klimas, N., Caralis, P. & Fletcher, M. A. (1990). Exercise intervention attenuates emotional distress and natural killer cell decrements following notification of positive serologic status for HIV-1. *Biofeedback and Self-Regulation, 15,* 229-242.

LaPerriere, A.R., Fletcher, M.A., Antoni, M.H., Klimas, N.G., Ironson, G. & Schneiderman, N. (1991). Aerobic exercise training in an AIDS risk group. *International Journal of Sports Medicine, 12,* S53-S57.

LaPerriere, A.R., Ironson, G., Antoni, M.H., Schneiderman, N., Klimas, N. & Fletcher, M. A. (1994). Exercise and psychoneuroimmunology. *Medicine and Science in Sports and Exercise, 26,* 182-190.

LaPerriere, A.R., Klimas, N., Major, P. & Perry, A. *(1997). Acquired immune deficiency syndrome. In ACSM's Exercise Management for Persons with Chronic Diseases and Disabilities* (pp. 132-136). Human Kinetics: Champaign, Ill.

Lavi, E., Kolson, D.L., Ulrich, A.M., Fu, L. & González-Scarano, F. (1998). Chemokine receptors in the human brain and their relationship to HIV infection. *Journal of Neurovirology, 4,* 301-311.

Lawless, D., Jackson, C.G.R. & Greenleaf, J. E. (1995). Exercise and human immunodeficiency virus (HIV-1) infection. *Sports Medicine, 19,* 235-239.

Legg, J.L. & Balano, K.B. (1997). Symptom management in HIV-infected patients. *Primary Care, 24,* 597-606.

Lewicki, R.H., Tchorzewski, H., Majewska, E., Nowak, Z. & Baj, Z. (1988). Effect of maximal physical exercise on T-lymphocyte cell populations and on interleukin 1 (IL-1) and interleukin 2 (IL-2) production in vitro. *International Journal of Sports Medicine, 9,* 114-117.

Macarthur, R.D., Levine, S.D. & Birk, T.J. (1993). Supervised exercise training improves cardiopulmonary fitness in HIV-infected persons. *Medicine and Science in Sports and Exercise, 25,* 684-688.

Mellors, J.W., Rinaldo, C.R.J., Gupta, P., White, R.M., Todd, J.A. & Kingsley, L.A. (1996). Progress in HIV-1 infection predicted by the quantity of virus in the plasma. *Science, 272,* 1167-1170.

McCullough, M.J., Firth, N.A. & Reade, P.C. (1997). Human immunodeficiency virus infection: A review of the mode of infection, pathogenesis, disease course and the general and clinical manifestations. *Australian Dental Journal, 42,* 30-37.

Moore, J.P. (1997). Coreceptors: Implications for HIV pathogenesis and therapy. *Science, 276,* 51-52.

Murray, J.F. (1996). Pulmonary complications of HIV infection. *Annual Review of Medicine, 47,* 117-126.

Nieman, D.C., Johanssen, L.M., Lee, J.W., Cermak, J. & Arabatzis, K. (1990). Infectious episodes in runners before and after the Los Angeles Marathon. *Journal of Sports Medicine and Physical Fitness, 30,* 316-328.

Nieman, D.C., Miller, A.R., Henson, D.A., Warren, B.J., Gusewitch, G., Johnson, R.L., Davis, J.M., Butterworth, D.E., Herring, J.L. & Nehlsen-Cannarella, S.L. (1994). Effect of high versus moderate intensity exercise on lymphocyte subpopulations and proliferative response. *International Journal of Sports Medicine, 15,* 199-206.

O'Brien, W.A., Hartigan, P.M., Martin, D., Esinhart, J., Hill, A., Benoit, S., Rubin, M., Simberkoff, M.S., Hamilton, J.D. & the Veterans Affairs Cooperative Study Group on AIDS. (1996). Changes in plasma HIV-1 RNA and CD4+ lymphocyte counts and the risk of progression to AIDS. *New England Journal of Medicine, 334,* 426-431.

Pantaleo, G., Graziosi, C., Demarest, F., Butini, L., Montoni, M., Fox, C.H., Orenstein, J. M., Kotler, D.P. & Fauci, A.S. (1993). HIV infection is active and progressive in lymphoid tissue during the clinically latent stage of disease. *Nature, 362,* 355-362.

Perelson, A.S., Neumann, A.U., Markowitz, M., Leonard, J.M. & Ho, D.D. (1996). HIV-1 dynamics in vivo: Virion clearance rate, infected cell life-span and viral generation time. *Science, 271,* 1582-1586.

Pothoff, G., Wasserman, K. & Ostmann, H. (1994). Impairment of exercise capacity in various groups of HIV-infected patients. *Respiration, 61,* 80-85.

Powderly, W.G., Landay, A. & Lederman, M.M. (1998). Recovery of the immune system with antiretroviral therapy. *Journal of the American Medical Association, 280,* 72-77.

Report of the NIH panel to define principles of therapy of HIV infection. (1998). *Annals of Internal Medicine, 128,* 1057-1078.

Rigsby, L.W., Dishman, R.K., Jackson, A.W., Maclean, G.S. & Raven, P.B. (1992). Effects of exercise training on men seropositive for the human immunodeficiency virus-1. *Medicine and Science in Sports and Exercise, 24,* 6-12.

Rosenberg, Y.J., Anderson, A.O. & Pabst, R. (1998). HIV-induced decline in blood CD4/CD8 ratios: Viral killing or altered lymphocyte trafficking. *Immunology Today,* 19, 10-17.

Smith, A.I. & Pigott, P.C. (1996). HIV and respiratory disease. *Medical Journal of Australia,* 164, 425-428.

Soppi, E., Varjo, P., Eskola, J. & Laitenen, L.A. (1982). Effect of strenuous physical stress on circulating lymphocyte number and function before and after training. *Journal of Clinical and Laboratory Immunology,* 8, 43-46.

Spence, D.W., Galantino, M.L.A., Mossberg, K.A. & Zimmerman, S.O. (1990). Progressive resistance exercise: Effect on muscle function and anthropometry of a select AIDS population. *Archives of Physical Medicine and Rehabilitation,* 71, 644-648.

Stringer, W.W., Berezovskaya, M., O'Brien, W.A., Beck, C.K. & Casaburi, R. (1998). The effect of exercise training on aerobic fitness, immune indices and quality of life in HIV+ patients. *Medicine and Science in Sports and Exercise,* 30, 11-16.

Stryer, L. (1995). *Biochemistry* (4th ed.). W. H. Freeman & Company: New York.

Tvede, N., Kappel, M., Halkjaer-Kristensen, Galbo, H. & Pedersen, B.K. (1993). The effect of light, moderate and severe bicycle exercise on lymphocyte subsets, natural and lymphokine activated killer cells, lymphocyte proliferative response and interleukin 2 production. *International Journal of Sports Medicine,* 14, 275-282.

Ullum, H., Lepri, A.C., Victor, J., Skinhøj, P., Phillips, A.N. & Pedersen, B.K. (1997). Increased losses of CD4+CD45RA+ cells in late stages of HIV infection is related to increased risk of death: Evidence from a cohort of 347 HIV-infected individuals. *AIDS,* 11, 1479-1485.

Ullum, H., Palmo, J., Halkjaer-Kristensen, J., Diamant, M., Klokker, M., Kruuse, A., LaPerriere, A. & Pedersen, B.K. (1994). The effect of acute exercise on lymphocyte subsets, natural killer cells, proliferative responses and cytokines in HIV-seropositive persons. *Journal of Acquired Immune Deficiency Syndrome,* 7, 1122-1133.

Watson, R.R., Moriguchi, S., Jackson, J.C., Werner, L., Wilmore, J.H. & Freund, B.J. (1986). Modifications of cellular immune functions in humans by endurance exercise training during b-adrenergic blockade with atenolol or propranolol. *Medicine and Science in Sports and Exercise,* 18, 95-100.

Wei, X., Ghosh, S.K., Taylor, M.E., Johnson, V.A., Emini, E.A., Deutsch, P., Lifson, J. D., Bonhoeffer, S., Nowak, M.A., Hahn, B.H., Saag, M.S. & Shaw, G. M. (1995). Viral dynamics in human immunodeficiency virus type 1 infection. *Nature,* 373, 117-122.

Yunis, N.A. & Stone, V.E. (1998). Cardiac manifestations of HIV/AIDS. *Journal of Acquired Immune Deficiency Syndrome and Human Retrovirology,* 18, 145-154.

Suggested Readings

Birk, T.J. (1996). HIV and exercise. *Exercise Immunology Review,* 2, 84-95.

Calabrese, L.H. & LaPerriere, A. (1993). Human immunodeficiency virus infection: *Exercise and athletics. Sports Medicine,* 15, 6-13.

CDC. (1986). Current trends classification system for human T-lymphotropic virus typ*e III/lymphadenopathy-associated virus infections. Morbidity and Mortality Weekly Report,* 35, 334-339.

CDC. (1992). 1993 revised classification system for HIV infection and expanded surveillance case definition for AIDS among adolescents and adults. *Morbidity and Mortality Weekly Report,* 41(no. RR-17).

Coffin, J.M. (1996). HIV viral dynamics. *AIDS,* 10 (suppl 3), S75-S84.

Evans, W.J., Roubenoff, R. & Shevitz, A. (1998) Exercise and the treatment of wasting: Aging and human immunodeficiency virus infection. *Seminars in Oncology,* 25, 112-122.

Lawless, D., Jackson, C.G.R. & Greenleaf, J.E. (1995). Exercise and human immunodeficiency virus (HIV-1) infection. *Sports Medicine,* 19, 235-239.

Report of the NIH panel to define principles of therapy of HIV infection. (1998). *Annals of Internal Medicine,* 128, 1057-1078.

Rigsby, L.W., Dishman, R.K., Jackson, A.W., Maclean, G.S. & Raven, P.B. (1992). Effects of exercise training on men seropositive for the human immunodeficiency virus-1. *Medicine and Science in Sports and Exercise,* 24, 6-12.

Spence, D.W., Galantino, M.L.A., Mossberg, K.A. & Zimmerman, S.O. (1990). Progressive resistance exercise: Effect on muscle function and anthropometry of a select AIDS population. *Archives of Physical Medicine and Rehabilitation,* 71, 644-648.

Stringer, W.W., Berezovskaya, M., O'Brien, W.A., Beck, C.K. & Casaburi, R. (1998). The effect of exercise training on aerobic fitness, immune indices and quality of life in HIV+ patients. *Medicine and Science in Sports and Exercise,* 30, 11-16.

CHAPTER 17

Selected Immunological/ Hematological Disorders

CONNIE B. SCANGA

Connie B. Scanga, Ph.D., earned her bachelor's degree in psychology from the University of Pennsylvania. After completing her doctorate in exercise physiology from Temple University, Scanga was an assistant professor at Temple University and, later, Eastern College, both located in southeastern Pennsylvania. Currently she is a research fellow at the Malaghan Institute of Medical Research in Wellington, New Zealand, pursuing research on the role of various components of the immune system in the disease process of atopic asthma.

Anemia
Chronic
Fatigue Syndrome
Lupus

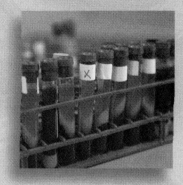

This chapter reviews three distinct disorders that are characterized by debilitating or disabling fatigue: chronic fatigue syndrome, systemic lupus erythematosus and anemia.

Fatigue is associated with various physiological states and conditions. For example, it is a normal and typical response to a particularly intense workout or to a period of sleep deprivation. Undue fatigue that is persistent or not relieved by sleep also is a common complaint. In fact, as many as 15 percent to 30 percent of patients seeing primary-care physicians report fatigue as a major problem (Hickie, 1995).

Chronic Fatigue Syndrome

What is Chronic Fatigue Syndrome?

Chronic fatigue syndrome (CFS) is a poorly understood condition characterized by severe and disabling fatigue that persists or recurs for six or more consecutive months, and is not relieved by rest (Fukuda et al., 1994). This condition often is accompanied by other symptoms, including mild fever and recurring sore throat, swollen lymph nodes, muscle weakness or soreness (**myalgia**), headaches, and disturbances of memory, concentration or mood. The syndrome first was recognized in the latter part of the 19th century and was named "neurasthenia" (i.e., nerve weakness). Throughout the 1900s, epidemics and isolated cases of chronic fatigue were recorded, although the condition was variously designated "neuromyesthenia," "postviral fatigue syndrome," "chronic Epstein-Barr virus syndrome" and "**fibromyalgia** syndrome" (Sabin & Dawson, 1993).

To standardize research on chronic fatigue, the Centers for Disease Control proposed the name "chronic fatigue syndrome" and developed a definition of the condition (Fukuda et al., 1994; Holmes et al., 1988). According to the CDC, CFS is defined by unexplained, persistent or relapsing chronic fatigue that:

- lasts at least six months
- is of new or definite onset
- is not the result of ongoing exertion, and is not significantly relieved by rest
- results in substantial reduction in previous levels of occupational, educational, social or personal activities

Additionally, four or more of the following symptoms must concurrently occur and cannot predate the fatigue:

- impairment of short-term memory or concentration
- sore throat
- tender cervical or axillary lymph nodes
- headache
- unrefreshing sleep
- muscle or multi-joint pain without swelling or redness
- post-exertion malaise lasting more than 24 hours

It is important to remember that the CDC criteria were established to delineate a controlled-subject population for research studies. As a result, these criteria are rather rigorous. Physicians in the primary-care setting are likely to be more liberal in applying the CFS diagnosis. Thus, your referred clients who have been diagnosed with CFS may not specifically meet the criteria described above.

Etiology and Pathophysiology of CFS

Epidemiology

Epidemiological reports on the prevalence of CFS in patients reporting severe fatigue vary from 0.002 percent to 3.3 percent, depending on the case definition used to define the illness. The illness is more likely to affect women than men, and typically has its onset when patients are in their late 20s to early 30s. In the majority of cases, but not all, the onset of CFS is immediately preceded by viral illness. It may be reassuring to patients to know that CFS is not fatal. The course of the disease is characterized by partial remissions and exacerbations of symptoms that usually persist for 2.5 to 7.5 years (Farrar, Locke & Kantrowitz, 1995).

Etiology of the Illness

CFS is a heterogeneous disorder; the duration and reported symptoms of the illness vary from case to case. Over the years, different models have been proposed to explain the events that trigger and sustain CFS. The major hypotheses include:

- *Persistent viral infection*

There are reports that CFS patients may have chronic infections by human herpesvirus-6, an enterovirus (e.g., a less virulent strain of poliovirus), the Epstein-Barr virus or a retrovirus (e.g., human T-lymphotropic virus type I or II) (Komaroff, 1993; Parker, Brukner & Rosier, 1996). Viral infection during a period of overtraining, and exercise training during and immediately after viral infection, may place athletes at increased risk of developing CFS (Parker, Brukner & Rosier, 1996). However, although many CFS patients report acute viral infection immediately prior to the onset of symptoms, nearly half of all CFS patients show no evidence of infection immediately prior to CFS onset. Further, no single infectious agent has been identified in all cases of CFS. Antiviral therapies are reported to be ineffective in treating the disease (Farrar et al., 1995).

- *Chronic immune dysfunction*

Abnormal cellular immune responses result in abnormal **cytokine** production and activity, mediating the persistent symptoms of CFS. Minor abnormalities in immune function have been reported in CFS patients. These include higher-than-normal levels of antibody to viral antigens, decreased natural killer cell number and cytotoxicity, suppressed lymphocyte proliferation response in *in vitro* assays, and abnormal cytokine activity. However, these results have not been standardized or reproduced (Farrar et al., 1995).

- *Neuropsychiatric disorder*

The frequency of depression, anxiety and **somatization** (i.e., attributing psychological distress to physical symptoms) is higher in CFS patients than in controls. A significant number of patients are reported to have had psychiatric problems before the onset of chronic fatigue (Katon, Buchwald, Simon, Russo & Mease, 1991; Kreusi, Dale & Straus, 1989). However, there also is evidence that the frequency of premorbid depression (Hickie, Lloyd, Wakefield & Parker, 1990) and psychosocial stress (Lewis, Cooper & Bennett, 1994) is similar in patients and controls. Many patients develop symptoms of depression and anxiety within one to two months of the onset of the disorder (Hickie et al., 1990). Although this may exacerbate other symptoms and play a role in sustaining the illness, there is no clear evidence that psychiatric factors alone are the triggering mechanism for CFS.

- *The "hybrid" model*

As noted previously, CFS is a complex disorder that manifests differently in each patient. This has led some experts to suggest a "hybrid" model of causation that includes both physical and psychological factors. Briefly, this model proposes that CFS results from a disturbance in immunologic function triggered by an external factor (e.g., stress, allergies, toxins, a mild defect in the hypothalamic-pituitary-adrenal axis). Once triggered, the interaction between the immunologic, virologic, neurologic and psychological factors sustains the array of CFS symptoms (Komaroff, 1993).

Clinical Evaluation and Treatment

People with chronic fatigue often are dismayed to find there is no definitive screening test for CFS. As a result, diagnosis essentially is a process of ruling out alternative conditions that may explain the symptoms typically experienced. Medical assessment of chronic fatigue patients typically includes a thorough history (mental and psychosocial), mental status examination, physical evaluation and basic laboratory screenings (including complete and differential blood counts; erythrocyte sedimentation rate; liver and renal function tests; serum levels of electrolytes, blood glucose, proteins and blood urea nitrogen; thyroid function tests; and urinalysis). Based on the symptoms presented and the results of these preliminary tests, additional studies also may be required (Fukuda et al., 1994; Hickie, Lloyd & Wakefield, 1995) before CFS is diagnosed.

No one treatment strategy can be applied to all patients. Rather, the treatment approach employed depends on specific symptoms and their intensity. Treatment may be aimed at restoring sleep or mood, relieving myalgia and **arthralgia**, and lifestyle management. The following medications and treatments often are employed:

- *nonsteroidal anti-inflammatory agents:* NSAIDS may be either over-the-counter or prescription strength, depending on the severity of muscle aches (fibromyalgia) and flu-like symptoms.

- *antidepressant medications:* Antidepressant drugs frequently are prescribed for CFS patients who may experience depression as either a premorbid condition or a consequence of their illness. Additionally, antidepressants may be prescribed in low doses to help control sleep patterns and to relieve muscle aches.

- *other medications:* Allergies (to inhalants, food or drugs) are common in patients with CFS, and antihistamines may be used for treatment. Additionally, anti-anxiety medication may be prescribed to alleviate acute anxiety and panic attacks.

- *cognitive behavior therapy:* Individual or group cognitive behavior therapy may be recommended to promote behavioral change and alter dysfunctional thought patterns. Although widely used, the benefits of this therapy have not been clearly demonstrated.

- *alternative approaches to treatment:* Many patients employ alternative therapies, including dietary and nutritional approaches, herbal remedies, detoxification therapies and avoidance of environmental toxins. These therapies often are expensive and, to date, their benefits have not been demonstrated in controlled studies.

Physiological Responses to Exercise in CFS Patients

CFS patients demonstrate a normal cardio-respiratory and metabolic response to aerobic exercise (Gibson, Carroll, Clague & Edwards, 1993; Sisto et al., 1996). Although there are reports of significantly lower VO_2max and reduced exercise tolerance in CFS patients versus controls (Riley et al., 1990), subsequent studies have reported only mildly decreased VO_2max in CFS patients (Gibson et al., 1993; Kent-Braun, Sharma, Weiner, Massie & Miller, 1993). Maffulli, Testa & Capasso (1993) investigated the changes in exercise capacity in eight male varsity athletes with post-viral fatigue syndrome over a 13-month period. They found a small (but statistically significant) reduction in absolute and relative VO_2max within a month after the onset of illness. Thirteen months after the end of the illness, VO_2max had recovered to near baseline values in all the athletes.

Individuals with CFS tend to exhibit alterations in perceived exertion, and are likely to have higher rating of perceived exertion scores at submaximal workloads than normal subjects. Interestingly, in their study with highly trained athletes, Maffulli et al. (1993) reported that prior to infection, the anaerobic threshold (defined by the authors as the exercise intensity at which there was a loss of linearity between heart rate and external work) occurred at approximately 82 percent of VO_2max; at one month and 13 months post-infection, the anaerobic threshold occurred at 71 percent and 79 percent, respectively. Endurance also was significantly reduced throughout the period of this study. The lowering of the anaerobic threshold and endurance could help to explain the reduced exercise tolerance in CFS patients. However, other studies have failed to show consistent abnormalities in skeletal muscle function (i.e., endurance and recovery) or in the biochemical and histological properties of skeletal muscle in people with CFS (Gibson et al., 1993; McCully, Natelson, Iotti, Sisto & Leigh, 1996; Wong et al., 1992) that might help account for their limited exercise tolerance.

It remains unclear to what extent physical deconditioning limits exercise tolerance in these subjects. However, it has been suggested that the early fatigue experienced by CFS patients is associated with a lowered threshold for sensation in skeletal muscle that results in increased afferent (sensory) activity. Thus, the fatigability of exercising CFS individuals may be due to central (i.e., neurological) factors, rather than deconditioning alone.

The physical and psychological benefits of exercise training in this population have been well documented. Fulcher & White (1997) recently reported a 13-percent improvement in

Table 17.1

Client Information to Obtain from Medical Professionals

1) Are there systemic manifestations that preclude or limit exercise?

2) Specifically, are you aware of cardiovascular conditions that may preclude or limit exercise?

3) Has this client had a graded exercise test? If so, were any abnormal cardiovascular responses observed?

4) Does this client have known musculoskeletal, neuromuscular or arthritic conditions that may be exacerbated by exercise?

5) What medications is the client currently taking?

6) Are there limitations on this client's activity?

7) Do you have recommendations regarding the level of supervision for exercise sessions?

VO$_2$max and a 26-percent improvement in isometric strength in CFS patients following 12 weeks of progressive aerobic exercise training. Their patients also reported improvements in fatigue and functional capacity following training — improvements that were maintained or exceeded at three- and 12-month follow-ups. Only one subject (out of 29 exercisers) withdrew from the study because the treatment worsened their symptoms. Therefore, physical activity is unlikely to be harmful. In fact, greater aerobic fitness and muscular strength may lead to decreased disability in CFS patients.

The Pre-exercise Screening & Assessment

Assessment

Mild- to moderate-intensity exercise is one of the treatment strategies recommended to CFS individuals by an increasing number of primary-care physicians. People with CFS can be excellent candidates for successful exercise programming in a community-based setting.

In most cases, people with CFS initiate exercise training on their physician's recommendation. Prior to the initial screening and fitness assessment, you should notify the primary-care physician of the client's intent to exercise and request pertinent medical information. This contact can be made in writing and should include a copy of your client's signed consent for the release of information. Obtain specific medical information that will be useful in planning a safe assessment and subsequent exercise program (Table 17.1).

To ensure your client's safety during subsequent fitness testing, have them complete the PAR-Q (Physical Activity Readiness Questionnaire) prior to the screening session.

As noted previously, medications commonly used in the treatment of CFS include analgesics (NSAIDS) and antidepressants. Specific medications prescribed vary depending on the type of symptoms experienced and their severity. Antidepressant medications have variable effects on resting and exercise heart rate and blood pressure responses, and you must be aware of these specific effects. Instruct your client to notify you when medication changes are made.

The initial pre-exercise screening allows you to review your client's medical history and form a positive relationship with them. During this session, it is helpful to gather information about the physical symptoms your client is experiencing (or has recently experienced) and the strategies they use to cope. Many people with CFS vacillate between the absolute avoidance of physical activity and intense efforts to achieve unrealistic physical goals. This behavior pattern tends to exacerbate their symptoms, and may reinforce a belief that exercise is harmful. The typical CFS individual has frequently experienced extreme fatigue and increased muscle soreness following exercise. Be prepared to talk about your client's misconceptions about exercise training, and provide information about the physiological effects of deconditioning and progressive exercise training.

Fitness Testing

The complete fitness evaluation may include assessments of body composition, cardiorespiratory endurance, muscular endurance and flexibility. Follow the guidelines in Chapter 2 of the *ACE Personal Trainer Manual* for assessing body composition, muscular endurance and flexibility.

Submaximal cycle ergometry tests are recommended for evaluating cardiorespiratory fitness and deriving an estimated VO$_2$max. CFS clients fatigue quickly and may be severely deconditioned due to prolonged periods of physical inactivity. The test should be limited to eight to 12 minutes (i.e., two to four three-minute stages).

Contraindications to Exercise

Chronic mild fever (i.e., oral temperature between 37.5° C and 38.6° C) is not uncommon in CFS clients. Those who experience intermittent fevers as a symptom of CFS should check their temperature before exercising. If your client's temperature is elevated, but below 38° C, limit exercise activity to gentle stretching. Instruct your client to avoid vigorous exercise when their temperature is over 38° C (100.4° F).

Exercise Programming

Exercise Guidelines

There are few reports on the effects of exercise programming on CFS patients. From the published reports available, however, exercise does not appear to be harmful to CFS patients or to prolong the course of the disease (Kantrowitz et al., 1995).

Keep in mind the following points when providing exercise guidelines for your CFS client:

1. The primary goal of exercise training is to prevent further deconditioning and progressive physical disability; initial phases of the exercise program should be more conservative and less intense than programming for a healthy person of the same age, gender and fitness level.

2. Following initial training sessions, your client is likely to experience greater fatigue and discomfort (delayed muscle soreness) than they are accustomed to; you may improve long-term participation and compliance by warning your client about this in advance.

3. Studies have reported that CFS patients have a tendency to overestimate their premorbid fitness levels, leading them to set unrealistic expectations for exercise performance after becoming ill; help your client develop realistic long-term fitness goals.

4. Typically, CFS clients will note a period during the day when their symptoms are less severe; encourage them to exercise at this time.

5. Fibromyalgia-like symptoms are most likely to affect the hip and shoulder-girdle region; exercise program modifications may be necessary if client discomfort warrants it.

The Aerobic Program

Mode: Walking is excellent during initial programming stages. Instruct clients using a treadmill to walk at no incline (0-percent grade), especially if hip discomfort is a problem. After several weeks, your client should be more comfortable with exercise training and adept at monitoring exercise intensity, and you can introduce alternate modes of activity (e.g., exercise bikes, ski exercisers, and water aerobics in a heated pool).

Intensity: Begin at 40 percent of estimated VO_2max, and progress incrementally over the initial 12 to 15 weeks of training to 60 percent of estimated VO_2max.

Duration: Initial sessions should last five to 15 minutes and increase to 30 to 45 minutes of aerobic activity per session.

Frequency: Initially, your client should exercise on alternate days, three to five days per week. After the initial two to three weeks, encourage them to exercise up to five days per week.

Progression: The main focus is on increasing duration, rather than intensity. Duration of aerobic sessions should be increased gradually (no more than two to three minutes per week). Once your client can sustain low-intensity aerobic activity for 30 minutes, exercise intensity may gradually be progressed.

Stretching and Flexibility

Instruct your client to complete slow, static stretching exercises at the beginning and end of the exercise session. Stretching exercises should focus on the hip/thigh and shoulder girdle. Prescribe one to three repetitions of each stretching exercise, and recommend that each stretch be held for 10 to 30 seconds. Gentle stretching may help relieve muscle discomfort, and also can be performed at home on rest days.

Resistance Training

The goal of resistance training is to improve muscular endurance. To this end, the American College of Sports Medicine (1995) recommendations for resistance training are applicable to CFS clients. Resistance training should incorporate eight to 10 exercises that train major muscle groups, and can be performed three days per week on alternate days. Prescribe one set of 12 to 15 repetitions for each exercise. Initially, be sure to use minimal to low resistance.

People with mild CFS and no other chronic diseases can participate in sports and other recreational activities as their tolerance allows. Your client should receive medical clearance to participate in contact sports. Stress the need to start with low-intensity activities.

Exercise Leadership

Although there are relatively few reports on the physiological responses to acute and chronic exercise in CFS, there is no reason to believe that the response will be significantly different than that observed in healthy adults who engage in low- to moderate-intensity training. When monitoring exercise, note the following:

- Planned rest is important and should be incorporated into the exercise program. Encourage your client to avoid inconsistent and variable activity.
- Reduce or discontinue exercise activities when clients have acute viral infections and/or when their temperature is elevated.
- Monitor your client's exercise, especially in the initial stages, to ensure that they follow the program and do not over-exert.
- Relapse is common in CFS. Depending on the severity of symptoms, exercise may need to be reduced or discontinued during these periods. Exercise can resume when symptoms abate, but begin at a lower intensity than that at which your client had been training prior to the relapse.
- Assist your client in monitoring relative levels of energy and fatigue, as well as their patterns of rest and refreshing sleep. Document this information on a weekly basis and use it to make appropriate recommendations about exercise progression and to avoid overtraining.

Provide written follow-up reports to the referring physician every three months. These reports should summarize the modes of exercise employed, exercise progression since the last report, and information regarding your client's response to exercise programming.

Case Study 1

Anne Russell is a 34-year-old woman who works as a regional manager for a national healthcare corporation, and is active in parent organizations at her children's

school. Although she travels frequently on business, she says that prior to the CFS diagnosis she maintained a healthy lifestyle that included exercise four to five times per week.

Anne's first symptoms of CFS began approximately eight months ago, and included fatigue and unrefreshing sleep. The fatigue was so extreme that after work she was unable to fulfill home and family responsibilities. After two weeks of persistent exhaustion, Anne developed swollen lymph nodes and aches in her muscles and joints. She also began to experience headaches and an inability to concentrate at work. Most of her symptoms seemed to recur sporadically – except fatigue, which was persistent.

Over the next three to four months, Anne was evaluated several times by her physician. Initially, he prescribed rest/relaxation and medications to relieve her symptoms. When the symptoms persisted, he ran a series of diagnostic tests to help identify her disease. All of the test results were negative. During this time, Anne tried to maintain regular exercise by walking during lunch. However, these sessions left her exhausted for several days and intensified the aches in her muscles and joints. Five months after the onset of symptoms, Anne changed physicians. After reviewing her case and repeating a series of tests, this doctor diagnosed her condition as CFS. He provided Anne with educational information about the disease, and prescribed lifestyle modifications, including exercise training, to help her more effectively cope with her symptoms.

During Anne's initial session you review her responses to the PAR-Q and determine there are no immediate contraindications to her involvement in an exercise program. It becomes obvious during the interview that Anne is impatient with her illness and depressed by her physical limitations.

The initial fitness assessment includes a three-stage cycle ergometry test (with resting and exercise blood pressures), modified push-ups, body composition assessment (skinfold measures), and evaluation of flexibility (sit-and-reach test). Anne's estimated

Table 17.2

Typical Activity Guidelines

- Activity as tolerated
- No vigorous exercise during viral illness or periods of acute infection

VO_2max (approximately 26.5 ml/kg^{-1}/min^{-1}) and muscular endurance are low.

Anne's exercise program emphasizes flexibility and endurance training, and consists of 10 minutes of aerobic training (treadmill walking) at an intensity of 40 percent to 45 percent VO_2max, with stretching prior to and after aerobic exercise. You instruct her to exercise three times the first week (on alternate days), and since she usually feels less lethargic in the late morning, you encourage her to exercise at that time. You both agree to meet at the end of the first week to review her progress and modify the program.

At the first follow-up meeting (and subsequent follow-ups), exercise progression is determined based on Anne's report of how she felt immediately before and after exercise sessions, and on the day after exercise. After one week of training, Anne is not experiencing any increase in symptoms, so the duration of the aerobic phase of exercise is progressed (to 12 minutes). In subsequent weeks, you continue the progression in the duration of the aerobic phase of training. Motivation to continue exercise is a significant problem for Anne and you frequently must reinforce the goal of this stage of training (i.e., stop further deconditioning and increase Anne's ability to perform daily activities).

You introduce resistance training in the third week of exercise (two upper-body and two lower-body exercises initially, one set of 12 to 15 repetitions for each activity), and in the fourth week, four additional exercises are added to the resistance phase of her training.

Systemic Lupus Erythematosus

What is Systemic Lupus Erythematosus?

Systemic lupus **erythematosus** (SLE) or "lupus" is a chronic inflammatory, autoimmune disease that affects multiple organ systems and most commonly occurs in women of childbearing age. Typically, the organ systems involved do not become affected simultaneously. Rather, disease manifestations in organs become apparent over time. The severity of lupus symptoms is highly variable, ranging from mild (requiring no treatment) to severe (potentially fatal loss of organ function) (Braden, McGlone & Pennington, 1993; Schroeder & Euler, 1997).

Epidemiology

Sex, race, age and socioeconomic status influence the expression of SLE. The disease is eight to nine times more common in women than men, although it is only three times more common in women outside childbearing age (Rasaratnam & Ryan, 1997). In the United Kingdom, the incidence of SLE was found to be approximately two-and-one-half times greater in Asian women and five times greater in Afro-Caribbean women than Caucasian (Johnson, Gordon, Palmer & Bacon, 1995). In the U.S., the incidence of SLE among blacks was reported to be three times greater than among whites. The mean age at diagnosis was significantly lower for black women than for white, and lower in all women than in men. The prognosis of the disease also was found to be less favorable in blacks (Hochberg, 1985). Pediatric-onset SLE tends to be more severe, while SLE in the elderly is milder and not as debilitating (Rasaratnam & Ryan, 1997).

Despite the increase in survival rate in recent decades, patients with SLE still die at a rate three times greater than the general population. Deaths early in the disease course are likely to be related to the disease itself. However, those late in the course of the disease may be attributed either to the disease or to the cumulative effects of SLE treatment. Infection, either directly or indirectly, is the primary cause of death (Gladman, 1996).

Classification and Diagnosis of SLE

Because SLE symptoms are so broad and variable, clinical diagnosis usually is not clear-cut. To aid classification of SLE, the American College of Rheumatology (ACR) established and revised criteria that helps to distinguish lupus from other related diseases. According to ACR criteria (Tan et al., 1982), individuals must fulfill four of the following 11 criteria at some point in the course of the disease to be diagnosed with SLE:

1. malar rash: an erythemic rash that covers both cheeks and the bridge of the nose, often called "butterfly rash"
2. discoid rash: erythematosus raised patches that may result in scarring
3. photosensitivity: a skin rash that results from an unusual reaction to exposure to sunlight

4. oral ulcers
5. arthritis
6. serositis: either pleuritis or pericarditis
7. renal disorder: proteinuria or cellular casts
8. neurological disorder: seizures or psychosis (in the absence of offending drugs or metabolic disorder)
9. hematological disorder: hemolytic anemia, **leukopenia** or **lymphopenia** (low white-blood-cell or lymphocyte count, respectively) or **thrombocytopenia** (low platelet count)
10. immunological disorder
11. presence of **antinuclear antibodies**

Etiology and Pathophysiology of SLE

Etiology of the Illness

The specific etiology of lupus is unknown. However, the consensus is that it is an autoimmune disorder characterized by production of autoantibodies (antibodies reactive to "self" peptides) that are directed against several antigens, including nuclear antigens. Some of the autoantibodies do not appear to be pathogenic, but they do have high diagnostic specificity and serve as serological markers for the disease in clinical tests. Others (antiphospholipid antibodies that cause increased blood clotting and increased rates of arterial and venous thromboses) contribute in clearly identified ways to the disease process itself (Rasaratnam & Ryan, 1997; Schroeder & Euler, 1997).

The mechanism through which most autoantibodies induce the SLE disease process is unknown. There is no evidence that antinuclear antibodies are able to penetrate cell membranes or bind to intracellular receptors (Kotzin, 1996). It is known that some autoantibodies bind to extracellular antigens, forming immune complexes that then produce inflammation. Tissue damage can result from either the inflammatory process or from other dysfunction caused by the autoantibodies (Rasaratnam & Ryan, 1997).

Epidemiological evidence exists for the role of genetic factors in the etiology of SLE. Family studies report that approximately 5 percent to 12 percent of relatives of SLE patients also develop the disease (Rasaratnam & Ryan, 1997). Further, Deapen and colleagues (1992), who studied the prevalence of SLE in monozygotic and dizygotic twins, reported a concordance of 24 percent of 45 monozygotic twins and 2 percent of 62 dizygotic twins. The genetic basis for SLE in animal models has been shown to be quite complex. Evidence indicates that in animals, different genetic contributions may underlie the same phenotype. This same phenomenon also may be true in humans. Therefore, it is likely that environmental triggers also play some role in the etiology of SLE. One hypothesis is that genetic susceptibility underlies the etiology of SLE, but environmental factors activate the immune system. The specific environment factors involved in immune activation are as yet unknown. However, this dysfunctional activation of the immune system causes both T- and B-lymphocytes to be activated, and B-lymphocytes begin the production and release of autoantibodies (Kotzin, 1996).

Pathophysiology of SLE

SLE is a complex disease that involves multiple organ systems. The manifestations of the disease are diverse and variable, and a wide range of symptoms and severity are possible. Some of the more common clinical features are described below.

Constitutional Features

Common nonspecific systemic features of SLE are malaise, fatigue, fever and weight loss. Malaise and fatigue are common presenting concerns (first signs/symptoms that send people to the doctor), and often recur during "flares" (periods of disease activity). The incidence of fibromyalgia in SLE is high, and may contribute to fatigue (Petri, 1995). Weight loss of up to 10 percent is most likely in the period immediately prior to diagnosis of the disease. In some patients, fever may be the only manifestation of the disease. Because no pattern of fevers is specifically associated with SLE, it often is difficult to distinguish infection-related fevers from those related to SLE. People with SLE are especially prone to infections, perhaps as a result of the immunomodulations associated with the disease. The use of corticosteroids and immunosuppressive agents in disease treatment also enhances this tendency (Pisetsky, Gilkeson & Clair, S., 1997; Rasa-ratnam & Ryan, 1997).

Cutaneous (dermatologic) Features

Approximately 80 percent of SLE patients exhibit cutaneous involvement. Clinical manifestations of SLE are quite variable, and include the classic "butterfly" rash, vasculitis (inflammation of blood vessels), discoid lesions, oral ulcers and alopecia. Between one- and two-thirds of SLE patients are photosensitive. For these patients, even brief exposure to sunlight can trigger dermal and systemic flares of the disease (Pietsky et al., 1997; Petri, 1995; Rasaratnam & Ryan, 1997).

Musculoskeletal Features

Almost all SLE patients experience some form of musculoskeletal symptoms. Arthritis and arthralgia, with morning stiffness, are the most common initial manifestations of the disease. Arthritis typically affects the small joints of the hands, wrists and knees. It can cause joint swelling and decreased range of motion, and can lead to deformation of joints (especially in the hands), but does not usually damage joint tissue. Fibromyalgia is commonly exhibited. Abnormalities have been noted in muscle biopsies of patients. These include vessel wall thickening and Type II fiber atrophy. Skeletal damage may occur as a result of avascular **necrosis,** increasing the risk of hip fractures and vertebral compression. There is evidence that long-term corticosteroid treatment is associated with an increased prevalence of osteoporosis in SLE patients, although this remains controversial (Pietsky et al., 1997; Petri, 1995; Rasaratnam & Ryan, 1997; Sims & Smith, 1996).

Hematological Features

Anemia is the most common hematological disorder of SLE. Although the anemia may have different etiologies, hemolytic anemia is the most common. Leukopenia and lymphopenia also may occur, usually during flares. Thrombocytopenia (decreased platelet number) occurs in as many as one-quarter of SLE patients, and can be problematic as it increases the risk for bruising and bleeding — either

spontaneously or following injury (Boumpas et al., 1995; Rasaratnam & Ryan, 1997; Sims & Smith, 1996).

Serositis

Serositis (inflammation of the serous membranes) is most likely to manifest as pleuritis or pericarditis (Pisetsky et al., 1997).

Cardiovascular Manifestations

Approximately 60 percent of SLE patients exhibit cardiovascular complications, with symptoms ranging from mild serositis to organ failure. Valvular complications occur in 20 percent of SLE patients. As mentioned previously, vasculitis is a common feature of SLE. The inflammation of vessel walls usually affects smaller vessels. As vessels in almost any organ can be affected, vasculitis can have a variety of manifestations. The constitutional manifestations of vasculitis include fever, myalgias and arthralgias, and malaise.

The most common cardiac manifestation is pericarditis. However, valvular disease, conduction disturbances, endocarditis and myocarditis, and premature atherosclerosis also are frequently observed in SLE patients. Coronary artery disease has become increasingly prevalent in the SLE population. Boumpas et al. (1995) report that 53 percent of SLE patients have at least three cardiac risk factors. Atherosclerosis in SLE patients is accelerated by long-term corticosteroid use, as well as by complications stemming from the SLE disease process in other organs (Boumpas et al., 1995; Petri, 1995; Rasaratnam & Ryan, 1997; Sims & Smith, 1996).

Respiratory Manifestations

The most common respiratory manifestation is pleuritis. Other acute and chronic features have been reported (e.g., alveolar hemorrhage, acute reversible hypoxemia, interstitial lung disease and pulmonary hypertension), but they are less common (Boumpas et al., 1995; Petri, 1995; Rasaratnam & Ryan, 1997; Sims & Smith, 1996).

Renal Features

Kidney abnormalities occur in virtually all cases of SLE, and the pattern and severity of renal manifestations differ among patients.

The disease process includes acute inflammation of renal tissue during periods of disease activity, as well as permanent damage associated with scarring and fibrosis (Pisetsky et al., 1997). Approximately 5 percent of SLE patients progress to chronic renal failure and require dialysis or renal transplant (Rasaratnam & Ryan, 1997). Hypertension and hyperlipidemia, both of which are frequent correlates of SLE, may be related to either renal disease or corticosteroid treatment (Schroeder & Euler, 1997).

Neuropsychiatric Features

Nervous system dysfunction occurs in at least 50 percent of SLE patients, with specific manifestations reflecting the pattern of tissue injury (Pisetsky et al., 1997). Most common are headaches and peripheral **neuropathy**. Other manifestations include seizures, **paresthesia**s (abnormalities of sensation), cognitive impairment and psychiatric disorders (e.g., depression, anxiety and psychosis). The etiology of nervous system disorders is unclear, but is likely due to vascular abnormalities (premature atherosclerosis or thrombosis) or immune-mediated injury (Pisetsky et al., 1997; Rasaratnam & Ryan, 1997).

Course of SLE and Common Treatments

The first symptoms of SLE commonly reported by adults are constitutional (fatigue, fever and weight loss), serositis, arthritis, photosensitivity and rashes. Fatigue is often the most disabling symptom of the disease. The course of the disease is marked by fluctuating intensity of symptoms, with flares (periods of inflammation and disease activity) occurring intermittently. Flares may be generalized, in which case systemic involvement and damage can occur, or discrete (involving only a single organ system). Flares may be precipitated by physical and psychological stress, infections and exposure to sunlight. An important component of disease management is awareness and avoidance of events that precipitate flares.

Management of active SLE is geared toward treating symptoms when they are present. Thus, the degree of therapeutic intervention at any given time in individual patients will be determined by the type and severity of the symptom. The following medications are typically employed in the treatment of SLE:

- *Nonsteroidal anti-inflammatory agents (NSAIDS):* NSAIDs are widely used to manage mild lupus manifestations, including arthritis and myalgia, constitutional symptoms (e.g., fever, headaches) and serositis.
- *Corticosteroids:* Topical corticosteroids may be used to treat cutaneous symptoms. Intermediate- and high-dose oral corticosteroids (prednisone and prednolisone) are routinely used to control constitutional, cutaneous and musculoskeletal symptoms, as well as serositis and certain central nervous system disorders. High-dose intravenous corticosteroids (methylprednisolone) may be used during periods of severe immunological, hematological, pulmonary and renal involvement. As noted earlier, the chronic use of corticosteroids is associated with immunosuppression, weight gain, increased incidence of hyperlipidemia, accelerated atherosclerosis and osteoporosis.
- *Antimalarials:* Antimalarials (chloroquine, hydroxychloroquine and quinacrine) are used to treat mild to moderate cutaneous, musculoskeletal (arthritis and arthralgias) and constitutional symptoms. Long-term antimalarial treatment has been associated with retinopathy which can, in extreme cases, lead to blindness.
- *Immunosuppressive agents:* These medications (azathioprine and cyclophosphamide) are used to treat resistant end-organ inflammation and lupus nephritis. The adverse side effects of these drugs include infections and malignancies (Rasaratnam & Ryan, 1997; Schroeder & Euler, 1997).

Physiological Responses to Exercise in SLE Patients

SLE patients have a significantly lower VO_2max than age- or sex-matched (Daltroy et al., 1995; Sakauchi et al., 1995). Reductions in maximal exercise capacity may be attributable to various causes, depending on the individual's disease manifestations. Reduced exercise capacity may be attributable to deconditioning, limited increase in the (a-v)O_2 difference associated with abnormalities in muscle microcirculation or reduced extraction of oxygen by muscle tissue (Sakauchi et al., 1995), or cardiorespiratory abnormalities (Hellman et al., 1994; Winslow et al., 1993).

The benefits of exercise for SLE patients parallel those derived by healthy individuals. Specifically, the reduced risk of coronary artery disease, improved cardiovascular function and work capacity, increased flexibility and improved quality of life have been demonstrated in those with rheumatic diseases, including mild- to moderate SLE (Beals et al., 1985; Daltroy et al., 1995; Harkcom et al., 1985; Nordemar, 1981; Robb-Nicholson et al., 1989). Although the effects of exercise on lipid profile and bone density have not been studied to date, it is expected that exercise training in SLE patients would also provide benefits in these areas.

The Pre-exercise Screening & Assessment

The Assessment

Prior to the initial screening and fitness assessment, notify the client's rheumatologist of their intent to exercise and request pertinent medical information. Contact can be made in writing and should include a copy of the client's signed consent for the release of information. Obtain specific medical information that will be useful in planning a safe assessment and subsequent exercise program (Table 17.3).

To ensure your client's safety during subsequent fitness testing, have them complete the PAR-Q (Physical Activity Readiness Questionnaire) prior to the screening session.

As noted previously, medications commonly used in the treatment of SLE per se include NSAIDS, antimalarial agents and corticosteroids. Specific medications prescribed vary depending on the type and severity of symptoms experienced. Remember that the risk of accelerated atherosclerosis in this population increases with the duration of the disease (especially with renal disease) and/or cumulative corticosteroid treatments. SLE clients also may be taking medications for chronic conditions that develop secondary to SLE (e.g., anti-

hypertensive agents). Be aware of the specific effects induced by the medications prescribed, and instruct your client to notify you when medication changes occur.

Fitness Testing

The complete fitness evaluation may include assessments of body composition, cardiorespiratory endurance, muscular endurance and flexibility. Follow the guidelines in Chapter 2 of the *ACE Personal Trainer Manual* for assessing body composition, muscular endurance and flexibility.

Submaximal cycle ergometry tests are recommended for evaluating cardiorespiratory fitness and deriving an estimated VO_2max. Exercise capacity is typically reduced by approximately 30 percent to 40 percent in SLE subjects, as a result of the disease process itself and/or deconditioning. The test should be limited to eight to 12 minutes (i.e., two to four three-minute stages).

Contraindications to Exercise

Infections are particularly problematic for SLE patients, and may precipitate a disease flare. Additionally, infection is a major cause of mortality in SLE patients, especially in those receiving high-dose corticosteroid or immunosuppressive agents. Instruct your client to monitor fevers and flu-like symptoms, and to avoid vigorous exercise when infection is suspected.

Exercise Programming

Exercise Guidelines

Remember the following points when providing exercise guidelines for your SLE client:

1. Expect a range of symptom severity and disease manifestations (e.g., hypertension and hyperlipidemia, fibromyalgia, non-eroding arthritis, coronary artery disease, etc.) in this population, and tailor exercise according to the symptoms presented.
2. The primary goal of exercise training should be to prevent further deconditioning; initial phases of the exercise program should be more conservative and less intense than programming for a healthy person of the same age, gender and fitness level.
3. Typically, SLE clients note a period during the day when their symptoms are less severe; encourage them to exercise at this time.

4. Exposure to sunlight triggers flares in a significant number of SLE patients; avoid prescribing outdoor exercise.

Aerobic Program

Mode: Walking and cycle ergometry are excellent during initial programming stages. Introduce alternate modalities after your client becomes more comfortable with exercise training and adept at monitoring exercise intensity.

Intensity: Begin at 50 percent of predicted VO_2max, and progress incrementally over the initial 12 to 15 weeks of training to 60 percent to 70 percent of predicted VO_2max.

Duration: Initial sessions should last 10 to 15 minutes, increasing to 30 to 45 minutes of aerobic activity per session.

Frequency: Initially, your client should exercise on three to five days per week on alternate days. After two to three weeks encourage them to exercise up to five days per week.

Progression: The main focus is on increasing duration, rather than intensity. Increase exercise duration gradually until your client can sustain low-intensity aerobic activity for 30 minutes, then gradually progress exercise intensity.

Stretching and Flexibility

Instruct your client to complete slow, static stretching exercises at the beginning and end of the exercise session. Tailor these per instructions for CFS clients (Table 17.2).

Resistance Training

The goal of resistance training is to improve muscular endurance. To this end, the American College of Sports Medicine (1995) recommendations for resistance training are applicable to SLE clients. Resistance training should incorporate eight to 10 exercises that train major muscle groups, and can be performed three days per week on alternate days. Prescribe one set of 12 to 15 repetitions for each exercise. Initially, be sure to use minimal to low resistance.

Clients with mild to moderate SLE and no other chronic diseases can participate in sports and other recreational activities as their tolerance allows.

Exercise Leadership

When monitoring exercise, note the following:
- Clients should reduce or discontinue exercise activities when they have acute viral infections.
- During a flare (depending on symptoms and severity), it may be necessary to reduce or discontinue exercise. When symptoms are under control, resume exercise at an intensity lower than that at which the client had been exercising prior to the flare.
- Monitor your client's exercise and their response; if any manifestation of their lupus worsens, or if new symptoms develop, instruct your client to discontinue exercise until they have discussed the symptoms with their physician.
- Remind any client who has a history of Reynaud's phenomenon, which is not uncommon in SLE, to wear adequate clothing to protect fingers and toes during cold-weather outdoor exercise.

Provide written follow-up reports to the referring physician every three months. Summarize the modes of exercise employed, exercise progression since the last report and information regarding your client's response to exercise programming.

Case Study 2

Melanie Petrowski, a 25-year-old woman who works as a textile designer, has SLE. She experienced what may have been her first symptoms of the disease (fatigue, dry and reddish skin on her face and neck, morning stiffness in her fingers, toes and knees) when she was in her late teens, but these were dismissed as "growing pains." Symptoms recurred several times over the next few years. A few months ago, Melanie experienced a period of relatively severe arthritis and fibromyalgia, along with fatigue and oral ulcers. It was during this flare that the disease was diagnosed. Disease manifestations were brought under control with oral corticosteroid therapy (prednisone), and Melanie continues on low-dose prednisone treatment. She is hoping to discontinue corticosteroid treatment in the near future, in part because of the weight gain she has experienced while on the medication.

Your initial fitness assessment of Melanie includes a three-stage cycle ergometry test (with resting and exercise blood pressures), modified push-ups, body composition assessment (skinfold measures) and evaluation of flexibility (sit-and-reach test). Melanie's estimated VO$_2$max (approximately 26.5 ml/kg^{-1}/min-1) and muscular endurance are low, and her body fat is approximately 26 percent.

Melanie's exercise program emphasizes endurance training. She knows that longer-duration activity is the best way for her to use excess calories and lose weight. However, her low level of conditioning and fatigability prevent prolonged continuous activity. Her initial program consists of 15 minutes of aerobic training (treadmill walking or cycling) at an intensity of 50 percent to 55 percent VO$_2$max, with stretching at the beginning and end of the exercise session. You introduce resistance training exercises in stages at Melanie's first two exercise sessions (one set of 12 to 15 repetitions, three times per week). Melanie feels that her best time to exercise is early afternoon, and she is able to flex her work schedule to accommodate midday workouts.

In the initial months of training, the duration and intensity of the aerobic phase of Melanie's workout are gradually increased. She walks or cycles for 30 minutes at 55 percent to 60 percent VO$_2$max, five days per week. Unfortunately, Melanie experiences a viral infection that precipitates a flare and necessitates a three-week break in training. When Melanie returns to the health club, you advise her to gradually resume her previous level of aerobic training beginning with 20 to 30 minutes at 50 percent to 55 percent VO$_2$max, three to four days per week.

Anemia

What is Anemia?

Anemia is defined as reduced hemoglobin content in the blood. Hemoglobin, which is packaged in red blood cells, carries oxygen from the lungs to the body's tissues. The hematocrit measures the percentage of red blood cells in a vol-

ume of whole blood. In men the normal hematocrit range is 42 percent to 50 percent, while in women the normal range is 36 percent to 45 percent. When the blood hemoglobin level falls, the oxygen-carrying capacity of the blood also decreases. Normal hemoglobin concentration of whole blood is 14 to 18 g/dL^{-1} in men and 12 to 15 g/dL^{-1} in women. Anemia is diagnosed when an individual's blood hemoglobin concentration falls below this range.

Anemic individuals may feel weak and lethargic, experience excessive fatigue, have a pale appearance, become short of breath with exertion, and be prone to bruising. Interestingly, some anemic individuals do not experience any symptoms. Conversely, not all people who experience fatigue are anemic.

Pathophysiology and Treatment of Anemia

In adults, red blood cells are produced in the red bone marrow. Development begins when myeloid stem cells differentiate and develop into erythroblasts that synthesize hemoglobin as they grow and develop. After a few days, erythroblasts eject their nucleus and become reticulocytes. Reticulocytes continue to synthesize hemoglobin for up to two more days before becoming mature erythrocytes (red blood cells). Both reticulocytes and mature erythrocytes are released from the red marrow into circulation. Reticulocytes account for approximately 1 percent of the circulating red blood cell population. The rate of erythrocyte synthesis is regulated by the hormone erythropoietin.

The normal red blood cell has a life span of approximately 120 days. When an erythrocyte becomes old, damaged or defective, it is removed from circulation by macrophages in the spleen or liver. It is estimated that normally, about 2.5 million erythrocytes are destroyed every second. Thus, to maintain hematocrit and hemoglobin

Table 17.3

Typical Activity Guidelines

- Activity as tolerated
- No vigorous exercise during viral illness or periods of acute infection

concentrations within normal ranges, an equivalent number of normal red blood cells must be produced in the red marrow to replace those that die. Anemia, an abnormally low blood hemoglobin content, results when there is an imbalance between the rate of normal erythrocyte production and destruction. This can occur when there is inadequate erythrocyte or hemoglobin production, or premature erythrocyte death (Steinberg, 1982).

Anemias Associated with Inadequate Nutrition

Iron Deficiency

This is the most common cause of anemia worldwide. Iron is an essential component of heme (and other enzymes, including myoglobin). Most (70 percent to 95 percent) of the 2 to 4 grams of iron in the adult body is contained in hemoglobin; much of the remaining iron is held in a storage pool (in the form of ferritin or hemosiderin). Iron, which is bound to the transport protein transferrin, is transferred from storage sites to the red marrow in the blood. Normally transferrin is approximately one-third saturated (approximately one-third of the iron-binding sites are occupied). The clinical measure of total iron-binding capacity (TIBC) represents the unsaturated iron-binding capacity (UIBC) plus the serum iron content. Both UIBC and TIBC are commonly increased in iron-deficiency anemia, while transferrin saturation is significantly decreased. Serum ferritin levels are positively correlated (although not linearly) with total-body iron stores (normal serum ferritin is 20 g/L^{-1}). Serum ferritin is characteristically decreased with iron-deficiency anemia (serum ferritin <12 gL^{-1}). Serum ferritin may be elevated in certain chronic disease states (e.g., rheumatoid arthritis). Thus, serum ferritin values alone may not provide a totally reliable index of iron storage in these patients.

The human body is remarkably efficient in conserving its iron content. Adults lose approximately 1 mg of iron from the body daily, primarily through feces. Perspiration and exfoliation of the skin and mucosae also contribute to iron loss, although the effect is generally minimal. Only a small percentage of dietary iron is absorbed. However, the average American diet contains 10 mg to 15 mg of iron per day, which is normally adequate to balance the 1-mg-per-day iron loss.

Manifestations of iron deficiency become more severe as negative iron balance is sustained for prolonged periods. In the initial stage of iron deficiency (iron depletion stage), the body's iron stores are depleted or significantly reduced. Blood hemoglobin, hematocrit and serum ferritin levels are all within normal range during this stage. As iron depletion progresses, serum ferritin concentration, iron concentration and transferrin saturation begin to fall. This condition is clinically termed iron deficiency without anemia because, although storage iron is decreased, serum hematocrit and hemoglobin levels are still within the clinically normal range. In the most advanced stage, when hemoglobin level also falls below normal, the patient is diagnosed with iron-deficiency anemia.

Women with heavy menstrual flow can lose so much iron that they must absorb 3 mg to 4 mg of dietary iron per day to maintain iron balance. In fact, the most common cause of iron deficiency in women is blood loss through abnormally heavy menstrual flow. Also, during pregnancy and lactation, iron requirements increase two- to five-fold. Interestingly, approximately 25 percent of adult American women have depleted iron storage (Linker, 1996), and as many as 90 percent of pregnant women may be iron-depleted (Beutler et al., 1995). Thus, while iron deficiency is relatively rare in men, it is not uncommon in younger women, and iron supplementation may be required to correct the condition. However, serious health effects are associated with chronic iron overload (including hepatic fibrosis, cardiac disease and diabetes). Thus, caution is advised regarding the use of iron supplementation.

Bleeding is another important cause of iron-deficiency anemia. Because iron-deficient diets are rare in Western countries, iron-deficiency anemia is usually viewed as an indication of occult blood loss (especially in the gastrointestinal tract). Stomach or duodenal ulcers and chronic aspirin use (e.g., in rheumatoid arthritis patients) are common causes of iron-deficiency anemia. Obviously, successful treatment of an iron deficiency due to bleeding must be directed toward the underlying cause of blood loss, as well as restoration of body iron.

Endurance exercise training may modulate iron metabolism. There are reports of higher incidences of iron deficiency and iron-deficiency anemia in endurance-trained men and women versus controls (Mouton et al., 1990; Pate, Miller, Davis, Slentz & Klingshirn, 1993). Additionally, serum ferritin levels in previously sedentary subjects who begin endurance exercise training programs may decrease at least transiently (reflecting a decrease in storage iron). However, these effects are obscure (Bourque, Pate & Branch, 1997; Lukaski, Hoverson, Gallagher & Bolonchuk, 1990; Rajaram et al., 1995). Although the impact of endurance exercise on iron balance has not been fully explained, it is suspected that intravascular hemolysis (associated with foot striking during running) and greater iron loss through sweat may lead to greater rates of iron excretion in physically active people (Lamanca, Haymes, Daly, Moffatt & Waller, 1988; Mouton et al., 1990; Waller & Haymes, 1996).

Folic Acid (folate) Deficiency

Folate is a vitamin present in most fruits and vegetables. One of its key roles in the body is as a coenzyme used in DNA synthesis. Folate deficiency is associated with **megaloblastic** anemia, a condition in which lack of DNA prevents cell division in immature erythrocytes. As a result, fewer mature erythrocytes, and mostly immature megaloblasts, are released from the bone marrow.

The primary cause of folate deficiency is an inadequate diet. In Western countries, those most likely to develop folate deficiency are the poor, the elderly, alcoholics and hemodialysis patients.

Folate deficiency also may occur due to impaired absorption or increased requirements. Since most folate is absorbed in the duodenum, deficiencies of this nutrient may be caused by small intestinal disease, surgical resection and malabsorption syndromes. Also, certain medications (dilantin and methotraxate) are known to interfere with absorption. Folate requirements are increased during pregnancy and in conditions where there is increased cell turnover (e.g., psoriasis and hemolytic anemias) (Linker, 1996; Steinberg, 1982; Beutler, Lichtman, Coller & Kipps, 1995).

Vitamin B_{12} Deficiency

Vitamin B_{12} is present in all foods of animal origin. Dietary deficiency is seen only in vegans and is very rare. During digestion, vitamin B_{12} binds with intrinsic factor, a protein secreted by the gastric glands, in the stomach. The intrinsic factor-vitamin B_{12} complex actually is absorbed in the terminal portion of the ileum by cells with specific receptors for the complex.

The most common cause of vitamin B_{12} deficiency is malabsorption that may result from conditions such as gastrointestinal surgeries (removal of large portions of the stomach) or Crohn's disease. The most common cause of vitamin B_{12} deficiency, however, is pernicious anemia. Pernicious anemia is a hereditary autoimmune disease in which intrinsic factor secretion (and thus, vitamin B_{12} absorption) is reduced due to inflammation and atrophy of the gastric mucosa. The progression of the disease may span several decades, so the diagnosis is more common in the elderly.

Vitamin B_{12} is required for activation of folate coenzymes. Therefore, vitamin B_{12} deficiency can contribute to folate deficiency. Also, vitamin B_{12} plays a role in maintaining myelin. Deficiency of this vitamin can lead to various neurological symptoms (peripheral neuropathy, poor balance and impaired mental function). It is important to distinguish between folate deficiency and vitamin B_{12} deficiency as the cause of a nutritional anemia to prevent the progressive neurological damage associated with untreated vitamin B_{12} deficiency.

Deficiency usually is successfully treated with regular (and lifelong) injections of vitamin B_{12}. This therapy will stop the progression of neurological damage, but usually will not completely reverse damage that ensued prior to diagnosis and treatment (Ban-Hock, Van Driel & Gleeson, 1997; Linker, 1996; Steinberg, 1982).

The Hemolytic Anemias

Hemolysis is the breakdown or destruction of red blood cells, with a resulting release of hemoglobin. Hemolytic anemias are disorders characterized by premature erythrocyte death. Bone marrow can normally increase red blood cell production by six- to eight-fold. Hemolytic anemia, then, only occurs when the marrow's ability for erythrocyte production is outpaced by erythrocyte destruction. Because the first three types of anemias (sickle cell anemia, thalassemia and glucose-6-phosphate deficiency) discussed in this section have a common etiology in abnormal hemoglobin structure or function, some basic information will be reviewed about hemoglobin prior to discussing the specific hemolytic anemias.

Hemoglobin is a complex molecule with a quaternary structure. It is composed of four polypeptide chains, two of one kind and two of another. Each polypeptide contains an iron-containing heme group that can reversibly bind to oxygen. Hemoglobin A (HbA) comprises approximately 97 percent of hemoglobin in healthy adults and is made up of two alpha (α) chains and two beta (β) chains. The remaining 2 percent to 3 percent of adult hemoglobin is HbA2, a molecule composed of two α chains and two delta (δ) chains. Fetal erythrocytes contain fetal hemoglobin (HbF), a molecule composed of two alpha (α) chains and two gamma (γ) chains. Normally almost all fetal hemoglobin is replaced by adult hemoglobin during the first year of life. Each of the different types of polypeptide chains (α, β, δ and γ) has a slightly different amino acid composition that determines the chain's conformation and noncovalent interactions within the hemoglobin molecule.

Sickle Cell Anemia and Sickle Cell Trait

Sickle cell anemia is an autosomal recessive disorder. It results from a single nucleotide base change in DNA that leads to a single amino acid substitution in the β chains of hemoglobin. The resulting hemoglobin contains two α chains and two β^S chains and is designated HbSS. Due to the amino acid composition of β^S chains, deoxygenated HbSS aggregates to form large polymers. These polymers have a rigid elongated structure that deforms the red blood cell, producing the "sickle" shaped erythrocyte characteristic of this disease. The polymers, and the early membrane damage they induce, are reversible. However, repeated sickling leads to permanent membrane damage and deformation of the cell. Damaged erythrocytes are removed prematurely from the circulation (i.e., they have an average life span of 17 days), primarily in the spleen. As a result of this hemolysis, the marrow has to replace ap-

proximately 6 percent of the total erythrocyte population rather than the normal 0.9 percent per day. Functional adaptation to the chronic anemia of this condition is facilitated by the low O_2 affinity of HbSS, which facilitates O_2 unloading in the tissues.

Factors which enhance the sickling response include:

- *The hydration state of red blood cells.* Dehydration makes the cells more vulnerable to sickling. Unfortunately, the membrane damage resulting from sickling increases the erythrocyte tendency to dehydrate, creating a vicious cycle of cellular damage.

- *The relative amounts of other types of Hb in red blood cells.* HbF cannot participate in polymer formation. When the proportion of HbF in the cells is increased, sickling is inhibited. Certain populations are homozygous (i.e., they have inherited the sickle gene from both parents) for the sickle cell mutation, yet exhibit only mild clinical manifestations of the disease due to their relatively high proportion of HbF. However, the most common forms of sickle cell anemia in America are associated with low proportions of HbF.

- *Hypoxemia and acidosis (within the erythrocyte).* Both of these factors promote sickling.

The course of sickle cell disease is marked by acute episodes associated with vaso-occlusion. Acute episodes (sickle crisis) occur when sickled cells aggregate and occlude the microvasculature. Although small blood vessels in any part of the body may be affected, common sites of vaso-occlusion are vessels in the bones (especially in the back, and the long bones of the arms and legs) and the chest. Acute episodes may last hours to days, and are accompanied by excruciating pain and low-grade fever. Repeated episodes result in permanent organ damage. The most common debilitating conditions that occur are enlargement and infarct of the spleen and liver, kidney infarcts and nephron dysfunction, bone infarcts and ischemic necrosis of the bone, nonhealing ulcers of the lower leg, gallstones, retinopathy, pulmonary emboli and strokes. Almost all individuals with sickle cell anemia develop cardiomegaly and have systolic murmurs due to chronic anemia. Sickle crisis may be precipitated by the following factors:

- infection
- dehydration — a special problem because kidney damage may interfere with the ability to concentrate urine
- hypoxia
- cold exposure — promotes vasoconstriction, making vaso-occlusive episodes more likely

In their recent investigation of blood pressure and sickle cell disease, Pegelow et al. (1997) found significantly lower blood pressures in those with sickle cell anemia versus NHANES II norms for age, race and sex. The blood pressure difference increased with age, and the risk for occlusive stroke increased in sickle cell anemia subjects with increased systolic (but not diastolic) blood pressure. They conclude that blood pressure values that would be considered normal or only slightly elevated in adults with HbA (blood pressure greater than 140/90) should be medically evaluated for treatment.

Although therapeutic approaches have been proposed and developed to mitigate the sickling process, to date there is no specific treatment for sickle cell anemia. Individuals with this disorder regularly take folate supplements to help sustain their high rate of erythrocyte production. Individuals should try to maintain adequate hydration and avoid hypoxia — factors that may precipitate acute episodes. During aplastic and hemolytic crises, transfusions may be necessary.

The sickle gene is most commonly found in those of African ancestry, and less often in those of Mediterranean, Indian or Middle Eastern descent. The genetic mutation responsible for sickling is generally thought to have conferred protection against malaria. The sickle gene is found in 8 percent of American blacks. However, only about 1 percent are homozygous for the trait and, thus, have sickle cell anemia. More commonly, individuals are heterozygous (they have inherited the mutated gene from only one parent) for the trait. These people are said to have sickle cell trait.

Individuals with sickle cell trait (heterozygous for the sickle gene mutation, HbAS) are clinically normal, and may go through life unaware that they have a genetic mutation. Since they have one copy of the S gene, they do make abnormal hemoglobin. However, the proportion of defective hemoglobin in the blood is relatively low. These people have acute episodes only under extreme circumstances (e.g., vigorous exertion at high altitudes or flying in unpressurized aircraft). It is recommended that those with sickle cell trait avoid factors (i.e., dehydration, hypoxia, acidosis and exposure to extreme cold) that can precipitate sickle crisis. Unfortunately, sickle cell trait can be inherited along with thalassemia or other hemoglobin abnormalities (Bunn, 1997; Linker, 1996; Steinberg, 1982; Beutler, Lichtman, Coller & Kipps, 1990).

Thalassemia

Thalassemia affects millions of people worldwide and may be one of the most common inherited disorders. Originally discovered in those of Mediterranean descent (Italians and Greeks), it is now also known to affect (albeit to a lesser extent) Chinese, Indians and African Americans. Thalassemia is a heterogeneous group of disorders, ranging in severity from mild to fatal. Fortunately, the mildest forms are the most common.

Thalassemia is characterized by decreased synthesis of one or more of the globin chains, leading to decreased Hb production. It eventually results in a chronic anemia, in which erythrocytes are small and have a low hemoglobin content. When there is a decreased synthesis of α-globin chains, the condition is known as α-thalassemia; decreased β-chain production leads to β-thalassemia. The imbalance in α- and β-chain synthesis leads to an excess of polypeptides within red blood cells, producing cellular damage. This erythrocyte damage results in both destruction of developing erythrocytes within the red marrow and premature erythrocyte death in the circulation. The bone marrow attempts to compensate for the resulting anemia, but is ineffective in doing so.

Alpha-thalassemia is caused by a gene deletion. The condition is most common in individuals from Southeast Asia and China, and less common in blacks. Normal adults have four α-globin genes. When only three α-globin genes are present, the individual is a silent carrier (i.e., they have normal blood but can pass the genetic defect to offspring). When two α-globin genes are present, the individual has α-thalassemia trait; these people have mild anemia, but are considered clinically normal and have a normal life expectancy. When only one α-globin gene is present, the individual is diagnosed with HbH disease, and will have chronic hemolytic anemia of mild to moderate severity. Alpha-thalassemia is a frequent complication in those with sickle cell trait.

Beta-thalassemia is common in persons of Mediterranean ancestry and, to a lesser extent, Chinese, Asians and blacks. The etiology of the disease is attributed to point mutations, rather than gene deletions. As a result of the genetic mutation, β-chain synthesis is markedly reduced (β^+) or absent altogether (β°). The variants of β- thalassemia are as follows:

- *β-thalassemia major (homozygous for β°)*

This is a severe hemolytic anemia. Newborns with this disease are normal until about six months of age, when sufficient HbF is replaced by the defective HbA. Children are treated with transfusion therapy and folate supplementation, but they may still experience growth failure, bone deformities (due to expansion of marrow cavities), enlarged liver and spleen, increased incidence of infection, and leg ulcers. By puberty, consequences of chronic iron overload start to become apparent, and the prevalence of resulting cardiomyopathy, damaged liver, spleen and/or pancreas, and endocrine dysfunction is quite high. Iron-chelating agents (e.g., deferoxamine) are routinely administered to delay or avoid permanent organ damage. Cardiac failure and death usually occur between the ages of 20 and 30.

- *β-thalassemia intermedia (homozygous for β^+)*

Since some β-chain synthesis occurs, these people have a milder form of the disease. They have chronic hemolytic anemia, but usually only require transfusions during periods of stress. Individuals with thalassemia intermedia are also prone to iron overload. These people survive into adulthood, but may have bony deformities and enlargement of the liver and/or spleen.

- *β-thalassemia minor*

These individuals are heterozygous for a mild form of the disease. They develop mild anemia, but it is not clinically significant (Linker, 1996; Steinberg, 1982; Beutler, Lichtman, Coller & Kipps, 1995).

Glucose-6-phosphate Dehydrogenase (G6PD) Deficiency

G6PD is an enzyme involved in the reaction sequence that detoxifies the hydrogen peroxide produced as a byproduct of intracellular erythrocyte metabolism. When G6PD is absent from the cells, Hb becomes oxidized, resulting in denaturation and precipitation. Thus, G6PD deficiency results in membrane damage and premature erythrocyte destruction in the spleen.

G6PD is an X-linked recessive disorder that affects 10 percent to 15 percent of American black males. Its prevalence also is quite high in the Mediterranean region, China and Southeast Asia, and certain populations in the Middle East.

Many variants of the G6PD enzyme have been described. The variant most common in affected American blacks exhibits activity levels about 15 percent of normal. Its activity begins to rapidly decline even further when the red blood cells are more than 40 days old, resulting in cellular damage and premature death. The Mediterranean variants of G6PD have dramatically lower activity levels, and result in chronic hemolytic anemia and severe-to-fatal hemolytic crises. Women who are heterogeneous for G6PD deficiency are carriers. One gene is inactivated in each cell. The inactivation process is random, and the extent of the enzyme deficiency depends on the percentage of normal genes inactivated. Thus, the expression of G6PD deficiency is extremely variable in women. Women who are homozygous for G6PD deficiency are quite rare.

People with G6PD deficiency usually are healthy and treatment is unnecessary. However, when their erythrocytes are exposed to abnormal oxidative stress, an acute hemolytic episode may be precipitated. Acute hemolytic anemia following drug ingestion is the most common manifestation of the disease. Common precipitating drugs are the sulfanomides, sulfones and antimalarials (Linker, 1996; Steinberg, 1982; Beutler, Lichtman, Coller & Kipps, 1995).

Autoimmune Hemolytic Anemia

Autoimmune hemolytic anemia is an acquired disorder in which one's own immune system produces autoantibodies against proteins in the erythrocyte membrane. As a result of this inappropriate immune activity, erythrocytes are destroyed prematurely and removed from the circulation by the spleen. In nearly half the people who have autoimmune hemolytic anemia, the underlying cause is unknown, although it is sometimes seen in conjunction with other chronic diseases (e.g., SLE and chronic lymphocytic leukemia).

Typically, this anemia is severe and has a rapid onset. The treatment of choice is corticosteroids such as prednisone. The long-term prognosis for those with the disorder is good.

Anemias Resulting from Decreased Bone Marrow Production

Anemia of Chronic Disease

Many chronic systemic diseases (e.g., rheumatoid arthritis, other inflammatory diseases, cancer, liver and renal disease) are associated with mild to moderate anemia. Generally, these anemias develop gradually as a result of the bone marrow's failure to increase erythrocyte production to compensate for the moderate decrease in erythrocyte life span. This imbalance can be at least partially attributed to a blunted erythropoietin production by the kidney. These anemias are rarely severe enough to require treatment.

The anemia of chronic renal disease seems to be more complex in its pathogenesis. Not only is erythropoietin production severely compromised by renal disease, but other factors commonly associated with chronic renal disease (e.g., uremia and hypertension) contribute to a dramatic reduction in erythrocyte life span. Therapy for the anemia of chronic renal disease includes folate and iron supplementation. Additionally, recombinant human erythropoietin (rEPO) is administered to stimulate red blood cell production. Due to the expense of rEPO therapy, it is only prescribed for patients with more severe anemia of chronic disease (Linker, 1996; Means, 1995; Steinberg, 1982; Beutler, Lichtman, Coller & Kipps, 1995).

Aplastic anemia

Not only are erythrocytes derived from the hematopoietic stem cell in the bone marrow, but granulocytes and platelets are as well. Aplastic anemia results from injury to or suppression of hematopoietic stem cells. As a result, this anemia is characterized by pancytopenia (abnormally low blood concentrations of erythrocytes, granulocytes and platelets) and a fatty or "empty" bone marrow cavity. The condition can vary in severity, depending on the extent of the marrow damage. Severe aplastic anemia is potentially fatal, due to the patient's increased risk of infection and bleeding associated with decreased granulocytes and platelets, respectively.

There are numerous causes of aplastic anemia. They include radiation and chemotherapy, adverse reactions to various drugs, SLE, autoimmune suppression of blood cell production and environmental toxins (e.g., benzene and insecticides). Although the aplastic anemia induced by radiation and chemotherapy is transient, it is probably the most common form of the disease.

Treatment of aplastic anemias varies based on the pathogenesis and severity of the condition. Supportive therapies (e.g., transfusions and antibiotics for infection) are prescribed as needed. In many cases, bone marrow damage can be corrected with immunosuppressive agents. The success of immunosuppressive therapies depends on the extent of the marrow damage and the capacity to regenerate functional hematopoietic stem cells. Very severe cases are treated through bone marrow transplant when an appropriate donor is available (Linker, 1996; Steinberg, 1982; Beutler, Lichtman, Coller & Kipps, 1995; Young & Maciejewski, 1997).

Physiological Responses to Exercise in Anemia

The anemic patient has a reduced O_2- and CO_2-carrying capacity due to low blood hemoglobin content. Compensatory mechanisms that help maintain O_2 delivery at rest include increased respiration rate and increased cardiac output. Additionally, increased levels of 2, 3-DPG (associated with a high proportion of young erythrocytes and/or with chronic stress) and decreased pH within erythrocytes may cause a right shift of the oxyhemoglobin dissociation curve, facilitating oxygen delivery to the tissues (Loria, Sanchez-Medal, Lisker, de Rodrigues & Labardini, 1967; Magazanik et al., 1991; Sproule, Mitchell & Miller, 1959).

Both submaximal exercise endurance and VO_2max are reduced in anemia. This lower exercise tolerance is primarily associated with the reduced O_2-carrying capacity of the blood, which is only partially compensated by hemodynamic adjustments. Specifically, cardiac output, heart rate and ventilation are higher in anemic individuals than normal controls at any given submaximal workload. Additionally, there appears to be increased redistribution of blood flow to working muscles, which helps to compensate for the reduced O_2 content of arterial blood. As a result of the rapid increase in heart rate and cardiac output during progressive exercise, peak aerobic power (VO_2max) is always reduced in anemia. The magnitude of the reductions in VO_2max and submaximal exercise endurance is proportional to the severity of the anemia. It has been suggested that chronic anemia also may be associated with altered endocrine profiles. For example, Celsing et al. (1986) suggest that the reduced maximal heart rate they reported in anemic subjects may be associated with reduced β-adrenergic receptor activity associated with chronically elevated catecholamine levels (Celsing, Nyström, Pihlstedt, Werner & Ekblom, 1986; Gregg, Willis & Brooks, 1989; Koskolou, Roach, Calbet, Rådegran & Saltin, 1997; Sproule, Mitchell & Miller, 1959; Woodson, 1984; Woodson, Wills & Lenfant, 1978; Zhu & Haas, 1997).

Angina and myocardial infarction have been reported in individuals who have sickle cell anemia (HbSS) without coronary artery disease (Hamilton, Rosenthal, Berwick, & Nadas, 1978; Martin, Cobb, Tatter. Johnson & Haywood, 1983). Furthermore, the incidence of S-T segment depression during exercise in people with sickle cell anemia may be as high as 16 percent, although the exact cause of this ischemia is unknown (Alpert, Dover, Strong, & Covitz, 1984; Alpert, Gilman, Strong, Ellison, Miller & McFarlane, 1981). However, people with sickle cell trait (HbAS) appear to exhibit a normal exercise and recovery response. Exercise performance and adaptations to exercise training are apparently inversely related to the severity of anemia in those with sickle cell disease (Alpert et al., 1984; Gozal et al.,

1992; McConnell, Daniels, Lobel, James & Kaplan, 1989; Robinson, Stone & Asendorf, 1976).

The anemia of end-stage renal disease can now be at least partially corrected with rEPO therapy. However, the increased blood hemoglobin content does not result in proportionately increased exercise capacity, perhaps because uremia limits peripheral O_2 uptake and utilization (Brautbar, 1983; Lazaro & Kirschner, 1980; Moore, Parsons, Stray-Gundersen, Painter, Brinker & Mitchell, 1993). Increases in VO_2 peak of 20 percent to 45 percent following three or more months of endurance exercise training have been reported in this population. The improved exercise capacity following training can occur independent of improvements in serum hematocrit and hemoglobin concentrations (Painter et al., 1986; Ross et al., 1989). Interestingly, it has been reported that trained anemic animals had lower VO_2max, but greater muscle oxidative capacity and greater endurance than untrained controls (Gregg, Willis & Brooks, 1989). Taken together with data from studies of those with chronic renal disease, this suggests that training-induced improvements in muscle oxidative capacity could be important functional adaptations for all anemia clients.

It should be noted that anemia itself is not a disease, but rather a sign of an underlying condition that may (or may not) be resolved with treatment. The conditions underlying or associated with anemia may themselves create exercise risks. For example, the chronic iron overload associated with moderate to severe hemolytic anemias (e.g., β-thalassemia and sickle cell anemia) may result in cardiomyopathy, premature atherosclerosis or other organ damage that could result in reduced exercise tolerance. And, as a consequence of abnormally low O_2 content in the blood, anemic adults with no previous history of cardiac symptoms may experience angina during intense exercise.

The Pre-exercise Screening & Assessment

The Assessment
Prior to the initial screening and fitness assessment, notify the primary-care physician of

the client's intent to exercise and request pertinent medical information. This contact can be made in writing and should include a copy of the client's signed consent for the release of information. Obtain specific medical information that will be useful in planning a safe assessment and subsequent exercise program (see Table 17.4).

Have your client complete the PAR-Q prior to the screening session to ensure their safety. As noted previously, medications and/or therapies will be directed toward conditions that underlie the anemia, as well as the anemia itself. Specific medications will vary depending on the etiology of the anemia and its severity. Instruct your client to notify you when medication changes are made.

Fitness Testing

The complete fitness evaluation may include assessments of body composition, cardiorespiratory endurance, muscular endurance and flexibility. Follow the guidelines set forth in Chapter 6 of the *ACE Personal Trainer Manual* for assessing body composition, muscular endurance and flexibility.

Submaximal cycle ergometry tests are recommended for evaluating cardiorespiratory fitness. People with anemia fatigue quickly and will have a VO_2max lower than predicted norms based on age, gender and heart-rate response to submaximal workloads. The test should be limited to eight to 12 minutes (i.e., two to four three-minute stages).

Contraindications to Exercise

Both infections and dehydration may precipitate a sickling crisis, which should be considered potentially fatal. Clients with sickle cell anemia or sickle cell trait should avoid exercise during infections. Additionally, following an illness, they should allow adequate time for full recovery and rehydration before resuming exercise.

Clients with sickle cell anemia and resting blood pressures above 140/90 should be medically evaluated for treatment prior to beginning an exercise program.

Exercise Programming

Exercise Guidelines

The primary goal of exercise training for anemic clients is to improve cardiorespiratory endurance.

Aerobic Program

Mode: Exercise should emphasize large muscle groups for the greatest aerobic training effect.

Intensity: Begin at 40 percent to 50 percent of (estimated) VO_2max, and progress incrementally over the initial 12 to 15 weeks of training to 60 percent to 70 percent of (estimated) VO_2max.

Duration: Initial sessions should last 15 minutes, increasing to 30 to 45 minutes of aerobic activity per session.

Frequency: Your client should exercise three to five days per week.

Progression: The main focus is on increasing duration, rather than intensity. Gradually progress exercise intensity once your client can sustain mild-intensity aerobic activity for 30 minutes.

Stretching and Flexibility

Clients should be instructed to complete slow, static stretching exercises at the beginning and end of the exercise session.

Table 17.4

Client Information to Obtain from Medical Professionals

1) Are there known medical problems that would preclude or limit exercise? (Bear in mind that there is an underlying cause for the reported anemia.)

2) Are you aware of cardiovascular conditions that may preclude or limit exercise?

3) What medications is the client currently taking?

4) Are there limitations on this client's activity?

5) Are there recommendations regarding the level of supervision for exercise sessions?

Resistance Training

The goal of resistance training is to improve muscular endurance. To this end, the American College of Sports Medicine (1995) recommendations for resistance training are applicable to clients with anemia. Resistance training should incorporate eight to 10 exercises that train major muscle groups, and should be performed three days per week on alternate days. Have your client perform one set of 12 to 15 repetitions for each exercise.

Clients with anemia and no other complications or chronic diseases can participate in sports and other recreational activities as their tolerance allows.

Exercise Leadership

Relatively few reports exist on the physiological responses to exercise training in individuals with anemia. However, it is likely that the profile of adaptations to chronic exercise will be similar in anemic and healthy adults, although maximal aerobic power (even after training) will be limited by the severity of the anemia. When monitoring exercise in anemic clients, note the following:

- Intense exercise may trigger a sickle crisis, as a result of either hypoxia or acidosis, in those with sickle cell anemia or sickle cell trait.
- Clients with sickle cell anemia or sickle cell trait should reduce or discontinue exercise activities when they have acute viral infections and/or when their temperature is elevated.
- Clients with sickle cell anemia or sickle cell trait should ingest fluids liberally before, during and after endurance exercise to maintain adequate hydration.

Provide written follow-up reports to the referring physician every three months. These reports should summarize the modes of exercise employed, exercise progression since the last report and information regarding your client's response to exercise programming.

Case Study 3

Marcus Johnson, a 43-year-old man who provides technical support for a large computer firm, has sickle cell anemia (hematocrit 23.6%, hemoglobin 8.1 g/dl^{-1}). At his recent annual physical, Marcus was advised to begin regular exercise. The only medication he takes is a folate supplement.

During his initial session, you review his responses to the PAR-Q and determine there are no immediate contraindications to Marcus' involvement in an exercise program. As is typical for those with anemia, Marcus reports shortness of breath due to relatively mild exertion. His resting blood pressure at the initial session is 110/68.

The initial fitness assessment includes a three-stage cycle ergometry test (resting and exercise blood pressures included), push-ups, body composition assessment (skinfold measures) and evaluation of flexibility (sit-and-reach test). Marcus' estimated VO$_2$max (approximately 26.5 mL/kg^{-1}/min^{-1}) and muscular endurance are low.

You design an exercise program that emphasizes cardiorespiratory endurance, and initially consists of 15 minutes of aerobic training (treadmill walking and cycling are recommended) at an intensity of 45 percent to 50 percent VO$_2$max, and flexibility training prior to and after exercise. You discuss the importance of drinking fluids during endurance exercise to avoid dehydration. You also incorporate resistance training into Marcus' program.

In the initial months of training, you gradually increase both the duration and intensity of the aerobic phase of Marcus' workout until he is performing 30 to 40 minutes at 60 to 65 percent VO$_2$max, five days per week. After three months of consistent participation,

Table 17.5

Typical Activity Guidelines
■ Activity as tolerated.
■ Clients with sickle cell anemia or sickle cell trait should avoid exercise during periods of acute infection.
■ Clients with sickle cell anemia or sickle cell trait should maintain adequate hydration.

Marcus' fitness parameters are reevaluated and his program is adjusted to appropriate levels.

References

Chronic Fatigue Syndrome

American College of Sports Medicine. (1995). *ACSM's Guidelines for Exercise Testing and Prescription* (5th ed.). Baltimore, Md.: Williams & Wilkins.

Farrar, D.J., Locke, S.E. & Kantrowitz, F.G. (1995). Chronic fatigue syndrome 1: Etiology and pathogenesis. *Behavioral Medicine, 21,* 5-16.

Fukuda, K., Straus, S.E., Hickie, I., Sharpe, M.C., Dobbins, J.G. & Komaroff, A. (1994). The chronic fatigue syndrome: A comprehensive approach to its definition and study. *Annals of Internal Medicine, 121,* 953-959.

Fulcher, K.Y. & White, P.D. (1997). Randomised controlled trial of graded exercise in patients with the chronic fatigue syndrome. *British Medical Journal, 314,* 1647-1652.

Gibson, H., Carroll, N., Clague, J.E. & Edwards, R.H.T. (1993). Exercise performance and fatigability in patients with chronic fatigue syndrome. *Journal of Neurology, Neurosurgery, and Psychiatry, 56,* 993-998.

Kantrowitz, F.G., Farrar, D.J. & Locke, S.E. (1995) Chronic fatigue syndrome 2: Treatment and future research. *Behavioral Medicine, 21,* 17-24.

Katon, W.J., Buchwald, D.S., Simon, G.E., Russo, J.E. & Mease, P.J. (1991). Psychiatric illness in patients with chronic fatigue and those with rheumatic arthritis. *Journal of General and Internal Medicine, 6,* 277-285.

Kent-Braun, J.A., Sharma, K.R., Weiner, M.W., Massie, B. & Miller, R.G. (1993). Central basis of muscular fatigue in chronic fatigue syndrome. *Neurology, 43,* 125-131.

Komaroff, A.L. (1993). Experience with sporadic and "epidemic" cases. In T.D. Sabin & D.M. Dawson (Eds.), *Chronic Fatigue Syndrome* (pp. 25-43). Boston, Mass.: Little, Brown and Co.

Kruesi, M.J., Dale, J. & Straus, S.E. (1989). Psychiatric diagnoses in patients who have chronic fatigue syndrome. *Journal of Clinical Psychiatry, 50,* 53-56.

Hickie, I., Lloyd, A.R. & Wakefield, D. (1995). Chronic fatigue syndrome: Current perspectives on evaluation and management. *The Medical Journal of Australia, 163,* 314-318.

Hickie, I., Lloyd, A., Wakefield, D. & Parker, G. (1990). The psychiatric status of patients with chronic fatigue syndrome. *British Journal of Psychiatry, 156,* 534-540.

Holmes, G.P., Kaplan, J.E., Gantz, N.M., Komaroff, A.L., Schonberger, L.B., Straus, S.E., Jones, J.F., Dubois, R.E., Cunningham-Rundles, C., Pahwa, S., Tosato, G., Zegans, L.S., Purtilo, D.T., Brown, N., Schooley, R.T. & Brus, I. (1988). Chronic fatigue syndrome: A working case definition. *Annals of Internal Medicine, 108,* 387-389.

Lewis, S., Cooper, C.L. & Bennett, D. (1994) Psychosocial factors and chronic fatigue syndrome. *Psychological Medicine, 24,* 661-671.

Maffulli, N., Testa, V. & Capasso, F. (1993). Post-viral fatigue syndrome. A longitudinal assessment in varsity athletes. *The Journal of Sports Medicine and Physical Fitness, 33,* 392-399.

McCully, K.K., Natelson, B.H., Iotti, S., Sisto, S. & Leigh Jr., J.S. (1996). Reduced oxidative muscle metabolism in chronic fatigue syndrome. *Muscle & Nerve, 19,* 621-625.

Parker, S., Brukner, R. & Rosier, M. (1996). Chronic fatigue syndrome and the athlete. *Sports Medicine Training and Rehabilitation, 6,* 269-278.

Riley, M.S., O'Brien, C.J., McCluskey, D.R., Bell, N.P. & Nicholls, D.P. (1990). Aerobic work capacity in patients with chronic fatigue syndrome. *British Medical Journal, 301,* 953-956.

Sabin, T.D. & Dawson, D.M. (1993). History and epidemiology. In T.D. Sabin & D.M. Dawson (Eds.) *Chronic Fatigue Syndrome* (pp. 1-24). Boston, Mass.: Little, Brown and Co.

Sisto, S.A., LaMance, J., Cordero, D.L., Bergen, M.T., Ellis, S.P., Drastal, S., Boda, W.L., Tapp, W.N. & Natelson, B.H. (1996). Metabolic and cardiovascular effects of progressive exercise tests in patients with chronic fatigue syndrome. *American Journal of Medicine, 100,* 634-640.

Wong, R., Lopaschuk, G., Zhu, G., Walker, D., Catellier, D., Burton, D., Teo, K., Collins-Nakai, R. & Montague, T. (1992). Skeletal muscle metabolism in the chronic fatigue syndrome: In vivo assessment by 31P nuclear magnetic resonance spectroscopy. *Chest, 102,* 1716-1722.

Systemic Lupus Erythematosus

American College of Sports Medicine. (1995). *ACSM's Guidelines for Exercise Testing and Prescription* (5th ed.). Baltimore, Md.: Williams & Wilkins.

Beals, C.A., Lampman, R.M., Banwell, B.F., Braunstein, E.M., Albers, J.W. & Castor, C.W. (1985). Measurement of exercise tolerance in patients with rheumatoid arthritis and osteoarthritis. *Journal of Rheumatology, 12,* 458-461.

Boumpas, D.T., Austin, H.A., Fessler, B.J., Balow, J.E., Klippel, J.H. & Lockshin, M.D. (1995). Systemic lupus erythematosus: Emerging concepts. *Annals of Internal Medicine, 122,* 940-950.

Braden, C.J., McGlone, K. & Pennington, F. (1993). Specific psychosocial and behavioral outcomes from the systemic lupus erythematosus self-help course. *Health Education Quarterly, 20,* 29-41.

Daltroy, L.H., Robb-Nicholson, C., Iversen, M.D. & Wright, E.A. (1995). Effectiveness of minimally supervised home aerobic training in patients with systemic rheumatic disease. *British Journal of Rheumatology, 34,* 1064-1069.

Deapen, D., Escalante, A., Weinrib, L., Horivitz, D., Bachman, B., Roy-Burman, P., Walker, A. & Mark, T.M. (1992). A revised estimate of twin concordance in systemic lupus erythematosus. *Arthritis and Rheumatism, 35,* 311-318.

Gladman, D.D. (1996). Prognosis and treatment of systemic lupus erythematosus. *Current Opinion in Rheumatology, 8,* 430-437.

Harkcom, T.M., Lampman, R.M., Banwell, B.F. & Castor, C.W. (1985). Therapeutic value of graded aerobic exercise training in rheumatoid arthritis. *Arthritis and Rheumatism, 28,* 32-39.

Hellmann, D.B., Kirsch, C.M., Whiting-O'Keefe, Q., Simonson, J., Schiller, N.B., Petri, M., Gamsu, G. & Gold, W. (1995). Dyspnea in ambulatory patients with SLE: Prevalence, severity, and correlation with incremental exercise testing. *Journal of Rheumatology, 22,* 455-461.

Hochberg, M.C. (1985). The incidence of systemic lupus erythematosus in Baltimore, Maryland, 1970-1977. *Arthritis and Rheumatism, 28,* 80-86.

Johnson, A.E., Gordon, C., Palmer, R.G. & Bacon, R.A. (1995).The prevalence and incidence of systemic lupus erythematosus in Birmingham, England. *Arthritis and Rheumatism, 38,* 551-558.

Kotzin, B.L. (1996). Systemic lupus erythematosus. *Cell, 85,* 303-306.

Nordemar, R. (1981). Physical training in rheumatoid arthritis: A controlled long-term study. II. Functional capacity and general attitudes. *Scandinavian Journal of Rheumatology, 10,* 25-30.

Pisetsky, D.S., Gilkeson, G. & St. Clair, E.W. (1997). Systemic lupus erythematosus. Diagnosis and treatment. *Medical Clinics of North America, 81,* 113-128.

Petri, M. (1995). Clinical features of systemic lupus erythematosus. *Current Opinion in Rheumatology, 7,* 395-401.

Rasaratnam, I. & Ryan, P. F. (1997). Systemic lupus erythematosus. *Medical Journal of Australia, 166,* 266-270.

Robb-Nicholson, C., Daltroy, L., Eaton, H., Gall, V., Wright, E., Hartley, L.H., Schur, P.H. & Liang, M.H. (1989). Effects of aerobic conditioning in lupus fatigue: A pilot study. *British Journal of Rheumatology, 28,* 500-505.

Sakauchi, M., Matsumura, T., Yamaoka, T., Koami, T., Shibata, M., Nakamura, M., Watanabe, R., Kaneko, K., Kato, S., Seguchi, H., Ohishi, A., Fukuda, K., Aosaki, N. & Katsu, M. (1995). Reduced muscle uptake of oxygen during exercise in patients with systemic lupus erythematosus. *Journal of Rheumatology, 22,* 1483-1487.

Schroeder, J.O. & Euler, H.H. (1997). Recognition and management of systemic lupus erythematosus. *Drugs, 54,* 422-434.

Sims, G.N. & Smith, H.R. (1996). Outpatient management of systemic lupus erythematosus. *Cleveland Clinic Journal of Medicine, 63,* 94-100.

Tan, E.M., Cohen, A.S., Fries, J.F., Masi, A.T., McShane, D.J., Rothfield, N.F., Schaller, J.G., Talal, N. & Winchester, R.J. (1982). The 1982 revised criteria for the classification of systemic lupus erythematosus. *Arthritis and Rheumatism, 25,* 1271-1277.

Winslow, T.M., Ossipove, M., Redberg, R.F., Fazio, G.P. & Schiller, N.B. (1993). Exercise capacity and hemodynamics in systemic lupus erythematosus: A Doppler echocardiographic exercise study. *American Heart Journal, 126,* 410-414.

Anemia

American College of Sports Medicine. (1995). *ACSM's Guidelines for Exercise Testing and Prescription* (5th ed.). Baltimore, Md.: Williams & Wilkins.

Alpert, B.S., Dover, E.V., Strong, W.B. & Covitz, W. (1984). Longitudinal exercise hemodynamics in children with sickle cell anemia. *American Journal of Diseases of Childhood, 138,* 1021-1024.

Alpert, B.S., Gilman, P.A., Strong, W.B., Ellison, M.F., Miller, M.D. & McFarlane, J. (1981). Hemodynamic and ECG responses to exercise in children with sickle cell anemia. *American Journal of Diseases of Childhood, 135,* 362-366.

Ban-Hock, T., Van Driel, I.R. & Gleeson, P.A. (1997). Pernicious anemia. *The New England Journal of Medicine, 337,* 1441-1448.

Beutler, E., Lichtman, M.A., Coller, B.S. & Kipps, T.J. (1995). *Williams Hematology* (5th ed.). New York: McGraw-Hill Publishing Co.

Bourque, S.P., Pate, R.R. & Branch, J.D. (1997). Twelve weeks of endurance exercise training does not affect iron status measures in women. *Journal of the American Dietetic Association, 97,* 1116-1121.

Brautbar, N. (1983). Skeletal myopathy in uremia: Abnormal energy metabolism. *Kidney International, 24,* S81-S86.

Bunn, H.F. (1997). Pathogenesis and treatment of sickle cell disease. *The New England Journal of Medicine, 337,* 762-769.

Celsing, F., Nyström, J., Pihlstedt, P., Werner, B. & Ekblom, B. (1986). Effect of long-term anemia and retransfusion on central circulation during exercise. *Journal of Applied Physiology, 61,* 1358-1362.

Gozal, D., Thiriet, P., Mbala, E., Wouassi, D., Gelas, H., Geyssant, A. & Lacour, J.R. (1992). Effect of different modalities of exercise and recovery on exercise performance in subjects with sickle cell trait. *Medicine and Science in Sports and Exercise, 24,* 1325-1331.

Gregg, S.G., Willis, W.T. & Brooks, G.A. (1989). Interactive effects of anemia and muscle oxidative capacity on exercise endurance. *Journal of Applied Physiology, 67,* 765-770.

Hamilton, W., Rosenthal, A., Berwick, D. & Nadas, A. S. (1978). Angina pectoris in a child with sickle cell anemia. *Pediatrics, 61,* 911-914.

Koskolou, M.D., Roach, R.C., Calbet, J.A.L., Rådegran, G. & Saltin, B. (1997). Cardiovascular responses to dynamic exercise with acute anemia. *American Journal of Physiology, 273,* H1787-H1793.

Lamanca, J.J., Haymes, E.M., Daly, J.A., Moffatt, R.J. & Waller, M.F. (1988). Sweat iron loss of male and female runners during exercise. *International Journal of Sports Medicine, 9,* 52-55.

Lazaro, R.P. & Kirschner, H.S. (1980). Proximal muscle weakness in uremia: Case reports and review of the literature. *Archives of Neurology, 37,* 555-558.

Linker, C.A. (1996). Blood. In L.M. Tierney Jr., S.J. McPhee & M.A. Papadakis (Eds.) *Current Medical Diagnosis and Treatment 1996* (pp. 434-488). Stamford, Conn.: Appleton & Lange.

Loria, A., Sanchez-Medal, L., Lisker, R., de Rodrigues, E. & Labardini, J. (1967). Red cell life span in iron deficiency anemia. *British Journal of Haematology, 13,* 294-298.

Lukaski, H.C., Hoverson, B.S., Gallagher, S.K. & Bolonchuk, W.W. (1990). Physical training and copper, iron, and zinc status of swimmers. *American Journal of Clinical Nutrition, 51,* 1093-1099.

Magazanik, A., Weinstein, Y., Abarbanel, J., Lewinski, U., Shapiro, Y., Inbar, O. & Epstein, S. (1991). Effect of an iron supplement on body iron status and aerobic capacity of young training women. *European Journal of Applied Physiology, 62,* 317-323.

Martin, C.R., Cobb, C., Tatter, D., Johnson, C. & Haywood, L.F. (1983). Acute myocardial infarction in sickle cell anemia. *Archives of Internal Medicine, 143,* 830-831.

McConnell, M.E., Daniels, S.R., Lobel, J., James,

F.W. & Kaplan, S. (1989). Hemodynamic response to exercise in patients with sickle cell anemia. *Pediatric Cardiology,* 10, 141-144.

Means Jr., R.T. (1995). Erythropoietin in the treatment of anemia in chronic infectious, inflammatory, and malignant disease. *Current Opinion in Hematology,* 2, 210-213.

Moore, G.E., Parsons, D.B., Stray-Gundersen, J., Painter, P.L., Brinker, K.R. & Mitchell, J.H. (1993). Uremic myopathy limits aerobic capacity in hemodialysis patients. *American Journal of Kidney Diseases,* 22, 277-287.

Mouton, G., Sluse, F.E., Bertrand, A., Welter, A., Cabay, J.L. & Camus, G. (1990). Iron status in runners of various running specialties. *Archives Internationales de Physiologie et de Biochimie,* 98, 103-109.

Painter, P.L. Nelson-Worel, J.N., Hill, M.M., Thornbery, D. ., Shelp, W.R., Harrington, A.R. & Weinstein, A.B. (1986). Effects of exercise training during hemodialysis. *Nephron,* 43, 87-92.

Pate, R.R., Miller, B.J., Davis, J.M., Slentz, C.A. & Klingshirn, L.A. (1993). Iron status of female runners. *International Journal of Sport Nutrition,* 3, 222-231.

Pegelow, C.H., Colangelo, L., Steinberg, M., Wright, E.C., Smith, J., Phillips, G. & Vichinsky, E. (1997). Natural history of blood pressure in sickle cell disease: Risks for stroke and death associated with relative hypertension in sickle cell anemia. *American Journal of Medicine,* 102, 171-177.

Rajaram, S., Weaver, C.M., Lyle, R.M., Sedlock, D.A., Martin, B., Templin, T.J., Beard, J.L. & Percival, S.S. (1995). Effects of long-term moderate exercise on iron status in young women. *Medicine and Science in Sports and Exercise,* 27, 1105-1110.

Robinson, J.R., Stone, W.J. & Asendorf, A.C. (1976). Exercise capacity of black sickle cell trait males. *Medicine and Science in Sports and Exercise,* 8, 244-245.

Ross, D.L., Grabeau, G.M., Smith, S., Seymour, M., Knierim, N. & Pitetti, K.H. (1989). Efficacy of exercise for end-stage renal disease patients immediately following high-efficacy hemodialysis: A pilot study. *American Journal of Nephrology,* 9, 376-383.

Sproule, B.J., Mitchell, J.H. & Miller, W.F. (1960). Cardiopulmonary physiological responses to heavy exercise in patients with anemia. *Journal of Clinical Investigation,* 39, 378-388.

Steinberg, D. (1982). *Anemia.* New York: Holt, Rinehart and Winston.

Waller, M.F. & Haymes, W. M. (1996). The effects of heat and exercise on sweat iron loss. *Medicine and Science in Sports and Exercise,* 28, 197-203.

Woodson, R.D. (1984). Hemoglobin concentration and exercise capacity. *American Review of Respiratory Disease,* 129, S72-S75.

Woodson, R.D., Wills, R.E. & Lenfant, C. (1978). Effect of acute and established anemia on O_2 transport at rest, submaximal and maximal work. *Journal of Applied Physiology,* 44, 36-43.

Young, N.S. & Maciejewski, J. (1997). The pathophysiology of acquired aplastic anemia. *The New England Journal of Medicine,* 336, 1365-1372.

Zhu, Y.I. & Haas, J.D. (1997). Iron depletion without anemia and physical performance in young women. *American Journal of Clinical Nutrition,* 66, 334-341.

Suggested Readings

CFS

Fukuda, K., Straus, S.E., Hickie, I., Sharpe, M.C., Dobbins, J.G. & Komaroff, A. (1994). The chronic fatigue syndrome: A comprehensive approach to its definition and study. *Annals of Internal Medicine,* 121, 953-959.

Fulcher, K.Y. & White, P.D. (1997). Randomised controlled trial of graded exercise in patients with the chronic fatigue syndrome. *British Medical Journal,* 314, 1647-1652.

Gibson, H., Carroll, N., Clague, J.E. & Edwards, R.H.T. (1993). Exercise performance and fatigability in patients with chronic fatigue syndrome. *Journal of Neurology, Neurosurgery, and Psychiatry,* 56, 993-998.

Gordon, N.F. & Cooper, K.H. (1992). *Chronic Fatigue Syndrome: Your Complete Exercise Guide.* Champaign, Ill.: Human Kinetics.

Kantrowitz, F.G., Farrar, D.J. & Locke, S.E. (1995). Chronic fatigue syndrome 2: Treatment and future research. *Behavioral Medicine,* 21, 17-24.

Lewis, S., Cooper, C.L. & Bennett, D. (1994). Psychosocial factors and chronic fatigue syndrome. *Psychological Medicine,* 24, 661-671.

Sharpe, M., Chalder, T., Palmer, I. & Wessely, S. (1997). Chronic fatigue syndrome: A practical guide to assessment and management. *General Hospital Psychiatry,* 19, 185-199.

SLE

Daltroy, L.H., Robb-Nicholson, C., Iversen, M.D. & Wright, E. A. (1995). Effectiveness of minimally supervised home aerobic training in patients with systemic rheumatic disease. *British Journal of Rheumatology,* 34, 1064-1069.

Pisetsky, D.S., Gilkeson, G. & St. Clair, E.W. (1997). Systemic lupus erythematosus: Diagnosis and treatment. *Medical Clinics of North America,* 81, 113-128.

Robb-Nicholson, C., Daltroy, L., Eaton, H., Gall, V., Wright, E., Hartley, L.H., Schur, P.H. & Liang, M.H. (1989). Effects of aerobic conditioning in lupus fatigue: A pilot study. *British Journal of Rheumatology,* 28, 500-505.

Sakauchi, M., Matsumura, T., Yamaoka, T., Koami, T., Shibata, M., Nakamura, M., Watanabe, R., Kaneko, K., Kato, S., Seguchi, H., Ohishi, A., Fukuda, K., Aosaki, N. & Katsu, M. (1995). Reduced muscle uptake of oxygen during exercise in patients with systemic lupus erythematosus. *Journal of Rheumatology,* 22, 1483-1487.

Schroeder, J.O. & Euler, H.H. (1997). Recognition and management of systemic lupus erythematosus. *Drugs,* 54, 422-434.

Tan, E.M., Cohen, A.S., Fries, J.F., Masi, A.T., McShane, D.J., Rothfield, N.F., Schaller, J.G., Talal, N. & Winchester, R.J. (1982). The 1982 revised criteria for the classification of systemic lupus erythematosus. *Arthritis and Rheumatism,* 25, 1271-1277.

Anemia

Celsing, F., Nyström, J., Pihlstedt, P., Werner, B. & Ekblom, B. (1986). Effect of long-term anemia and retransfusion on central circulation during exercise. *Journal of Applied Physiology,* 61, 1358-1362.

Gozal, D., Thiriet, P., Mbala, E., Wouassi, D., Gelas, H., Geyssant, A. & Lacour, J.R. (1992). Effect of different modalities of exercise and recovery on exercise performance in subjects with sickle cell trait. *Medicine and Science in Sports and Exercise,* 24, 1325-1331.

Gregg, S.G., Willis, W.T. & Brooks, G.A. (1989). Interactive effects of anemia and muscle oxidative capacity on exercise endurance. *Journal of Applied Physiology,* 67, 765-770.

McConnell, M.E., Daniels, S.R., Lobel, J., James, F.W. & Kaplan, S. (1989). Hemodynamic response to exercise in patients with sickle cell anemia. *Pediatric Cardiology,* 10, 141-144.

Nieman, D.C. (1995). *Fitness and Sports Medicine: A Health-Related Approach.* Mountain View, Calif.: Mayfield Publishing.

Robinson, J.R., Stone, W.J. & Asendorf, A.C. (1976). Exercise capacity of black sickle cell trait males. *Medicine and Science in Sports and Exercise,* 8, 244-245.

Sproule, B.J., Mitchell, J.H. & Miller, W.F. (1960). Cardiopulmonary physiological responses to heavy exercise in patients with anemia. *Journal of Clinical Investigation,* 39, 378-388.

Woodson, R.D., Wills, R.E. & Lenfant, C. (1978). Effect of acute and established anemia on O transport at rest, submaximal and maximal work. *Journal of Applied Physiology,* 44, 36-43.

Uthman, E. (1998). *Understanding Anemia.* Jackson, Miss.: University Press of Mississippi.

Section Six

Neurological Disorders

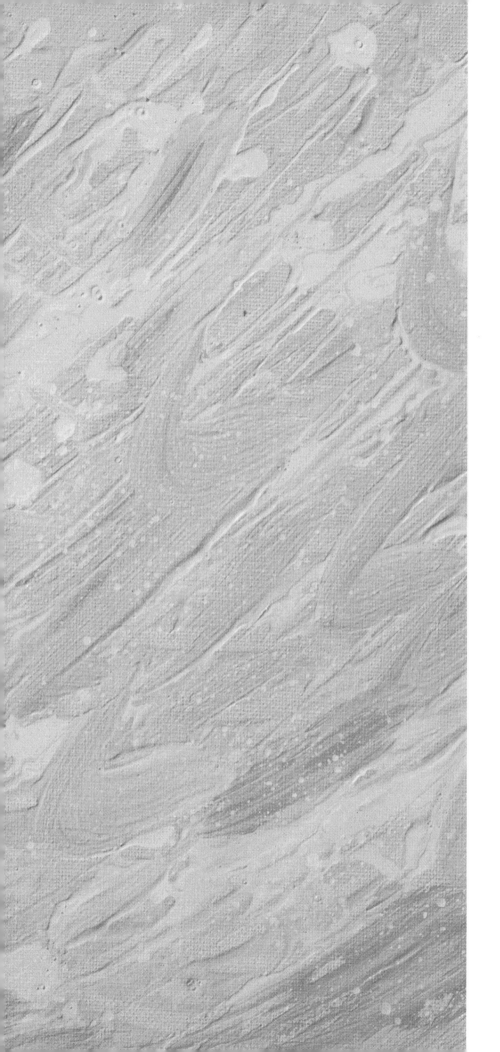

CHAPTER 18

Fibromyalgia

BRAD A. ROY

Brad A. Roy, Ph.D., F.A.C.S.M., is the director of The Summit, Kalispell Regional Medical Center's facility for health promotion and fitness in Kalispel, Mont. Dr. Roy has more than 20 years experience working with clinical patients in the rehabilitation setting and has successfully consulted with numerous world-class athletes. He received his master's degree in exercise physiology from San Diego State University and his doctorate in the same subject from Columbia Pacific University.

Relaxation Techniques
Posture
Evaluation

Stretching

Fibromyalgia (pro- nounced "fie-bro-my-al-jia") is classified not as a disease but as a syndrome. The term "fibromyalgia" comes from the Latin roots "fibro" (connective tissue fibers), "my" (muscle), "al" (pain) and "gia" (condition of), and the term syndrome refers to a group of signs and symptoms that occur together and characterize a particular abnormality (Clayton, 1979). Fibromyalgia is neither progressive nor deadly.

Chronic pain syndromes such as fibromyalgia syndrome (FS) present some of the most challenging and frustrating therapeutic dilemmas in medicine today. Characterized by widespread musculoskeletal aches and pains, stiffness, fatigue, muscle spasms and paresthesis, FS frequently remains un-diagnosed for a number of years as patients undergo a battery of exclusionary tests. It is estimated that 10 to 11 million Americans manifest symptoms characteristic of FS, most frequently females. The median age at onset of FS is between 29 and 37, while the median age of medical presentation is between 34 and 53. This suggests that many patients endure symptoms for several years before receiving an appropriate diagnosis (Wolfe, Ross, Anderson, Russell & Herbert, 1995; Goldenberg, Simms, Geiger & Komoroft, 1990).

Fibromyalgia syndrome is not new. Centuries ago, Hippocrates described a condition he observed in patients with diffuse, musculoskeletal pain that resembled FS, while in 1816 William Balfour, a surgeon at the University of Edinburgh, described similar symptomatology in his patients. In 1904 William Gowers labeled this collection of symptoms "fibrositis," a somewhat misleading term because FS is not characterized by inflammation. In 1976 Dr. P. Kahler Hench coined our current term, "fibromyalgia syndrome" to better reflect the true nature of the condition.

Etiology

Though myriad mechanisms have been proposed in literature (Goldenberg, 1989; Reiffenbeiger & Amundson, 1996; Ffan & Blanton, 1992; Bennett, 1993), there is no conclusive evidence identifying the etiology of FS. Most likely the underlying mechanisms of FS are multifactorial and typically have been classified as peripheral and central mechanisms. Proposed peripheral mechanisms consist mainly of abnormalities in muscle energy metabolism such as local hypoxia, excessive muscle tension leading to increased excitability of nociceptors, and disturbances in muscle microcirculation and in creatine and adenosine monophosphate levels (Reiffenbeiger, 1996; Bengtsson & Henriksson, 1989; Drews, Andreasen & Schjroder, 1993; Elert, Rantopan-Dahlquist, Henriksson-Larson, Lorentzon, Gerdle, 1992). Central mechanisms include abnormalities in regional cerebral blood flow, hormonal changes, stage-four sleep abnormalities, disordered serotonin metabolism and other neurobiochemical abnormalities (Simms, 1996; Mountz, Bradley & Modell, 1995; Bennett, 1993; Bennett, Clark, Campbell & Burckhardt, 1992; Moldofsky, 1989; Russell, 1989). Psychological disturbances and stress also have been proposed as possible mechanisms (Boissevain & McCain, 1991; Goldenberg, 1989). In fact, until recently, FS often was regarded as a psychological illness because no physical evidence for its cause could be identified. Unfortunately, minimal scientific evidence exists to support any of these theories.

A number of other medical problems associated with FS make it almost impossible to pinpoint an etiology. Twenty percent of patients with rheumatoid arthritis also have FS, while both migraine and nonmigraine headaches have been shown to occur in up to 58 percent of patients with FS. Irritable bowel syndrome, Raynaud's phenomenon, chronic fatigue syndrome, dysmenorrhea, mitral valve prolapse, temporomandibular joint syndrome, yeast infections, anxiety and clinical depression also have been associated with symptoms of FS (Krsnich-Schriwise, 1997).

A number of patients with FS cannot identify a single factor that initiated their condition because the onset is gradual. Others can identify physical trauma, viral illness and other events as precipitating factors, however there is no evidence that infectious agents are directly responsible for the symptoms of FS.

Common Symptoms

In many ways, FS is a sensitivity-amplification syndrome, leading more than one clinician to refer to it as the "Irritable Everything Syndrome" (Starland & Copeland, 1996). It's as if the brain is getting the wrong messages, resulting in hypermobilization of defenses and associated anxiety.

The most frequently reported symptoms include 1) aches and pains similar to flu-like exhaustion, 2) multiple tender points, 3) stiffness, 4) decreased exercise endurance, 5) fatigue, 6) muscle spasms and 7) paresthesis. Aches and pains generally are described as widespread and diffuse, fluctuating in intensity, and frequently are accompanied by marked stiffness. Tender points, frequently accompanied by muscle spasms, are clustered in the neck and shoulders, upper chest wall, and lower back (Goldenberg, 1992).

Other common symptoms described by FS patients include excessive fatigue, disruptive sleep patterns, numbness of the extremities, bowel and bladder irritability, anxiety, and depression. Many FS patients also describe difficulty performing simple mental tasks, poor concentration and short-term memory lapses.

Many individuals with FS wake up tired, even after sleeping through the night; some feel as though they've been hit by a truck when they awaken. Stiffness frequently occurs when individuals with FS have been in one position for some time, especially overnight, and can make exercise painful. As a result, daily tasks frequently are left undone because patients feel "tired" and "down."

Relationships, particularly within families, sometimes become strained as family members do not understand the pain and fatigue cycles that challenge FS patients. Pain and fatigue also make it difficult to participate in social activities, leaving some people with FS feeling isolated and lonely. Thus many individuals become depressed. In addition, symptoms make it impossible for some patients to work, resulting in financial worries and increased stress. In Sweden the FS diagnosis is associated with a 50 percent disability rate (Wolfe, 1995).

Diagnostic Criteria

Based on nonspecific, generalized symptoms, such as pain, fatigue and sleep disturbance, FS historically has been diagnosed through a process of elimination – resulting in extensive investigational costs and patient/physician frustration. Most FS patients feel relief when they finally learn they have a recognized condition that is neither deadly nor generally progressive.

The Copenhagen Declaration in 1992 defined FS as a "painful, but not articular (present in the joints) condition predominantly involving muscles, which is the most common cause of chronic, widespread musculoskeletal pain" (Csillag, 1992). In 1990 the American College of Rheumatology (ACR) published classification criteria for FS (Wolfe, Smythe & Yunus, 1990). Table 18.1 presents the ACR diagnostic criteria, which is characterized by a history of widespread pain occurring for longer than three months in combination with pain on palpation of 11 of 18 standard tender point sites. The criteria originally were developed for classification purposes in research studies but have proved useful in the clinical setting. Currently there is no single routine laboratory test or imaging procedure that is of diagnostic or prognostic value for FS (Wolfe, 1996).

Throughout the literature, the terms "tender points" and "trigger points" frequently are used interchangeably. While the terms are similar, there are specific differences. Trigger points are localized spots that elicit a characteristic pattern of radiating pain, tingling or numbness in response to sustained pressure. The ACR diagnostic criteria for FS defines tender points as localized points in muscle, ligaments, tendons or periosteal tissue that hurt in response to pressure but do not refer pain elsewhere. Tender points are palpated bilaterally using the thumb or first two fingers to apply steady, uniform pressure of 4 kg/cm2 (enough pressure to blanch the examiner's thumbnail). Generally, the clinician increasingly applies pressure until the patient requests the exam stop, withdraws and/or grimaces.

The ACR definition also states that tender points must be present in all four quadrants of

Etiology

Table 18.1
American College of Rheumatology Diagnostic Criteria for Fibromyalgia

History of Widespread Pain

Pain is considered widespread when all of the following are present:
Pain in the left side of the body
Pain in the right side of the body
Pain above the waist
Pain below the waist
In addition, axial skeletal pain (in the cervical spine or anterior chest, or thoracic spine or low back) must be present. Shoulder and buttocks pain is divided into left and right sides and considered pain for each involved side. "Low-back" pain is considered lower-segment pain.
Pain on digital palpation in 11 of 18 tender-point sites:
1. Occiput: bilateral, at the suboccipital muscle insertions
2. Low cervical: bilateral, at the anterior aspects of the intertransverse spaces at C5-C7
3. Trapezius: bilateral, at the midpoint of the upper border
4. Supraspinatous: bilateral, at origins, above the scapular spine and near the medial border
5. Second rib: bilateral, at the second costochondral junctions, just lateral to the junctions on upper surfaces
6. Lateral epicondyle: bilateral, 2 cm distal to the epicondyles
7. Gluteal: bilateral, in upper, outer quadrants of buttocks in anterior fold of muscle
8. Greater trochanter: bilateral, posterior to the trochanteric prominence
9. Knee: bilateral, at the medial fat pad proximal to the joint line

the body, (upper right and left, lower right and left). Because tender points can vary from day to day, tests sometimes are given on multiple visits to confirm an FS diagnosis. Tenderness at sites not specified by the ACR criteria does not exclude the diagnosis of FS (Simms, 1996). Patients who have fewer than the required number of tender points also may be diagnosed as having FS if they have other characteristic symptoms (e.g., fatigue, sleep disturbance).

A detailed medical history and physical examination are important to accurately diagnose FS and rule out other conditions that may cause chronic pain and fatigue. Recommended laboratory studies include a complete blood count, erythrocyte sedimentation rate, and measurement of muscle enzymes and thyroid stimulating hormone; rheumatoid factor, antinuclear antibody determinations, radiographs and electromyography are recommended in selected cases (Reiffenbeiger et al., 1996). Generally, such laboratory tests primarily are of value in proving (or disproving) the presence of other conditions, such as hypothyroidism. However, the presence of a second clinical disorder does not necessarily exclude the diagnosis of fibromyalgia.

Management Strategies for Fibromyalgia

Because of the wide array of symptoms, no single medication or therapeutic modality has been found to be completely effective in treating a majority of FS patients. The clinical complexity and lack of a well-defined pathogenesis make the effective treatment of FS patients difficult and often frustrating. Management strategies must take into account the reality that the condition is chronic and treatment is more palliative than curative. In other words, treatment is aimed at reducing symptoms instead of curing the underlying cause, which is unknown in the case of FS. A multidisciplinary approach that combines a variety of therapeutic modalities may be most effective in relieving symptoms.

The primary components of a multidisciplinary treatment program include education about FS (such as diagnosis, prognosis, prevalence, sleep physiology, medications, physical conditioning, physical-activity pacing strategies, etc.), exercise training, relaxation techniques

and other cognitive behavioral techniques. The program also should include one or more outcome measures such as Quality of Life questionnaires, Fibromyalgia Impact Questionnaire (FIQ), depression inventories and exercise testing.

Medications

Medications have limited usefulness in the treatment of FS patients and generally are prescribed for pain and poor sleep patterns. The most common medications used include nonsteroidal analgesics (NSAIDs), tricyclic antidepressants such as amitriptyline and doxepin, and muscle relaxants such as cyclobenzaprine, which is similar in composition to the tricyclic antidepressants. Tricyclic medications can precipitate side effects such as weight gain, grogginess, dry mouth and even short-term memory loss. Heart rate also may be elevated and ST-T wave changes can occur on the ECG in the absence of ischemia. Ambien, a short-acting hypnotic medication, also is commonly prescribed for sleep enhancement. Occasionally narcotic analgesics are prescribed, but these medications are not highly recommended and must be carefully controlled. Ultram (a member of a relatively new class of analgesics called centrally acting binary agents, CABP), recently has been shown to be effective in decreasing pain and improving sleep patterns in FS patients.

Relaxation Techniques

Because of the amplified pain and fatigue response associated with FS, individuals frequently hypermobilize defenses. This results in increased muscular tightness and sympathetic nervous system activity, and worsening of symptoms. Therefore, relaxation techniques frequently are incorporated into treatment to reduce the sympathetic stress response. Biofeedback, yoga, tai-chi and other stretching/ breathing exercises, along with cognitive therapy strategies, commonly are prescribed. Proper physical activity also may serve as an effective relaxation technique for selected individuals.

Physical Conditioning

Many individuals with chronic pain syndromes significantly decrease their levels of physical activity, resulting in deconditioning and loss of function. This decrease in skeletal muscle fitness may make the musculature more susceptible to microtrauma and pain caused by any given exercise activity, further reducing activity levels. Furthermore, epidemiological data indicates that individuals who do not participate in a minimal dose of daily physical activity are at increased risk for a number of other chronic health problems such as diabetes and cardiovascular diseases. It is crucial to encourage patients with FS to remain physically active to lessen the risk of secondary disabling disorders.

Unpublished studies in our laboratory suggest that more than 80 percent of patients with FS are not aerobically fit as assessed with peak oxygen uptake (mean values of 22.6ml/kg/ min) and ventilatory threshold (mean of 60.7 percent of predicted) measurements. These findings are consistent with the published literature that suggests aerobic capacity, flexibility and muscle strength are significantly reduced in FS patients (Deuster, 1996; Mannerkorpi, Burckhardt & Bjelle, 1994; Mengshoel, Forre & Komnaes, 1990; McCain, Bell, Mai & Halliday, 1988; Nichols & Glenn, 1994).

Bennett and co-workers (1989) found that 80 percent of their patients had reduced oxygen-uptake values and reduced blood flow in exercising muscle as assessed by xenon-133 clearance studies. Clark et al. studied 95 women (mean age = 43.2 years) with FS and reported mean oxygen uptake values of 22.23 ml/kg/min (Clark, Burckhardt, Campbell, O'Reilly & Bennett, 1994). Sixty-four percent of Clark's subjects engaged in no physical exercise prior to the study, 18 percent exercised occasionally and only 11 percent exercised at a level considered adequate to produce health-related benefits. These findings emphasize the fact that a majority of individuals with FS are physically inactive and deconditioned.

Individuals with FS also have significantly reduced muscular strength and endurance as well as limited range of motion, especially in the upper extremity. Mannerkorp and co-workers (1994) documented significantly impaired upper-extremity flexion and abduction and decreased muscular endurance in 97 FS subjects. While the primary limiting factor was pain and decreased

muscular strength, one-third of the subjects also had active abduction mobility below the 1200 required for ADL performance. Overall, the group's flexibility was markedly below age-specific norms. The pattern of reduced upper-extremity strength and limited range of motion in FS significantly influences an individual's ability to not only perform basic functional activities but also to comfortably carry out vocational tasks. Many individuals with FS alter their careers and in some cases quit working entirely. Appropriate exercise training, combined with correct body mechanics and other management techniques, may allow FS patients to continue working and contributing.

Regular exercise is a critical part of the FS treatment program because a physically inactive lifestyle compounds the effects of the syndrome itself, resulting in a vicious circle of symptoms, inactivity and further loss of function. While it also is well known that physical inactivity increases the risk of developing a variety of chronic diseases, poor endurance, reduced muscular strength and limited range of motion also negatively impact functional ability and ultimately personal independence. This loss of autonomy can further promote depression and other symptoms found in many FS patients.

Potential Benefits of Exercise Training

Physical fitness has been defined as the ability to carry out activities of daily living without undue fatigue, with ample energy reserves to enjoy leisure-time pursuits and meet unforeseen emergencies, and to respond to physical and emotional stress without an excessive increase in heart rate and blood pressure (Caspersen, Powell & Christenson, 1985). As has been previously discussed, most individuals with FS are deconditioned and often barely have enough reserve energy to "get through the day" much less participate in enjoyable leisure pursuits. Addition-ally, people with FS often have an accentuated response to both physical and emotional stress. Therefore, exercise training that promotes improvement in the physiological variables that pertain to physical fitness (such as oxygen delivery and utilization, sympathetic response, and skeletal muscle function) is important in FS. Such improvements enhance an FS patient's quality of life.

Health-related fitness refers to the capacity to perform daily activities with vigor and demonstrate low risk of development of hypokinetic (inactivity-related) disease (Gauvin, Wall & Quoney, 1994). Physical activity improves health-related variables such as body composition, metabolic control, lipid profiles, blood pressure and bone mineral density, thus lowering the risk of developing other chronic diseases.

Physical activity also promotes improvement in muscle strength, balance, coordination and range of motion, which serves as a protective mechanism from falls and other potential orthopedic problems. Current research also suggests that appropriate exercise training assists in reducing symptomatology and functional disability associated with FS. Furthermore, the literature supports the beneficial effects of physical activity on relieving depression and anxiety, and improving mood – common problems for people with FS.

Potential Adverse Effects of Exercise

Most special precautions and limitations relative to exercise training in people with FS have been discussed previously. However, a number of points bear repeating. Acute stress from sudden forceful movements, jarring and/or bouncing movements, repetitive motions, improper body mechanics, and inappropriate intensity/duration can cause increased pain, severe fatigue and musculoskeletal injuries. Overtrained individuals may be at increased risk of infection and illness. Strenuous activities in individuals with other chronic health problems, such as diabetes, cardiovascular disease or pulmonary disease, may precipitate symptoms and even life-threatening events.

Though a wide spectrum of adverse events can occur with physical activity, most are preventable with appropriate planning and education. Instruct clients to gradually progress to their physical activity goal and avoid excessive amounts of activity and/or high intensity levels.

Exercise Programming

While exercise is an important therapeutic approach, proper instruction regarding the type, intensity, frequency and duration of the activity is vital to prevent further exacerbation of symptoms. Many individuals with FS currently do not exercise due to prior painful experiences related to improper techniques and/or intensity/duration. Carefully monitor and instruct clients to ensure compliance and reduce the risk of exacerbating symptoms.

A log book provides excellent feedback regarding the activity program and its effect on symptoms. One such log book, the *MemoryMinder Personal Health Journal,* has been specifically designed for individuals with FS, and has served as an excellent tool in our program (Wilkins & Wilkins, 1997). The key is entering information daily.

Client Assessment

Carefully gather information and assess the FS client to ensure a safe and effective exercise program. It is strongly recommended that the FS client undergo a medical checkup by their physician prior to beginning the exercise program. This will identify possible underlying medical problems and/or risk factors that may necessitate modification of the exercise prescription or, in rare instances, contraindicate participation. Obtain and review the client's medical history, test results (i.e., tender point evaluation, lab work) and current medication list prior to the initial meeting. Information from other allied health professionals such as physical therapists can assist in evaluating pain, tender points, range of motion, muscular strength and aerobic fitness. See Table 18.2 for a list of questions you may want to ask the client's healthcare professional.

Initial Interview

Strong interviewing skills are essential for working with the FS population. The initial meeting should focus on gaining a clear understanding of the client's past and current activity patterns, symptomatic response, likes/dislikes, and other motivational factors and potential barriers. These factors may impact long-term compliance, available support systems and other issues that may influence the design of the program. Consider asking the questions presented in Table 18.3.

It is important to assess previously inactive individuals' readiness to change, because as difficult as it is to motivate FS patients to exercise, it is more difficult for an FS patient to begin a full-blown program if they haven't even considered starting to exercise. Research suggests that effective, meaningful activity programs are successful when clients gradually progress through the various stages of change.

It is critical to carefully review the importance of physical activity to general health and, more specifically, its ability to improve the symptoms of FS, with individuals identified as precontemplators (those not yet considering physical exercise). The objective is to start the precontemplator thinking about the benefits of physical activity and the barriers that frequently interfere with being physically active.

The initial session with individuals who have moved from the precontemplation stage to one of contemplating starting an exercise program should focus on the program's design, monitoring techniques and potential barriers that impact compliance.

The first thing all FS patients need to understand is that muscle is living tissue that, when not used, becomes short and stiff, and progressively declines in function. FS patients cannot afford sedentary living despite the musculoskeletal pain and severe fatigue that perpetuates inactivity. Explain to FS clients that the focus

is on "health training" not "sports training." Fibromyalgia patients must realize that the "no pain, no gain" mindset and past experience/achievements must be set aside.

Second, FS clients must be taught that the secret to improvement is consistency over time, not how long or how hard one works in any particular session. Backing off or even resting during severe flare-up periods is okay if the long-range pattern is consistent. Teach clients that exercise should not be viewed as a short-term, six- to 12-month program, but as part of a daily lifestyle.

Third, remind clients that exercise does not have to take place in expensive facilities that utilize fancy equipment. Many individuals list cost as a primary deterrent to participating in exercise training — a factor that should not be limiting. Provide clients with a home program consisting of stretching, gentle strengthening and aerobic conditioning exercises. Other forms of exercise may enhance the program and further benefit select individuals, but are not absolutely necessary. Individuals who are not currently exercising may best be served simply by increasing day-to-day activities prior to formalizing an exercise program.

Posture Evaluation

During the initial interview, perform a thorough posture evaluation to assess body asymmetry imbalances that may unnecessarily load the musculoskeletal system and cause

Table 18.2

Client Information to Obtain from Medical Professionals

1) Describe your symptoms. (e.g., Do you have full-body aches, extreme fatigue, stiff muscles?)

2) How active are you? What types of physical activity do you enjoy? Describe how your body feels after participating in physical activity (both acutely and chronically). Do you frequently experience low-back pain, lower-leg cramps or foot pain, or have "jumpy muscles"?

3) Do you experience motor coordination problems? Do you have a painful, weak grip that sometimes releases?

4) How do you treat your symptoms of fatigue and pain?

5) How would you describe your sleep habits? How do you feel upon waking in the morning? Does it take a long time to "get going"?

6) Do you frequently experience a stiff neck or numbness/tingling in your extremities?

7) Do you ever experience tightness in the chest, a rapid pulse or shortness of breath? If so, at rest or during exertion?

8) What medications are you taking?

9) Do you have diabetes? Do you frequently feel lightheaded and/or dizzy?

10) Do you smoke or use any form of tobacco?

increased pain and early fatigue. Clinical exercise specialists not familiar with postural evaluation techniques may want to consult with a trained physical therapist, athletic trainer or exercise physiologist.

Evaluate the left and right sides, and front and back of the body, from head to toe. Ideally, the body should be symmetrical. Shoulders, shoulder blades, arms, elbows, hips, knees, ankles and heels should be even and level on both sides. Imbalances, such as internal rotation of the knees, shoulders or hips, result in tightness of the musculature. Check shoes for wear patterns and stability along arches and toes.

Specific stretching and strengthening exercises can improve problems. For individuals with hypermobile joints, emphasize gentle strengthening, not lengthening, exercises. Discourage prolonged sitting and encourage ergonomically correct work stations and home furniture.

Fitness Testing

Information gathered from aerobic fitness tests is useful in planning the aerobic conditioning program and providing feedback to the FS client regarding current fitness levels and improvement. Positive feedback regarding improvements is a strong motivator for FS clients to maintain compliance.

A variety of submaximal protocols have been utilized to evaluate FS patients. The six-minute walk and submaximal bike tests are most common. Because many individuals with FS are unfamiliar with cycling, and to avoid the localized leg fatigue associated with cycling, walking tests may be the best choice. Pay close attention to detail and maximize reproducibility by following the exact same procedures for each test within the series. Ideally, the same trainer will conduct each test. In some instances the individual may require a symptom-limited maximal exercise test to evaluate symptoms and/or other risk factors prior to initiating the exercise program. Such testing should be carried out under the supervision of the client's physician.

While few facilities have the equipment to measure cardiopulmonary gas-exchange variables, such testing considerably increases the quality of information available to the clinical exercise specialist and client. Participants in our FEET (Fibromyalgia Education and Exercise Training) program undergo a two-part cardiopulmonary exercise evaluation that begins with a five-minute steady-state submaximal walk at 1.3 mph and 8 percent grade to assess oxygen kinetics. Following a short rest period the participant then undergoes a graded exercise test using a ramping protocol (Table 18.4). Gas exchange, ECG and symptoms are continuously monitored, while blood pressure and Rating of Perceived Exertion (RPE) measures

Table 18.3

Activity Guidelines

- Physical activity is essential for maintaining function. Patients should be encouraged not to give in to symptoms and undergo extended periods of inactivity but to adjust duration and intensity according to symptoms.

- Activity levels should be gradually increased using ADL's and low impact physical activities. Warm water therapy/exercise is highly recommended for the fibromyalgia population.

- Gentle stretching should become part of the daily routine, with extra care being taken not to "over stretch".

- Fibromyalgia patients do not have to train hard. Low to moderate intensities of fairly light to somewhat hard (Borg 11-13) are recommended.

- Intensity and/or duration should be reduced during periods of flare-up and increased fatigue/pain resulting form previous activity.

- Variety is important. Patients should be encouraged to participate in a variety of activities rather than one particular type of activity. Repetitive motion trauma can become a major problem in this population.

- Using correct technique and maintaining appropriate posture should be stressed. Individuals with fibromyalgia should maintain an acute awareness of their posture and movement techniques.

- Consistency over time is the key. Infrequent and especially over-intense exercise should be avoided.

are obtained every two minutes. In addition to deriving objective information regarding the individual's response to exercise and current fitness level, the ventilatory threshold (VT) serves as an excellent training-intensity marker. The exercise intensity preferably should be kept at or below the ventilatory threshold in FS patients.

Exercise Programming and Leadership

Exercise programs for individuals with FS are designed to promote health, not athleticism. Therefore, be flexible and willing to adapt the program to meet the client's current health status and symptomatology. Exercise professionals, in their enthusiasm to help people improve, occasionally push clients too hard and/or progress individuals too quickly. This is disastrous when working with FS clients and frequently results in increased pain and fatigue, and discontinuation of the activity program. Fibromyalgia clients do not have to train hard, but do have to train smart. Remember that the objective is to become moderately physically active and maintain consistency over a period of time.

Type of Exercise

Generally, physical activities for FS clients should be low- or non-impact, such as aquatic exercise, walking, cycling and use of a variety of non-impact cross training devices. Walking is an excellent low-impact activity that requires minimal instruction and equipment. Aquatic therapy is highly recommended for the FS population, especially those who have significantly reduced fitness levels, or orthopedic injuries and/or are overweight. The aquatic environment allows a significant amount of both upper- and lower-body work without the jarring and trauma that is characteristic of many land-based activities. Many experts believe that the water environment also helps minimize the embarrassment and self-consciousness that some people experience when beginning to participate in land-based activities. Water provides excellent resistance to promote strength gains and allows for a variety of range-of-motion activities. Accessories such as fins and kick boards gradually can be added to progressively increase resistance, and deep water walking/ jogging utilizing a flotation device is an excellent activity for selected FS clients to progress to. Because individuals with FS rarely tolerate cold water, a warm-water environment (84 to 90 degrees) is ideal. Aquatic workouts lend themselves well to individual and/or group workouts, and group classes that are individually paced provide an added social benefit, which can be therapeutic.

Resistance training that utilizes very light weights, elastic bands and/or gravity, and emphasizes proper technique and full range of motion also is recommended. Teach proper technique and stress moderation in resistance-training activities. Design exercises to improve postural imbalances, range of motion and generalized strength, especially in the upper extremity. Resistance loads should be kept at a minimum, and in many instances no-load activities may be most appropriate. One set of eight to 12 repetitions should be adequate; in fact, additional sets are discouraged. Complete the resistance-training phase of the program in 20 to 30 minutes to maximize compliance.

Generally, encourage individuals with FS to begin their exercise program by increasing activities of daily living and supplementing with low-level aquatic activities. Short (five- to 10-minute) activity breaks can be scheduled throughout the day without emphasizing intensity. Based on the Surgeon General's report, the goal is to accumulate 30 minutes of physical activity each day. There is no need to rush the progression into higher levels of activity, and individuals can gradually progress to other low-impact, land-based exercises and resistance

Table 18.4. Rite Treadmill Protocol (Lewalter, 1995)

TIME	VELOCITY (mph)	PERCENT GRADE
1:00	1.0	4
1:00	1.3	5
1:00	1.6	6
1:00	1.9	7
1:00	2.2	8
1:00	2.5	9
1:00	2.8	10
1:00	3.1	11
1:00	3.4	12
1:00	3.7	13
1:00	4.0	14
1:00	4.3	15
1:00	4.6	16

training over time. Consistency over time will develop an active lifestyle and a clear understanding of how to pace oneself on a daily basis. Highly conditioned, currently active FS clients may be able to start with land-based activities.

Intensity

Individuals with fibromyalgia should exercise at low to moderate ranges of intensity, defined as 85 percent of the target heart rate for their age (120 to150 bpm for most individuals) (Bennett & McCain, 1995). The American College of Sports Medicine recommends the training intensity be set at 40 to 85 percent of functional capacity, depending on an individual's current exercise habits and medical background (ACSM, 1995). Thus, Bennett and McCain's recommendation would place people with FS in the range of 40 percent to 70 percent of the maximum heart rate (Bennett & McCain, 1995).

Perceived effort (RPE) may be the best tool for determining and monitoring exercise intensity. Utilization of RPE allows for day-to-day variations in symptoms that may be reflected in heart rate. The use of RPE also eliminates problems associated with individuals who do not accurately count their pulse, and the effect of a variety of medications on the heart rate response.

Ideally, exercise intensity should remain at or below the VT, which is easily determined if a cardiopulmonary exercise test has been performed. This level of exercise intensity also can be estimated using RPE. Data suggests that an RPE of 11 to 13 on the Borg Scale (6 to 20) is frequently reflective of the VT region (Roy, Grove & Christie, 1993). Since the objective of the exercise program is to promote health-related fitness and to stretch and mobilize tight and weak muscles, it is best to be conservative when prescribing an intensity, especially for previously sedentary individuals.

Duration, Frequency and Progression

Encourage clients who have been physically inactive and are starting a home-based activity program to participate in five to 10 minutes of activity three or more times per day. Severely deconditioned individuals may have to start with as little as two to three minutes three times daily to keep from escalating post-exertion pain and

fatigue. As conditioning gradually improves, the duration of the activities can be lengthened and the daily frequency may be cut back to one to three times per day. Individuals able to participate in structured exercise training generally may start with single sessions of 15 to 20 minutes and gradually progress to 30 to 40 minutes three to four times per week. Sessions lasting longer than 40 minutes are not necessary to provide health improvements and lengthening sessions beyond this duration may produce diminishing returns in individuals with FS.

Stretching

People with FS frequently feel tight and stiff, especially after sleeping or sitting or standing for prolonged periods. Encourage participation in a simple program of static stretching exercises to improve and maintain mobility. Stretching activities should be encouraged during the warm-up and cool-down periods of exercise training as well as periodically throughout the day. Gentle stretching of major muscle groups is recommended; avoid ballistic activities.

Summary

Fibromyalgia syndrome is a complex, multifactorial chronic pain condition with an unknown etiology that demands palliative, rather than curative, treatment. Because the primary goal of treatment is to improve function, exercise training is an important component of the therapy program. However, proper prescription and education in regard to intensity, frequency and duration are essential. Low-impact activities such as walking, cycling and aquatics supplemented with gentle stretching and light resistance training are most helpful.

Clinical exercise specialists must become familiar with the background of each client with FS and carefully guide them through appropriate activities that the client can consistently use and enjoy. The appropriate program will be individualized and adaptable to day-to-day variations in symptoms. The goal of an exercise program for FS clients should be 30 to 40 minutes of continuous, comfortably-paced aerobic activity three to four times per week, supplemented with daily activities and stretching breaks at home and work.

Physical activity also appears to influence the psychological well-being of FS patients, as does the supportive environment of group exercise and education sessions. Physical activity, when performed on a consistent basis, significantly improves the quality of life enjoyed by people with fibromyalgia syndrome.

Case Studies

Case Study I

Client is a 49-year-old female who suffered a shoulder injury in an industrial accident in 1988. She subsequently underwent physical therapy with apparent ROM improvement, but developed chronic pain in the upper extremity. Over the next six years she suffered chronic symptoms of fatigue and upper-extremity pain, especially in the neck and shoulder areas. In 1995 she changed physicians and underwent a physical exam that produced the following findings:

Height: 65"

Weight: 206 pounds (approximately 159 percent over ideal weight)

- Hypertension with a blood pressure of 150/98
- Arthritic changes noted in right shoulder; left shoulder was slightly elevated compared to the right
- Described trouble sleeping at night, even though tired all day
- Tests revealed moderate depression
- Tested positive on 18 of 18 tender points
- Taking the following medications: Synthroid, Zoloft, Flexeril, melatonin

Based on the physical exam, the physician made the following diagnosis and referred the client for exercise counseling: 1) Fibromyalgia with chronic fatigue and pain, 2) Hypertension, 3) Moderate depression, 4) Insomnia.

Upon receiving the physician's referral, the clinical exercise specialist requested copies of the client's medical history and physical examination results. The physician granted permission for the clinical exercise specialist to administer treadmill fitness testing under the supervision of an ACLS-trained clinical exercise physiologist.

The exercise test, which included an analysis of expired air, was repeated four months later to document the effectiveness of the exercise conditioning program. Both a steady-state submaximal walk for five minutes and a graded exercise protocol were utilized. Additionally, the Zung Depression Inventory and Belza Fatigue Inventory were given to assess changes in the client's mental outlook. Results from both tests are reported in Table 18.5.

Following exercise testing, the clinical exercise specialist met with the client to review results and develop an individualized training program. Warm-water aquatic exercise training consisting of low-to-moderate aerobic exercise, and range-of-motion activities were recommended for three times per week. Intensity was set at an RPE of 10 to 11. Following one month of aquatic training, 20 to 30 minutes of walking twice a week at an RPE of 11 was added to the program. At six weeks the client began light resistance training, placing emphasis on proper technique and slow, controlled movements. The client also was encouraged to meet with other FS clients one evening per week for group education.

Throughout the program, the clinical exercise specialist met with the FS client twice per week to review her log book for any changes and/or worsening in symptoms, and other responses to the activity program. Modifications in the program periodically were made to alleviate symptom aggravation.

Testing was repeated after four months of training and 10 educational group sessions taught by various medical professionals. The results (see Table 4) showed a significant decrease in resting heart rate and blood pressure and a 6-pound weight loss. Oxygen uptake slightly improved as did ventilatory threshold VO_2. Heart rate and RPE at the ventilatory threshold were similar on both tests. Fatigue improved from severe to moderate and there also was a concurrent improvement in the depression score. A summary detailing outcome results was sent to the client's physician.

Case Study II

This client is a 37-year-old, 65-inches tall, 116-pound mother of two who was quite active prior to having

Table 18.5
Case I - Test Results

Variable	Initial Test (Sept)	Follow-up (Dec)
Resting HR	117	100
Resting BP	140/90	122/88
Submax Mean Response Time	62sec	50sec
VT V02 ml/min	1062	1342
VT HR	130	128
VT RPE	11	11
Peak HR	168	171
Peak BP	190/110	188/92
Peak V02 ml/min	1615	1953
Peak V02 ml/kg/min	19.8	21.5
Belza Fatigue	Severe	Moderate
Zung Depression	Mod-Severe	Moderate

children. She ran four to five times per week for 30 to 40 minutes, and her health history was unremarkable. Following the birth of her first child she began experiencing chronic symptoms of muscle aches and pains, and significant fatigue. She curtailed her exercise to walking or deep-water aerobics one or two times per week, depending on her fatigue levels. She believed her symptoms were the result of being a working mother with an active toddler. Other than an annual Pap screen no medical evaluations were done.

Three years after the birth of her first child, a second child was born and the fatigue and pain increased. It became a struggle to complete everyday chores, and upon relocating to a new community, she stopped working. The client rarely slept through the night and frequently would awake in the morning – even after a good night's sleep – feeling tired, stiff and achy.

Seven years after her symptoms originally manifested, she underwent a complete physical exam. Results revealed no musculoskeletal injuries or trauma related to her symptoms. However, the ROM in the upper extremity (shoulder flexion and abduction) and hip flexors was decreased. Laboratory blood and urine testing was normal, and resting HR, BP and ECG were within normal limits even though a systolic click was heard and a subsequent echocardiogram revealed mild mitral valve prolapse. A tender point evaluation revealed 13 of 18 positive tender points while the fatigue inventory revealed moderate fatigue. Depression scores were normal.

The following diagnosis was made: 1) Fibromyalgia, 2) Insomnia and 3) Mild mitral valve prolapse.

Table 18.6
Case II - Test Results

Variable	Initial Test (Sept)	Follow-up (Dec)
Resting HR	117	100
Resting BP	108/60	104/64
Submax Mean Response Time	46sec	47sec
VT VO$_2$ ml/min	1231	1369
VT HR	142	144
VT RPE	13	13
Peak HR	180	184
Peak BP	160/82	164/78
Peak VO$_2$ ml/min	1578	1825
Peak VO$_2$ ml/kg/min	30.1	34.7
Belza Fatigue	Moderate	Moderate
Zung Depression	Normal	Normal

Ambien was prescribed for sleep assistance and Ibuprofen PM for pain. The client was referred to a fitness facility for exercise testing and development of an individualized exercise program. The cardiopulmonary exercise test consisted of a submaximal steady-state walk and a graded exercise test to voluntary termination. The exercise evaluation was supervised by an ACLS-trained clinical exercise physiologist. Results for both the pre- and post-training test are presented in Table 18.6.

Following exercise testing, the clinical exercise specialist developed a walking program consisting of three to four sessions per week for 30 minutes at an RPE of 11 to 13. The walking program was supplemented by warm-water mobility exercises and light resistance training. A log book was given to the client to record daily activities, symptoms and general fatigue levels, and was reviewed weekly by the clinical exercise specialist. Adjustments were made to the training program based on the client's responses.

Five-minute increments were added to the client's walking program over the four-month training period until she progressed to 45 minutes of continuous walking at an RPE of 11 to13. Early in the program, resistance training provoked increased muscular fatigue and stiffness; consequently the workload was reduced to minimize symptoms. The resistance then gradually was increased to more strenuous levels, though the workload remained light and repetitions were held constant at 10 to 12 for one set of each exercise.

The client was fairly compliant with the exercise program, but participation in educational sessions was low. Testing was repeated four months after the initial tests, and showed a slightly improved VO$_2$ and ventilatory threshold. There was no change in the fatigue and depression inventories. The clinical exercise specialist encouraged the client to remain as active as possible and to continue the exercise training program, and she received instruction on how to monitor her symptoms and adjust activities on days of increased fatigue and muscular pain. Though the four-month program produced small fitness improvements, the primary emphasis of the long-range plan is to maintain her current level of conditioning.

References

American College of Sports Medicine. (1995). *ACSM's Guidelines for Exercise Testing and Prescription.* (5th Ed.). Baltimore, Md.: Williams and Wilkins.

Bengtsson, A. & Henriksson, K.G. (1989). The muscle in fibromyalgia - a review of Swedish studies. *Journal of Rheumatology (Supplement),* 19, 144-149.

Bennett, R.M. (1993). Fibromyalgia and the facts: sense or nonsense. *Controversies in Clinical Rheumatology*, 19, 1, 45-49.

Bennett, R.M. & McCain, G. (1995). Coping successfully with fibromyalgia. *Patient Care*, 29, 29-39.

Bennett, R.M. (1993). The Origin of Myopain: An Integrated Hypothesis of Focal Muscle Changes and Sleep Disturbance in Patients with Fibromyalgia Syndrome. *Journal of Musculoskeletal Pain*, 1, 3-4, 95-112.

Bennett, R.M., Clark, S.R., Campbell, S.M. & Burckhardt, C.S. (1992). Low levels of somatomedin C in patients with fibromyalgia syndrome: a possible link between sleep and muscle pain. *Arthritis Rheumatology*, 35, 1113-1116.

Bennet, R.M., Clark, S.R., Goldberg, L., Nelson, D., Bonafede, R.P., Porter, J. & Specht, D. (1989). Aerobic fitness in patients with fibromyalgia syndrome: A controlled study of respiratory gas exchange and 133xenon clearance from exercising muscle. *Arthritis/Rheumatism*, 32, 454-460.

Boissevain, M.D. & McCain, G.A. (1991). Toward an integrated understanding of fibromyalgia syndrome, II: Psychological and phenomenological aspects. *Pain*, 44, 239-248.

Caspersen, C.J., Powell, K.E. & Christenson G.M. (1985). Physical activity, exercise and physical fitness: Definitions and distinctions for health related researches. *Public Health Reports*, 100, 126-131.

Clark, S.R., Burckhardt, C.S., Campbell, S., O'Reilly, C. & Bennett R. (1994). Fitness Characteristics and Perceived Exertion in Women with Fibromyalgia. Musculoskeletal Pain, *Myofascial Pain Syndrome and Fibromyalgia*, 7, 123-129.

Clayton, L.T. (1979). *Taber's Cyclopedic Medical Dictionary*. Philadelphia, Pa.: F.A. Davis Company.

Csillag, C. (1992). Consensus Document on Fibro-myalgia: The Copenhagen Declaration. Second World Congress on Myofascial Pain and Fibromyalgia. *Lancet,* 340.

Deuster, P.A. (1996). Exercise in the Prevention and Treatment of Chronic Disorders. *Women's Health Issues*, 6, 6, 320-331.

Drews, A.M., Andreasen, A., Schroder, H.D., Hogsaa, B., Jennum, P. (1993). Pathology of skeletal muscle in fibromyalgia: a histo-immuno-chemical and ultrastructural study. *British Journal of Rheumatology*, 32, 479-483.

Elert, J.E., Rantopan-Dahlquist, S.B., Henriksson-Larson, K., Lorentzon, R. & Gerdle B. (1992). Muscle performance, electromyography and fibre type composition in fibromyalgia and work-related myalgia. *Scandanavian Journal of Rheumatology*, 1, 28-34.

Fan, P.T. & Blanton, M.E. (1992). Clinical features and diagnostics of fibromyalgia. *The Journal of Musculoskeletal Medicine*, 9, 4, 24-42.

Gauvin, L., Wall, T.A.E. & Quoney H.A. (1994). Physical Activity, Fitness and Health: Research and Practice. In: Brouchard, C. (Ed.). *Toward Active Living: Proceedings of The International Conference on Physical Activity, Fitness and Health.* Champaign, Ill: Human Kinetics.

Goldenberg, D.L. (1989). Diagnostic and therapeutic challenges of fibromyalgia. *Hospital Practice,* 24, 39-52.

Goldenberg, D.L., Simms, R.W., Geiger, A. & Komoroft, A.L. (1990). High frequency of fibromyalgia in patients with chronic fatigue seen in a primary care practice. *Arthritis Rheumatology,* 33, 381-387.

Goldenberg, D.L. (1989). Psychiatric and psychologic aspects of fibromyalgia syndrome. *Rheumatology Disease Clinics of North America,* 15, 105-114.

Goldenberg, D.L. (1992). Controversies in fibromyalgia and myofascial pain syndrome. In: Arnoff, G.M. (Ed.). *Evaluation and Treatment of Chronic Pain.* Baltimore, Md.: Williams and Wilkins.

Krsnich-Shriwise, S. (1997). Fibromyalgia syndrome: An overview. *Physical Therapy*, 77, 1, 68-75.

Lewalter, T., MacCarter, D., Jung, W., Schimpf, R., Manz, M. & Luderitz, B. (1995). Heart Rate to Work Rate Relation Throughout Peak Exercise in Normal Subjects as a Guideline for Rate-Adaptive Pacemaker Programming. *American Journal of Cardiology*, 76, 812-816.

Mannerkorpi, K., Burckhardt, C.S. & Bjelle A. (1994). Physical performance characteristics of women with fibromyalgia. A*rthritis Care Research*, 7, 123-129.

McCain, G.A., Bell, D.A., Mai, F.M. & Halliday, P.D. (1988). A controlled study of the effects of a supervised cardiovascular fitness training program on the manifestations of primary fibromyalgia. *Arthritis Rheumatology*, 31, 1135-1141.

Mengshoel, A.M., Forre, O. & Komnaes, H.B. (1990). Muscle strength and aerobic capacity in primary fibromyalgia. *Clinics in Experimental Rheumatology,* 8, 5, 475-479.

Moldofsky, H. (1989). Sleep and fibrositis syndrome. *Rheumatology Disease Clinics of North America,* 15, 91-103.

Mountz, J.M., Bradley, L.A., Modell, J.G., Alexander, R.W., Triana-Alexander, M., Aaron, L.A., Stewart, K.E., Alarcon, G.S. & Mountz, J.D. (1995). Fibromyalgia in women: abnormalities of regional cerebral blood flow in the thalamus and the caudate nucleus are associated with low pain threshold levels. *Arthritis Pheumatology*, 38, 926-938.

Nichols, D.S. & Glenn, T.M. (1994). Effects of aerobic exercise on pain perception, affect, and level of disability in individuals with fibromyalgia. *Physical Therapy,* 74, 327-332.

Reiffenbeiger, D.H. & Amundson, L.H. (1996). Fibromyalgia syndrome: A review. *American Family Physician*, 53, 5, 1698-1704.

Roy, B.A., Grove, M.A. & Christie, L.G. (1993). A New Formula for Determining Exercise Intensity in Coronary Artery Disease Patients. *Journal of Cardiopulmonary Rehabilitation,* 13, 271-276.

Russell, I.J. (1989). Neurohormonal aspects of fibromyalgia syndrome. *Rheumatology Disease Clinics of North America,* 15, 149-167.

Simms, R.W. (1996). Fibromyalgia Syndrome: Current Concepts in Pathophysiology, Clinical Features, and Management. *Artihritis Care and Research*, 9, 4, 315-328.

Starland, D. & Copeland, M.E. (1996). *Fibromyalgia and Chronic Myofascial Pain Syndrome: A Survival Manual.* Oakland, Calif. New Harbinger Publications.

Wilkins, F. & Wilkins, D. (1997). *MemoryMinder Personal Health Journal.* P.O. Box 23108, Eugene, Oregon 97402-0425.

Wolfe, F., Aarflot, T., Bruusgaard, D., Henriksson, K.G., Littlejohn, G., Moldofsky, H., Raspe, H. & Vaeroy, H. (1995). Fibromyalgia and Disability: Report of the Mass International Working Group on Medical-Legal Aspects of Chronic Widespread Musculoskeletal Pain Complaints in Fibromyalgia. *Scandinavian Journal of Rheumatology,* 24, 112-118.

Wolfe, F., Ross, K., Anderson, J., Russell, I.J. & Herbert, L. (1995). The prevalence and characteristics of fibromyalgia in the general population. *Arthritis Rheumatology,* 38, 19-28.

Wolfe, F. (1996). The fibromyalgia syndrome: A consensus report on fibromyalgia and disability. *Journal of Rheumatology,* 23, 534-539.

Wolfe, F., Smythe, H.A., Yunus, M.B., Bennett, R.M., Bombardier, C., Goldenberg, D.L., Tugwell, P., Campbell, S.M., Abelex, M. & Clark, P. (1990). The American College of Rheumatology 1990 Criteria for the Classification of Fibromyalgia: a report of the multicenter criteria committee. *Arthritis Rheumatology,* 33,160-172.

CHAPTER 19

Gait and Balance

GREGORY L. WELCH

Gregory Welch, M.S., is an exercise physiologist and president of SpeciFit, An Agency of Wellness, a company located in Seal Beach, Calif., that primarily focuses on enhancing the physical well-being of special-needs populations. Welch has written many articles and delivered presentations on special populations across the country. He is on the advisory board of the Lifespan Wellness Center at California State University, Fullerton, and assists in the development and teaching of a certificate course for fitness professionals working with seniors.

Falling
Gait
Mechanics
Spotting

In the simplest of terms, the human gait pattern is the way people walk and balance, and is responsible for our ability to maintain an upright posture. The components of gait and balance are fundamental to physical function. Together, normal gait and balance enable ambulation, also known as mobility. Personal mobility is essential to effective functioning, which, for the older adult, is commonly referred to as the ability to perform activities of daily living (ADL). Although the hierarchy of ability for this population will vary tremendously, the older adult must pay close attention to maintaining an upright posture. Controlling postural balance is a prerequisite to performing many ADLs, and emphasizes the ability to maintain a mobile and independent lifestyle (Black et al., 1993).

For most individuals, independent functioning

presupposes the ability to walk (Bohannon, 1997). While it appears relatively simple, walking is actually a complicated physiological process. A successful gait pattern is dependent on sufficient control at three levels: 1) basic reflexive **stride** and support patterns; 2) postural and equilibrium control; and 3) mechanisms that allow the body to adapt to unexpected changes in the environment (Spirduso, 1995). Tinetti et al. (1988) state that balance impairment, which is common among the elderly, is one of the most important risk factors for falls and injuries. Additionally, falls, instability and immobility are among the most common reasons for medical intervention for the older adult.

As our society places more emphasis on maintaining an independent lifestyle, more attention must be given to maintaining mobility as the population ages. The intent of this chapter is twofold: to educate the clinical exercise specialist with regard to current information on gait and balance, and to help them implement a gait and balance training strategy.

Defining the Population

For years, older adults were lumped into the general category of special populations. However, as we learn more about the elderly we realize there are often special subpopulations. This is especially true with regard to gait and balance, since the mechanisms leading to reduced mobility are complex. While age-related changes in the neural, sensory and musculoskeletal systems can lead to balance impairments that have a significant impact on the ability to maneuver safely (Maki & McIlroy, 1996), some older adults maintain normal gait into their ninth decade, suggesting that a disordered gait is not an inevitable component of aging (Bloem et al., 1992). Additional challenges occur when immobility is the result of a multifactorial etiology. Multiple chronic diseases, cognitive impairment, upper- and lower-extremity disabilities, and medication also contribute to the instability of the elderly. Attempting to define a population with gait and balance disorders based on any one problem would be difficult at best. The most effective approach in dealing with a gait and balance disorder is to communicate directly with a client's attending physician to obtain precise information specific to each individual.

Etiology

The root of the problem for gait and balance disorders is multifactorial. There may be many independent reasons for an affliction, as well as several issues undermining posture and ambulation. The effects of aging, deterioration caused by disease and alterations due to medication all are contributing factors.

Age-related changes occur in all of the sensory systems that support postural control (Maki & McIlroy, 1996). In a study of the healthy elderly, it was determined that progressive, functionally evident, age-related quantitative balance changes occur independent of typical geriatric pathological changes (Camicioli et al., 1997). Gait velocity slows, **stride length** shortens and double-support time increases due to the effects of aging (Judge et al., 1997).

Nutt et al. (1993) have classified gait and balance dysfunction by way of the following pathophysiological scheme:

- ➤ lower level disorders due to problems with sensation or strength
- ➤ middle level disorders due to problems within the spinal cord or brainstem
- ➤ higher level disorders due to problems with the cerebellum basal ganglia or cortical spinal tracts
- ➤ highest level disorders due to problems in the frontal cortex.

Sherlock (1996) adds identification of three categories causing balance disorders:

- ➤ peripheral causes of balance disorders such as vestibular neuronitis, an abrupt onset of severe vertigo
- ➤ disease processes of the central nervous system such as stroke and traumatic brain injury
- ➤ degenerative neurological diseases such as multiple sclerosis.

Be aware of these classifications should they be included on a physician's report.

Table 19.1 lists common medical conditions that cause gait and balance disorders in elderly persons (Tinetti et al., 1986).

Table 19.1
Medical Conditions that Cause Gait and Balance Disorders in the Elderly

Cardiovascular Conditions

orthostatic hypotension	vertebrobasilar insufficiency intermittent claudiction	chronic LE edema

Neurological Conditions

Parkinson's disease stroke etat lacunaire peripheral neuropathy dementia chronic subdural hematoma	normal pressure hydrocephalus cerbellar ataxia posterior column degeneration cervical spondylosis vitamin B_{12} myelopathy deficiency frontal lobe syndrome	encephalopathy progressive supranuclear palsy peripheral neuropathy spinal cord lesions

Musculoskeletal Conditions

osteoarthritis osteoarthroses	osteomalacia status post-ortho surgery	foot problems unsuspected fractures

Psychological Conditions

depression	fear of falling

Endocrinological Conditions

hypothyroidism

Other Conditions

general weakness drug intoxication/overdose	benzodiazepines tricyclic antidepressants	anticonvulsants salicylates	antivertigo agents senile gait

Tinetti, M.E., Williams, T.F., Mayewski, R. (1986). Fall risk index for elderly patients based on number of chronic disabilities. *American Journal of Medicine*, 80, 429-434.
Cunha, U.V. (1988). Differential diagnosis of gait disorders in the elderly. *Geriatrics*, 43, 34.

Components of Balance

In the broadest sense, balance involves an individual's capability to control upright posture under a variety of conditions and to sense their stability limitations (Berg & Norman, 1996). Postural control can be defined as the process by which the central nervous system (CNS) generates the patterns of muscle activity required to regulate the relationship between the center of gravity (COG) and the base of support (BOS) (Maki & McIlroy, 1996). In a study conducted to determine the relationship of postural balance to self-reported functional ability and general physical activity, Era et al. (1997) concluded that good balance is one of the prerequisites for mobility and **activities of daily living.** To maintain stability, the body's center of gravity must be positioned vertically over the base of support. The latitude of stability where the COG is still within the BOS is considered the area of sway. Controlling postural sway while standing is called static balance. Normal units of sway are approximately 12.5 percent for anterior/posterior sway and 16 percent for lateral sway (Sherlock, 1996). A study by Lucy and Hayes (1985) determined that sway in the anteroposterior direction was 52 percent greater in subjects 70 to 80 years old than in subjects 30 to 39 years old. Thus, postural stability, normally considered to be under automatic control processes, requires more conscious attention in the elderly than in younger individuals (Spirduso, 1995).

The act of processing internal and external information to react to destabilizing forces and cause the muscles to anticipate balance changes is called dynamic balance (Spirduso, 1995). Three different sensory systems derive the information necessary to maintain balance: 1) the visual system, 2) the vestibular system and 3) the somatosensory system.

The Visual System

Visual information provides feedback regarding the changing environment, and movement of the head with respect to surrounding objects (Sherlock, 1996).

Location, direction and speed of movement also are discerned through vision. Age-related changes in the visual system include reduced acuity, contrast sensitivity, depth perception and dark adaptation (Verrillo & Verrillo, 1985). Sekuler and Hartman (1980) state the importance of the need for up to three times more contrast to compensate for a loss in the ability to discriminate low spatial frequencies.

The Vestibular System

Located in the inner ear, the vestibular system is a network of receptors that provides information about position and movements of the head, with respect to gravity (Spirduso, 1995). Regardless of whether the head is upside down, tilted or changing positions, this system activates motor neurons, leading the muscle tissue to contribute substantially to maintaining balance. Both the size and number of vestibular neurons begins to decrease after the age of 40 (Rosenhall & Ruben, 1975). Because many postural reflexes triggered by the vestibular system also may be triggered by visual stimulation, vision can compensate for some loss of vestibular function (Spirduso, 1995).

The Somatosensory System

Somatosensory information on the position and motion of the body's support surface is gained from receptors in skin, muscles and joints (Sherlock, 1996). Pressure receptors in the skin and proprioceptors in the muscles,

joints and ligaments provide information about weight shifts and joint angles. While sense of joint position in the arms and legs does not markedly decline in the elderly, cutaneous or skin sensation does decrease with age (Kokmen et al., 1978; Brocklehurst et al., 1982).

Characteristics of Gait

Generally speaking, walking is the most common activity of daily living. It can be defined as the process of transferring the center of gravity of one foot to the other by alternately moving the legs forward. This performance of gait creates a continuous disturbance of the mechanical equilibrium as it forms new bases of support (Spirduso, 1995). Normal gait is dependent on the capacity of multiple-organ systems, specifically the neurologic (sensory, motor control), musculoskeletal (muscle force, joint range of motion and posture), and cardiovascular systems (Judge et al., 1996).

Although many individuals may take the simplicity of gait mechanics for granted, approximately 50 percent of falls occur during walking (Patla & Winter, 1990).

Gait Mechanics

It is necessary to understand the mechanics of the normal **gait cycle** to better comprehend assessment and training procedures. Following is an explanation of the normal gait cycle

Figure 19.1
The Subdivisions of Stance and Their Relationship to the Bilateral Floor-Contact Pattern

Vertical dark bars are the periods of double-limb stance (right and left feet). Horizontal shaded bars represent single-limb support (single stance). Total stance includes three intervals: the initial double stance, single-limb support and the next (terminal) double stance. Swing is the clear bar that follows terminal double stance. Note that right single-limb support is the same time interval as left swing. During right swing there is left single-limb support. The third vertical bar (double stance) begins the next gait cycle.

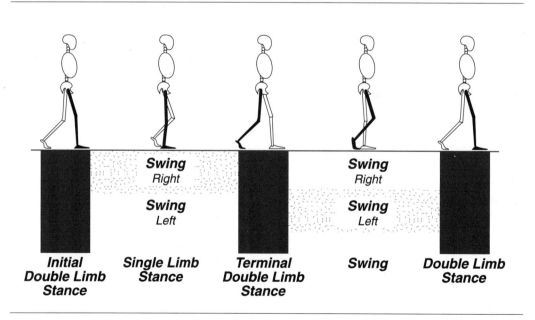

| Initial Double Limb Stance | Single Limb Stance | Terminal Double Limb Stance | Swing | Double Limb Stance |

by Perry (1992). The corresponding graphic description of a normal gait cycle is provided in Figure 19.1.

The mechanics of walking are referred to as the gait cycle, which is defined as a sequence of events between two sequential contacts by the same limb. There are two phases that make up the gait cycle: stance and swing. The stance phase, which constitutes approximately 60 percent of the normal gait cycle, is the interval in which the foot of the reference extremity is in contact with the ground. The swing phase, which makes up the remaining 40 percent of the gait cycle, is the interval in which the reference extremity does not contact the ground. Stance is further subdivided into three intervals, according to the sequence of floor contact by the two feet:

1) Initial double stance, also known as double-limb support, begins the gait cycle (GC). It is the time both feet are on the floor after initial contact (10 percent GC).

2) Single-limb support begins when the opposite foot is lifted for swing. The word "support" is preferred over "stance" to emphasize the functional significance of floor contact by just one foot. During the single-limb support interval, the body's entire weight is resting only on one extremity. The duration of single stance is the best index of the limb's support capability (40 percent GC).

3) Terminal double stance begins with floor contact by the other foot (**contralateral** initial contact) and continues until the original stance limb is lifted for swing (**ipsilateral** toe-off) (10 percent GC). The term "terminal double-limb support" has been avoided because weight bearing is asymmetrical.

Stride is the equivalent of a full gait cycle. The duration of a stride is the interval between two sequential initial floor contacts by the same limb. Stride length and cadence are the basic determinants of gait velocity. Of the two, stride length is the stronger factor. Stride length averages 1.5 meters in normal adults. Step refers to the timing between the two limbs. The interval between an initial contact by each foot is a step. When gait is symmetric, **step length** is 50 percent of stride length; when gait is asymmetric, the right and left step will differ, but right and left stride lengths will be identical. Step width is the distance between the foot contact of the left and right foot (Figure 19.2).

Gait and Balance Changes in Older Adults

Physical changes associated with aging directly affect an older adult's ability to maintain postural stability and normal gait mechanics. Normal functioning depends on free, passive joint mobility, appropriate timing and intensity of muscle action, and normal sensory input (Perry, 1987). Aging can lead to several physical changes that affect these basic pro- cesses: 1) stiffening of connective tissue; 2) decreased muscle strength; 3) prolonged reaction times; 4) decreased visual acuity; 5) impaired vibratory and proprioceptive sensation, and 6) increased postural sway (Trueblood & Rubenstein, 1990).

There is a close relationship between gait, balance and muscular tissue. This relationship is especially important because much can be done to retard and even reverse age-related changes in muscle tissue. It is commonly known that muscle mass, muscle strength and muscle contractility decline with advancing age (Klitgaard et al., 1990). Cross-sectional and longitudinal studies have found that muscle strength is directly associated with gait velocity (Fiatarone et al., 1990). Spirduso (1995) offers the following explanations for the preference by the older adult toward a reduced gait velocity: 1) endurance of weaker muscles in the lower limbs is maximized with the use of shorter strides, and the energy cost of walking is minimized; 2) less flexible ankle and knee joints constrain the stride length. Muscle strength also is associated with measures of static and dynamic balance (Judge et al., 1995). Studenski & Rigler (1996) add that gait stability relies upon an adequate support structure that consists of the musculoskeletal elements responsible for the mechanical work of holding the body upright while in motion. Therefore, it is logical to assume that maintaining the normal function of muscle tissue via exercise will help an individual maintain a successful gait pattern.

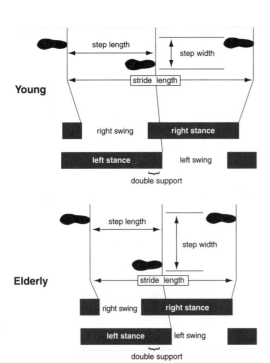

Young

Elderly

Adapted with permission from Chao, E.Y.S. (1986). Biomechanics of the Human Gait. In G.W. Schmid Schonbein, S.L.Y. Woo & B.W. Zweifach (Eds.) *Frontiers in Biomechanics* (p.226). New York: Springer-Verlag.

Figure 19.2

Age-related differences in step length, step width, period of double-support stance, and swing phases during walking

that the most common causes of falling are gait and balance disorders, weakness, arthritis, dizziness, environmental hazards, confusion, visual impairment and postural hypotension. Furthermore, the most important underlying risk factors for falls and injuries include some of these causes, as well as leg weakness, gait and balance instability, poor vision, cognitive and functional impairment, and sedating and psychoactive medications.

Approximately one-third of people older than 65 who live in the community fall each year (King & Tinetti, 1996). Major injuries, including head trauma, serious soft-tissue injuries, fractures and dislocations occur as a result of 5 percent to 15 percent of falls in any given year (Malmivaara et al., 1993). Seventy-five percent of serious fall injuries cause fractures (Nevitt et al., 1991). Specifically, fractures of the hip account for approximately 280,000 fall injuries per year in the U.S. in people older than 65. Two-thirds of these injuries occur in individuals 75 and older (Verfaillie et al., 1997).

Mechanisms of Falling

A fall occurs in the presence of two specific conditions. Maki and McIlroy (1996) state that there must be: 1) a **perturbation** (destabilizing force), and 2) a failure of the posture control system to compensate for the perturbation. Furthermore, they explain that in a small proportion of cases, a fall results when an internal physiologic perturbation momentarily disrupts the operation of the postural control system by interfering with perfusion of postural centers in the brain or brainstem (e.g., transient ischemic attacks, postural hypotension, cardiac arrhythmias or occlusion of vertebral arteries during neck movement), or by disrupting the sensorimotor systems (e.g., episode of dizziness or vertigo).

Maki and McIlroy (1996) continue their dissection of the mechanism of falling by explaining that there are two forms of external perturbation: mechanical and informational. Mechanical perturbations involve a change in the forces acting on the body that either displaces the center of gravity beyond the base of support (i.e., a push or collision) or prevents the BOS from being aligned beneath the COG (i.e., a slip or trip). Perturbations can be imposed by the environment (i.e., impact from a swinging

Aging, however, is still a factor regarding hip flexor power, as was suggested in a comparison study between a group of younger and older adults. The older adults were thought to be compensating for a reduction in ankle plantar flexor power by increasing hip flexor power. Therefore, it is possible that the reductions in ankle power found in several cross-sectional studies are responsible for at least part of the reduction in step length associated with advancing age (Judge et al., 1996).

Falling

The most severe consequences of poor balance are accidental falls that occur in connection with normal daily activities such as walking indoors or outside, climbing stairs, using the bathroom or changing posture (Era et al., 1997). Falling constitutes a significant risk to the health, function and independence of elderly people. Falls are particularly problematic in the nursing-home setting where their incidence is approximately three times greater than in community-based living. This is due in part to a higher degree of frailty (Rubenstein et al., 1996). The causes and risk factors associated with falls in nursing homes, however, are similar to those in community living. Rubenstein et al. (1996) state

door, a jostle from a crowd, standing in a moving vehicle) or may be self-induced, arising during volitional movements, such as walking, rising from a chair, bending over, reaching forward or pushing on a door. Informational perturbations change the nature of the orientation information available from the environment. This may create conflicts between the visual, vestibular and somatosensory input (e.g., moving visual fields that create an illusion of self-motion or carpets that distort proprioceptive information from the foot and ankle), or may change the quality of sensory input (e.g., dim lighting or glare that can interfere with visual input).

Characteristics of People who Fall

Individuals who are likely to fall or have a history of falling possess certain attributes. It is possible to identify older persons at risk of falling based on chronic age-associated and disease-related characteristics, acute illness and degree of mobility impairment (King & Tinetti, 1995). Risk factors for major injury or fracture have been identified in prospective cohort studies; however, they are not always consistent with other studies, due to differences in populations studied, risk factors examined and outcomes measured (King & Tinetti, 1996). In one study, for example, the risk of falling was predicted by slow hand-reaction time, decreased grip strength, previous fall with fracture and cognitive impairment (Nevitt, 1991). In another study, history of stroke or respiratory disorder and recent limitation in activity were used as predictable criteria (O'Loughlin et al., 1993).

In terms of certain physical characteristics, MacRae et al. (1992) identified incidents of falling due to unusually weak hip adductors, knee extensors, knee flexors and ankle dorsi-flexors. According to Lipsitz et al. (1991) people who fall tend to be those who take more steps to turn 360 degrees, who cannot rise from a chair without pushing off and who have difficulty determining their body position.

Fear of Falling

It has been reported by Tinetti et al. (1990) that some elderly persons develop symptoms or behaviors in response to a fall, regardless of physical trauma. Changes in gait cited as risk factors for falling may in fact be stabilizing adaptations related to fear of falling (Maki, 1997). Healthcare providers, family members and elderly persons all have acknowledged that in addition to loss of function due to physical trauma, psychological trauma may result from a self-imposed decline in activity and function not necessitated by physical disabilities or injury (Vellas et al., 1987). The older adult may express an enhanced or increased fear of falling that may result in deleterious emotional, psychological or social changes (Vellas et al., 1997).

Fear of falling also is associated with self-efficacy and confidence with regard to carrying out various ADL. Bandura (1986) refers to self-efficacy as an individual's perception of capabilities within a particular domain of activities. Older people's perception of their degree of ability and, more importantly, what they feel they cannot achieve, is instrumental in regulating their activity level. Depression also may be linked to the activity restriction, social withdrawal and loss of independence that often occur as a result of a fear of falling (Arfken et al., 1994).

Fear related to falling can manifest itself in artificial corrections in posture and gait. Spirduso (1995) states that due to an exagger-

Table 19.2

Client Information to Obtain from Medical Professionals

1) What health condition related to gait and balance does the client currently have?

2) What medications does the client take and how do they affect gait and balance?

3) Has the client ever fallen?

4) Does the client have any prosthetic joints or limbs?

5) What limitations are placed on the client's ability to participate in gait and balance training?

6) Has this person seen a physical therapist?

7) Should this person see a physical therapist?

ated fear of falling backward, the elderly may bias their posture so that if a fall occurs, they fall forward and break the fall with their arms. This flexed posture places a higher muscular load at the hips and knees, and shifts the base of support to the front of the feet over the toes. The main gait changes found to be associated with a fear of falling are increased double-support time and reduced stride length and velocity (Winter et al., 1990). Maki (1997) explains that the increase in double-support time is thought to increase gait stability by reducing the amount of time spent balancing on one leg. The slowing of the gait may have the benefit of allowing more time to react to obstacles or other changes in environment. It also may improve the probability of successful balance recovery in the event of loss of balance that results from reduced momentum of the body. The decreased stride length may promote stability by minimizing the forward excursion of the center of mass beyond the base of support provided by the stance foot.

Assessment of Gait and Balance

One of the key factors in the assessment of gait and balance is the progression of information gathering that takes place prior to any physical-performance tests. For every individual, there are a myriad of potential roadblocks that must first be identified (Welch, 1998). Because of the multifactorial nature of gait and balance disorders, it is necessary to acquire both a complete medical history and consent from a primary-care physician. A clear

diagnosis, precise medications, contraindications and information on whether the individual is prone to falling all should be obtained from the client's physician.

The Pre-exercise Interview

The pre-exercise interview is a simple, non-threatening way to acquire valuable information regarding an individual's history of physical activity. Likewise, present activities, goals and objectives, and likes and dislikes can be determined during the interview. Discussions of interests, hobbies, work regimen (professional as well as personal), involvement in the community, etc., can shed light on what an individual perceives they can successfully accomplish.

Begin the interview with a simple statement regarding the individual's ADL: Tell me about a typical week in your life (Welch, 1998). Follow with questions more specific to the work objective. For example, if a client included gardening within her typical week, you can assume she has the mobility to move about the yard successfully. However, to further scrutinize the information, a follow-up line of inquiry might be: 1) How often do you work in the garden? 2) How long do you spend in the garden at one time? 3) What kinds of foliage do you plant? 4) Do you ever get light-headed, dizzy or nauseated or have trouble with balance when standing after you've been planting? 5) What types of things do you lift when you're in the garden? 6) Have you ever stumbled or fallen?

Since mobility level can vary greatly in the elderly, answers to these types of questions based on other ADL scenarios can provide additional insight into your selection of the most

Table 19.3

Typical Activity Guidelines

- Total-body transitions: Support transitional movements, such as getting in and out of the car, bed, bath, chair and toilet, with personal assistance, or encourage the use of stabilizing objects, such as bars, walkers and quad canes.
- Ambulatory transitions: Provide assistance when moving from one floor

surface to another (e.g., carpet to hard floor, carpet to throw rug), and when stepping onto raised thresholds and stairs, or into narrow hallways.

- Pathway obstacles: Remove all obstacles from walking areas, including throw rugs, ottomans, pillows, toys, clothing, etc.

appropriate assessment tools. Information also may be elicited through questioning on why the individual stopped their usual activities, what aspects of the activity made them nervous or fearful, and what aspects of their performance had deteriorated (Berg & Norman, 1996). Similarly, description of a typical day in the life of a person who relies on a walker for safe ambulation generates information that would suggest a more basic assessment protocol. The point, however, is to identify the present level of mobility the individual possesses prior to engaging in physical activity.

Functional Assessment of Balance

In general, dynamic balance measures that assess the ability to maintain equilibrium in response to either self-motivated or external perturbation are superior to static tasks (Duncan et al., 1990). The following are assessment tools that address a wide variety of abilities. Each of the tests is adequate in determining functional ability. Though there is some degree of subjectivity, the tests are quantifiable so that measurements can be taken after a training period to identify improvement. Unfortunately, normative data has not yet been established to allow for comparison. However, Rikli and Jones (1997) are close to releasing such data.

Table 19.4 describes a field interpretation of the Functional Reach protocol (Duncan et al., 1990). In Table 19.5, Tinetti et al. (1986) offer an evaluation of balance that incorporates a series of challenges and a corresponding scoring system. Table 19.6 displays a measure of balance that was developed from a series of eight independent studies, collectively known as the FICSIT (Frailty and Injuries: Cooperative Studies of Intervention Techniques) (Buchner et al., 1993; Rossiter-Fornoff et al., 1995). Berg and Norman (1996) state that these tests were designed to examine the effect of diverse interventions in older adults with various ability, including active healthy individuals living in the community and disabled nursing home residents. Figure 19.3 is a test of stepping on and off objects of varying height (Williams & Greene, 1995). In addition to the timed component of this test, there are what the authors refer to as notable characteristics. These are

subjective evaluations that can further help to determine real-life function, issues of fear and areas of body weakness.

Table 19.7 is a series of dynamic balance tests that I developed to test the ability of establishing and maintaining rhythm or cadence, specifically without the use of a metronome. The SpeciFit Rhythm Series Tests challenge dynamic balance while testing the anticipatory timing component simultaneously. Successful completion of the maneuver suggests the ability to rhythmically correct for an anticipated weight shift.

Functional Assessment of Gait

Similar to maintaining balance in a standing position, gait involves the maintenance of upright posture and control over the projection of the center of gravity (Berg & Norman, 1996). Judge et al. (1996) explain that for an older person to feel safe while walking, periods of single-leg support cannot be perceived as dangerous. Stability while walking, during both single- and double-leg support, is enhanced by the ability to control the muscle movements at all lower-extremity joints. Furthermore, smooth progression and stability during walking are possible through power generation and absorption at all lower-extremity joints.

The first assessment of gait (see Figure 19.2) is to establish the individual's stride and step length, and step width. Have the individual walk on a dry surface immediately after placing the feet in a wet area. Measure distance according to foot patterns. Further assess gait with the evaluation by Tinetti et al. (1986) (Table 19.8). Gait speed is another test that is easy to perform. Have the individual walk as fast as possible for a specified distance, (6, 10 or 12 meters). Williams and Greene (1995) add a series of variations to the straight-line gait-speed evaluation. Figures 19.4, 19.5 and 19.6 display those variations.

Gait and Balance Training

There is mounting evidence that exercise training (strength, aerobic and balance exercise) can improve performance in individuals who demonstrate moderate gait and balance deficits. Likewise, research involving the very frail suggests exercise may delay fur-

Table 19.4
Functional Reach

1. Secure a yardstick to a wall horizontally at right acromion height.

2. The subject stands next to the wall with their right acromion aligned at beginning of yardstick.

3. With feet approximately shoulder-width apart, trace the subject's foot position to ensure identical foot placement for each trial.

4. Have the subject extend their right arm parallel to the yardstick with a clenched fist. Position one is measured at the third metacarpal.

5. Ask the subject to reach forward as far as possible without losing their balance or taking a step (which

represents position two), and again record the placement of the third metacarpal.

6. Do not allow the subject's upper extremity to contact the wall during this maneuver. If the subject touches the wall or takes a step during testing, repeat the trials.

7. Do not make any attempt to control the subject's method of reach.

8. Functional reach is defined as the mean difference between positions one and two after three trials.

9. Guard or spot subjects during the testing procedure to avoid loss of balance.

ther loss of function (Chandler & Hadley, 1996). In a study to test the effectiveness of a home-based exercise program, Campbell et al. (1997) concluded that strength and balance retraining exercises improved physical function and were effective in reducing falls in 116 women aged 80 years and older. Likewise, Shumway-Cook et al. (1997) reported that multidimensional exercise improved balance and mobility function in 105 community-dwelling older adults with a history of two or more falls within six months.

Sherrington and Lord (1994) discuss specificity as the focal point to skill acquisition, muscle strengthening and postural control, which makes it vital to selecting appropriate physical training strategies. Nugent et al. (1994) were successful in improving the gait in a group of stroke patients by utilizing a specific leg extensor exercise. Additionally, Chandler et al. (1998) concluded that while lower-extremity strength gain is associated with chair-rise performance, gait speed and stair climbing, there is no association with improved balance or endurance. The role of specificity

Table 19.5
Tinetti Balance Evaluation

Sitting Balance	Leans or slides in chair*	=0
	Steady, safe	=1
Rising	Unable without help	=0
	Able but uses arm to help	=1
	Able without use of arms	=2
Attempts to rise	Unable without help	=0
	Able but requires more than one attempt	=1
	Able to rise with one attempt	=2
Immediate standing balance (first 5 sec.)	Unsteady (staggers, moves feet, marked trunk sway)	=0
	Steady but uses walker or cane, or grabs other objects for support	=1
	Steady without walker, cane or other support	=2
Standing balance	Unsteady (staggers, moves feet, marked trunk sway)	=0
	Steady but wide stance (medial heels more than 5 in. apart)	=1
	Narrow stance without support	=2
Nudged (subject with feet close together; examiner pushes lightly on subject's sternum with palm of hand)	Begins to fall	=0
	Staggers, grabs, but catches self	=1
	Steady	=2
Eyes closed with feet close together	Unsteady	=0
	Steady	=1
Turning 360 degrees	Discontinuous steps	=0
	Continuous steps	=1
	Unsteady (grabs, staggers)	=0
	Steady	=1
Sitting down	Unsafe (misjudged distance, falls into chair)	=0
	Uses arms or not a smooth motion	=1
	Safe, smooth motion	=2

* Subject is seated in hard armless chair.
Maximum Balance Score is 16.

Table 19.6
The FICSIT

1) feet together
2) in stride stance (the heel of the front foot is ahead of the toe of the back foot)
3) with feet tandem (the heel of the front foot is placed at the toes of the rear foot)
4) standing on one leg

This four-item scale tests the subject for 10 seconds in one of three standing positions:
Record the best of three timed trials. Add additional challenge by repeating the four items while blindfolded.

training was further supported by the research of Verfaillie et al. (1997). They stated that older individuals can make significant gains in muscular strength and gait speed through resistance training, but that resistance training alone will not sufficiently improve balance and other gait parameters to significantly reduce risk factors for falls. Furthermore, to maximize the likelihood of reducing these risk factors, balance and gait training should be included with resistance training programs for the elderly.

Balance-training Techniques

To train clients for better balance, first determine the appropriate level of challenge. It is always wise to err on the conservative side by selecting an exercise for which the level of confidence is high for both the trainer and trainee.

One-legged balance

Support is optional. Switch legs after 10 to 15 seconds; repeat for three to five sets.

Level 1
- Subject stands on one leg.

Level 2
- Subject stands on one leg on a mini-trampoline.

Level 3
- Subject stands on one leg on a mini-trampoline and gently rebounds without breaking contact with the trampoline bed.

Level 4
- Subject stands on one leg and attempts to balance on a wobble board.

Level 5
- Standing on one leg, the subject intentionally rocks the board laterally. Repeat for anterior/posterior.

Level 6
- Divide the mini-trampoline with a line and have the subject hop over it laterally. Repeat for anterior/posterior.

Two-legged balance

Support is optional. Each work bout should last 15 to 30 seconds, followed by a rest period of the same length. Repeat for three to five sets.

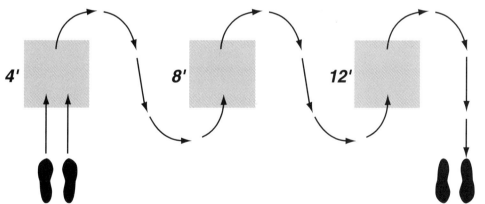

Figure 19.3

Stepping On and Off Objects

1. Subject stands in front of object with both feet together. On signal, the subject steps onto the first object and places both feet together.
2. Objects should be stable, square blocks of graduating height (e.g., 4 inches, 8 inches and 12 inches).
3. The subject steps down from the first object and places both feet together.
4. The subject immediately continues to the next two objects in turn, and repeats task.

5. Score is an average of three timed trials.

Process characteristics:
- Steps on or off objects with assistance.
- Trunk is erect when stepping on or off object.
- Easily maintains balance when stepping on and off objects.
- Moves from object to object easily and continuously.

Table 19.7
The Rhythm (Cadence) Test

1. This test requires a proprioception board, also known as a wobble board. The disc generally is about 12 inches in diameter with two 1-inch knobs or balls fastened to the bottom that allow it to tip anteriorly/posteriorly and laterally.

2. To test laterally, the subject stands on the board in ready position with body weight shifted to one side. On "go," the subject begins to shift body weight side to side, attempting to sustain the movement in a rhythmic motion. The subject may hold on to a support device; this would be noted as a process characteristic. Speed is not important and, in fact, should be discouraged. A slow cadence at about one sequence (a sequence equals a right and left touch) per second is recommended as a target.

3. Calculate the subject's score by counting the touches of one side of the board that are made in a rhythmic sequence, up to 20 touches, and take the best of three trials.

4. Test anterior/posterior rhythm by turning the board 90 degrees and repeating steps one through three.

5. Repeat steps one through four for the single-leg test.

Level 1
- Subject attempts to balance on a wobble board with one 1-inch knob (as opposed to two) in the middle of the bottom of the board.

Level 2
- Standing on a rocker board, subject shifts body weight side to side. Repeat for anterior/posterior.

Level 3
- Divide the mini-trampoline with a line and have the subject attempt to hop over it laterally. Repeat for anterior/posterior.

Hip and Torso Stabilization

Level 1
- Subject sits on a chair with upright back support and both feet on floor.
- Subject leans against back support, holds arms out to sides and extends one leg straight out.
- Have client alternate leg lifts for a count of seven to 10 repetitions.

Table 19.8
Tinetti Gait Evaluation

Initiation of gait after told to "go"*	Any hesitancy or multiple attempts to start	=0
	No hesitancy	=1
Step length and height	a) Right swing foot	
	Does not pass left stance foot	=0
	Passes left stance foot with step	=1
	Right foot does not clear floor completely with step	=0
	Right foot completely clears floor	=1
	b) Left swing foot	
	Does not pass right stance foot	=0
	Passes right stance foot with step	=1
	Left foot does not clear floor completely with step	=0
	Left foot completely clears floor	=1
Step symmetry	Right and left step length not equal (estimate)	=0
	Right and left step appear equal	=1
Step continuity	Stopping or discontinuity between steps	=0
	Steps appear continuous	=1
Path**	Marked deviation	=0
	Mild/moderate deviation or uses walking aid	=1
	Straight without walking aid	=2
Trunk	Marked sway or uses walking aid	=0
	No sway but flexion of knees or back, or spreads arms while walking	=1
	No sway, no flexion, no use of arms and no use of walking aid	=2
Walk stance	Heels apart	=0
	Heels almost touching while walking	=1

*Subject stands with examiner, walks down hallway or across room, first at their usual pace, then back at rapid but safe pace (using usual walking aid such as a cane or walker).
**Estimate path in relation to floor tiles. Observe excursion of one foot over about 10 feet of the course.
Maximum Gait Score is 12.

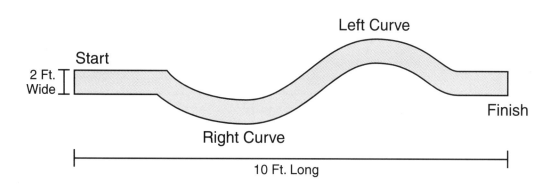

Figure 19.4

Body Agility with Wide Curve

1. On signal the subject walks as fast as possible through a curved pathway measuring 10 feet long and 2 feet wide.
2. Record the time; the score is the average of three trials.

Process Characteristics
- Steps are continuous.
- Arms swing while walking.
- Subject does not stop or slow down at curves.
- Length of right and left steps is equal.

- Wait for subject to recover, then repeat sequence for two to three sets.

Level 2
- Repeat level-1 sequence without back support.

Level 3
- Repeat level-1 sequence with a peanut-shaped physio-roll ball.

Level 4
- Repeat level-1 sequence with a stability ball.

Strength-training Techniques

Lower-extremity Strength (squats)
Support device is optional.

Level 1
- Subject sits in a chair, then stands and sits repeatedly for three to five repetitions.
- Recover and repeat for two to three sets.

Level 2
- Repeat level-1 sequence and increase to five to seven repetitions.

Level 3
- Repeat level-1 sequence holding two- to five-pound dumbbells in each hand.

Level 4
- Repeat level-3 sequence and increase to five to seven repetitions.

Lower-extremity Strength (heel lifts)

Level 1
- Subject faces a wall at arm's length away.
- With arms outstretched and body leaning slightly against the wall, the subject raises their heels and transfers total body weight to the balls of the feet for three to five repetitions.
- Recover and repeat for two to three sets.

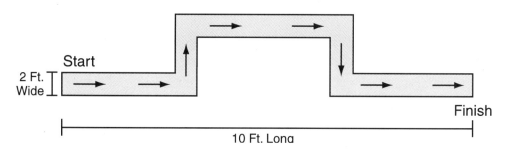

Figure 19.5

Body Agility with Two Changes of Direction

1. On signal the subject walks as fast as possible through a path with two sharp angles.
2. Record the time; the score is the average of three trials.

Process Characteristics
- Subject has difficulty turning corners.
- Subject stops or slows down to adjust for corners.
- Step length is equal and continuous.
- Subject uses cane or walker.

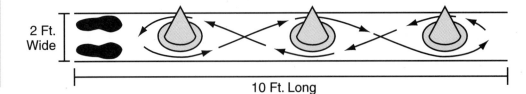

Figure 19.6

Body Agility/Moving around Objects

1. Three 2-foot-high cones are placed at equal distances over a 10-foot-long, 2-foot-wide path.
2. On signal the subject walks as fast as possible through the pathway and around the cones. The subject returns to the starting point by traversing the path in reverse, utilizing the cones.
3. Record the time; the score is the average of three trials.

Process Characteristics
* Subject moves easily around cones.
* Length of step is equal throughout trial.
* Subject stops or slows down to maneuver around cones.
* Subject walks close to cones.
* Subject looks at feet.

Level 2
* Repeat level-1 sequence and increase to five to seven repetitions.

Level 3
* Repeat level-1 sequence and increase to seven to ten repetitions.

Level 4
* Repeat level-1 sequence using only one leg and continue progress as detailed in levels 2 and 3.

Pelvic Girdle Stabilization and Hip Strength
(multi-hip machine)

Level 1
* Subject performs hip flexion, hip extension, hip adduction and hip abduction.
* Use lightest possible weight to surpass learning curve.
* Increase number of repetitions over a 12-week period from three to five, to five to seven, to seven to 10.
* Do not allow individuals with hip replacements to cross the midline of the body when adducting.
* Levels 2 and higher should be based on each individual.

Gait-training Techniques

Treadmill

The treadmill is one of the most beneficial training devices available for gait training. All variables can be manipulated and controlled to keep the individual safe at all times. Cardiovascular benefits also may be realized.

Recommendations:
* Subjects probably will experience a lack of stability in the early stages of treadmill work. Holding the handrails helps alleviate this problem.
* As soon as possible, encourage the individual to let go of the handrails. Progress to this by encouraging the client to hold on with one hand for 10 seconds, then return to two hands.
* Monitor activity with a wireless heart monitor, modified rate of perceived exertion (RPE) scale and weak link index (WLI) scale.
* At the conclusion of treadmill activity, have the subject hold handrails for 30 seconds with the treadmill stopped. Have the subject continue to hold the handrails when stepping off the machine.

Spotting

It is imperative that close spotting techniques be practiced when working with an individual affected by problems of gait and balance. All testing and exercise protocols for gait and balance should not be carried out unless you are experienced in effective spotting. Some individuals will need more attention than others. However, the fact that they have a gait and/or balance disorder suggests they might need assistance without warning, regardless of their level of function.

The spotting techniques utilized may vary from person to person, depending on their individual health issues. Sometimes a hand on the back at the waist will suffice because it reminds the client that you are there. Others may require support provided by holding a hand or arm. Some individuals may feel invalidated by their need for you to provide assistance in order for them to complete the evaluation. However, safety is more important and spotting can easily be noted in the process characteristics.

Communication also is an effective spotting technique. Frequent, reassuring comments can help alleviate apprehension and motivate the individual to new levels. Creating positive yet accurate perceptions of the work accomplished may even stimulate the individual's own self-efficacy.

Guidelines from the Physician

For gait and balance disorders, guidelines from a physician and/or physical therapist must be specific to the etiology and are, therefore, too difficult to place in a categorical list. A cane or walker, which does nothing to further gait and balance training, would most likely be prescribed. See Table 19.2 for information to obtain from the client's physician.

Conclusion

Gait and balance training is a vital link to maintaining autonomy for many individuals. It is not difficult to see that a loss of mobility would curtail even the simplest ADL. The problem, however, is that disorders of gait and balance are multifactorial. A variety of diseases can lead to gait and balance anomalies as can frailty, medication, fear or any combination thereof. Nevertheless, training the components of gait and balance will always be a prudent endeavor. This is because physical conditioning brings positive physiological changes to the individual even if gait and balance are only affected minimally. Therefore, it is wise to become knowledgeable in gait and balance program design in order to provide a more complete wellness offering to a rapidly growing population.

The Weak-link Index (Welch, 1998)

The weak-link index (WLI) is a subjective evaluation based on the same zero-to-10 scale used in the revised rating of perceived exertion (RPE) scale (Borg, 1998). The weak-link index is valuable because it directly addresses the issue of pain in specific body areas during an assessment or work session. For instance, a person on the treadmill may be walking at a comfortable pace but begin to experience slight discomfort in the left knee. This could be unimportant, or it could be a precursor to a more serious injury. Unless you ask, you may never know until it's too late. Your inquiry should be specific to any level of pain or discomfort in a particular area of the body, not general fatigue. The pain may be good reason for curtailing the activity even though the individual reports a low RPE value. Perceived exertion and perceived pain are different sensations and can be clearly delineated with the addition of the WLI scale. You are responsible for the well-being of your clients. If you do not monitor areas of discomfort, you will not be able to truly evaluate an individual's performance, and you will not be able to design the most effective exercise program.

Ask the following questions approximately every one to two minutes: 1) Is there any part of your body where you feel discomfort? 2) If so, where is the pain and how would you rate it on a scale from zero to 10 if zero means no discomfort at all and 10 indicates maximal pain? The individual should not be allowed to continue if the discomfort level is above two or three. Be sure to note when the test or work bout ended. Wait 24 to 48 hours, applying ice for 15 to 20 minutes every two to four hours, then ask the client if the pain is still present. It may have subsided after discontinuing the exercise, yet may return later in the form of soreness and/or point tenderness in the affected area. If pain is still present, wait another 24 hours. If the client is still experiencing pain, referral to a physician would be appropriate.

If the pain does not return, attempt the exercise again at a reduced intensity, i.e., slower pace, less elevation, more gradual ascent, etc. Do not exceed the length of the previous test in which discomfort was first discovered, regardless of whether the client experiences pain. Curtail the exercise at or before the previous work duration and note the successful parameters (i.e., time, distance, pace, elevation). Repeat this work four to six times before increasing the workload.

References

Arfken, C.L., Lach, H.W., Birge, S.J., et al. (1994). The prevalence and correlates of fear of falling in elderly persons living in the community. *American Journal of Public Health,* 84, 565-570.

Bandura, A. (1986). *Social Ffoundations of Thought and Action: A Social Cognitive Theory.* Englewood Cliffs, N.J.: Prentice Hall.

Berg, K. & Norman, K.E. (1996). Functional assessment of gait and balance. *Clinics in Geriatric Medicine,* 12, 4, 705-723.

Black, S.E., Maki, B.E. & Fernie, G.R. (1993). Aging, imbalance and falls. In *Vestibulo-ocular Reflex, Nystagmus and Vertigo.* New York: Raven Press.

Bloem, B.R., Haan, J., Lagaay, A.M., et al. (1992). Investigation of gait in elderly subjects over 88 years of age. *Journal of Geriatric Psychiatry and Neurology,* 5, 78-84.

Bohannon, R.W. (1997). Comfortable and maximum walking speed of adults 20-79 years: Reference values and determinants. *Age and Aging,* 26, 15-19.

Borg, G.B. (1982). Psychological basis of perceived exertion. *Medicine & Science in Sports & Exercise,* 14, 377-381.

Brocklehurst, J.C., Robertson, D. & James-Groom, P. (1982). Clinical correlates of sway in old age: Sensory modalities. *Age and Aging,* 11, 1-10.

Buchner, D.M., Hornbrook, M.C., Kutner, N.G., et al. (1993). *Journal of the American Geriatric Society,* 41, 297.

Camicioli, R., Panzer, V.P. & Kaye, J. (1997). Balance in the elderly. *Archives of Neurology,* 54, 976-981.

Campbell, A.J., Robertson, M.C., Gardner, M.M., Norton, R.N., Tilyard, M.W. & Buchner, D.M. (1997). Randomized controlled trial of a general practice program of home based exercise to prevent falls in elderly women. *British Medical Journal,* 25, 315, (7115), 1065-1069.

Chandler, J.M. & Hadley, E.C. (1996). Exercise to improve physiologic and functional performance in old age. *Clinics in Geriatric Medicine,* 12, 4, 761-784.

Duncan, P.W., Wiener, D.K., Chandler, J. & Studenski, S. (1990). Functional reach: A new clinical measure of balance. *Journal of Gerontology: Medical Sciences,* 45, 6, M192-197.

Era, P., Avlund, K., Jokela, J., Gause-Nilsson, I., Heikkinen, E., Steen, B. & Schroll, M. (1997). Postural balance and self-reported functional ability in 75-year-old men and women: A cross-national comparative study. *Journal of the American Geriatrics Society,* 45, 1, 21-29.

Fiatarone, M.A., Marks, E.C., Ryan, N.D., et al., (1990). High-intensity strength training in nonagenarians: Effects on skeletal muscle. *Journal of the American Medical Association,* 263, 3029-3034.

Judge, J.O., Ounpuu, S. & Davis, R.B. (1996). Effects of age on the biomechanics and physiology of gait. *Clinics in Geriatric Medicine,* 12, 4, 659-677.

King, M.B. & Tinetti, M.E. (1995). Falls in community-dwelling older persons. *Journal of the American Geriatric Society,* 43, 1146.

King, M.B. & Tinetti, M.E. (1996). A multifactorial approach to reducing injurious falls. *Clinics in Geriatric Medicine,* 12, 4, 745-759.

Klitgaard, H., Monatoni, M., Schiaffino, S., et al. (1990). Functional, morphology and protein expression of aging skeletal muscle: A cross-sectional study of elderly men with different training backgrounds. *Acta Physiol Scand,* 140, 42-54.

Kokmen, E., Bossemeyer, R.W. & Williams, W.J. (1978). Quantitative evaluation of joint motion sensation in an aging population. *Journal of Gerontology,* 33, 62-67.

Lipsitz, L.A., Jonsson, P.V., Kelley, M.M. & Koestner, J.S. (1991). Causes and correlates of recurrent falls in ambulatory frail elderly. *Journal of Gerontology: Medical Sciences,* 46, M114-M122.

Lucy, S.D. & Hayes, K.C. (1985). Postural sway profiles: Normal subjects and subjects with cerebellar ataxia. *Physiotherapy Canada,* 37, 140-148.

MacRae, P.G., Lacourse, M. & Moldavon, R. (1992). Physical performance measures that predict faller status in community-dwelling older adults. *Journal of Occupational and Sports Physical Therapy,* 16, 123-128.

Maki, B.E. (1997). Gait changes in older adults: Predictors of falls or indicators of fear. *Journal of the American Geriatrics Society,* 45, 313-320.

Maki, B.E. & McIlroy, W.E. (1996). Postural control in the older adult. *Clinics In Geriatric Medicine,* 12, 4, 635-656.

Malmivaara, A., Heliovaara, M., Knekt, P., et al. (1993). Risk factors for injurious falls leading to hospitalization or death in a cohort of 19,500 adults. *American Journal of Epidemiology,* 138, 384.

Nevitt, M.C., Cummings, S.R. & Hudes, E.S. (1991). Risk factors for injurious falls: A prospective study. *Journal of Gerontology: Medical Sciences,* 46, M164-M170.

Nugent, J.A., Schurr, K.A. & Adams, R.D., A dose-response relationship between amount of weight-bearing exercise and walking outcome following cerebrovascular accident. *Archives of Physical Medicine and Rehabilitation,* 75, 399-402.

Nutt, J.D., Marsden, C.D. & Thompson, P.D. (1993). Human walking and higher-level gait disorders, particularly in the elderly. *Neurology,* 43, 268-279.

O'Loughlin, J.L., Robitaille, Y., Boivin, J., et al. (1993). Incidence of and risk factors for falls and injurious falls among the community-dwelling elderly. *American Journal of Epidemiology,* 137, 342.

Patla, A. & Winter, D. (1990). Assessment of balance control in the elderly: Major issues. *Physiotherapy Canada,* 42, 89.

Perry, J. (1992). Gait analysis. *Normal and Pathological Function.* New Jersey: Slack.

Perry, J. (1987). Gait characteristics. *Therapeutic Considerations for the Elderly.* New York: Churchill Livingstone.

Rikli, R.E. & Jones, J.C., (1997). Assessing physical performance in "independent" older adults: Issues and guidelines. *Journal of Aging and Physical Activity,* 5, 244-261.

Rosenhall, U., Rubin, W. (1975). Degenerative changes in the human vestibular sensory epithelia. *Acta Otolaryngologica,* 79, 67-81.

Rossiter-Fornoff, J.E., Wolf, S.L., Wolfson, S.L., et al. (1995). Cross-sectional validation study of the

FICSIT common data base static balance measures. *Journal of Gerontology,* 50a, M291.

Rubenstein, L.Z., Josephson, K.R. & Osterweil, D. (1996). Falls and fall prevention in the nursing home. *Clinics in Geriatric Medicine,* 12, 4, 881-902.

Sekuler, R. & Hartman, L.P. (1980). Spatial vision and aging. *Journal of Gerontology,* 35, 692.

Sherlock, J. (1996). Getting into balance. *Physical Therapy,* Dec/Jan, 33-36.

Sherrington, C. & Lord, S.R., (1997). Home exercise to improve strength and walking velocity after hip fracture: A randomized controlled trial. *Archives of Physical Medicine and Rehabilitation,* 78, 208-212.

Shumway-Cook, A., Gruber, W., Baldwin, M. & Liao, S. (1997). The effect of multidimensional exercise on balance, mobility, and fall risk in community-dwelling older adults. *Physical Therapy,* 77,1, 46-57.

Spirduso, W.W. (1995). *Physical Dimensions of Aging.* Champaign, Ill.: Human Kinetics.

Studenski, S. & Rigler, S.K., (1996). Clinical overview of instability in the elderly. *Clinics in Geriatric Medicine,* 12, 4, 679-688.

Tinetti, M.E., Richman, D. & Powell, L. (1990). Falls efficacy as a measure of fear of falling. *Journal of Gerontology: Psychological Sciences,* 45, P239-P243.

Tinetti, M.E., Williams, T.F. & Mayewski, R. (1986).

Fall risk index for elderly patients based on number of chronic disabilities. *American Journal of Medicine,* 80, 429-434.

Tinetti, M.F., Speechly, M. & Ginter, S. (1988). Risk factors for falls among elderly patients living in the community. *New England Journal of Medicine,* 319, 1701-7.

Trueblood, P.R. & Rubenstein, L.Z. (1991). Assessment of instability and gait in elderly persons. *Comprehensive Therapy,* 17, 8, 20-29.

Vellas, B., Cayla, F., Bocquet, H., dePemille, E. & Albarede, J.L. (1987). Prospective study of activity in old people after falls. *Age and Aging,* 16, 189-193.

Vellas, B., Wayne, S.J., Romero, L.J., Baumgartner, R.N. & Garry, P.J. (1997). Fear of falling and re-striction of mobility in elderly fallers. *Age and Aging,* 26, 189-193.

Verfaillie, D.F., Nichols, J.F., Turkel, E. & Hovell, M.F. (1997). Effects of resistance, balance and gait training on reduction of risk factors leading to falls in elders. *Journal of Aging and Physical Activity,* 5, 213-228.

Verrillo, R.T. & Verrillo, V. (1985). *Aging and Human Performance.* New York: John Wiley & Sons.

Welch, G.L., (1998). Pre-exercise screening and assessment. In *Exercise for Older Adults.* Champaign, Ill.: Human Kinetics.

Winter, D., Patla, A., Frank, J. et al. (1990). Biomechanical walking pattern changes in the fit and healthy elderly. *Physical Therapy,* 71, 340-347.

CHAPTER 20

Selected Neuromuscular Disorders

MARY JO KORN

Mary Jo Korn, P.T., M.B.A., is vice president of business development for Edgewater Rehabilitation Associates Inc. (ERA). ERA is a private practice of 250-plus physical, occupational and speech therapists, alternative medical providers, and fitness specialists. First Fitness Personal Training Inc. (FFPT) is ERA's fitness division, providing personal and corporate fitness programs nationally. Korn earned a B.S. from Northern Illinois University, a certificate in physical therapy from Northwestern University, and an M.B.A. from Loyola University, and completed certificate course work in the Hospital and Health Service Management program at Northwestern University's Kellogg School of Management. She has more than 20 years' experience as a physical therapist and healthcare administrator.

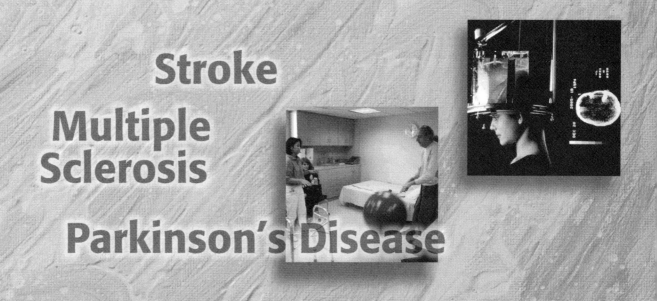

Stroke
Multiple Sclerosis
Parkinson's Disease

PART 1: NEUROANATOMY, PATHOPHYSIOLOGY AND MOVEMENT DISORDERS

The neuromuscular system combines sensory integration and movement. This collaboration permits function — the ability to respond to the world around us in a continuous symphony of desires, thoughts and actions.

The term "neuromuscular disorder" refers to a variety of sensory and/or movement deficits resulting from a nervous system disease or injury that impairs an individual's ability to perceive environmental change and to respond voluntarily or involuntarily.

The nervous system works much like a computer, transmitting and analyzing information. Its ability to produce results is a team effort of the human system: body, mind and spirit. The nervous system is composed of two related parts, the central and peripheral nervous systems. The central nervous system comprises the brain and the spinal cord, and the peripheral nervous system comprises the cranial and spinal nerves. Understanding basic neuroanatomy is important because the site affected by the disease or disorder specifically relates to the neuromuscular symptoms affecting your client.

Currently, damage to the central nervous system is permanent, meaning the damaged tissue does not recover or regenerate. However, the human machine is remarkably adaptive and permanent damage often does not grossly impair function. In addition, research is being done to discover means to reverse damage to the central nervous system. New antibodies are being developed and tested in rats that allow for spinal cord tissue **regeneration** (*PT Bulletin,* May 29, 1998). Damage to the peripheral nervous system, by contrast, is repairable via nerve regeneration, although the healing process is not always absolute.

When working with a post-rehab client you should be able to identify neuromuscular disorders, be aware of their effect and make accommodations to the fitness program. Working collaboratively with members of the clinical healthcare team will result in the best combination of knowledge and skill on the client's behalf.

This chapter explains the pathophysiology of neuromuscular disorders, how to recognize movement deficits and other functional implications, and how to adapt fitness programs for clients affected by these disorders. Key disorders, including stroke, traumatic brain injury, multiple sclerosis, Parkinson's Disease and spinal cord injury are reviewed. Even the most impaired client will benefit from organized physical activity, motivation, personal attention and participation in fitness programs (Florance & Hagberg, 1984). It is not the client's deficits, but rather how they adapt, that truly maximizes their life's potential.

The Central Nervous System

The brain is divided into three parts: the cerebrum or cortex, the cerebellum and the brainstem. Each part has distinct but interdependent functions.

The cerebrum is responsible for cognitive and sensory functions and gross movement. Lesions of the cerebrum may result in a loss of voluntary movement, increased muscle tone (**spasticity**) and pathological reflexes, as seen following a stroke (**cerebral vascular accident**). The cerebrum is divided into two halves, the right and left hemispheres. The right hemisphere is responsible for sustaining or controlling movement and posture, while the left hemisphere is responsible for planning or sequencing movement (O'Sullivan & Schmitz, 1994).

The cerebellum coordinates movement. Disorders in the cerebellum usually result in **ataxia**, a disturbance of balance and equilibrium, as seen in multiple sclerosis.

The brainstem, more primitive than the cerebrum, subtly affects movement. Brainstem disorders usually result in **tremors** and **rigidity** as seen in Parkinson's disease, or in athetoid or choreic movements as seen in cerebral palsy.

The spinal cord is the nervous system's primary relay station, allowing messages to travel between the brain's central control and the trunk and extremities. Injury to the spinal cord can result in complete or **flaccid paralysis** (an absence of muscle tone), a loss of the sense of touch, disruption of proprioception or kinesthetic sense (awareness of position and movement), and visceral dysfunction, such as bowel and bladder incontinence.

The Peripheral Nervous System

Peripheral nerves are made of motor and sensory fibers and serve as the body's messengers. Motor fibers are either somatic (terminating in skeletal muscles) or autonomic (innervating the organs or glands). Sensory fibers carry messages from peripheral receptors such as muscle spindles (monitoring muscle length), Golgi tendon organs (monitoring muscle tension) and nociceptors (responding to noxious stimuli), and allow the perception of pain.

Cranial nerves are in part responsible for the senses of sight, hearing, taste and balance (vestibular system); the ability to chew, speak and swallow; facial expression; and vital functions such as breathing, cardiac output and digestion. The vestibular system coordinates reflexes of the eyes, neck and body for maintaining balance (equilibrium) in accordance with posture and movement of the head (Manter & Gatz, 1975).

Spinal nerves are related to in specific trunk or extremity regions, and are responsible for movement, the sense of touch and nutrition of the overlying tissue (skin). Disruption to a spinal nerve causes the following symptoms:

flaccid paralysis (loss of muscle tone); loss of light touch and deep pressure; and trophic or nutritional changes to the tissue. The analgesic area of the skin becomes dry and inelastic, and it ceases to sweat. In contrast to central nerve damage, adhesive and fibrous changes to the affected tendons, joints and muscles following a peripheral nerve injury result from lack of movement and can be prevented with massage and range of motion (Bannister, 1973).

In summary, disease or injury to the neuromuscular system can result in impairment of the following (*APTA, 1997*):
- ➤ affect or emotion
- ➤ arousal or attention
- ➤ balance and coordination
- ➤ autonomic function (involuntary visceral response)
- ➤ cognitive function (thoughts, memory, judgment, learning)
- ➤ expressive or receptive communication
- ➤ motor (movement) control and motor learning
- ➤ sensory integration (awareness and response)
- ➤ function of skeletal, respiratory, digestive and cardiac systems

Movement Disorders

Before delving into the specifics of key neuromuscular disorders, a general review of more typical movement deficits caused by disease or injury to the nervous system is necessary. Don't lose sight of the fact that cognitive and sensory deficits also are commonly associated with movement disorders and often complicate the clinical picture.

Muscle Tone Abnormalities

Muscle tone is governed by the muscle spindle, a receptor in the muscle that responds to stretch. The stretch response is relayed to the spinal cord, which returns a message to the muscle spindle, thereby affecting muscle length. This spinal reflex is influenced by higher levels of the nervous system such as the brainstem, cerebellum and cerebrum. Disruption of the spinal reflex and/or its higher levels of control results in a change in muscle tone.

Flaccid paralysis or hypotonia is the loss of, or decrease in, muscle tone that results from destruction of the spinal cord or the spinal nerve itself. Both voluntary movement and reflex response are lost. Within weeks the muscle begins to atrophy or waste, eventually leaving only connective tissue. This atrophy is much more pronounced than that caused by inactivity (such as when an extremity is casted to treat a bone fracture). In the case of nerve damage, loss of the motor neuron disrupts the trophic or nutritional status of the muscle fibers, which leads to their eventual wasting (Gatz, 1970).

Spasticity (hypertonia) is the increase in muscle tone, resulting from the loss of the brain's inhibition of the basic stretch reflex. The spinal cord is organized into nerve trunks (bundles) or tracks. The corticospinal track is responsible for carrying brain control messages to the nerves via the spinal cord. The track crosses as it enters/exits the brain. Damage on the right side of the brain elicits paralysis on the opposite or left side of the body and vice versa. The damage may be the result of an injury or trauma (crushing or penetrating), a tumor (compression), or a vascular accident (loss of blood supply or a stroke). Spasticity can be seen in clients with a stroke, cerebral palsy, multiple sclerosis, spinal cord injury and traumatic brain injury (TBI).

Spasticity is a resistance to passive or voluntary movement. As the muscle is stretched, resistance is strong initially and then eventually gives way. A quick stretch of a spastic muscle results in **clonus** or a sustained series of rhythmic jerks (Gatz, 1970). Spasticity usually occurs in a synergistic pattern. Synergistic patterns are named for the dominant muscle groups involved, either flexor or extensor synergy. Flexor synergy most commonly occurs in the upper extremity, and extensor synergy most commonly occurs in the lower extremity. Any movement or stress — even a sneeze — can elicit a spastic response in the involved muscles.

Spastic paralysis is a lack of movement. The joint or extremity is fixed in one dominant position. Occasionally some voluntary effort can elicit movement in a spastic joint, but the result is most likely incomplete. Great effort is required to produce functional movement. Often persons with a spastic extremity use their limb as only a gross assist to movement as they lack the motor control needed for more refined use. Medical treatment of spasticity ranges from pharmaceuticals, and nerve and motor point blocks, to intermuscular injections such as botulinum toxin (BTX) (Spedinoff & Cava, April 1995). Surgical interventions include tenotomy and tendon transfers. In addition, the science of therapeutic exercise is designed to decrease spasticity and elicit functional movement.

Cerebellar Dysfunction

Disease or injury to the cerebellum interferes with its control of voluntary movement. Movement is still possible and no paralysis occurs, but the quality of movement is impaired. The muscle groups are not able to work together in a coordinated fashion.

Ataxia, or lack of coordination, affects balance, especially during walking. An ataxic gait often is mistaken for a drunken stumble. Individuals suffering from ataxia find it challenging to walk in a straight line. Their arms or legs appear uncoordinated as they attempt purposeful movement. You can differentiate the balance disturbances associated with ataxia from those caused by a disorder of the proprioceptive nervous system by asking the client to close their eyes during a dynamic task. If the disorder worsens, there likely is a proprioceptive dysfunction. Closing the eyes has little or no effect on ataxia.

Dysmetria is an inability to stop a movement. During movement, individuals will overshoot the goal and look clumsy. For instance, asking a client with dysmetria to point at their nose may result in an accidental poke in the eye.

Dysdiadochokinesia or **adiodochokinesia** are impressive words for the inability to smoothly reciprocate movement. The typical test involves asking a person to hold their hands in front of their trunk and then to repeatedly pronate and supinate their forearms. As the speed of movement increases, their lack of coordination will be evident.

Cerebellar lesions can also cause hypotonia (a decrease in muscle tone but not flaccid paralysis);

Table 20.1
Client Information to Obtain from Medical Professionals

Questions To Ask	Examples of Conditions for Concern or Program Restriction
Are there any movement restrictions?	**CVA:** shoulder may be subluxed restricting range of motion
	CVA: client may suffer from orthostatic hypotension
	PD: poor postural control may significantly increase risk of falling
	SCI: unstable spine may preclude spinal movements or stress positions
Are there weight-bearing restrictions?	**SCI:** osteoporosis may make standing contraindicated
Are there exercise restrictions?	**CVA:** vascular status may limit exertion parameters (heart rate, blood pressure)
	MS or Post Polio: fatigue contraindicated
	TBI or Epilepsy: seizure precautions may prevent work at maximal level
Are there skin or sensory deficits that need to be considered?	**CVA:** may lack sensation of touch, awareness, etc.
	CVA, PD or MS: balance may be impaired
	SCI or CVA: pressure sore may be present
Are there cognitive deficits?	may lack learning or judgment skills
Are there any other recommendations for exercise guidelines?	**CVA or MS:** increased spasticity or cognitive difficulties
	PD: increased rigidity or tremor

asthenia, or weak, easily fatigued muscles; and intentional tremors that are evident during movement and absent at rest. Intentional tremors usually affect the head and upper extremities. Unlike cerebral injury and spasticity, lesions to the cerebellum are **ipsilateral**, meaning a lesion to the right side of the cerebellum elicits symptoms on the right side of the body.

Brainstem Dysfunction

Severe trauma or disease to the brainstem often results in severe, life-threatening disability, inhibiting participation in a fitness program. More subtle brainstem dysfunction typically results in movement disorders that are bothersome, but not totally debilitating, such as in Parkinson's disease.

Tremors from damage to the brainstem are defined as resting tremors because they occur during relaxation or rest and disappear or lessen with intentional movement. The most classic resting tremor is the pill-rolling tremor that is most often seen in clients with Parkinson's disease. The fingers and thumbs move alternately in a rhythmic pattern to mimic a pill-rolling movement.

Rigidity also commonly occurs in Parkinson's disease. Rigidity, like spasticity, manifests in increased muscle tone, but the response to stretch is different. Rigidity affects both the agonist and the antagonist muscle groups equally without synergistic patterns. A rigid muscle's response to stretch is to give way in incremental bouts, causing a cogwheel sensation. The muscle relaxes, allowing movement, and then, within a few degrees of motion, tightens again. This alternating **muscle tone** causes a jerky movement pattern, making it difficult to initiate movement. The client may seem stuck in a particular posture.

Chorea is an involuntary purposeless movement — usually quick, nonrhythmic and jerky. Facial grimaces are one example of choreiform movements (Chusid, 1976).

Athetosis results in movement that is slower and more writhing or worm-like in nature. In the extremities, athetosis involves more peripheral joints than proximal. Athetoid movements always are exaggerated by voluntary movements or other stress. They too diminish or disappear when at rest (Bannister, 1973).

Neuromuscular Disorders and the Training Program

Now that you have a basic understanding of neuroanatomy and neuromuscular dysfunction, let's relate what you have learned to specific disease or injury conditions. Then, you can begin to appreciate how fitness programs need to be adapted for clients with these disabilities.

The symptoms of neuromuscular disorders can be subtle, and the cause of those symptoms can be life-altering. Treating the involved body parts is best left to specialists, and coordinating your efforts with them is essential. Seek out individualized guidelines for fitness programs for your clients who have neuromuscular disorders. An ounce of prevention is always worth a pound of cure!

If your client has a neuromuscular disorder, functional retraining of the involved extremities is best left to the clinical rehabilitation team. Physical or occupational therapists have specialized training in therapeutic exercise techniques that use very specific movement patterns, as well as sensory feedback facilitators. Monitoring and managing a therapeutic exercise program is an art and a science. Many therapists go through years of additional training to perfect their skills and knowledge of therapeutic exercises.

If your client has recently completed a clinical rehabilitation program, confer with the therapists involved. Be sure you understand the principles behind the home exercise program they provide. If your client has not had clinical rehabilitation for some time, it may be necessary to arrange for a collaborative session with a therapist. In some states, the therapist will need a physician's referral. This is governed by the state's practice act for the specific discipline (physical or occupational therapy), as well as by what the third party payor (insurance companies and Medicare) demands as criteria for reimbursement. Most third party payors will pay for a therapist's visit if it is designed to establish or upgrade a home program. Your client always has the option of paying out of pocket for this service. The going rate for a home visit by a therapist ranges from

$100 to $150 per visit. Rates for visits that are paid for privately can be negotiated. Evaluate your client first, and have a general plan of how you would like to proceed. Then you can ask specific questions and get the therapist's input on adapting the program to maximize your client's potential. Of course, physician endorsement of your plan is always a good idea. Some physicians may set specific guidelines; others may want to know what guidelines you intend to follow and how your client's response to your program will be monitored.

General Pre-training Screening and Program Planning

Before working with any client with a neuromuscular disorder, ask their physician or therapist about their status. Routine preassessment questions and condition-specific concerns are addressed in Table 20.1. In addition, conduct your own assessment of their status.

Assess your client's voluntary control over their movements. Can they hold or maintain a posture, such as keeping their arms out to the side or overhead without tremor or drifting? Do they recognize where their limbs are in space? Can they smoothly and consistently alternate movements, such as pronation and supination of their forearm or reciprocal drumming of their fingers? Can they rise from a chair unassisted, stair climb and walk on their toes/heels? Watch for the quality and quantity of the movement. If disability is limited to one part of their body, think about how you will isolate that part from your routine to prevent it from inhibiting other functional movement. You can accomplish this through positioning and equipment adaptation. Also, consider how you will support that part to maintain or improve its function.

Check your client's overall flexibility. Ask your client to move their trunk and extremities through a full range of motion. Remember that norms for geriatric clients will vary (Lewis, 1997a). Functional range is more important than absolute anatomical range. Some clients with neuromuscular disorders may have developed protective or functional tightening of their muscles and/or joints. This is part of the adaptation process. It would be best to consider the client's functional use of the body part before stretching solely for flexibility. Discuss this with your client and the therapist

if in doubt. Remember, stretching should be slow and sustained. Research indicates that muscle tissue needs to be stretched for at least 20 to 30 seconds to be effective (Lewis, 1997b).

Look for bony or soft tissue abnormalities; deformed postures such as winging of the scapula; abnormalities of spinal alignment (may be the result of spastic or weak muscles); swelling of the joints in the hands and feet especially the ankles (may indicate cardiac problems). Bruising or other skin lesions may indicate trauma due to poor coordination or lack of sensory feedback. Long-term postural changes, especially with paralysis, can result in and/or cause weakened elongated muscles, loss of joint mobility, pinched nerves in the neck or back, or even protruding disks of the spine. Poor posture can either be habitual or pathologic in nature. Create awareness through feedback, and facilitate correction with strengthening and flexibility exercises.

Assess any reported or perceived pain. Ask your client for specific feedback. Pain is one of the body's best feedback mechanisms and should never be ignored or tolerated without a medical checkup to determine its cause.

If a body part has been nonfunctional over time, consider the implications of disuse muscle atrophy and the risk of **osteoporosis**.

Check for normal sensation including touch, sense of movement (vestibular) and **proprioception**. Simple sensation is tested by lightly touching a body part and asking for feedback. Was the touch felt, was sensation diminished or did the touch cause pain? Vestibular or movement sense can be tested with your client's eyes closed. Place one of your client's limbs into a position and ask them either to copy that position with the opposite limb or to describe the position. Vestibular sense can be tested by moving the big toe. While your client closes their eyes, move their big toe up or down and ask them to identify the direction of movement. You also can use the thumb for this test (Allen, 1971).

Test your client's static and dynamic balance. Challenge their balance in more than one static position (seated, hands and knees, kneeling, standing) by applying a quick force in multiple directions. If standing balance is impaired, check to see if closing the eyes improves or worsens the condition. Vision compensates for some nervous system damage.

Also test balance or control problems during dynamic activities, such as tandem walking (heel to toe along a straight line), stepping over and around objects, changing direction and hopping. Guard carefully.

If balance or falls are of particular concern, you may wish to test your client's balance more thoroughly. Therapists use a variety of validated balance tests that are good predictors of falls in the elderly or infirm population. The one-legged stand test is the easiest. Ask your client to stand on one leg and record how long they can do so. They should be able to sustain the position for 20 seconds or more if their balance is intact. If this test is too demanding, try the functional reach test. Place a yard stick on the wall perpendicular to the client's trunk. Your client stands with arms extended in front of them and leans as far forward as possible. A reach exceeding 10 inches is considered normal. Unwillingness or inability to reach at all puts the risk of falling at 28 times a normal individual's risk. A reach of 1 to 6 inches signifies a four-times higher likelihood of a fall. These tests can be repeated throughout the training program to document dynamic balance improvements (Cocchi, 1997; Lewis, 1996).

Check which medications your client is taking and be alert for drugs that alter their alertness and/or cardiac status. Your client may be well versed on their medication's effects and can serve as a valuable resource.

Interview your client to assess their judgment, learning deficits, overall perception of their disability and, most importantly, their goals.

General Fitness Guidelines

"First do no harm" is a maxim embraced by the medical community and is good advice for any professional working with a population that has dysfunction or disability. Listen and observe, watch for abnormal signs, and hear what your client is telling you about their abilities and how they feel. Innately, your client knows what is best for their circumstance. Examples of condition-specific activity restriction guidelines are outlined in Table 20.1.

- Begin strength training at a submaximal level while you assess your client's response. High-intensity resistance training programs appear to offer no advantages over moderate programs for clients with neuromuscular disease (Kilmer, 1994). Apply the four S's for decreasing exercise intensity: Slow down, use Smaller moves, Stabilize and Substitute with a modified move if needed (Sanders & Maloney-Hills, 1998).
- Perform flexibility training within a pain-free range and be mindful that some joint/muscle restrictions may be protective or functional in nature.
- Modify balance activities to prevent falls. Clients with neuromuscular disorders have impaired response and protective reflexes. They fall harder and often suffer greater injury due to osteoporosis and other deficits.
- Understand that endurance activities fatigue individuals with neuromuscular disorders, such as multiple sclerosis, Parkinson's and epilepsy. Many neuromuscular disorders are related to cardiac disease. Recognize the dif-

Table 20.2

Typical Activity Guidelines

- Wear upper-extremity arm sling at all times and avoid quick changes in position
- Hands-on guarding during all standing activities
- Avoid excessive head and neck extension
- Weight-bearing only with lower-extremity orthotics
- Work at submaximal level parameters (heart rate, blood pressure)
- Allow frequent rest periods

- Do not use treadmill; avoid overhead weightlifting
- Watch for neglect of left arm
- Use fall precautions
- Avoid weight bearing on buttocks during exercise
- Guard for safety at all times

Note: The doctor or therapist may be aware of other issues; you should monitor to alert them to impending medical concerns.

ferences between working with a healthy system and a compromised system.

- Bowel and bladder incontinence may be an issue, and fear of embarrassment may make some clients unwilling to leave home. Matter-of-fact acceptance, frequent voiding and the use of a diaper or pad will help your client adjust to these challenges. Stress incontinence can be an issue, so warn your client of your strength-training plans to help them prepare and possibly avoid an embarrassing situation. For your safety, have rubber gloves on hand in the event you need to clean equipment or handle soiled material.

- General well-being is profoundly affected by disease and/or disability. Mental, emotional and social implications need to be considered. Be prepared to address issues of the whole person to effectively train these clients.

- Being realistic is essential in any fitness program design, but even more so when your client's own judgment may be impaired or when they may be unwilling to accept their limitations. Use your good sense, experience and feedback from the healthcare team to monitor your expectations and those of your client. No one will be well served if goals are set too high. Most importantly, be patient and focus on what is working, and be thankful for small incremental improvements. Recovery and adaptation are time-honoring processes.

PART II: SPECIFIC DISEASE OR INJURY CONDITIONS RESULTING IN NEURO-MUSCULAR DISORDERS

Stroke

Stroke is the common name for a cerebral vascular accident (CVA), the third most common cause of death (Springhouse Corp., 1996). Strokes can occur at any age and are caused by a sudden impairment of cerebral circulation. The blood supply to a particular area of the brain is either interrupted or diminished. Brain tissue without oxygen via the blood supply will die (necrose) quickly, so it is essential to begin cardiopulmonary resuscitation (CPR) immediately when an individual's heart or breathing has stopped. Research tells us we have four minutes or less to restore blood supply to the central nervous system to prevent or diminish permanent brain damage.

Warning Signs and Early Treatment

Much is being done to educate the public about the early warning signs of stroke. The old belief that we can't do anything for stroke patients during the acute process is wrong.

The early signs of an impending stroke are the acute or sudden onset of the following:

- ➤ impaired cognitive skills (confusion)
- ➤ blurred vision, dimness or loss of vision especially in one eye
- ➤ dizziness or an unexplained fall
- ➤ severe headache
- ➤ slurring or other speech difficulties
- ➤ numbness or tingling (even minor) in the face or an extremity
- ➤ loss of movement or weakness in the face or extremity.

It is possible that a client may suffer a stroke while exercising. In fact, there is an increased risk of the onset of stroke during early morning hours, especially between 6 a.m. and noon — a prime time for training (*PT Bulletin,* May 29, 1998). Be aware of stroke symptoms and be sure your client understands the importance of reporting any abnormal feelings, sensations or difficulties to you. Remind them that they alone can give you this valuable feedback, and frequently ask your client how they are feeling throughout the session.

Should they experience any of the warning signs, stop the exercise. Get your client to a safe resting position, monitor their symptoms, and take their blood pressure and compare it to their pre-exercise or normal values. If symptoms worsen or persist while at rest, call for emergency support. A person who suffers a stroke generally will not lose consciousness and will not need CPR. Their heart and breathing continues unless the damage is severe, such as with a major **intracranial bleed**.

Even if symptoms subside, strongly encourage your client to discuss them with their physician as soon as possible. **Transient Ischemic Attacks** (TIAs) are small strokes from a temporary compromise to the blood flow. Your client might ignore these events because the symptoms don't persist for more than a few minutes (less than 24 hours by definition) and don't result in permanent deficits. TIAs more commonly occur in people who have cardiac problems. Recurring TIAs are obvious warning signs of compromised cerebral blood flow and should not be ignored. Never attempt to work through or self-treat these symptoms.

Immediate treatment at the first warning signs is very effective and may include drugs or surgery depending on the cause of the stroke. A loss of blood supply causes swelling (**edema**) in the surrounding tissue. This increase in fluid volume creates pressure that can cause further damage and restriction to blood flow. Drugs control the edema and reduce blood pressure to allow the healing process to proceed without further damage. Drugs should be administered within minutes or hours, hence the need for emergency support. Surgery also may be needed to stop the bleeding or extract pooled blood or other tissue that is compromising blood flow. Early intervention is the key to saving a life and preventing disability.

Etiology of a Stroke

The basic causes of a stroke are a narrowing or blockage of a cerebral artery, **hemorrhage,** or compression. Each results in different symptoms depending on where it occurs. Precursors to stroke include prolonged hypertension, cardiac arrhythmia, rheumatic heart disease, diabetes, gout, **postural hypotension**, cardiac enlargement, high serum triglycerides, obesity, lack of exercise, use of oral contraception, cocaine and/ or cigarettes, and family history.

Atherosclerosis is a narrowing of the blood vessels by fatty tissue that occurs over time. Symptoms may be transient and/or gradual in onset, and this condition usually occurs in older adults. Blood vessels already compromised by atherosclerosis can be further restricted by a **thrombus** or embolism.

A thrombus is a stationary clot that forms in an artery and blocks blood flow. This is the most common cause of stroke. Like atherosclerosis, thrombosis develops over time and may result in a transient and/or gradual onset of symptoms.

An embolism is a wandering blood clot or other material, carried from elsewhere in the circulatory system, that lodges in an artery.

Embolisms are the second most common cause of strokes. An embolism can be a blood clot, tumor, fatty deposit, bacteria or simply an air bubble, and may result from cardiac disease, trauma or surgery. An embolism develops rapidly and can occur at any age.

Hemorrhage or bleeding also is sudden and can occur at any age. Hemorrhages usually are related to trauma, ongoing hypertension or an **aneurysm** (a weakened outpocketing of the blood vessel). They cause pooling of blood that creates further compression and restriction of blood flow. The ability to stop the bleeding and control the pooling often is a matter of life and death, and contributes to a long-term prognosis.

A compression of the blood supply can be caused by any external force, pooled blood, a tumor or tissue edema resulting from disease or injury to the brain. The brain is confined and protected by the skull, a relatively uncompromising container. Therefore, cerebral edema is the most common cause of death in an acute stroke (O'Sullivan & Schmitz, 1994). Edema needs to be controlled quickly to prevent further damage.

Traumatic Brain Injury (TBI):

Traumatic brain injury often results in symptoms similar to those occurring during a stroke. Injury may be caused by a crushing force such as a blow to the head, a penetrating wound such as a gunshot or jarring of the brain tissue inside the skull (closed-head injury), which can occur in a traffic accident when the head is bounced or severely shaken. Jarring also occurs in abused infants who are forcibly shaken. Brain tissue bruises, which results in edema and further tissue damage. About 500,000 new cases of TBI occur each year in the U.S., making TBIs the most common cause of brain disorder (Katz, 1998).

Even mild head injuries such as those sustained during sporting events can cause brain tissue damage. Should your client sustain a mild head injury, they will need at least three days of rest to heal. Returning to competition too soon can result in secondary impact syndrome, which causes loss of brain function and can lead to respiratory arrest. Half of those individuals who develop the syndrome die, and survivors have some degree of permanent brain damage (*PT Bulletin,* September 12, 1997).

The brain, for all its fragility, is remarkably adaptive. Although specific tissue may be damaged or destroyed, the surrounding blood vessels expand to reroute blood to the area. In addition, the brain has an abundance of clever brain cells. Healthy cells often take over the function of damaged cells so that function is minimally or not at all compromised. This is particularly true when damage occurs early in life, making it easier to relearn functional activities. This, in part, accounts for the gradual recovery noted in some stroke/TBI victims that can continue for months and even years after the initial insult.

Rehabilitation Programs

Clinical rehabilitation programs for stroke/TBI clients focus on functional return of movement (i.e., the skills and ability to resume typical **activities of daily living**). Therapists are most concerned with basic functions including: the ability to transfer from one position to the next (such as from bed to a chair or on and off the toilet); the ability to dress and perform other self-care activities; and, if possible, the ability to walk, speak and perform higher levels of cognitive function.

As the resources for prolonged rehabilitation services lessen, more emphasis is put on these essential quality-of-life issues and less time is spent on other obvious fitness concerns, such as overall strength, flexibility, cardiac endurance and general well-being. The therapist also often works with clients who are acutely ill or injured. Much of their recovery occurs over time. You may be working with a client who has had a stroke or TBI years ago. Their recovery stage may be different from when they initially completed their clinical rehabilitation program. Long-term disabilities and overall health determine a post-rehab client's ability to participate in a fitness program; however most, if not all, can participate on some level. Conditioning programs yield significant improvement in fitness parameters, prevent recurrence and promote disability adaptation (Daviddoff et al., 1991; Tangeman, Banaitis & Williams, 1990).

Movement Disorders
Following a Stroke or TBI

The most common movement disorder you will encounter with these clients is some form of paralysis. Spastic paralysis in the form of hemiplegia (affecting one side of the body) is common. Remember that spasticity usually is increased by stress (sometimes something as minor as a sneeze or cough) or by attempts at voluntary movement. For example, you may encounter a client whose upper extremity is spastic. The arm may be nonfunctional, used as a gross assistance to movement and stability, or mildly impaired where the signs of spasticity are evident only with moderate stress. Whatever the level of dysfunction, the principles of adaptation remain the same. Make use of whatever function the client has without jeopardizing their safety or the health status of their neurologically impaired body parts.

Flaccid paralysis most likely will require supportive devices to protect the client's involved extremities and to promote overall stability. Some clients will use upper-extremity slings or orthotic supports to disperse the weight of the flaccid arm to prevent further damage, such as a subluxed shoulder. Some may wear a brace on their lower extremity to promote a more normal gait pattern, holding a flaccid foot in a neutral position to prevent tripping or helping to control a spastic knee to prevent **hyperextension**. In addition to support, an orthotic device promotes normal range of motion by preventing contracture of soft tissue. For instance, a cock-up splint for the wrist can hold the hand in a functional position. In general, leave these devices in place during your exercise program. Specific questions can be referred to the therapist or orthotist who supplied the device.

Shoulder **subluxation** and/or the development of a shoulder-hand pain syndrome is not atypical in clients who have paralysis of the upper extremity. This occurs when the head of the humerus is displaced from the shoulder joint, creating a syndrome of pain and impaired function for the entire extremity (Calliets, 1981).

Motor control is governed by the two halves or hemispheres of the brain. A stroke/TBI in the left hemisphere (affecting the right side of the body) will affect the sequencing of movement. Clients may have problems initiating movements and learning new exercises or activities, especially if they involve a complex sequence. Also, in general, their movements will be slower, so keep things simple. Use a limited number of tasks. A stroke/TBI in the right hemisphere (affecting the left side of the body) results in more problems with movement control and posture, and clients will have difficulty sustaining a position (O'Sullivan & Schmitz, 1994). Use stabilizing postures and guard carefully.

Stroke/TBI victims suffer from poor or absent support reactions, resulting in difficulty sustaining an extremity in an extended or support position. This is most noticeable in the lower extremity when attempting to stand and/or walk, but also can be seen in the upper extremity, for example in the hands-and-knees position. Weak support reactions result in flexion of the key joints during weight-bearing activities. The reaction also may be abnormally sustained so that the involved extremity does not relax when unloaded to allow the leg to swing forward during stepping. The response may be inconsistent, which requires you to be vigilant during standing or walking activities, as the client's knee may buckle unpredictably. If the reaction is absent or weak, practice weight shifting while the client stands with their back supported by a wall or kitchen counter. To encourage the support reaction, your client can perform exercises that require a diagonal movement pattern that causes them to shift their weight from one side to the other. For example, have them lift a weight from a low position on the right side up across the body to over the left shoulder. They should move slowly and hold the weight for a few seconds at each end of the range. By performing the movement slowly and holding contractions, your client benefits from the proprioceptive feedback provided by their working muscles.

Functional Impairments Following a Stroke or TBI

Some stroke/TBI clients have a loss of sensation in their affected extremities and may be unaware of their affected side to the point that they ignore or neglect it completely. In these cases, guard against injuries during positioning from crushing, pinching or abrasions to the skin.

Apraxia is the inability to carry out a purposeful movement. Although your client understands, and may be physically able to perform, the task, they cannot translate their will to action. Apraxia most commonly is seen in the speech muscles following injury to the left hemisphere. This causes

an individual great difficulty in speaking at will, but they can spontaneously recite or sing. Apraxia also is seen in clients who suffer from lesions to the right hemisphere. Although these clients cannot lift their arm to don a shirt, they can reflexively catch a ball.

Visual deficits may influence your client's balance, and thus their safety, when working with equipment or when exercising outside their typical environment. Because the optic nerves cross to the opposite side of the brain, damage in one hemisphere causes blindness of the nasal half of one eye and the temporal half of the other. This symptom is called **hemianopsia** and causes the client to ignore one side of the body, or even their dinner plate or a page of written material. Clients must learn to compensate for this deficit by turning their heads to scan for the whole picture.

Proprioceptive (awareness of position and movement) deficits impair your client's ability to react. For example, adjustments to walking on uneven surfaces, such as those commonly found outside the home, are not automatic. Clients will need to be guarded carefully.

Impairments in dynamic balance are an issue when making positioning decisions and when asking your client to get on and off exercise equipment. Instruct your client to approach the equipment on their unimpaired side so that they can use their functional limbs to lead the movement. Remind them to be mindful of what they are attempting to do and to mentally plan the movement before attempting it. Break down the task into steps, give them a demonstration, and then provide verbal and tactile cues as they proceed.

Impairment of judgment is an issue, especially with right-hemisphere damage. Clients may seem impulsive or may overestimate their ability. Be particularly attentive to their response to exercise and their attempts to accomplish new movements or tasks.

Motor learning, or the ability to repeat an activity, also may be impaired, especially with left-hemisphere damage. Clients may display negativity or over-anxiousness when presented with a new task. In these cases, use repeated demonstrations and verbal and tactile (touching) cues throughout the activity. Relate each component of an activity to the whole task.

Don't assume that a movement learned at one session will be retained; repetition often becomes essential and should be offered in a way that the client doesn't perceive your frustration. After all, the client lives with their deficits daily; you, on the other hand, are exposed to their limitations for a very finite period. Be physically and emotionally supportive, and together you will accomplish your goals.

Adaptations to a Fitness Program for Clients with Stroke or TBI

Strength Training

Don't overload an extremity during weight training, and be cautious when accommodating for balance or stability deficits. Be sure a possible change in muscle tone can be accommodated by your client before you ask them to perform a specific movement. For example, clients performing biceps curls in a standing position with their uninvolved extremity may experience an increase in tone in their involved extremities. This increased tone may disturb their balance and cause them to fall. Therefore, begin the exercise in a more cautious position (e.g., sitting). Watch for the response and provide hands-on support when they attempt the standing movement.

Because hypertension is a cause and/or an underlying symptom of stroke, care must be taken to monitor and control the client's blood pressure during strength training. Always avoid a Valsalva maneuver, an exerted force while breath is being held, that occurs when lifting more than 85 percent of maximal voluntary contraction (Lewis, 1998). Be sure your client understands the importance of proper breathing during exercise, and be sure they comply with your instructions to breathe. In addition, if necessary, modify their strength program to stay within maximum heart rate or blood pressure guidelines. Because taking a client's blood pressure during exercise may be impractical, research is being conducted to test the viability of using a heart-rate monitor to measure cardiovascular response during strength testing (Westcott & O'Grady, 1998).

Flexibility

Just as functional moving parts need to be stretched, so do nonfunctional parts, whether they are spastic or flaccid extremities. Range-of-motion exercises for nonfunctional limbs or joints should be performed at least daily, as loss of motion causes muscle contractions or shortening. Passive range-of-motion exercises can be performed by the client who has learned the proper techniques, or by the trainer or family member when range of motion is outside the client's capabilities. Passive range of motion implies no active voluntary participation by your client for the movement of that joint; however, your client may use their opposite extremities to assist in the movement. Active or volitional movement always is preferable, though, it is not always possible with nonfunctional muscles and joints. Discuss this issue with the client and determine their needs and willingness to participate.

Passive range-of-motion exercises of a severely spastic extremity can be difficult and painful, and should be performed carefully to prevent tissue damage. Participate in additional training with your client and a therapist to learn specific techniques unique to your client's needs. Touch, movement, speed and range can increase spasticity. Learn to moderate. As always, slow, sustained stretching is preferable. Quick, bouncing movements will increase spastic tone and are counterproductive. Rotational movement may help to reduce spasticity. Moving the extremities in diagonal patterns versus straight anatomical planes may facilitate fuller range of motion. Proprioceptive Neuromuscular Facilitation (PNF) is a therapeutic exercise technique that details the use of diagonal patterns (Voss, Ionta & Myers, 1985).

Range-of-motion exercises of flaccid extremities are much easier. When performed by a therapist, passive range-of-motion exercises can be combined with proprioceptive techniques that may facilitate the return of muscle tone and movement. Such techniques include joint approximations, therapeutic use of stretch and diagonal movement patterns, and positioning the body part to encourage facilitation of movement during other activities. You will need additional training to incorporate these methods, but simple range-of-motion exercises or moving extremities through normal movement patterns are essential for maintaining the health of the muscle and joint tissues and promoting good posture and circulation.

Don't forget the all-important trunk muscles when designing the stretching program. Emphasize trunk extension and rotation. A classic therapeutic exercise for the trunk is lower-trunk rotation. The client lies supine with hips and knees flexed, feet flat on the floor. With arms at their sides, they rotate both knees together to one side and then the other as far as possible. Advance this basic exercise by rotating the upper extremities, upper trunk, and head and neck in the opposite direction. Add weights to the upper extremities or manual resistance at the knees. Trunk rotation is a simple activity that dramatically affects overall muscle tone, posture and visceral responses such as breathing. This exercise is an important warm-up activity for a client with spasticity.

Cardiac Conditioning

Clients who have suffered a stroke as the result of cardiac disease may demonstrate significant cardiac limitations (O'Sullivan & Schmitz, 1994). However, if a post stroke/TBI client has physician clearance, cardiac training can be performed. Monitor your client's pulse and blood pressure. Converse directly with the client's physician to review your exercise program. Ask for recommended precautions. Depending on your client's medical status, ask the physician for specific heart rate and/or blood pressure maximum guidelines. Physicians may be conservative in setting guidelines, especially if they have not worked with you in the past. Be respectful of the physician's perspective, understanding the significant liability risk that they take when referring their patient for your services. If you find the guidelines too restrictive, negotiate more progressive guidelines by providing the physician with data on your client's response to exercise and/or copies of recent research findings. Be patient, open and nonthreatening, and avoid being perceived as too aggressive. Strive to align your agenda with that of the physician's. Both of your goals are to provide the client with a safe and effective means of maintaining or improving overall well-being.

Posture

Clients with **hemiplegia** typically assume a stooped posture when sitting and standing. Posture retraining is not only essential, but therapeutic to restoring normal movement patterns. Because of changes in muscle tone, balance and sometimes vision, clients may seem to curl up. A challenge to **equilibrium** or stability, impaired senses and/or an altered emotional state may elicit a natural response to guard, tighten up and curl inward. Emphasize extension of the head, neck, hip and knee, as well as spinal rotation. Begin with your client lying flat or sitting or standing while supported, and provide them with visual, verbal and active feedback. Assist them in attaining correct posture to reinforce what it feels like and to promote motor learning. Don't forget that their normal feedback systems may be impaired and you may serve as a substitute with your eyes, hands and other tactile cues. Ask them if they can feel the difference when they assume a better posture. Put your hand on the back of your client's head and ask them to push their head back (extending, not rotating, to flatten the cervical spine curve). Give mild resistance to this movement as tactile feedback. Providing feedback that enhances postural awareness goes a long way toward improving the client's ability to recognize and subsequently correct postural deficits.

Nutrition

Changing eating habits may be life-sustaining for a stroke victim, especially if the stroke was the result of clotting in arteries. Excessive weight on compromised joints also puts the client at risk for injury or long-term arthritic changes and strains the cardiovascular system. It is appropriate to refer your client to a nutritionist or licensed dietitian.

General Well-being

If your client has been restricted in their ability to bear weight (stand or walk), they are at a high risk for osteoporosis. Help your client avoid falling or overloading their joints, substituting exercises such as bench leg presses to simulate weight bearing. The involved extremity sometimes can be positioned and supported to perform a bilateral exercise. It may be more effective to isolate the involved extremity, particularly if an increase in muscle tone interferes with the successful movement of the uninvolved extremity. For example, if extensor spasticity of one leg prevents your client from performing a pedaling activity, isolate the involved extremity. Seat your client behind an exercise bike so that while pedaling, the involved leg can be positioned off to the side. Watch carefully to be sure the involved leg doesn't wander too close to the rotating pedal. Remember, exercise stress increases spastic tone. Your client might pedal with their arms if they are unable to do so with their legs. Call your client's therapist for suggestions on equipment adaptations.

Stroke/TBI victims can experience emotional changes caused by damage to the brain or resulting from the frustration associated with chronic disabilities. Respect these changes, and support your client's need to express their emotions. Your client may not have emotional control and may cry, laugh or get upset easily. They may have bouts of bad temper, feel apathetic, have a shortened attention span, or be depressed or anxious. They also may be self-centered and focus on controlling their environment or possessions. These behavioral changes are real symptoms of the injury to their brain. If they persist and interfere with the fitness program, first discuss them with your client and then with their physician. Sometimes medication and/or psychotherapy can help.

Multiple Sclerosis

Multiple sclerosis (MS) is a **demyelinating disease** of the central nervous system. **Myelin** is a lipoprotein that forms a protective sheath or cover for individual nerves. Plaques or patches, like small scars, form in the nerve tissue, causing a disruption in their function and leading to an array of symptoms depending on their location.

Etiology and Progression of MS

Why the myelin sheath breaks down is unknown; in fact, some breakdown is asymptomatic and only can be seen during an autopsy. Viral infections, an autoimmune response, trauma, exposure to toxins or other undue stress may precipitate the onset of symptoms. How these events are related to the disease is unknown (Eliasson, Prensky & Hardin, 1978).

MS usually is first diagnosed in young adults but may occur at even younger ages. The course of the disease is variable and often unpredictable. It usually begins with local symptoms relating to damage in a specific area of the nervous system, and progresses to more generalized disability in severe or recurring cases. Typically the symptoms occur in a course of **exacerbation** and remission. Some patients flux between dramatic disability and complete remission.

The onset of symptoms, or more commonly a single symptom, usually is rapid and initially present only for a few days or weeks followed by months or even years of remission. As the disease progresses, multiple symptoms occur. Remission occurs with less frequency, is less complete and lasts for a shorter duration. Increases in core body temperature have proven to elicit dormant symptoms or increase the occurrence of symptoms (Eliasson, Prensky & Hardin, 1978), including: visual disturbances (loss of central vision or blurred or double vision); tingling or numbness (paresthesia); clumsiness or loss of proprioceptive sense; spasticity, weakness **(paresis)**; poor balance and loss of coordination (ataxia).

Rehabilitation Programs

Because MS is an ongoing and progressive disease, clients may have had a series of clinical rehabilitation episodes (with each exacerbation) or may be experiencing symptoms that are not severe enough to warrant rehabilitation referral. Early symptoms usually are managed by the physician. Because these symptoms are transient in nature, they may not persist long enough to result in significant or chronic disability. Also, because MS can begin at a young age, you may be the first member of the healthcare team to interact with a client with MS. Be observant of mild symptoms, and be prepared to discuss them with your client and/or their physician, but remember that undue alarm at the first sign of a twitch is not serving. Look for recurring or persistent symptoms that may worsen as your client fatigues or as their core body temperature increases. Often, visual disturbances are the first to occur. Ask your client if they have noticed similar symptoms at other times or if any of the other symptoms noted above are present.

If symptoms warrant clinical rehabilitation, program design is similar to that outlined for stroke/TBI victims (i.e., restoring functional skills). Because balance often is a major issue for clients who are more severely affected by MS, emphasis is placed on adapting activities of daily living for safe performance. This might include training with adaptive equipment, such as a cane or wheelchair. Recent research has demonstrated that clients with progressive MS benefit from an ongoing, comprehensive outpatient maintenance rehabilitation program (De Fabio, Choi, Soderberg & Hansen,1997).

Movement Disorders Associated with MS

Spasticity often is the most disabling symptom and usually occurs as spastic **paraplegia** involving the lower extremities. During acute exacerbation of the disease, clients may be forced to use a wheelchair for mobility. It is imperative that their lower-extremity muscles and joints are exercised through their range of motion to keep them healthy as the disease may go into remission. Cold packs or pool therapy may temporarily reduce spasticity. Incorporating rotational versus straight anatomical plane movements reduces spasticity. Sometimes stroking or applying light pressure to the antagonist muscle group helps to relax a spastic muscle so that active or passive movement can occur.

Ataxia is the other primary disabling movement disorder associated with MS. Gait most often is affected, and requires the client to walk with an ambulatory aide, such as a cane or walker, or with physical assistance. MS clients usually use a wide-based stance and feel most secure when they are seated. Modify your program to increase their sense of security with proper positioning and/or support.

Clients also may be affected by weakness or **paresis**. Unlike individuals who have had a stroke or TBI, clients with MS may demonstrate progressive weakness vs. complete paralysis. They lose the ability to orderly recruit muscle activity and may display modulations in strength so that an activity can be performed well in one circumstance but not in another. Clients also may experience disuse atrophy from prolonged inactivity (O'Sullivan & Schmitz, 1994). Strength training can improve all of these symptoms as long as it is moderated to prevent fatigue.

Clients may experience intention tremors that vary from mild to severe and result from damage to the cerebellum. Usually these are most bothersome for performance of fine motor activities such as personal hygiene, eating, writing or even tying shoes, but they may not dramatically affect your program.

Functional Impairments Associated with MS

Clients with MS, especially during acute exacerbation, are easily fatigued. Often they will start the day refreshed, but by early afternoon they are nearly exhausted. Plan your session around this symptom, as excessive physical activity, muscle strain, depression and even an elevated core body temperature may increase your client's fatigue (Lechtenberg, 1988).

Increases in core body temperature are followed by increased symptoms, so your client will perform best in a cool environment. Pool therapy often is effective for its cooling properties.

Visual disturbances are common but generally do not limit physical function, as they tend to subside early in the course of the disease. However, reading and visually tracking activities may remain difficult (Lechtenberg, 1988). Blurred vision might be improved with tinted lenses that reduce glare, and an eye patch can be worn to reduce the effects of double vision. Let your client know there may be treatment options for visual disturbances, and encourage them to discuss these problems with their physician.

Sensory disturbances include tingling, overall numbness of an area, and loss of position and vibratory sense. Clients without position sense need to use vision and other proprioceptive feedback. Give your client additional feedback through touch or approximation (gently bearing down on proximal joints). For example, if a client is sitting, gently push down on both shoulders to give approximation feedback to the spine and pelvis.

Pain is a problem in some cases due to hypersensitivity to normal stimuli, such as touch, pressure or even a light breeze. Often, clients with MS complain of a burning sensation felt along a nerve's path. Pain also is caused by muscle spasms and contractures. Work around pain issues by avoiding touching or putting pressure on painful areas, or by padding bony areas during exercise. If pain persists, ask the client to consult with their physician.

Fitness Program Adaptations for Clients with MS

Strength Training

Loss of strength and endurance in involved muscles usually occurs quickly and can be dramatic. Muscle atrophy becomes visually apparent (O'Sullivan & Schmitz, 1994). You may work with a client who is experiencing their first period of symptom exacerbation. If you notice a dramatic change in strength or endurance, don't assume it is related to your client's motivation. And don't overload muscles or joints, especially those with disuse atrophy. Use the same guidelines and judgment that you would follow for any client in progressing resistance and repetitions, and remember the role fatigue plays in MS. Because your client's endurance is reduced, carefully choose exercises so that you can maximize their functional effect. Exercise to the point of fatigue is contraindicated; it can make your client feel worse and negatively affect motivation (Pal Brar & Wangaard, 1985).

As signs of weakness occur, focus on exercises that improve or maintain your client's functional status. Stepping or stair climbing can be substituted for lower-extremity bench presses if your client's balance permits. Stepping using a stairwell with bilateral hand rails provides added support. Change the frequency and/or flow of workouts as it will take the client longer to recover. Plan according to their feedback. Self-pacing overrules tough motivational tactics in these cases.

Ataxic clients require proximal or trunk stabilization to help control their movements. A stabilized weight-bearing position causes co-contraction of the proximal muscles to better control distal movements. This can be accomplished through positioning. In fact, if ataxia is particularly bothersome, assuming a stabilizing position may be therapeutic. For example, lying prone supported on bent elbows is a good position for practicing shoulder movements and/or head and neck posture. Assuming a hands-and-knees position may allow your client to better control the exercising extremity. In general, ataxic clients perform better in a low-stimulus environment that allows them to concentrate fully on movement control. They require feedback (knowledge of results and performance)

and high degrees of repetition to learn motor tasks (O'Sullivan & Schmitz, 1994). Slowing reciprocal movements and placing isometric contractions at each end of a range of motion is effective. Asking a client to hold a position before reversal in the range is a very helpful technique.

Flexibility

As with stroke or TBI, clients with MS may require passive range of motion of nonfunctional joints to prevent fibrous changes or ankylosis. You may find **range-of-motion** losses if **spasticity** is present. Isolate and check each involved joint.

Cardiac Conditioning

MS does not affect cardiac status other than the deconditioning that generally occurs from prolonged inactivity. An aerobic program tailored to your client's capabilities is important. Combining a cardiac workout with a social aspect, such as training for wheelchair sports, may prove to be an invaluable spirit booster for your client if and when the disease progresses.

Posture

Because MS causes the body to curl inward, prolonged inactivity allows the extensor muscles of the trunk to overstretch. Clients with MS who normally are active and functional may need focused intervention to promote postural awareness. Those who are particularly weak may require support to sustain good posture when sitting, such as a pillow behind the low back. A tennis ball at the mid-thoracic spine level may remind a slouching client to sit erect. Head and neck posture should not be ignored, as visual disturbances may lead to unusual posturing of the head. Frequent range-of-motion exercises and stretching remind the client of the normal orientation, and prevent muscle tightness that encourages bad posture.

Nutrition

Inactivity, depression, pain and stress affect appetite and influence nutrition. Talk to your client about their eating habits and whether they have experienced changes. Sometimes eating small but frequent portions helps, especially if digestive function is slowed or impaired. Eating when least fatigued also is beneficial. Because lack of coordination affects your client's ability to feed themselves and/or eat in social situations, the disease may be socially isolating. Recognize these issues and, if possible, provide companionship and empathy to reduce stress and frustration. A referral to a dietitian or nutritionist would be appropriate.

General Well-being

Mild-to-moderate impairment of cognitive function is often seen in clients with MS. Cognitive function impairments include recall and memory deficits, problems with attention and concentration that affect learning, and conceptual reasoning (Peterson & Kokmen, 1989; Franklin et al., 1989). Repetition, feedback and patience all are required to overcome or adapt to these problems.

Affective or emotional disorders are common. Euphoria or the exaggerated feeling of well-being is typical and may be demonstrated by what seems to be poor judgment of physical capabilities.

Any disease or disability affecting a person in their prime of life may lead to depression, and the unpredictable course of MS can leave a client in despair. Concentrate on what they can accomplish. Clients with MS are known to engage in fewer social and recreational activities than would be expected based on their level of disability (Stables & Lincoln, 1979). Working out in groups, team activities or simply taking the session outside can help.

If coordination or weakness affects the client's tongue and other head and neck muscles, your client may experience dysphagia (slurred speech) and problems with swallowing and breath control. Change activity when there is a communication block to help diffuse frustration and stress, and to allow your client to communicate more clearly later in the session. If the individual has good upper-extremity control, writing may be an alternative form of communication. If you don't understand, just say so. Empathize with their frustration, then try to get them to move to another activity. Explain that switching the focus may help and that you intend to come back to the issue at hand later in the session. It is important that they know you want to understand them and that you are not dismissing them or their needs.

Parkinson's Disease

Parkinson's disease (PD) is a degenerative neurochemical condition that involves a specific area of the brainstem, the **basal ganglia**. PD is the second most common neurodegenerative disease (Alzheimer's is first), afflicting approximately 500,000 Americans (*PT Bulletin,* August 1, 1997). Symptoms are chronic and progressive and include rigidity, **bradykinesia** (slowing of movements), loss of automatic movements, tremors, **dementia**, increase in reaction time, poor balance and postural changes. Classic signs of PD include a "masked face" that makes the client seem emotionless, a "pill-rolling" tremor of the fingers and thumb (seen at rest), a shuffling (maybe festinating) gait, hesitance in beginning any movement, and a stooped posture. Symptoms usually become evident in the mid 50s, but it now is believed that the disease process begins earlier in life with milder symptoms that often are ignored.

Etiology and Progression of PD and Treatment Options

The cause of Parkinson's disease is unknown and may in part be genetic (*PT Bulletin,* August 1, 1997). PD results from the brain's inability to properly process **dopamine,** a neurotransmitter, in the **substantia nigra**, which is part of the basal ganglia. Change in dopamine's production, or in the number or function of its receptors, results in PD symptoms. Symptoms also can occur following an infection such as the influenza epidemic that occurred in the early 1900s. Exposure to toxins (including cytotoxins such as free radicals) and drug side-effects also have been thought to lead to PD (Ciccone, 1998). Drugs that may cause PD include heavy tranquilizers and blood pressure medications. Symptoms usually subside when drug use is terminated or reduced.

Diagnosis usually is made when a multitude of symptoms are present and when other causes have been excluded. With early treatment, including a fitness program and medication, the effects of the disease can be controlled but not eliminated. Drug therapy may include anticholinergic drugs, neuroprotective drugs and Levadopa (**L-dopa**) which is a metabolic precursor to dopamine and has been found to be effective in controlling symptoms. With medication, the initial improvement may be dramatic, decreasing with continued use. Clients with decreased response are often put on a "drug holiday" for seven to 10 days to reduce side effects and enhance future response. A sudden improvement often leads to clients' overstressing their muscular or cardiac system, so be cautious and encourage temperance.

Stereotaxic surgery, which destroys particular areas of the brain, can be used in select clients to control tremor or rigidity. Microsurgery developments have made this a more reliable treatment option, but it remains ineffective in controlling bradykinesia. New techniques, such as implantation of deep brain stimulators, are being tested at research centers such as the University of Chicago Hospitals. Transplantation of fetal brain tissue also is believed to help regenerate damaged nerve cells. Dr. James Schumacher in Sarasota, Fla., is experimenting with the transplantation of pig cells. His results on a limited number of patients show up to 20 percent improvement over time (*PT Bulletin,* April 24, 1998).

Rehabilitation Programs

PD often is managed medically, and patients are seen by a therapist only when their symptoms are grossly impairing functional skills. Medical management may require fine-tuning of medication. A patient might be unable to perform activities of daily living before medication, but, they can function with proper drug control, provided they have maintained their strength and flexibility. The clinical rehabilitation team is primarily concerned with functional skills and teaching the patient to cope with the progressive disease. Long-term programs stress balance, mobility and posture. Therapeutic exercises and techniques "unlock" rigid movements, prevent falls and subsequent injury, and facilitate postural awareness. Severe cases require transfer and gait training, primarily to teach patients to be aware of their deficits and how to accommodate for them. As resources for clinical rehabilitation decline, PD outpatient programs are being designed to allow patients to participate in short-duration group classes to upgrade or refresh their skills. These programs also provide a revised home-exercise program as the disease process progresses. Our current medical delivery system is poorly designed to meet the needs of those who suffer from chronic progressive conditions such as PD. It allows for treatment on an acute basis, but does little to support maintenance of functional skills that prevent long-term disability. When patients most need clinical expertise to ensure prolonged function, they are left to manage on their own. This is why many patients seek alternative support services.

Movement Disorders Associated with PD

PD causes an overwhelming "poverty of movement" that affects the ability to execute, respond to and control movement speed and range. Rigidity often is the biggest problem, affecting both gross and fine motor function. Gross motor function includes activities such as standing and walking that require major-muscle-group cooperation and sensory support. Fine motor function includes refined movements such as writing, playing the piano or picking up utensils. Rigidity causes the muscles to feel heavy or sluggish and results in an increased resistance to movement in any direction. Spasticity, on the other hand, usually limits movement only in one direction. Stress, movement or attempts at volitional control can increase rigidity, which may begin in one body part or affect the entire body.

Rigidity is characterized by a masked face. Look at your client's eyes and you can see their pain or emotion, but their face often gives few clues. Automatic or spontaneous laughter can elicit a smile, but without the joke, there is minimal response. Another key sign of rigidity is the loss of rhythmic motions that accompany normal activities, contribute to sensory feedback, and promote balance and stability. Observe your client as they approach you from a distance. A loss of rhythmic arm swing, a stiff trunk and/or small hesitant steps are all clues. Because of its effect on movement, prolonged rigidity can lead to muscle contracture and loss of joint mobility (Jankovic, 1987). Rigidity also interferes with balance and coordination and grossly impairs function.

Some other terms you may encounter with PD are bradykinesia, **akinesia** and **festination**. Bradykinesia is slowness of movement, resulting from the PD client's difficulty in initiating movements. If you ask your client to do something and they sit motionlessly, don't assume they don't understand or lack motivation. Their reaction time is impaired, causing a significant delay between their will to move and actual results. This is very frustrating, and emotional stress may only make the condition worse. Akinesia is severe bradykinesia, resulting in a complete state of immobility. This freezing of movement can last for moments or hours (Jankovic, 1987).

Coping techniques include breaking down a big task into smaller components by isolating volitional activity to one small body part. For example, if your client is having trouble beginning walking, instruct them to think only of bringing their toe off the floor. Isolating this small movement may allow them to pick the entire foot off the floor and begin walking. Rocking or assisting a client to do reciprocal movements of the trunk or an extremity also may help them get started. For example, instruct your client who seems "stuck" in their chair and unable to stand to scoot to the edge of the chair first. This can be accomplished by having them lean back and slide/push their buttocks forward, then rock from side to side as you manually assist in pulling their hips and thighs forward. Once they are forward in the chair, assist them in producing a forward-rocking motion. Once rocking, they can then stand. Movements, even once initiated, will be slow. Sometimes playing music may help your client increase their tempo. Carefully guard your client so they do not get ahead of themselves and trip and fall.

Festination is the display of poverty of movement in the lower extremities, causing short, shuffling steps. Coupled with poor balance and a flexed posture, clients appear as if they are falling forward while shuffling to maintain their balance. A festinating gait can and should be interrupted. Have the client stop, regroup and begin again. Continued festination usually worsens and results in a fall before the client reaches their intended destination. Continually remind them that it is far better to stop and start multiple times so that they arrive uninjured and upright.

Presence of the typical pill-rolling resting tremor often is the first visible sign of PD, leading to diagnosis and early treatment. Watch for this tremor in your clients who are aged 40 to 50-plus. The tremor often is mild and you may be the first to observe its presence. It is easily observed during a posture evaluation if you pay particular attention to the hands. Observe your client when they are relaxed and standing with their arms hanging at their sides.

PD clients also may suffer from postural tremor. Posture requires a continual modulation of muscle tone to oppose gravity. Unlike resting tremors, postural tremors are less obvious during rest but worsen with voluntary effort, are heightened by stress (Cohen, 1991), and are usually evident in proximal body parts, especially during standing.

Functional Impairments Associated with PD

Balance reactions of PD clients are impaired or absent, and are poorly compensated for, because **righting reactions** (the ability to recover a loss of balance) are impaired. In addition, because they lack the natural ability to "catch" themselves, fall injuries often are worse for individuals with PD. Sometimes they fall backward (Cohen, 1991). Always be alert to the potential of a fall. Because their balance ability may change as the disease progresses, retest your client's balance periodically. The one-legged-stand and functional-reach tests are good predictors of your client's likelihood of falling (Smithson, Morris & Iansek, 1998).

Clients with PD fatigue easily, even during speech. They might begin with normal cadence and volume, but their voice drops off and words become less clear as they continue. This can be socially isolating. Encourage them to speak up, and incorporate this as part of their fitness program. You should see their neck extend and head lift as they improve their voice volume. If posture and voice deteriorate during sessions, give continual reminders and insist on eye contact as the client speaks to you.

Research has verified that PD also results in functional weakness apart from rigidity and bradykinesia. The weakness may be due to the slowing rate of muscle torque development. Therefore, the weakness is not typically displayed during isometric muscle-strength tests, but is more evident while performing functional activities. Trunk muscle weakness may be the primary contributing factor to the stooped posture that seems to progress in severity with PD. Postural and strength training for trunk extensors and rotators, especially during early stages of PD, can contribute to your client's long-term well-being (Bridgewater & Sharpe, 1998).

PD clients must increase their cognitive effort to accomplish even simple tasks. Motor planning deficits require more effort to learn or to repeat tasks (Berger, 1995). Keep exercise programs simple and repetitive. **Dementia** or impaired cognitive function occurs in about 40 percent of advanced cases of PD, and medication toxicity may cause delusions and visual hallucinations (Bowen, 1976).

Autonomic nervous system dysfunction may impair appetite, digestion, temperature regulation (excessive perspiration), bowel and bladder control, and salivation. PD clients may have unusually low resting blood pressures and suffer from orthostatic hypotension or the sudden drop in blood pressure that occurs when assuming an upright posture (from lying to sitting, or sitting to standing). Be sure your client takes a moment to adjust between changes in position.

Fitness Program Adaptations for Clients with PD

Strength Training

Concentrate on postural muscles used in trunk extension, chest wall expansion, shoulder external rotation, scapular adduction, lower-extremity extension of the hips and knees, and ankle dorsiflexion. Keep exercises simple and functional (e.g., going from sitting to standing, and stair climbing). Expect strength to decrease more rapidly than normal as repetitions increase. Loss of strength due to inactivity may be a PD patient's primary disability. Research shows that the moderately disabled PD client's symptoms improve after as few as four weeks of exercise. However, consistent participation is a must, as improvements return to baseline in as few as six months without regular exercise (Comella, 1994).

Slow rhythmic movements reduce rigidity. Rocking in a chair or on a gym ball, and shifting weight while standing can be effective (Pederson, 1975; Stockmeyer, 1967). Passively initiate a movement and repeat its rhythmic reversal several times before your client takes over and does it on their own (Voss, Ionta & Meyers, 1985).

Use visual cues, such as masking-tape markings on the floor, to encourage stepping. Promote large, rhythmic steps to break out of a festinating gait pattern. Mark a start and stop point and have the client count the steps from one to the other. They should try to decrease the number of steps required each time they travel between the points.

Auditory cues, such as clapping, a metronome or music, can help your client keep up the pace. Research has demonstrated the positive effects of music therapy with this population (Macintosh, Brown, Rice & Thaut, 1997).

Flexibility

PD clients usually will become stiff and immobile in their proximal joints first. Encourage active motion and passive stretch that is gentle and prolonged to avoid tissue damage and pain. Deep breathing exercises that encourage chest expansion and extension are valuable. When possible, incorporate rotation and reaching activities to encourage muscle elongation for the spine and upper trunk. Pay close attention to the head and neck to improve posture, decrease drooling and allow the client to be more sociably acceptable in their appearance and demeanor. Teach your client bridging (lying supine, hips and knees flexed, and lifting buttocks from the floor) to emphasize trunk mobility. When performing floor activities, encourage your client to work without a pillow under their head, allowing the neck and upper trunk muscles to stretch. This may be accomplished in graduated stages. Reducing dependence on a pillow is important during sleep as well. Encourage your client to perform a stretching routine each morning before getting out of bed and beginning their daily activities, and to stop and stretch frequently during the day. Wall push-ups from a corner stretch tight chest muscles.

Cardiac Conditioning

Often, PD patients will have been inactive long before they are debilitated from the disease. Rigidity affects vital capacity as it affects thoracic expansion, even more so if a kyphotic posture is evident. Substitute cycling for walking if festination grossly impairs walking. Swimming may not be an option in advanced cases of rigidity. The challenge is to increase heart rate before the client is fatigued. Simple activities that have functional overtones, like bending and lifting small weights from the floor to a tabletop or tossing a ball at a target, may prove effective. Completion of a routine task gives your client focus and reduces the effort spent on planning the activity; the more automatic the task, the better.

Posture

The stooped or flexed posture associated with PD affects not only the head, neck and upper trunk, but also hip and knee extension and ankle dorsiflexion. As PD clients attempt to assume a normal, erect posture, you may see postural tremors in their lower extremities. Some walk on tiptoes, further disturbing their balance and safety. Kyphosis is common, characterized by a marked drooping of the head and neck. Feedback that enhances postural awareness goes a long way to improving your client's ability to recognize and correct postural deficits. Improved posture allows for better socialization; lets your client better scan their visual horizon to prepare for environmental challenges; helps to inhibit festination; promotes trunk rotation which frees extremity movement; and helps prevent falls.

Nutrition

Social implications of PD isolate the client. Problems with eating and swallowing, and loss of appetite, usually lead to weight loss. Poor nutrition contributes to osteoporosis, lack of energy and general lethargy. Encourage consultation with a dietitian or nutritionist. Often, PD clients are on a high-calorie, low-protein diet; however, protein may interfere with dopamine processing or the effects of L-dopa, and should be consumed during the evening meal when activity is lessening. Good nutrition maximizes an individual's response to drug therapy and the fitness program.

General Well-being

Depression is a related symptom of PD caused by the impairment of dopamine processing, as well as the debilitating effects of the dis-

ease. Some clients may appear apathetic or seem to lack motivation due to the rigidity and slowed response time. The best way to discern between lack of interest and disability is to ask your client for feedback and involve them in goal development.

Stooped posture, a tendency to fall, slurred speech, drooling and loss of appetite all contribute to making PD a socially isolating disease. Your visit may be the only frequent contact your client has with the outside world, so engage them in discussion of current events. This can be done while practicing postural activities. Play music to loosen them up. Singing is a great voice and breathing activity.

Relaxation also is key. Tapes that encourage relaxation and deep breathing while in an extended posture (lying supine, no pillow is best) are an important part of a fitness program. Yoga and Feldenkrais are effective techniques that emphasize relaxation and breathing (Schenkman, 1989; Feldenkrais, 1972).

Spinal Cord Injury (SCI)

Injury to the spinal cord, either by disease or trauma, can produce permanent neuromuscular disorders. Adaptation to an SCI requires significant levels of fitness and a continually vigilant program to maintain overall health and function.

Etiology of SCI

Spinal cord injury is most frequently the result of trauma from a car/motorcycle accident (39 percent), jumps and falls (16 percent), gunshot wounds (13 percent) and diving accidents (9 percent) (O'Sullivan & Schmitz, 1994). Nontraumatic injuries to the spine are caused by a vascular malfunction (a bone or joint subluxation) due to overriding disease such as rheumatoid arthritis, an infection such as syphilis or a tumor. Nontraumatic SCIs account for only 30 percent of the total number of injuries (O'Sullivan & Schmitz, 1994). The majority are related to trauma from reckless behavior.

Spinal cord lesions result in two primary disabilities. Quadriplegia refers to loss of movement in the trunk and all four extremities that results from lesions in the cervical cord. Paraplegia

Spinal Cord Injury

affects only a part of the trunk and the lower extremities, resulting from lesions below the cervical section of the spinal cord. A complete lesion results in no motor or sensory function below the level of the injury. Injuries that occur from bruising or crushing create a mixture of symptoms and are followed by some level of recovery that usually begins after the spinal shock stage (24 to 48 hours). Spinal shock occurs immediately following injury and is evidenced by a loss of all reflexes, flaccid paralysis and loss of sensation below the level of injury. Following this phase, there is a consistent progression in improvement that eventually plateaus within months. When no improvement is noted for several weeks the plateau has been reached, and additional spontaneous recovery is not common. However, the client's functional status can improve as they learn adaptive skills. Discussion in this chapter is limited to paraplegia that does not include primary respiratory impairment.

Rehabilitation Programs

Acute injuries require an intense rehabilitation program to stabilize the patient, and to prevent further injury or disability. The therapist works to facilitate deep breathing, provide range-of-motion and strengthening exercises, teach skin care and transfer techniques, and provide and instruct in the use of assistive devices to facilitate activities of daily living. Emphasis is on restoring function and/or teaching adaptation techniques. If your client has recently sustained an SCI, you will need to be more vigilant about their response to a program and work closely with the rehabilitation team. Clients who have completed a progressive rehabilitation program may access your services to maintain their fitness level much like any other "able-bodied" client. In fact, many individuals with SCI consider themselves able-bodied, and work, raise families, and participate in sports and recreational activities.

Movement Disorders with SCI

Spasticity occurs in SCI because the stretch reflex is released from central nervous system control. Spasticity tends to occur after the initial spinal shock subsides, gradually increases for a few months after injury and usually peaks within the first year following the injury. Severe spasticity is managed with drug therapy and, in some extreme cases, surgery to release muscles and tendons or to destroy nerve tissue (rhizotomy). Refer to previous discussion of spasticity for management recommendations.

Flaccid paralysis also may occur and should be managed with support and range of motion as discussed previously.

Functional Impairments with SCI

Clients with SCI may suffer from bladder and bowel dysfunction, sexual dysfunction, pressure sores and **autonomic dysreflexia**. Autonomic dysreflexia is an abnormal autonomic reflex that occurs when the spinal cord has been injured above the sixth thoracic level. It usually subsides over time but can be life-threatening. Usually the reflex is initiated by bladder distension but can be caused by other noxious stimuli from the bladder or bowel, skin and kidneys. Symptoms of autonomic dysreflexia include hypertension, slowed heart beat, headache, sweating, increased spasticity, flushing, restlessness, nasal congestion, constricted pupils, goose bumps and blurred vision. These symptoms are signs of a medical emergency and require immediate relief and monitoring. If your client experiences any of these symptoms, call for emergency support.

Long-term inactivity can lead to heterophic bone formation, usually near large joints, which results in acute swelling, decreases in range of motion, and redness and warmth around the joint. Formation of heterophic bone usually does not cause significant functional limitations but requires routine range-of-motion exercise to maintain flexibility.

Inactivity also may cause a deep-vein thrombosis or clot that forms in the blood vessels of the lower extremities. If the clot breaks free, it becomes an **embolus**, which can be life-threatening. Clots form because blood flow is decreased without normal lower-extremity muscle activity. Also, prolonged pressure can damage a vessel and result in a clot. Signs of a deep-vein thrombosis (DVT) are local swelling, redness and heat. Watch for these symptoms and report them to your client's physician immediately. Most DVTs occur early in recovery but onset is not limited. Never exercise or perform range-of-motion exercises with an extremity if you suspect the presence of DVT.

Pain associated with SCI, other than that caused in the initial trauma, usually is the result of damage to a nerve root. Nerve root pain is described as sharp, stabbing, burning or shooting pain along the area innervated by the nerve. It most commonly occurs after injuries to the **cauda equina**, the lowest portion of the spinal cord where there is a high density of nerve roots (Nepomuceno et al., 1979). Pain management includes drugs, electrical stimulation and surgery if it is intractable. Pain associated with **dysesthesia** (unusual sensations) also is common, and occurs in body parts otherwise lacking sensation as a feeling of numbness, tingling, burning or "pins and needles." The cause of this pain is unknown, making it difficult to treat. Involved body parts must be handled gently and positioned to diminish the sensations if possible.

Osteoporosis and subsequent bone fractures are ongoing concerns for SCI clients. Most of the osteoporotic changes occur in the first year after injury (Hancock, Reed & Atkinson, 1979). Care should be taken not to overstress a paralyzed limb.

Fitness Program Adaptations for Clients with SCI

Strength Training

It is foolish and inappropriate to try to strengthen paralyzed muscles after the initial recovery period. You can dramatically influence function, however, by maximizing your client's remaining muscle strength. Upper-extremity and trunk strength are essential for transfers, wheelchair mobility and for those clients who can walk with braces. Use common strength-training principles with the following restrictions.

- Keep in mind the danger of osteoporosis of the nonfunctional limbs.
- Don't overload or create unnecessary spinal joint stress.
- Never attempt to "stand" a client or dramatically change a weight-bearing position for a client who has been non-weight-bearing for a significant time.
- Protect the involved lower extremities from trauma. Even a dropped medicine ball or free weight could cause a fracture.
- Place the legs under a tabletop or guard your client when they are performing upper-extremity free-weight activities. Many wheelchairs come with detachable tabletops that can be used for protection.

Flexibility

Paralyzed joints should be moved through their pain-free range of motion. Don't forget the importance of spine extension and rotation in the range-of-motion sequence. Clients confined to a wheelchair need to pay particular attention to spine and hip extension.

Cardiac Conditioning

An SCI should not reduce a client's incentive to perform cardiac fitness activities. Exercise bikes and other equipment can be adapted to provide a sufficient cardiac workout. Pushing a wheelchair in laps, much like running or race walking, is a good option for a cardiac workout. Wheelchair basketball and volleyball leagues are fun and provide a vigorous workout. If you can't find enough SCI participants to make a full team, get your friends and associates to try playing while confined to a chair (you can immobilize their legs with straps to increase the difficulty)!

Posture

All the standard principles apply to areas above the level of injury. Good posture is essential for good respiration and digestion, so incorporate deep-breathing and postural exercises in your warm-up routines.

Nutrition

It is recommend that SCI clients eat a diet restricted in calcium and generous in protein. It also is recommended they consume additional fluids to prevent renal stones. After SCI, substantial bone loss leads to an excess of calcium in the urinary system, which creates a predisposition to stone formation (Maynard & Imai, 1977).

General Well-being

SCI clients face a life-long challenge to maintain their health. They must consistently avoid bone fractures, urinary infections, respiratory infections and pressure sores. Despite these setbacks, most embrace life and adapt to their disabilities. Should one of the above problems lead to hospitalization, a SCI client will be deconditioned on discharge. Even a few days of inactivity can have an effect, and they will need your services to regain their full function.

Pressure sores (**decubitus ulcers**) are one of the biggest challenges facing individuals with SCI. They result from prolonged pressure or shearing force especially over a bony prominence. Damage can occur in a relatively short period, but take a long time to heal. Pressure sore treatment is a major reason for hospitalization of SCI clients. Lack of sensory function and sometimes the inability to move lead to tissue breakdown. Continually remind clients with SCI to shift their weight. Many use special seating devices to redistribute weight. Be aware of their lack of sensation and the need to protect their involved body parts, and be cautious of shearing forces caused by tight clothing, orthotic devices or simply dragging a body part across a surface, e.g., when SCI clients are moved passively from one position to the next.

As part of the rehabilitation program, patients are taught to inspect their skin daily, watching for areas of abrasion or bruising, and adapting posture or movement to relieve stress.

Miscellaneous Disorders

Cerebral Palsy

Cerebral Palsy (CP) is a diagnosis applied to a wide group of disabilities. CP is caused by cerebral dysfunction that occurs during gestation, birth or the neonatal period (Rusk, 1964). The **etiology** of CP includes developmental deficits, vascular accidents, infections, toxins (e.g., chemical abuse by the mother), trauma and genetic factors. Symptoms are so varied that each client is unique. Thanks to modern medicine, many children with CP who would not have survived in the past are now able to lead productive lives. You may encounter a client with a history of mild or moderate CP who is affected with the movement disorders noted above. Since CP is associated with birth, these clients have had ample time to adapt. Most have had extensive therapy in a mandated, federally funded school program.

Much of the science and art of therapeutic exercise owes its roots to the study of treatment for the child with CP. These clients may teach you what works best for them, which may be invaluable when treating other clients with similar symptoms.

Post-polio Syndrome

The polio epidemic that occurred in the U.S. during the 1940s and '50s left an estimated 1.6 million survivors who may suffer from post-polio syndrome. Thanks to mass immunization that began in the mid 1960s, new cases are rare in the U.S. Comments in this section are limited to post-polio syndrome.

Polio is caused by an acute viral infection that attacks the central nervous system in the spinal cord. The primary neuromuscular disorder is muscle weakness and sometimes total paralysis. Polio survivors may have normal muscle mass and strength, despite a loss of more than 50 percent of the motor units involved (Trojan, 1997). Post-polio clients may note new symptoms, including muscle atrophy and loss of strength over time. Studies have demonstrated that the average polio survivor has 50 percent normal strength in the quadriceps (Agre, 1998). Post-polio clients have difficulty performing endurance activities because they lack an enzyme involved in aerobic metabolism (Trojan, 1997). In addition, they have deficits in muscle-work capacity and strength recovery after activity. However, research supports the use of fitness programs for improving muscle strength, flexibility and cardiac endurance in post-polio clients.

Post-polio clients who monitor their fatigue level and adjust their workout accordingly can participate in all types of activities without risk of injury. If excessive fatigue or fibromyalgic complaints limit participation, clients can benefit from a short course of reduced activity with frequent rest periods. In fact, the exercise program may differ for each limb depending on its functional capabilities and disease status. Table 20.3 portrays a classification system that can be applied to each limb, with exercise guidelines for each classification.

Investigation of pharmacological treatment of post-polio syndrome is being conducted. Drugs are being used to improve neuromuscular-tissue exercise recovery and pain relief. Drugs used to treat Parkinson's disease have shown merit in enhancing post-exercise recovery (Bamford, 1993) in individuals with post-polio syndrome.

Peripheral Neuropathies

Injury of a peripheral nerve or nerve root results in paralysis of the muscle supplied, loss of sensation, and trophic or nutritional changes to the tissue surrounding the innervated area.

Usually a peripheral neuropathy is caused by pressure, trauma or entrapment. Prolonged pressure, such as from a **herniated disk** or bony formation in the spine, a cast, or an ill-fitted ski boot, can cause peripheral neuropathy. Most of the symptoms subside when the pressure is released. Long-term damage will result in localized dysfunction in the form of paralysis, sensory loss and eventual muscle contractures.

Carpal Tunnel Syndrome (CTS) is an example of a peripheral neuropathy caused by entrapment of the median nerve at the wrist. Clients with CTS should avoid weightlifting during acute flare-up. They should also avoid wrist flexion, forearm supination and pressure to the base of the palm such as when leaning on the handle bars of a bike or treadmill.

Causalgia is another example of a peripheral neuropathy and usually occurs in the median or sciatic nerve (Bannister, 1973). Causalgia symptoms are intense burning pain; pink, sweating, tight skin; and loss of sensation. Clients are protective of the involved body part as any movement or touch may elicit more pain. Nerve blocks and occasionally medication are the treatments of choice.

Epilepsy

Epilepsy is a seizure disorder caused by the misfiring of electrical impulses in the brain. The electrical impulses may misfire due to neurochemical disorders. Symptoms depend on the area of the brain affected, but may include a loss of consciousness, changes in muscle tone and sensory disturbances. Symptoms may last for seconds or minutes. Summon emergency support if a seizure is severe or prolonged or if your client has no known history of seizures. Epileptic seizures range from petit mal (minor) to grand mal. Seizures may begin with an aura or warning of the attack. Usually, a symptom is perceived by the individual before the seizure begins. Examples of auras are a specific odor, a visual disturbance, a taste or a feeling such as fear. Sometimes these warnings are perceived enough in advance to allow the individual to warn others that a seizure is pending.

Epilepsy is caused by a variety of conditions including a lack of blood supply or oxygen to the brain, low blood sugar or other metabolic imbalances, a high fever especially in children, trauma, exposure to toxins, drug or alcohol abuse, or a tumor.

Most epilepsy can be controlled with medication. Surgery is an option for rare and severe

Table 20.3
Post-polio Classifications

Class	Description	Intensity	Duration	Frequency
I	no clinical pathology in the limb	6-9 METS	15-30 min./session	3-5/wk
II	EMG evidence, but no clinical symptoms in the limb	5-7 METS	15-30 min./session, paced at 4-5 min. of exercise to 1 min. rest periods	3-4/wk
III	clinically stable polio, no new dysfunction noted	4-5 METS	15-20 min./day, paced in 2-3 min. of exercise and 1 min. rest periods	3-4/wk
IV	clinically unstable	stretching, activities of daily living and gentle nonfatiguing exercise	to tolerance	daily
V	severe polio	activities of daily living and support	to tolerance	as needed

Source: Agre, 1998

cases. Aside from the risk of injury, controlling seizures is important because repeat seizures can cause long-term neurological deficits most commonly in cognitive functions (especially memory and learning skills). A ketogenic diet is rich in lipids and oils and low in protein and carbohydrates, and may increase the seizure threshold in some individuals (usually children), but should only be attempted with medical supervision.

If a seizure occurs in your presence, follow these guidelines:

➤ Stay calm so that you can best support or protect your client.
➤ Get your client to a safe position. The floor is best. Don't try to lift them alone. Instead, attempt to roll or lower them to a safe position. Get help if possible.
➤ Remove any restrictive clothing, and clear away any items that might fall, hit or otherwise injure your client during the seizure.
➤ Don't place anything in your client's mouth, including your fingers. Swallowing the tongue is anatomically impossible.
➤ Once the seizure has subsided, gently turn your client on their side or stomach with their face turned to one side to let saliva and possibly vomit run freely from the mouth. Quietly reassure your client that everything is fine.
➤ Your client will be groggy, weak and possibly confused following a seizure. Be sure to allow adequate recovery time before moving them from the resting position.

There are no movement disorders specific to epilepsy. If your client has a history of seizures, discuss this history with them carefully. Do they typically have an aura or warning sign? Have they been able to warn others of a seizure onset in the past? Are there sensory stimuli such as flashing lights or loud noises that have initiated a seizure in the past? How long do their seizures usually last? Do they want you to notify someone if they have a seizure during your session? Are there activities or pieces of equipment that they would consider unsafe given their experiences? Record the answers to these questions and be sure to review them with any trainer who substitutes for you. Always guard your clients with a history of seizures carefully, being close by to intervene if necessary.

Most epileptics lead normal lives and their seizures are under control with medication. However, some seizures may be exercise induced. This has been hypothesized to be due to renal drug clearance (Borchert, 1997). If the frequency or severity of your client's seizures increase during or following an exercise session, consult with their physician.

Summary

Neuromuscular disorders can cause a wide array of symptoms and movement deficits. Adaptation is the key for both the client and the trainer. Success often is measured in small pleasures and gains, and what may seem insignificant to you may be inspiring to your client. Be patient, caring and continuously on the alert for positive change. Focus on what they can do and support the spirit of their effort. Champions are unique in their abilities, but they share the desire and the determination to maximize every potential.

References

Agre (1998). Exercising judgment. *Advance for Directors in Rehabilitation.* February.

American Physical Therapy Association (1997). Guide to Physical Therapy Practice. *Physical Therapy,* 77, 11, 1371.

Bamford (1993). Post polio syndrome response to deprenyl. *International Journal of Neuroscience,* 71, 183-88.

Bannister (1973). *Brains Clinical Neurology.* New York: Oxford University Press.

Berger (1985). Impaired swallowing and excessive drooling in Parkinson's Disease. *Parkinson Report.* Miami, Fla.: National Parkinson Foundation.

Borchert (1997). Exercise-induced exacerbation of partial seizures due to enhanced gavapentin clearance. Valhalla, N.Y.: Department of Neurology, New York Medical College.

Bowen (1967). Behavioral alterations in patients with basal ganglia lesions. Yahr (Ed.) *The Basal Ganglia.* New York: Raven Press.

Bridgewater & Sharpe (1998). Trunk muscle performance in early Parkinson's Disease. *Physical Therapy,* 78, 6, 566-575.

Calliets, R. (1981). *Shoulder Pain.* Philadelphia, Pa.: F.A. Davis Co.

Chusid (1976). *Correlative Neuroanatomy & Functional Neurology,* 16th ed. Los Altos, Calif.: Lange Medical Publications.

Ciccone (1988). Free radical toxicity and antioxidant medications in Parkinson's Disease. *Physical Therapy,* 78, 313-319.

Cocchi (1997). Putting mobility to the test. *Advance for Directors in Rehabilitation.* October.

Cohen (1991). Tremors and the Parkinson patients. *Parkinson Report.* Miami, Fla.: National Parkinson Foundation.

Daviddoff et al. (1991). Acute stroke patients long-term effects for rehabilitation and maintenance of gains. *Archives of Physical and Medical Rehabilitation,* 72, 869.

Di Fabio, Choi, Soderberg & Hansen (1997). Health-related quality of life for patients with progressive multiple sclerosis: Influence of rehabilitation. *Physical Therapy,* 77, 1704-1715.

Eliasson, Prensky & Hardin (1978). *Neurological Pathophysiology,* 2nd ed. New York: Oxford University Press.

Feldenkrais (1972). *Awareness Through Movement: Health Exercises for Personal Growth.* New York: Harper & Row.

Florance & Hagberg (1984). Effect of training on the exercise response of neuromuscular disease patients. *Medicine and Science in Sports and Exercise,* 16, 460-465.

Franklin, et al. (1989). Cognitive loss in multiple sclerosis. *Archives of Neurology,* 46,162.

Gatz (1975). *Manters Essentials of Clinical Neuroanatomy and Neurophysiology,* 5th ed. Philadelphia, Pa.: F.A. Davis Co.

Hancock, Reed & Atkinson (1979). Bone and soft tissue changes in paraplegic patients. *Paraplegia,* 17, 267.

Jankovic (1987). Pathophysiology and clinical assessment of motor symptoms in Parkinsons disease. Koller (Ed.) *Handbook of Parkinsons Disease.* New York: Marcel Dekker.

Katz (1998). Neurorehab and TBI. *Rehab Management,* Feb/March.

Kilmer (1994). *Archives of Physical and Medical Rehabilitation,* 75, 560-563.

Lechtenberg (1988). *Multiple Sclerosis Fact Book.* Philadelphia, Pa.: F.A. Davis Co..

Lewis (1996). Testing and treating static and dynamic balance problems. *Advance for Physical Therapists,* Dec.

Lewis (1997b). Using modalities in stretching of elderly. *Advance for Physical Therapists,* June 2.

Lewis (1998). Using strength training as treatment post stroke. *Advance for Physical Therapists,* May.

Mayeux (1987). Mental state. Koller(Ed.) *Handbook of Parkinsons Disease.* New York: Marcel Dekker.

Maynard & Imai (1977). Immobilization hypercalcemia in spinal cord injury. *Archives of Physical and Medical Rehabilitation,* 58, 16.

McIntosh, Brown, Rice & Thaut (1997). Rhythmic auditory-motor facilitation of gait patterns in patients with Parkinson's Disease. *Journal of Neurology, Neurosurgery and Psychiatry,* 62, 22-26.

Nepomuceno, et al. (1979). Pain in patients with spinal cord injury. *Archives of Physical and Medical Rehabilitation,* 60, 605.

O'Sullivan & Schmitz (1994). *Physical Rehabilitation Assessment and Treatment,* 3rd ed. Philadelphia. Pa.: F.A. Davis Co.

Pal Brar & Wangaard (1985). Physical therapy for patients with multiple sclerosis. Maloney, Burks & Ringel (Eds.) *Interdisciplinary Rehabilitation of Multiple Sclerosis and Neuromuscular Disorders.* Philadelphia, Pa.: JB Lippincott.

Pederson (1995).The soothing effects of rocking as determined by the direction and frequency of movement. *Canadian Journal of Behavioral Science,* 7, 237.

Peterson & Kokmen (1989). Cognitive and psychiatric abnormalities in multiple sclerosis. *Mayo Clinical Procedures,* 64, 657.

PT Bulletin (August 1, 1997). Scientists identify Parkinson's Gene. American Physical Therapy Association. Alexandria, Va.

PT Bulletin (September 12, 1997). Recent Study Shows Three Days Rest Necessary after a Mild Head Injury. American Physical Therapy Association. Alexandria, Va.

PT Bulletin (April 24, 1998). Early Results Promising in Parkinson's Research. American Physical Therapy Association. Alexandria, Va.

PT Bulletin (May 29, 1998). Nerve Fibers Regrown in Rats; Hope Seen for Spinal Injuries; and Many Strokes Occur in Morning. American Physical Therapy Association. Alexandria, Va.

Rusk (1964). *Rehabilitation Medicine,* 2nd ed. St. Louis, Mo.: C.V. Mosby Co.

Schenkman et al. (1989). Management of individuals with Parkinson's Disease: Rationale and case studies. *Physical Therapy,* 69, 944.

Smithson, Morris & Iansek (1998). Performance on clinical tests of balance in Parkinson's disease. *Physical Therapy,* 78,6, 577-592.

Spedinoff & Cava (1995). BTX: Miracle drug for managing muscle spasticity. *Advance/Rehabilitation,* April.

Stables & Lincoln (1979). Intellectual impairment in multiple sclerosis and its relation to functional abilities. *Rheumatology and Rehabilitation,* 18, 153-160.

Stockmeyer (1967). An interpretation of the approach of Rood to the treatment of neuromuscular dysfunction. *American Journal of Physical Medicine,* 46, 900.

Tangeman, Banaitis & Williams (1998). Rehabilitation of chronic stroke patients: Changes in functional performance. *Archives of Physical and Medical Rehabilitation,* 71, 876.

Torance & Hagberg (1984). Effect of training on the exercise response of neuromuscular disease patients. *Medicine and Science in Sports and Exercise,* 16, 460-465.

Van Allen (1971). *Pictorial Manual of Neurologic Tests.* Chicago, Ill.: Year Book Medical Publishers Inc.

Voss, Ionta & Myers (1985). *Proprioceptive Neuromuscular Facilitation,* 3rd ed. New York: Harper & Row.

Suggested Reading:

O'Sullivan & Schmitz (1994). *Physical Rehabilitation Assessment and Treatment*. 3rd ed. Philadelphia, Pa.: F.A. Davis Co.
   A comprehensive text on rehabilitation management of adults that serves as a reference for rehabilitation professionals and provides trainers working with post-rehabilitation clients a thorough understanding of rehabilitation topics as they apply to specific conditions.

Umphred, D. (Ed.) (1985). *Neurological Rehabilitation*. St. Louis, Mo.: Mosby.
   A comprehensive text specifically addressing neurologic conditions.

Voss, Ionta & Myers (1985). *Proprioceptive Neuro-muscular Facilitation*. 3rd ed. New York: Harper & Row.
   A text addressing a therapeutic exercise model that is particularly effective in dealing with neurologically impaired patients. Basic techniques of therapeutic exercise are explained, and the use of diagonal movement patterns that are especially effective in working with clients with spasticity is demonstrated.

Section Seven

Exercise Following Orthopedic Rehabilitation

CHAPTER 21

Low-back Pain

M. DARRYL ANTONACCI
STEPHEN I. ESSES
HAROLD W. KOHL, III

M. Darryl Antonacci, M.D. graduated from Georgetown University School of Medicine in 1992. He completed six years formal surgical residency training in Orthopedic Surgery at the Baylor College of Medicine in Houston, Texas. In addition to his surgical interest in disorders of the spine, Dr. Antonacci has published several research articles about the spine, and has been awarded the Paul Harrington Award for excellence in research on two different occasions. Currently, Dr. Antonacci is the Fellow in spine surgery at the University of Miami-Jackson Memorial Hospital.

Stephen I. Esses, M.D., is a professor of clinical orthopedic surgery at Baylor College of Medicine in Houston, Texas, where he is deputy chief of the Department of Orthopedic Surgery. Dr. Esses also serves on the staff of several Houston hospitals and in 1991 was the recipient of a Cervical Spine Research Society Award.

Harold W. Kohl III, Ph.D., is director of research at Baylor Sports Medicine Institute in Houston, Texas. Dr. Kohl was the principal investigator and founder of the Baylor Outcomes in Orthopedic Medicine Study. He is on the editorial staff of Medicine and Science in Sports and Exercise and the Clinical Journal of Sport Medicine, and is a member of the Bone, Muscle and Exercise Integrated Product Team of the NASA/Johnson Space Center Space Medicine Project.

Sciatica
Chronic
Low-back Pain
Program Design

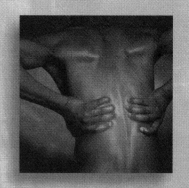

I n the United States, musculoskeletal complaints are the most common reason for patients to seek consultation from their primary care physician. Back-related symptoms are among the most expensive musculoskeletal afflictions, and low-back pain is the most common symptom in that group of patients. It is estimated that 80 percent of adults in North America will have at least one episode of low-back pain sufficiently severe that they lose time from work. In Americans younger than 45 years of age, the most common cause of disability is back complaints. The cost of low-back pain in the United States as a result of time lost from work and permanent disability is estimated to be $75 billion per year

(Esses, 1995; Macnab, 1977; Garfin & Vaccaro, 1977).

Back complaints can generally be categorized into one of three presentations: **acute low-back pain, chronic low-back pain** and back pain in association with leg pain, or **sciatica**. Rehabilitation of patients with back complaints includes accurate diagnosis and comprehensive early intervention. The goals of intervention are primarily directed toward improvement of function, rather than just treating pain. Frequently, return of function minimizes the associated complaints of pain (Hansen et al., 1993; Malmivaara et al., 1995; Manniche et al., 1991).

The following chapter will first discuss the most common causes of low-back pain and their interventions. It will conclude with a more specific discussion of the exercise considerations and select case studies.

Acute Low-back Pain

Acute low-back pain is nonspecific low-back pain of six weeks duration or less. It is not usually necessary to make a specific diagnosis for those patients presenting simply with acute low-back pain. It is important, however, to determine if there is radiation of the back pain into the legs, or to determine that the patient does not have any systemic symptoms indicative of an infective or neoplastic process. In most instances, the pain is the result of musculoskeletal strain (Esses, 1995; Macnab, 1977; Garfin & Vaccaro, 1977). Acute back pain is typically mechanical in nature. That is, it is activity related. Patients feel better at rest, and bending, twisting and lifting exacerbates symptoms. On further questioning, it is often possible to elicit a history of back strain or a preceding strenuous activity not typically performed by the patient.

Additionally, a history of trauma or low-back pain that is not activity related are causes for physician referral. Diagnosis of an acute exacerbation of back pain includes a physical, a thorough neurologic examination, and evaluation of the hip, sacroiliac and knee joints.

Many studies have shown that acute low-back pain is usually a limited process. Symptoms can be expected to resolve in 80 percent of patients within four to six weeks. It is not certain whether any specific modality can accelerate this process

(Macnab, 1977; Hansen et al., 1993; Malmivaara et al., 1995; Deyo et al., 1986). There is inadequate data to define which patients and what type of interventions are effective. The purpose of initiating treatment is to provide symptomatic relief and to prevent retardation of the healing process.

The triad of treatment is activity modification, physical modalities and medication. Whereas activity modification often consisted of prolonged bed rest in the past, it is now generally agreed prolonged bed restriction can slow recovery and may lead to debilitation (Malmivaara et al., 1995; Deyo et al., 1986). Certain postures may aggravate their condition. That is, sitting may place more stress on the low back than standing or lying (Esses, 1995; Garfin & Vaccaro, 1997), and forward flexion may increase low-back loads. Patients are encouraged to assume whatever position provides them with maximal comfort. The most beneficial treatment in the first six weeks may be preventive education (Garfin & Vaccaro, 1997).

Physical modalities have been advocated for the treatment of acute low-back pain. Most are not justified by scientific study (Garfin & Vaccaro, 1997). There is good evidence that cryotherapy and heat, in conjunction with exercise, are of some benefit. A short course of supervised physical therapy may be prescribed to specifically educate the patient how to use heat and cold options at home together with an exercise program (Garfin & Vaccaro, 1997; Hansen et al., 1993; Manniche et al., 1991). A physician or therapist only should initiate this treatment.

Three groups of medications may be of value in the treatment of acute low-back pain: analgesics, nonsteroidal anti-inflammatory agents and muscle relaxants. Side effects of these drugs vary. Up to 50 percent of patients taking muscle relaxants have significant complaints of drowsiness and fatigue.

Chronic Low-back Pain

An orthopedic surgeon specializing in spinal surgery commonly assesses patients with chronic symptoms. Most instances of chronic low-back pain in the adult are thought to be due to degenerative disk disease. Other causes include spondylolisthesis, spinal stenosis, herniated nucleus pulposus (herniated disc) and degenerative scoliosis. For the purpose of this discussion, only patients with isolated back pain are considered. Patients who have **radicular** symptoms (sciatica) are discussed under a separate heading. Some of the exercise information contained in this chapter does not apply to diagnosis of spondylolisthesis, spinal stenosis, herniated disc and degenerative scoliosis.

A thorough history and physical examination, including imaging modalities, are used in the work-up of the chronic low-back pain sufferer. After evaluation by a physician, most patients can be adequately treated similar to patients with acute back pain. That is, by the triad of lifestyle modification, physical modalities and medication. In terms of lifestyle modification, activities and work that require prolonged sitting, activities and work that require repetitive bending, and activities and work that involve vibration have been shown to be associated with an increased frequency of chronic low-back pain or recurrent acute exacerbations of pain. (Esses, 1995; Macnab, 1977) Therefore, low-back pain sufferers are encouraged to reduce these activities. In addition, the evidence is clear that smoking increases the risk for chronic low-back pain, and tobacco and nicotine use in any form is discouraged.

The mainstay of physical modalities for the patient with chronic low-back pain or recurrent episodes of acute pain is exercise (Hansen et al., 1993; Manniche et al., 1991). The frequency and severity of chronic low-back pain are decreased in individuals who exhibit good cardiovascular fitness, strong abdominal musculature and good paravertebral strength. Patients are usually made aware of this by their physician or therapist and instructed to carry out a balanced, organized and regular exercise program.

For those patients whose symptoms are not adequately controlled by the triad of treatment described, other nonoperative options are considered. These may include pain management techniques such as biofeedback, transcutaneous electrical nerve stimulation, acupuncture, lumbar orthoses and manipulation (Garfin & Vaccaro, 1997; Saal & Saal, 1989; Saal et al., 1990).

Low-back Pain and Sciatica

A clear distinction should be made between those patients presenting with back pain and those patients presenting with back and leg symptoms. If the leg complaints follow a specific pattern into the leg, it is most likely radicular. The term radicular refers to symptoms that are of nerve root origin. Consequently, the pattern of disturbance follows the path of enervation of the particular nerve root involved. Pain, sensory disturbances (e.g. numbness, tingling, cramping) and motor weakness along a particular radicular distribution are the hallmarks of nerve root irritation. This is commonly referred to as sciatica. An orthopedic surgeon should evaluate most patients with sciatica or significant radicular symptoms. The physical evaluation of the patient consists of a careful neurologic examination and peripheral vascular examination to rule out a circulatory origin of symptoms.

Leg pain from a herniated nucleus pulposus can almost always be treated nonoperatively, since over time, the herniated disk tends to resorb and/or cause a limited inflammatory reaction (Saal & Saal, 1989; Saal et al., 1990; Bush et al., 1992). Physical modalities including exercise, epidural steroids, nerve root block, and nonsteroidal anti-inflammatory agents can be useful in this regard. Nonoperative treatment is less successful in patients with leg complaints due to bony spinal stenosis (Johnsson et al., 1993). Patients who have significant neurologic deficit, have intractable pain and are functionally disabled are considered for surgery.

Exercise and Low-back Pain

Exercise, in addition to oral pharmacotherapy, injections, manipulation, physical agents, biofeedback and prolonged bed rest, has been the subject of some scientific inquiry for its role in rehabilitation of acute low-back pain. Typically however, exercise has been part of multifactorial approaches to rehabilitation that have included ergonomic education and motivation and counseling, making it difficult to specifically isolate any independent effects of the exercise regimens. There have been several randomized prospective studies conducted regarding exercise and spinal rehabilitation (Tuomey & Taylor, 1995). Most of the research in the literature supports the efficacy of exercise.

It is generally agreed that strong abdominal musculature and strong paravertebral musculature will decrease the instance of acute low-back pain. This is because there is no intrinsic structural integrity to the spinal column. Maintenance of posture and the ability to move in three planes is provided by the surrounding musculature. It is crucial, therefore, that the paravertebral muscles are healthy and strong. Weakness in the back extensor musculature has been associated with an increased incidence of chronic back pain (Campello et al., 1996).

Therefore, a regular organized exercise program is conducive to maintenance of function. A strengthening program has been shown to decrease pain frequency and pain scores in patients who have chronic back pain (Ljunggren et al., 1997). Movement has been shown to be of benefit to the nutrition of the intervertebral discs and influences the neurophysiologic perception of pain. In all cases, a physician or therapist should supervise this activity to ensure its appropriateness.

Some patients who suffer from a spinal malignancy or infectious process will not benefit from an exercise program. A physician should refer all individuals with complaints of low-back pain who are to be started on an exercise program. In this way conditions that can potentially be made worse by exercise and conditions that will not respond to mobilization can be identified.

The therapist should outline specific objectives of the exercise program for the trainer. In most instances the objectives will include relief of pain, increased muscular strength, increased range of motion, and improved functions such as walking, standing and bending. The principle of exercise training is to create a mobile and stable functional range of motion (Davies et al., 1979).

Physicians and therapists recommend two main programs of exercise: a program specifically designed to improve trunk, extensor and abdominal muscular strength, and a program of general cardiovascular endurance. The specific program design is aimed at decreasing the forces of the spinal column since many instances of low-back pain are due to intervertebral disc pathology. By strengthening the muscles surrounding the spinal column one can decrease the stress on these discs and, therefore, decrease pain. Small increases in abdominal muscular strength will result in large decreases in spinal column stress. The reason for this is that there is a moment arm from the spinal column to the anterior abdominal wall. Shortening this moment arm significantly decreases spinal load.

It has been shown that individuals with increased general fitness and endurance are less prone to back problems (Cady et al., 1979). Traditionally, both flexion and extension exercises have been investigated and recommended for low-back pain of both acute and chronic nature. Flexion exercises are designed to train and maintain the spinal flexor muscles, primarily those in the abdominal region, thus helping to prevent an anterior displacement of

Table 21.1

Typical Activity Guidelines

- Monitor all activity for complaints of pain, weakness and radicular symptoms.
- Sitting exercises may place more stress on the low back than standing or lying.
- Avoid prolonged sitting, repetitive bending or vibration.
- Emphasize cardiovascular conditioning, abdominal and paravetebral strength, and lower extremity flexibility.

- Educate clients on proper body mechanics, postural awareness and dynamic lumbar stabilization.
- Monitor body mechanics and postural position during all activities.
- Short-term goals are to reinforce skills and training exercises initiated in therapy.
- Long-term goals include functional flexibility and strength and adherence to a regular exercise program.

the center of gravity associated with sedentary living. Theoretically, this anterior displacement of the abdomen over time is compensated by a posterior shift in the thorax, results in an increasing force on the lumbosacral and posterior lumbar structures, and places a person at risk for a back impairment should a sudden or severe force be applied (Williams, 1955). Extension exercises, on the other hand, are designed to strengthen and maintain the back extensors, helping to maintain lumbar lordosis and alignment of the spine (McKenzie, 1979).

Safety is a concern for all participants in exercise programs and is of special concern to patients with low-back pain. Of primary interest are increases in mechanical stresses to the spine with various postures or loadings during exercise that will result in increased intradiscal pressures and potentially increased neurologic involvement. There is some evidence that hyperflexion can increase intradiscal pressures (Nachemson, 1976). When working with a low-back pain patient, the exercise professional should be aware of any changes or worsening of symptoms, especially those that may indicate neurologic involvement (radiculopathy). Patients with a spinal stenosis or herniated nucleus pulposus may be at risk for worsening symptoms. As the exercise protocol progresses, should any evidence of neurologic involvement occur, the patient should be referred to his or her physician for evaluation and possible imaging studies.

Program Design

The short-term goals for the personal trainer should focus on reinforcing the skills and training exercises that were begun by the therapist. The long-term objectives are soft tissue extensibility within functional limits, an ability to complete all functional activities without limitations, and achievement of a trunk strength and lower-extremity strength within functional limits. The program involves a recommended frequency of exercise regimens two to three times per week with a progressive increase in dose as appropriate.

Exercise programming involves a continuation of low-back and leg stretching and strengthening, postural stabilization, and endurance activities. Specific muscles on which to concentrate stretching activities are the iliopsoas, hamstrings, piriformis, gluteal complex, quadriceps and quadratus lumborum. Postural stabilization progressions include concentration on areas relevant to the low back and trunk musculature including hamstrings, quadriceps, low back extensors and trunk flexors. Submaximal strengthening and endurance activities should be continued (and progressed) as tolerated. These include weight circuits or possibly elastic resistance exercises and a continuation of aerobic training (walking program and/or stationary cycling). As a client progresses, occupational as well as functional demands should be integrated into the exercise routine.

An important role of the trainer working with a client with a history of low-back pain is that of an educator. In addition to the times spent with a trainer, most of the client's day, including many activities of daily living that may place a substantial stress on the lower back, will be spent unsupervised. The important knowledge and skills that must be reinforced during exercise consist of appropriate body mechanics (including movement transitions) and postural education (including dynamic lumbar stabilization techniques) in

Table 21.2

Client Information to Obtain from Medical Professionals

1) Are there any contraindicated exercises?

2) Are there any exercises specifically indicated?

3) Are there any range of motion or spinal loading limitations?

4) What signs and symptoms should be monitored for referral or program modification?

5) Are there any exercise-related side effects to the client's medication? (e.g. change in heart rate or blood pressure response or fatigue)

order to protect from relapse and allow for unimpeded progression.

Case Studies

Case Study 1

Lisa, a 45-year-old overweight female with chronic low-back pain has decided to begin an exercise program to lose weight on the advice of her physician and therapist. She has no previous exercise history and has become increasingly inactive due to her low-back pain. Physical therapy reduced her symptoms to localized discomfort and she is afraid of making her back worse again by doing the wrong things at the gym. Lisa was released from therapy with a home exercise program that included supine pelvic tilts, crunches, several dynamic stabilization exercise, wall squats, hamstring and piriformis stretches, and 10 minutes of cycling. She has requested the help of a trainer to help her achieve her weight-loss goal without exacerbating her low-back pain.

All the exercises on Lisa's home exercise program are clearly described with illustrations, verbal cues, intensity and frequency. Additional programming is developed by the trainer to address Lisa's conditioning and weight-loss goals. The trainer initially tried aerobic exercise on a recumbent cycle; however, Lisa reported some increased pain with prolonged sitting. Several other modes of activity are tested. Treadmill walking, on a cushioned deck, provides the most comfortable aerobic exercise and is primarily utilized. The speed is kept below Lisa's stride maximum to insure that she can maintain postural alignment throughout her workout. Incline is introduced as tolerated by her conditioning as well as her low back.

A total body strength program supplements the aerobic work for weight loss and promotes more complete conditioning. Initially weights are low and repetitions are moderate to high due to Lisa's deconditioned state and to promote her learning of exercise technique. Supine or standing exercises replace seated exercises whenever possible. In the event a seated exercise is used, posture is closely monitored. Strengthening of the abdominal muscles is emphasized. Back extension exercises are cautiously introduced because Lisa's therapist did not recommend them and it is not clear if they are appropriate. Any complaints of pain, weakness, radicular symptoms or increased low-back discomfort indicate that these exercises should be discontinued.

Stretching concentrates on the iliopsoas, hamstrings, piriformis, gluteal complex, quadriceps and quadratus lumborum.

As Lisa progresses, the frequency, intensity and time will increase as tolerated. Her low-back comfort is continuously monitored. More functional exercises will be introduces as her strength improves. Proper lifting techniques and postural maintenance are always a critical concern during Lisa's workout.

Case Study 2

Your 6 a.m. client woke up with an acute onset of low-back pain. He has had episodes of this in the past and has been prescribed analgesics for these situations. His pain is isolated in his low back and he feels comfortable with attempting his workout. You have never worked with him when he has had an episode and want to be cautious with his workout to ensure that you do no harm.

His normal program consists of 30 minutes of treadmill running with variable inclines followed by a complete free-weight strength program, then stretching. You modify this program to reduce impact, unstable lifting positions and spinal loading. Additionally, stretching and abdominal work are emphasized.

His cardio workout is changed to walking on a treadmill and elliptical cross-training. Stretching is conducted after a five-minute warm-up, immediately following his cardio workout and after his strength workout. His stretching focuses on the hamstrings, quadriceps, iliopsoas, piriformis, gluteal complex and quadratus lumborum. Leg press is substituted for squats and lateral raises are substituted for overhead press to reduce spinal compression. Machine lifts are used instead of free weights to increase the stability of the lifting position and make it easier to ensure proper posture is maintained. Additional abdominal exercises are begun and mechanics of proper lifting are reviewed for use during the exercise session and daily activities.

The client is monitored for increased pain, lower extremity weakness and radicular symptoms. If any of these signs are noted, the session is ended. The trainer advises the client to avoid prolonged sitting and repetitive bending and to contact his physician if the current symptoms increase or persist.

References

Bigos, S., Bowyer, O., Braen, G., et al. (1994). Acute low back problems in adults. Clinical Practice Guideline No. 14. *AHCPR Publication No. 95-0642.* Rockville, Md.: Agency for Health Care Policy and Research, Public Health Service, U.S. Department of Health and Human Services.

Bush, K., Cowan N., and Katz, D.E. (1992). The natural history of sciatica associated with disc pathology: A prospective study with clinical and independent radiologic follow-up. *Spine,* 17, 1205-1212.

Cady, L., Bischoff, D., O'Connell, E.R., Thomas, P.C. & Allan, S.H. (1979). Strength and fitness and subsequent back injuries in firefighters. *Journal of Occupational Medicine,* 21, 269-272.

Campello, M. Norida, M. & Weiser S. (1996). Physical exercise and low back pain. *Scandinavian Journal of Medicine Science & Sports,* 6, 63-72.

Davies, J.E., Gibson, T. & Tester, L. (1979). The value of exercises in the treatment of low back pain. *Rheumatological Rehabilitation,* 18, 243-247.

Deyo, R.A., Diehl, A.K. & Rosenthal, M. (1986). How many days of bed rest for acute low back pain? A randomized clinical trial. *New England Journal of Medicine,* 315, 1064-1070.

Elnaggar, E.M., Nordin, M., Sheikhzadeh, A., Parnianpour, M. & Kahanovitz, N. (1991). Effects of spinal flexion and extension exercises on low back pain and spinal mobility in chronic low-back pain patients. *Spine,* 16, 967-972.

Esses, S.I. (1995). *Textbook of Spinal Disorders.* Philadelphia, Pa.: J.B. Lippincott Company.

Friedrich, M., Gittler, G., Halberstadt, Y., Cermak, T. & Heiller, I. (1998). Combined exercise and motivation program: effect on the compliance and level of disability of patients with chronic low back pain: a randomized controlled trial. *Archives of Physical Medicine & Rehabilitation,* 79, 475-487.

Garfin, S.R. & Vaccaro, A.R. (Eds). (1997). Spine: Orthopaedic Knowledge Update. *Spine.* Rosemont: American Academy of Orthopaedic Surgery.

Hansen, F.R., Bendix, T. & Skov, P. (1993). Intensive, dynamic back-muscle exercises, conventional physiotherapy, or placebo-control treatment of low-back pain: A randomized, observer-blind trial. *Spine,* 18, 98-108.

Johnsson, K.E., Rosen, I. & Uden, A. (1993). The natural course of lumbar spinal stenosis. *Acta Orthop Scand,* 251(suppl.), 67-68.

Ljunggren, A., Weber, J., Kogstad, O., Thom, E. & Kirkesola, C. (1997). Leave due to low back pain. *Spine,* 22, 1610-1617.

Macnab, I. (Ed.) (1977). *Backache.* Baltimore, Md.: Williams and Wilkins.

Malmivaara, A., Hakkinen, U. & Aro, T. (1995). The treatment of acute low back pain: Bed rest, exercises, or ordinary activity? *New England Journal of Medicine,* 332, 351-355.

Manniche, C., Lundberg, E. & Christenson, I. (1991). Intensive dynamic back exercises for chronic low back pain: A clinical trial. *Pain,* 47, 53-63.

McKenzie, R.A. (1979). Prophylaxis in recurrent low back pain. *New Zealand Medical Journal,* 89:22-23.

Nachemson, A.L. (1976). The lumbar spine: An orthopaedic challenge. *Spine,* 1, 1, 59-71.

Saal, J.A. & Saal, J.S. (1989). Nonoperative treatment of herniated lumbar disc with radiculapathy: An outcome study. *Spine,* 14, 431-437.

Saal, J.A., Saal, J.S. & Herzog, R.J. (1990). The natural history of lumbar intervertebral disc extrusions treated nonoperatively. *Spine,* 15, 683-686.

Sham, S.M. & Taylor, T.K.F. (1971). Tension signs in lumbar disc prolapse. *Clinical Orthopaedics,* 75, 195-205.

Tuomey L. & Taylor, J. (1995). Exercise and spinal manipulation in the treatment of low back pain. *Spine,* 20, 615-619.

Williams, P.C. (1955). Examination and conservative treatment for disc lesions of the lower spine. *Clinical Orthopedics,* 5, 28-40.

CHAPTER 22

Musculoskeletal Challenges

CHRISTINE "CC" CUNNINGHAM
LISA A. BOURAZAK

Christine "CC" Cunningham, M.S., is a NATABOC-certified athletic trainer with extensive experience as a personal trainer. Formerly the director of programming for First Fitness, Inc., she is now a private consultant specializing in fitness program development and education. She is a frequent writer and lecturer and an American Council on Exercise Master Practical Trainer.

Lisa A. Bourazak, M.P.T., C.S.C.S., is the clinic manager and practicing therapist at NovaCare Outpatient Rehabilitation in Lincolnwood, Ill. She specializes in athletic rehabilitation of lower-extremity injuries and the development of sport-specific injury prevention programs.

Exercise Guidelines

Specific Musculoskeletal Challenges

Case Studies

Clients with musculoskeletal challenges will usually come to you one of two ways. Most will present with another health challenge that is their primary concern, and through the screening and assessment process you will discover the additional musculoskeletal concern. Other clients will come to you specifically for assistance with a home program designed by their rehab therapist. Their goal will be to advance their exercise beyond that of the home program to a level of optimal function.

A joint disorder can be a past or recent injury that has resulted in an alteration in joint range of motion, strength or functional capacity when compared to the opposite side or normal ranges. Diagnosis of the disorder should be left to your client's physician. If a joint disorder is suspected, but has not yet been diagnosed, refer the client back to their physician.

The key to working with a client with a musculoskeletal concern is to gather the necessary information to develop and lead a safe and effective exercise program. A physician's referral is required of all clients with health challenges. The most important step you take in working with a client is to perform a thorough screening and report your findings to a client's primary physician to obtain a referral and guidelines based on all of the reported health challenges. Remember, when working as an ACE-certified Clinical Exercise Specialist, you are supporting your client's efforts to return to a physically active lifestyle after they have completed their treatment and/or rehabilitation. This is in contrast to the treatment and/or rehabilitation focus of a physician or physical therapist. While every client who reports a musculoskeletal challenge will not require program modifications, it is your responsibility to report the results of your screening to their physician in order to receive clearance for the client to exercise without limitations.

Your goal is to create a program that helps the client achieve their fitness goals and follow a home exercise program without exacerbating the existing disorder. The exercises you choose must adhere to the guidelines provided by the client's healthcare professional. Exercise program design is based on the following factors:

➤ type of injury
➤ severity of injury
➤ phase of healing and rehabilitation
➤ extent and type of treatment, if any (surgery, physical therapy)
➤ client's pre-injury level of function (competitive athlete vs. sedentary individual)

These factors combine to create a profile of the disorder that determines the appropriate guidelines for exercises. Due to the complexity and number of variables related to each factor, exercise guidelines should be defined by your client's physician or, if appropriate, physical therapist. The 10-Step Decision-Making Process outlined in Appendix A is a model for screening, information gathering and program design.

Obtaining Exercise Guidelines

When you contact a healthcare professional to obtain the appropriate exercise guidelines, ask the following questions:

1. Are there any recommended or contraindicated exercises? A home exercise program provided by a healthcare professional will provide the current recommended exercises. If the program is old or is easily completed by the client, obtain an updated program. The home program must provide a detailed description of the desired exercise and equipment used. Check to make sure any equipment changes, such as a different type of resistance, are appropriate.

If the client is released without exercise restrictions, it is possible that the healthcare professional may not be aware of the various exercise techniques and equipment available in a fitness environment. Their assessment of the possible exercise activities may be limited to what they are familiar with, which may lead them to overlook a possible exercise contraindication. Conversely, advancements in exercise equipment may provide exercise options that are superior to those mentioned by the healthcare professional. Use the information obtained from the following questions to determine if specific exercises are safe and affective for the disorder.

Table 22.1

Client Information to Obtain from Medical Professionals

1) Are there any recommended or contraindicated exercises?	during strength training or cardiovascular exercise?
2) Is there a limitation in range of motion the joint can be worked through for strength training, stretching or cardiovascular exercise?	4) What are the expected gains in flexibility and strength, and the rate at which they are expected to occur?
3) Is there a limitation on loading of the joint	5) What joint-specific signs and symptoms should be monitored?

2. Is there a limitation in joint range of motion for strength training, stretching or cardiovascular exercise? Some disorders may require that the joint be limited to activity through less than the normal range of motion. These limitations are often designed to protect surgical repairs or to minimize the likelihood of additional damage to joint structures. If limitations are placed on the joint range of motion, adherence to the restrictions in all exercise activities is essential. Whenever possible, use mechanical methods to control range of motion (e.g., pin stops on knee extension), and spot the client closely.

3. Is there a limitation on loading of the joint during strength training or cardiovascular exercise? Load limits may refer to the amount of loading, the frequency of loading or the method of loading (open vs. closed-chain). Loading may also be restricted to a specific type of resistance such as elastic bands or weights. Weight-bearing activity can also be considered a load. Impact stress during activities such as running is considered a load in addition to the weight-bearing forces. If load limitations are placed on the joint, adherence to the restrictions in all exercise activities is essential.

4. What are the expected gains in flexibility and strength, and the rate at which they are expected to occur? Some musculoskeletal challenges may respond differently to exercise stimulus than a normal joint would. Gains in strength and flexibility may be slowed due to the condition. In some cases, gains to within normal limits may not be expected at all. This is especially true after some surgical procedures where the joint anatomy is significantly affected.

5. What joint-specific signs and symptoms should be monitored? During the execution of

an exercise program, the client is monitored for progress and any signs of exacerbation of the condition. If any such sign is observed, the client's healthcare professional should be contacted to obtain modified guidelines for exercise. General signs to watch for are:

- complaints of pain during or after exercise
- increases in joint swelling
- decreases in range of motion
- decreases in strength
- decreases in functional capacity

Depending on the client's condition and course of treatment, the healthcare professional may indicate additional or more specific signs.

Once the answers to the aforementioned questions are obtained, you can choose from appropriate and available equipment and exercise options to design a safe and effective program for the client.

Exercise Testing and Programming with a Joint Disorder

Exercise guidelines for individuals with musculoskeletal challenges apply to exercise testing as well as exercise programming, and limitations in range of motion and loading should be adhered to. During cardiovascular testing, the musculoskeletal challenge may cause a premature test end and invalidate the test results. To avoid this problem, choose a test mode that does not involve the injured joint. For example, a client with plantar fasciitis could be testing using cycle ergometry instead of a treadmill. Testing the flexibility of the injured joint should be limited to movement within the guidelines for range of motion. Record the amount of indicated flexibility the client possesses. Testing the strength of the involved joint is contraindi-

Table 22.2

Typical Activity Guidelines

- Avoid exercise that exacerbates the joint disorder.
- Monitor the client for signs of problems and refer when necessary.
- Work within the disorder-specific limitation given by the healthcare professional.

- Apply given limitations to all fitness activities.
- Follow-up with the healthcare professional regularly to obtain updated exercise guidelines.

cated in many phases of rehabilitation and for some conditions. Limitations in loading indicate this problem. If strength testing is appropriate, the chosen method must adhere to the range-of-motion guidelines.

The exercise program should be specific to the desired goal. If the client desires a general fitness program, all aspects of the program must adhere to the determined exercise guidelines for the joint disorder. Evaluate the cardiovascular mode and all strength and flexibility exercises to ensure the range of motion and loading are within any given limitations. Determination of frequency, intensity and time depends on the client's overall condition and the tolerance of the joint to exercise.

Follow-up Communication

Follow-up communication with the healthcare professional should be conducted at regular intervals. A written summary of the client's progress, in the form of a S.O.A.P. (Subjective, Objective, Assessment, Planning) note is the recommended method. (See Chapter 4 for information on writing S.O.A.P. notes.) Include information on the client's flexibility, strength and

functional capacity progress. If the client is making the expected progress, request advanced guidelines for exercise. If the client has experienced any signs of exacerbation or has not made the expected gains, indicate this and request the necessary modifications to their exercise program.

Specific Musculoskeletal Challenges

The following information provides a generalized review of some specific musculoskeletal challenges. These exercise guidelines are not designed to substitute for the guidance of a healthcare professional. Additionally, various philosophies regarding exercise guidelines for specific disorders exist. The information provided below may conflict with the philosophy of the client's healthcare professional. In the event that this occurs, you should adhere to the healthcare professional's guidelines.

Lateral Ankle Sprain

A lateral ankle sprain occurs when the foot is inverted forcefully during weight-bearing activity. Damage to the anterior talofibular ligament is most common; however, the calcaneofibular ligament can also be involved (Figure 22.1). Sprains range in severity from slight tears or stretching of the ligament to complete ruptures of one or more of the lateral ligaments (Malone & Hardaker, 1990). Lateral ankle sprains are commonly treated with R.I.C.E. and progressive exercise to return function. Surgical intervention is less common, but may be used to correct chronic instability. The prognosis for a lateral ankle sprain is very positive. Most individuals recover full range of motion, strength and function to pre-injury levels.

After a lateral ankle sprain, range-of-motion exercises include passive stretching of ankle dorsiflexion and plantar flexion and active movement such as ankle circles and "alphabets." Progressive strengthening for inversion, eversion, dorsiflexion and plantar flexion may be accomplished using rubber tubing as tolerated to increase the stability of the ankle. Single leg balance on a variety of surfaces and balance boards is used to assist the recovery of proprioception. Impact during cardiovascular exercise

Figure 22.1

Ankle Sprain

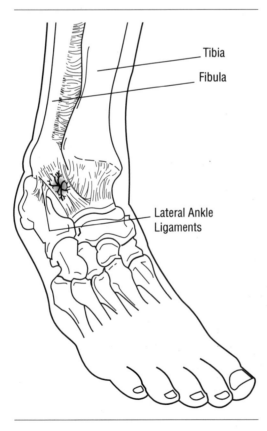

Tibia

Fibula

Lateral Ankle Ligaments

is reduced, and cycling with the heel on the pedal is a good way to get a workout if range of motion and weight bearing are limited.

Cutting, jumping and lateral movements are not recommended until full strength and pro-prioception have returned. Cardiovascular workouts may have to be divided among impact and nonimpact modes to minimize ankle discomfort. Closed-chain strengthening of the lower extremity will have to be loaded according to the tolerance of the ankle joint.

Monitor the client for the following signs of exacerbation of the disorder. If any are present, make changes to the exercise program and/or refer the client to their physician or therapist if signs persist:

- complaints of pain
- increased or return of swelling
- increased or return of limp or favoring of limb
- decreased range of motion
- decreased strength

Plantar Fasciitis

Plantar fasciitis is microtearing of the fascia at or near its attachment to the bone. Repetitive overloading of the tissue at its calcaneal attachment is believed responsible for the tearing (Figure 22.2) (Kibler, et al, 1991). Common treatment for plantar fasciitis is rest, ice massage, stretching, modifications in training intensity, and strengthening of the muscles of the foot and ankle (Seto & Brewster, 1994). Surgery and orthotics to correct abnormal foot mechanics are used in some cases of plantar fasciitis. Evaluation of exercise footwear to ensure proper fit and support is also recommended. Full return to pre-injury ROM, strength and function, including athletic participation, is expected in most cases of plantar fasciitis. However, the condition may recur in some individuals, especially if the exercise program is not carefully designed.

The exercise program should include stretching of the gastrocnemius, soleus and plantar fascia. Strengthening focuses on the muscles of the foot and lower leg. Many of the posterior lower leg muscles have tendons that attach on the plantar surface of the foot and therefore assist the plantar fascia in the absorption of

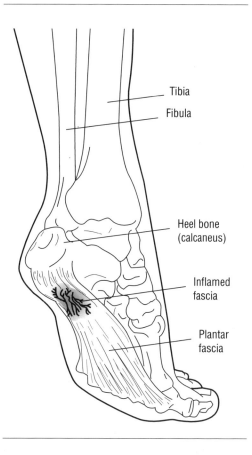

Tibia

Fibula

Heel bone (calcaneus)

Inflamed fascia

Plantar fascia

Figure 22.2

Plantar Fasciitis

impact force. These include toe flexors, plantar flexors and the peroneals.

Sudden increases in training intensity or frequency, especially in runners, is contraindicated. Plyometric exercises such as jumping or high-force loading of the foot should not be included until the client has full strength and range of motion and is pain-free. Progression of loading and close monitoring of total workout impact is always essential. Prior to any activity, a full warm-up and stretching of the involved foot is recommended.

Monitor the client for the following signs of exacerbation of the disorder. If any are present, make changes to the exercise program and refer the client to their physician or therapist if signs persist:

- complaints of pain during/after exercise or early in the morning
- increase or return of limp or favoring of limb
- decreased range of motion

Rotator Cuff Strain

A rotator cuff strain is the overstretching, overexertion or overuse of the musculotendonus unit of one or more of the rotator cuff muscles (Kisner & Colby, 1985). Rest, stretching and slowly progressive strengthening exercises are used to return the shoulder to pre-injury function. The prognosis for return to full range of motion, full strength and full functional capacity is good following a rotator cuff strain.

Frequently prescribed flexibility exercises following a rotator cuff strain include stretching of the posterior cuff, inferior cuff and chest musculature. Strength exercises for internal and external shoulder rotation and scapular stability are also prescribed. Additionally, strengthening of the pectoralis major, latissimus dorsi and deltoids are indicated. Closed-chain upper-extremity exercises are thought to be beneficial for returning the shoulder's kinesthetic and stabilizing function (Davies & Dickoff-Hoffman, 1993), and therefore can be included in an upper-extremity exercise program.

Contraindicated exercises include any loading of the shoulder joint that exceeds the tolerance of the rotator cuff to stabilize the shoulder. This might occur in the dumbbell press or pec flies,

where the rotator cuff is too weak to stabilize the shoulder against the load needed to effectively stimulate the chest muscles. Reducing the stabilizing requirement of the exercise by using a machine chest press can assist in developing a complete upper-body workout without compromising the rotator cuff. Do not fatigue the rotator cuff muscles prior to executing exercises that require their activity for stabilization. This is likely to exacerbate a strain.

Monitor the client for the following signs of exacerbation of the disorder. If any are present, make changes to the exercise program and refer the client to their physician or therapist if signs persist:

- complaints of pain
- decreased range of motion
- presence of accessory muscle activity
- decreased muscular strength or endurance

Rotator Cuff Impingement

Rotator cuff impingement is a common overuse syndrome of the shoulder in athletes who participate in overhead sports (swimming, baseball, volleyball) or individuals who perform repetitive overhead work (carpenters, painters). It is characterized as a pinching of the supraspinatus and/or long head of the biceps tendon under the coraco-acromial arch when the arm is abducted (Figure 22.3) (Roy & Irvin, 1983). Rotator cuff impingement is treated conservatively with rest, stretching and gradual strengthening exercises. Other treatments for impingement include various surgical techniques and anti-inflammatory injections. Each surgical technique is different in regards to its approach at relieving the disorder and the subsequent exercise guidelines. Impingement syndrome treated early, before anatomical damage has occurred, will likely return the individual to full functional capacity, including athletic competition (Jobe & Pink 1993).

Strengthening includes internal and external rotators, scapular stabilizers, pectorals, latissimus dorsi and deltoids. Closed-chain strengthening is also included to improve kinesthesia and promote stability. Stretching of the posterior cuff is encouraged, while stretching of the anterior structures is discouraged. Active ab-

Figure 22.3

Impingement of bursa and supraspinatus under the coracoacromial arch with abduction movement:
a. with arm adducted
b. with arm abducted

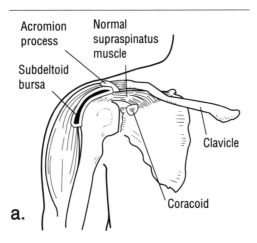

a.

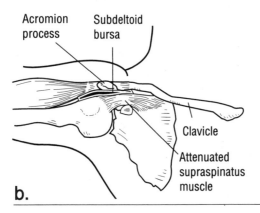

b.

duction and overhead activities should be avoided unless pain-free, and the repetition of this movement should always be closely monitored. Military press, triceps pull-overs, lat pull-downs behind the neck and pull-ups behind the neck are likely to exacerbate this problem (Litchfield et al., 1993).

The serratus anterior is thought to be a critical muscle in the coordination of shoulder movements. It should be exercised for improvements in both strength and endurance to prepare it for the demands of daily activities. This can be accomplished with the addition of scapular protraction to the push-up or machine or free-weight chest press.

Monitor the client for the following signs of exacerbation of the disorder. If any are present, make changes to the exercise program and refer the client to their physician or therapist if signs persist:

- complaints of pain
- decreased range of motion
- presence of accessory muscle substitution
- decreased muscular strength or endurance

Anterior Shoulder Instability

Anterior shoulder instability is a weakness in the anterior wall musculature (subscapularis, pectoralis major, latissimus dorsi and teres major) and/or stretching of the anterior capsule and ligaments that allows the humeral head to sublux or dislocate anteriorly (Jobe & Pink, 1993). The condition can be caused acutely from a fall or blow to the shoulder causing it to sublux or dislocate anteriorly. Chronic instability presents with gradual onset of muscle weakness and progressive damage of the anterior structures. Anterior shoulder instability is treated conservatively with rest, stretching and gradual strengthening of weak muscles. Significant anatomical damage to the anterior structures is repaired surgically. If conservative treatment is appropriate and started early, there is a high rate of return to full activity. Post-surgical prognosis is dependent upon the surgical procedure used and the adherence to rehabilitation guidelines (Jobe & Pink, 1993). Different surgical procedures result in varying losses in range of motion and function and therefore require exercise choices that reflect the limitations.

Strengthening for anterior shoulder instability is similar to shoulder impingement. Open- and closed-chain exercises for the internal and external rotators, scapular stabilizers, pectorals, latissimus dorsi and deltoid are included in most exercise programs. Motion is generally limited to avoid humeral abduction with external rotation or horizontal extension. Lat pull-downs behind the neck, pec flies, and full-range or wide-grip chest press should not be performed due to anterior shoulder stress (Litchfield et al., 1993). The shoulder musculature should be exercised for both strength and endurance. Stretching of the posterior cuff is encouraged, while stretching of the anterior structures is discouraged.

Monitor the client for the following signs of exacerbation of the disorder. If any are present, make changes to the exercise program and refer the client to their physician or therapist if signs persist:

- complaints of pain
- decreased range of motion
- lack of confidence in shoulder stability
- decreased muscular strength or endurance
- presence of accessory muscle substitution

Lateral Epicondylitis ("Tennis Elbow")

Lateral epicondylitis is an overuse injury affecting the musculotendonus junction of the wrist extensor muscles at the lateral epicondyle of the humerus. Repetitive activities involving the wrist, such as playing tennis, carpentry or pruning shrubs, result in microdamage to the tissue. (Figure 22.4) The cause is associated with inadequate wrist extensor strength, power, endurance and flexibility. The onset of lateral epicondylitis is usually gradual. Conservative treatment consists of rest, ice, and gradual stretching and strengthening of the wrist extensors. Cortisone injections and surgery are used when conservative management is not successful. Return to full activity is expected.

Stretching for all motions of the wrist is recommended. This includes flexion, extension, radial/ulnar deviation and pronation/supination. The wrist flexion stretch is performed with the elbow extended and wrist and fingers flexed (Hertling & Kessler, 1996). Perform wrist flexion stretching before all activities that involve the wrist (e.g., lat pull-downs, seated row). Strength exercises for the shoulder, wrist and fingers are recommended (Roy & Irvin, 1983). Loads must be carefully chosen to avoid overloading the tissue and causing pain during or after the exercise. Emphasis should be placed on the eccentric phase of the movement (Curwin & Standish, 1984). Design the client's exercise program to accommodate rest between exercises that involve the wrist to hold onto a bar, pull or push.

Monitor the client for the following signs of exacerbation of the disorder. If any are present, make changes to the exercise program and refer the client to their physician or therapist if signs persist:

Figure 22.4

Tennis Elbow

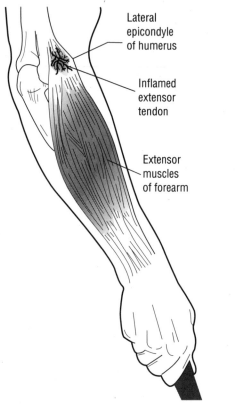

Lateral epicondyle of humerus

Inflamed extensor tendon

Extensor muscles of forearm

- complaints of pain during or after activity
- decreased range of motion
- decreased muscular strength or endurance
- increased or return of swelling

Anterior Cruciate Ligament Tear and Replacement

The anterior cruciate ligament (ACL) lies within the joint capsule of the knee (Figure 22.5). It attaches superiorly on the femur and inferiorly on the tibia. The ACL is instrumental in preventing the tibia from shifting forward on the femur especially during forceful quadriceps

contraction. Injuries to the ACL are commonly caused by rapid deceleration (such as a basketball player stopping suddenly) or by a direct blow to the knee causing the knee to hyperextend (Roy & Irvin, 1993). Knee instability, or the tendency for the tibia to shift during quadriceps contraction or weight bearing, is a concern when the integrity of the ACL is disrupted. This shifting can cause additional damage to the structures of the knee. The amount of instability is related to the extent of the damage to the ACL. ACL injuries range from a partial tear to a complete rupture of the ligament. Partial tears are frequently treated with R.I.C.E. and an extensive rehabilitation program to return the knee to full range of motion and strength. Throughout rehabilitation, and all activity thereafter, the ACL is protected to prevent additional damage to the ligament that may result in increased instability. Reconstructive surgery is often encouraged in the case of large tears and complete ruptures to restore the stability of the knee.

The most common reconstructive procedure is a patellar tendon autograft (Wilk & Andrews, 1992). The surgery involves the removal of a portion of the patellar tendon, with bone plugs on either end, to be used as a graft. Tunnels are drilled in the tibia and femur and the graft is carefully positioned through the tunnels and secured. Once secured, the graft mimics the function of the original ligament. The lengthy rehabilitation after an ACL reconstruction is a careful progression to return full range of motion, strength, proprioception and function to the knee without damaging the graft. Range-of-motion limitations are used to avoid premature stress on the graft, while quadriceps contraction force limits reflect the state of tissue healing and integrity of the graft during each phase of rehabilitation(Wilk & Andrews, 1992). Post-surgical complications include knee extension weakness, loss of range of motion and patellofemoral problems (McHugh et al., 1998). Successful ACL reconstruction results in the return to full activity, including athletic competition.

Lower-extremity flexibility is essential to allow proper functioning of the knee. Exercise guidelines after an ACL partial tear or reconstruction include stretching of all major muscles of the hip, knee and lower leg to encourage normal range of motion. Cardiovascular conditioning is important, especially if the client is to return to athletic participation. Swimming, biking, stair climbing and running are acceptable if approved by the healthcare professional. Advanced activities, such as cutting, jumping and pivoting, should be avoided until the client has been cleared to do them. The client's program should also include proprioception exercises such as balance board and single leg stance (Mangine & Noyes, 1992).

Strengthening of all motions of the knees, hips and ankles is appropriate following an ACL injury. Closed-chain exercises are recommended for lower-extremity strengthening due to the decreased stress on the ACL during loading (De Carlo et al., 1992; Fu et al., 1992; Hertling & Kessler, 1996; Lutz et al., 1993; Wilk & Andrews, 1992; Wilk et al., 1995; Yack et al., 1993). The contraction of the hamstrings during a closed-chain exercise counteracts the pull of the quadriceps and reduces tibial shifting. Thus, hamstring strengthening is emphasized to promote knee stability (Hertling & Kessler, 1992). Open-chain knee extension exercises place strain on the ACL and increased patellofemoral compression (Fu et al., 1992). Due to these factors, knee extension exercises may not be appropriate following operative or nonoperative treatment of an ACL injury depending on the condition of the ligament or graft and the presence of patellofemoral complications. If knee extension exercises are utilized, equipment fit

to ensure knee joint alignment with the machine axis of rotation is essential to minimize the deleterious effects on the joint.

Monitor the client for the following signs of exacerbation of the disorder. If any are present, make changes to the exercise program and refer the client to their physician or therapist if signs persist:

- complaints of pain
- complaints of the knee feeling "unstable"
- complaints of the knee "catching," "locking" or "giving out"
- decreased range of motion
- decreased muscular strength or endurance
- increased or return of swelling
- increased or return of limp or favoring of limb

Patellofemoral Pain Disorders

Patellofemoral pain disorders (PFPDs) may involve the patella, the femoral condyles, the quadriceps muscle and/or the patellar tendon (Figure 22.6). These components as a whole are referred to as the extensor mechanism. There are many conditions that affect the extensor mechanism including chondromalacia, patellar tendinitis, anterior knee pain and patellofemoral malalignment (Shelton & Thigpen, 1991). The majority of PFPDs are considered overuse syndromes and thus are associated with overload or repetitive microtrauma to the knee. Training errors, improper footwear, anatomical abnormalities and post-surgical complications all contribute to PFPDs (Rintala, 1990). While the conditions are similar and the exercise guidelines are generalized, each specific condition requires modifications that should be determined by a healthcare professional in order to ensure appropriateness.

Conservative treatment of PFPD is highly effective and generally used prior to surgical treatment. If nonoperative treatment fails, surgical management may be used. Rest, ice, lower-extremity strengthening emphasizing the quadriceps, lower-extremity stretching, and gradual functional progressions are all used in conservative management of PFPD. Non-steroidal anti-inflammatory medication and bracing or taping may also be included.

The exercise guidelines for PFPD are designed to increase the function of the extensor mecha-

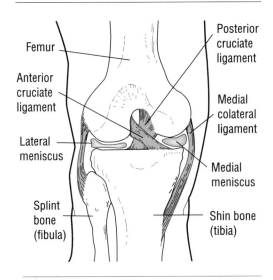

Figure 22.5

Anatomy of the knee

Femur

Anterior cruciate ligament

Lateral meniscus

Splint bone (fibula)

Posterior cruciate ligament

Medial colateral ligament

Medial meniscus

Shin bone (tibia)

nism while reducing patellofemoral joint compressive forces (PJCF) and facilitating the coordinated contraction of the vastus medialis obliquus (VMO) to promote patellar alignment. PJCF increase progressively as the knee is flexed from 0 to 90 degrees. Maximum PJCF during knee extension exercises have been reported between 30 and 90 degrees of flexion (Woodall & Welsh, 1990). Loading of the extensor mechanism between 30 and 0 degrees of knee flexion promote VMO contraction with minimal PJCF (Hertling & Kessler, 1996; Rintala, 1990; Woodall & Welsh, 1990). Open- and closed-chain exercises are appropriate.

Stretching of the lower extremity should include exercises for the quadriceps, hamstrings, gastrocnemius-soleus and tensor fascia latae/ IT band. Normal range of motion is essential for extensor mechanism function and the reduction of PFPD (Hertling & Kessler, 1996; Shelton & Thigpen, 1991; Woodall & Welsh, 1990). Cardiovascular training is recommended, especially if the client is to return to sport activity. Swimming and cycling are frequently the mode of choice due to the reduced lower-extremity stress. When cycling, the seat must be as elevated as possible to reduce the amount of knee flexion and the subsequent patellofemoral joint compression forces. Running and stair climbing also are recommended as tolerated by the client.

Monitor the client for the following signs of exacerbation of the disorder. If any are present, make changes to the exercise program and refer the client to their physician or therapist if signs persist:

- complaints of pain
- decreased range of motion
- decreased muscular strength or endurance
- increased or return of swelling
- increased or return of limp or favoring of limb

Conclusion

The key to designing safe and effective programs for your clients with musculoskeletal challenges is to perform a thorough screening and evaluation to gather the necessary guidelines to aid in the design of an exercise program. All clients with past musculoskeletal challenges may not require program modification, but those who have had recent treatment or continuing symptoms will need physician clearance along with guidelines for the appropriate healthcare professional.

Case Study #1

Shoulder Impingement

Eric, a 32-year-old carpenter, has come to the health club seeking guidance for an exercise program to decrease body fat and improve overall strength. After filling out the health history form, you discover Eric had a prior diagnosis of left-shoulder impingement. During the interview, Eric states that he has recently experienced increased difficulty with overhead lifting and endurance activities with the left shoulder. It is explained to Eric that he can immediately begin a lower-extremity exercise program, but more information needs to be obtained about his shoulder before he can begin any upper-extremity work.

You contact Eric's physician and gather the following information:

1) Resisted internal and external shoulder rotation and gentle stretching of the posterior cuff, chest and upper back are recommended.

2) All overhead exercises are contraindicated at this time.

3) Range of motion is limited to the pain-free range between 0 and 90 degrees of shoulder abduction.

4) No loading should be performed overhead, with gradual increases in loads through the pain-free range.

Figure 22.6

Patellar Anatomy

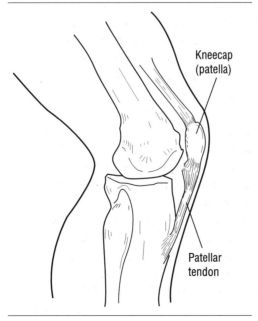

Kneecap (patella)

Patellar tendon

5) Eric is expected to be pain-free in the described range and achieve full strength in all allowed exercises within the next 4-6 weeks.

6) Eric should be monitored for any complaints of popping, clicking, increased pain, or further decreases in strength, pain-free range of motion or function.

Based on this information, you evaluate Eric's current pain-free shoulder flexibility and add exercises for the upper extremity to his exercise program. Loading for Eric's left shoulder begins conservatively and increases gradually as tolerated. Exercises such as lat pull-downs, military press and incline bench are avoided until Eric's physician lifts the overhead restriction. Eric progresses, as expected, without complication and after six weeks his physician is recontacted to change his exercise guidelines.

Case Study #2

ACL Reconstruction

Sara, a 17-year-old soccer player, is entering her senior year of high school in the fall. She had ACL reconstructive surgery on her right knee at the end of July. It is now November and Sara's therapist refers her to you to get her ready for the upcoming soccer season and possible college recruitment. The therapist informs you that Sara lacks 3 degrees of knee extension due to hamstring tightness, but has full flexion, and that her hamstring strength is still lacking. Sara's therapist also has given her a home exercise program with elastic resistance squats, hamstring curls and ankle exercises.

You contact the therapist for additional information regarding Sara's knee and the following exercise guidelines are established:

1) Hamstring strengthening is the main emphasis with continuation of her quadriceps work. Her ankle and hip strength and proprioception should also be improved.

2) Open-chain knee extensions are contraindicated.

3) All major muscles of the lower extremity should be stretched with an emphasis on gaining full knee extension.

4) Straight line running is O.K., but cutting, turning and stopping are contraindicated until the involved hamstring is stronger and bilateral quadriceps strength is even.

5) Plate-loaded machines and barbells are approved as a substitution for elastic resistance for the home exercises.

6) Sara should be monitored carefully for complaints of anterior knee pain, increased swelling, clicking or a sense of giving-out at the knee.

You design Sara's exercise program for development of her aerobic base through treadmill running and cycling. Her strength program includes seated hamstring curls, leg press, squats, calf raises, ankle dorsiflexion, hip ab/adduction, balance board and stork stands as well as a full upper-body workout.

Throughout Sara's program, resistance is gradually increased and contact with her therapist occurs every four weeks to continually progress her exercise guidelines.

References

Curwin, S. & Standish, W.D. (1984). *Tendonitis: Its Etiology and Treatment*. The Collator Press: Lexington, Mass.

Davies, G.J. & Dickoff-Hoffman, S. (1993). Neuromuscular testing and rehabilitation of the shoulder complex. *Journal of Orthopedic and Sports Physical Therapy*, 18, 2, 449-458.

DeCarlo, M.S., Shelbourne, K.D., McCarroll, J.R. & Rettig, A.C. (1992). Traditional versus accelerated rehabilitation following ACL reconstruction: A one-year follow-up. *Journal of Orthopedic and Sports Physical Therapy*, 15, 6, 309-316.

Fu, F.H., Woo, S. & Irrgang, J.J. (1992). Current concepts for rehabilitation following anterior cruciate ligament reconstruction. *Journal of Orthopedic and Sports Physical Therapy*, 15, 6, 270-277.

Hertling, D. & Kessler, R.M. (1996). *Management of Common Musculoskeletal Disorders*, 3rd ed. Philadelphia, Pa.: Lippincott

Jobe, F.W. & Pink, M. (1993). Classification and treatment of shoulder dysfunction in the overhead athlete. *Journal of Orthopedic and Sports Physical Therapy*,, 18, 2, 427-432.

Kibler, W.B., Goldberg, C. & Chandler, T.J. (1991) Functional biomechanical deficits in running athletes with plantar fasciitis. *American Journal of Sports Medicine*, 19, 1, 66-71.

Kisner, C. & Colby, L.A. (1990). *Therapeutic Exercise: Foundations and Techniques*, 2nd ed. Philadelphia, Pa.: F.A. Davis

Litchfield, R., Hawkins, R., Dillman, C.J., Atkins, J. & Hagerman, G. (1993). Rehabilitation for the overhead athlete. *Journal of Orthopedic and Sports Physical Therapy*, 18, 2, 433-441.

Lutz, G.E., Palmiter, R.A., An, K.N. & Chao, E.Y.S. (1993). Comparison of tibiofemoral joint forces during open-kinetic-chain and closed-kinetic-chain exercises.American *Journal of Bone and Joint Surgery*, 75, 5, 732-738.

Malone, T.R. & Hardaker, W.T. (1990). Rehabilitation of foot and ankle injuries in ballet dancers.*Journal of Orthopedic and Sports Physical Therapy*, 11, 8, 355-361.

Mangine, R.E. & Noyes, F.R. (1992). Rehabilitation of the allograft reconstruction. *Journal of Orthopedic and Sports Physical Therapy*,15, 6, 294-303.

McHugh, M.P., Tyler, T.F., Gleim, G.W. & Nicholas, S.J. (1998). Preoperative indicators of motion loss and weakness following anterior cruciate ligament reconstruction. *Journal of Orthopedic and Sports Physical Therapy,* 27, 6, 407-411.

Rintala, P. (1990). Patellofemoral pain syndrome and its treatment in runners. *Journal of Athletic Training,* 25, 2, 107-110.

Roy, S. & Irvin, R. (1983). *Sports Medicine: Prevention, Evaluation, Management and Rehabilitation.* Englewood Cliffs: Prentice-Hall

Shelton, G.L. & Thigpen, L.K. (1991). Rehabilitation of patellofemoral dysfunction: a review of literature. *Journal of Orthopedic and Sports Physical Therapy,* 14, 6, 243-249.

Wilk, K.E. & Arrigo, C. (1993). Current concepts in the rehabilitation of the athletic shoulder. *Journal of Orthopedic and Sports Physical Therapy,,* 18, 1, 365-378.

Woodall, W. & Welsh, J. (1990). A biomechanical basis for rehabilitation programs involving the patellofemoral joint. *Journal of Orthopedic and Sports Physical Therapy,* 11, 11, 535-542.

Yack, H.J., Collins, C.E. & Whieldon, T.J. (1993). Comparison of closed and open kinetic chain exercises in the anterior cruciate ligament-deficient knee. *American Journal of Sports Medicine,* 21, 1, 49-53.

Recommended Reading

Brukner, P. & Khan, K. (1993). *Clinical Sports Medicine.* Sydney, Australia: McGraw-Hill Book Co.

Garrick, J.G. & Webb, D.R. (1990). *Sports Injuries: Diagnosis and Management.* Philadelphia, Pa.: W.B. Saunders Co.

CHAPTER 23

Osteoporosis

KARA A. WITZKE

Kara A. Witzke, Ph.D,. is an assistant
professor in the Department of Health,
Physical Education, Recreation and Dance
at the University of Guam. She specializes
in research pertaining to the effects of high-
impact exercise on bone mass in
adolescents. Dr. Witzke is an ACE-certified
Personal Trainer and is also certified by the
ACSM as an exercise test technologist. She
has served the American Council on
Exercise through committee participation,
item-writing for certification exams, and as
an ACE FitnessMatters contributor and
media spokesperson.

Lifestyle Factors

General Mobility

The Resistance Program

Osteoporosis, which means "porous bones," is a systemic skeletal disease characterized by low bone mass and deterioration of bone strength, leading to bone fragility and an increased risk of fracture. An estimated 1.5 million fractures occur each year in the U.S. as a result of low bone mass, with someone suffering a hip fracture approximately every two minutes. (Chrischilles, Sherman & Wallace, 1994). Americans aged 50 and older have almost a 40 percent chance of suffering an osteoporotic fracture. Thus, one in three people — about 90 percent of them women — will suffer a fracture related to low bone mass (Cooper, Campion & Melton, 1992). According to the National Osteoporosis Foundation, the associated cost of osteoporotic fractures is approximately $10 billion annually.

Organization of the Skeleton

The human skeleton is composed of two types of bone: cortical (compact) and trabecular (spongy). **Cortical bone** forms a dense shell around all bones, and constitutes the thick shafts of long bones, while **trabecular bone** is found in the vertebrae and in the ends of long bones. Trabecular bone forms a lattice-like network, which greatly increases its surface area for metabolic activity. As a result, trabecular bone undergoes far more **remodeling** cycles during an individual's lifetime than does cortical bone (Marcus, 1987). A remodeling cycle consists of a bone **resorption** (bone removal) stage which is followed by a period of new bone formation. Through this coupled process, bone is constantly renewed.

During growth and young adulthood, the rate of bone formation is faster than the rate of bone resorption, leading to an overall gain in bone mineral. This is called bone **modeling**. Following growth, however, the continual process of bone resorption occurs at a slightly faster rate than bone formation, causing a steady, gradual decline in the amount of bone mineral in the skeleton of about 1 percent per year (Snow-Harter & Marcus, 1991). These age-related bone mineral decrements are not as pronounced in men, primarily because men reach a higher **peak bone density** and do not undergo rapid postmenopausal bone loss as women do (Figure 23.1). Bone resorption is rapid (if estrogen therapy is not implemented) during the first five years following menopause, and may ac-

count for a 3 percent to 5 percent loss of overall bone mass per year.

The three most common **osteoporotic** fracture sites are the wrist (distal radius), hip (femoral neck and greater trochanter) and spine (Figure 23.2). Wedge and compression fractures of the vertebrae are common in osteoporotic individuals, and are responsible for a loss of height and/or **kyphosis** (hunchback) (Figure 23.3). These fractures often go unnoticed until complications related to spinal deformity cause the individual to seek treatment. Vertebral fractures cause the center of gravity to shift forward, which may predispose the individual to falling. This, in turn, increases the chance of a subsequent hip fracture. In the case of multiple spinal fractures, the rib cage rests on the iliac crests and compromises proper lung function. Prolonged pain following a vertebral fracture may be caused by weak back extensor muscles.

Hip fractures are by far the most debilitating osteoporotic fracture, often causing a loss of independence, prolonged immobility and death due to complications from surgery or being confined to bed. Ninety percent of hip fractures occur due to a fall from standing height or less (Hayes et al., 1993). It is estimated that 50 percent of people who sustain a hip fracture due to a fall never become functional walkers again (Spirduso, 1995).

To provide an accurate prognosis for the osteoporotic patient, physicians identify four components:

- quantification of bone mass (see Screening and Measurement Techniques)
- identification of previous fractures
- identification of factors that influence the risk of fractures independent of bone mass (e.g., falls, hip geometry)
- assessment of the rate of bone loss (annual bone density scans)

The severity of the disease dictates possible treatment options. However, maintaining mobility and regular physical activity on some level is indicated (Kanis et al., 1997).

The remainder of this chapter focuses on the factors that affect bone and lifestyle-modification strategies for osteoporosis prevention. Since osteoporosis occurs nine times more fre-

Figure 23.1

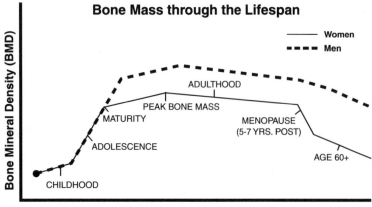

Bone Mass through the Lifespan

— Women
---- Men

Bone Mineral Density (BMD)

CHILDHOOD

ADOLESCENCE

MATURITY

PEAK BONE MASS

ADULTHOOD

MENOPAUSE (5-7 YRS. POST)

AGE 60+

Stage of Maturity

quently in women than in men, this chapter addresses the female client, although all training principles presented apply to men as well. Extreme care should be taken with the clinically osteoporotic client, and you will need to work closely with the client's physician and physical therapist to observe proper safety precautions and contraindications.

Factors that Affect Bone

While there is no cure for osteoporosis, a combination of genetic, dietary, age-related, hormonal and lifestyle factors help determine an individual's potential risk for the disease. As with other chronic diseases, prevention of osteoporotic fractures is the focus of much research and debate. Preventive measures include altering lifestyle factors, such as nutrition and exercise, and, in some cases, administering pharmacological agents (e.g., hormone replacement, amino **bisphosphonates**). Clearly, the best time to implement prevention strategies is in adolescence and young adulthood when peak bone mass is achieved (Recker et al., 1992). Between the ages of 30 and 50, reducing the rate of age-related bone loss with lifestyle modification is essential. Following menopause and into the seventh decade and beyond, individuals should strive to reduce their risk of falling by maximizing home safety and implementing a carefully designed exercise program.

Genetics

An individual's potential peak adult bone mass is largely determined by genetics. In fact, about 80 percent of an individual's adult bone density is preprogrammed into their genes (Sambrook et al., 1996). Genetic traits that may predispose a woman to osteoporosis include:

- Northern European or Asian descent
- fair complexion
- family history of osteoporosis
- small, thin frame

Since it is impossible to change genetic make-up, it is crucial to pay attention to the factors that can be controlled. (See the Osteoporosis Risk Profile.)

Estrogen

Besides genetics, the single most important factor affecting bone and the maintenance of bone mass throughout life is the presence of estrogen. This powerful sex hormone, which acts as an anti-resorptive agent in the body, controls the rate of bone removal from the skeleton. Without estrogen, the rate of removal exceeds

**Figure 23.2
Bone Fracture Areas**

Each year, osteoporosis leads to 1.5 million bone fractures, including more than 500,000 vertebral fractures, 300,000 hip fractures, 200,000 wrist fractures and 300,000 fractures of other bones.

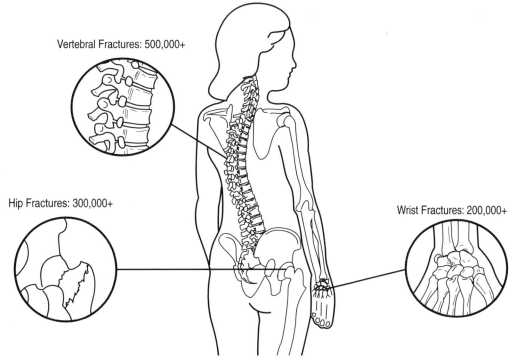

Vertebral Fractures: 500,000+

Hip Fractures: 300,000+

Wrist Fractures: 200,000+

Source: National Osteoporosis Foundation, 1993

the rate of formation, resulting in a net loss of bone mass.

Estrogen deficiency occurs most often in post-menopausal women and young, athletic amenorrheic women. Endogenous estrogen production falls to low levels at menopause, which typically occurs around the age of 50. Bone loss during the first five to seven years following menopause is rapid if estrogen is not replaced. After menopause, all women should consider whether estrogen replacement is right for them. It not only offers benefit to the skeleton by preventing rapid bone resorption, but also reduces the risk of heart disease. Women also may discuss with their physician the many new pharmaceutical therapies used to treat osteoporosis including bisphosphonates (e.g., alendronate, trade name Fosamax), calcitonin and a new class of pharmaceutical agents that act as selective **estrogen receptor modulators** (e.g., raloxifene, trade name Evista). These agents increase overall bone mass by inhibiting bone resorption. They do not carry the increased risk of breast cancer that estrogen replacement therapy may, but they also do not offer the cardiovascular benefits of estrogen.

Athletic women may be at increased risk for athletic **amenorrhea**, a condition where menstrual cycles become irregular or cease altogether, presumably due to a combination of high-intensity and high-volume physical training, stress hormones, and inadequate caloric intake. While many active women consider the loss of periods to be a convenience, research has shown irreversible bone loss in young women who have failed to menstruate for as little as 12 months. The risk of osteoporosis in these women is greatly increased. Young amenorrheic but otherwise healthy aerobics instructors, for example, have been shown to have bone density equal to that of 50-year-old women (Drinkwater, Nilson & Chesnut, 1994). Women with irregular or no menstrual cycles should seek the care of a physician, who may recommend a reduction in training volume and intensity, hormone replacement (often in the form of birth control pills containing estrogen) and/or an increase in caloric intake.

Dietary Calcium Intake

Dietary calcium provides the essential building blocks for bone formation. Calcium also plays an important role in muscle contraction and intra- and extra-cellular ion **homeostasis**. Without an adequate daily intake, calcium is withdrawn from the bones to maintain normal blood levels. Adequate calcium intake is especially important during growth while the skeleton is still forming, and during an important "window of opportunity" until age 30 in which peak bone mass may still be increased (Recker et al., 1992). The RDA currently recommends that children age 10 and younger and adults older than 25 consume 800 mg of calcium per day. Individuals between 10 and 24 should strive for 1,200 mg per day, as should pregnant and lactating women. The National Osteoporosis Foundation (NOF) recommends 1,500 mg per day for postmenopausal women not taking estrogen (Dawson-Hughes, 1996).

Calcium supplements should be evaluated on the basis of their elemental calcium content (usually 200 to 600 mg), and not the overall milligrams of calcium compounds such as calcium carbonate or calcium citrate. Calcium carbonate supplements (e.g., Tums®) are usually less expensive and are best taken with a meal, which promotes an acidic environment in the gastrointestinal tract that aids calcium absorption. Calcium citrate or calcium citrate malate supplements, while more expensive,

**Figure 23.3
Cause of Stooped
Posture and
Height Loss**

The spine is made up of a series of small connected bones called vertebrae (left). Healed vertebral fractures become compressed (flattened) or may mend in a wedge shape. Over time, multiple fractures can result in stooped posture, a loss of height and continual pain (right).

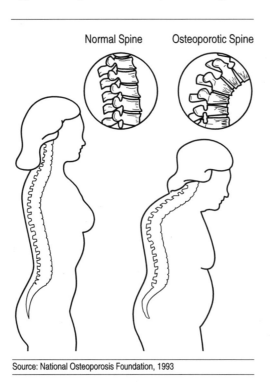

Source: National Osteoporosis Foundation, 1993

often do not cause constipation, a side effect experienced by some individuals using calcium carbonate. Many new calcium supplements also contain Vitamin D, which aids in the intestinal absorption of calcium.

Lifestyle Factors

Physical activity transmits mechanical forces to the skeleton via gravitational forces and muscular pull at bony attachment sites. Skeletal loading remains the only means to actually increase new bone formation in the mature skeleton (after the cessation of growth). Recall that estrogen, bisphosphonates, selective estrogen receptor modulators and calcitonin are classified as anti-resorptive agents that slow bone removal. Bone that is apparently gained using these drugs is actually not gained at all; instead, removal slows to a level where bone formation can catch up. These agents do help improve the overall strength of bone, but a comprehensive osteoporosis prevention program also should include physical activity.

While research has shown that physically active people typically have higher bone mass than their sedentary counterparts, the most profound support for exercise as a preventative measure for osteoporosis is the extraordinary bone loss that occurs with immobilization. Early bed-rest studies showed that the high levels of urinary calcium excretion that accompanies prolonged periods of non-load-bearing can be significantly reduced with a small amount of weight-bearing activity (Issekutz et al., 1966).

During the past decade scientists have sought to determine which type of exercise is most beneficial to bone, and whether or not a dose response exists, whereby a minimum amount of exercise to prevent loss and gain bone can be identified. Although many of these questions have yet to be answered, the overload principle seems to hold the key (Drinkwater, 1994).

It has been proposed that the magnitude of the load on the bone is more important than the number of load repetitions. The optimum exercise protocol must sufficiently overload the bone, and push it beyond the "lazy zone" to promote bone formation (Whalen & Carter, 1988). Exercises that produce stimuli below the bone's minimum threshold to promote new bone formation will not cause an increase in bone mass (Lanyon, 1987). Therefore, exercises such as walking and running, which produce low-force magnitudes but high-force repetitions, do not represent enough of a change in daily loading to signal an increase in bone mass. A landmark study showed that a regular program of brisk walking did not provide enough overload stimulus to bone to prevent age-related loss in postmenopausal women who were not on estrogen-replacement therapy (Cavanaugh & Cann, 1988). Therefore, while walking may benefit older individuals

Table 23.1

Client Information to Obtain from Medical Professionals

1) Does this client experience clinical conditions other than osteoporosis, e.g., cardiovascular disease?

2. What postures (especially in the person with kyphosis) are recommended for this individual?

3. Does this individual have postural hypotension that may result in dizziness when changing postures?

4. Is this person taking medications that will alter the exercise response. If so, what are the medications and how will they affect the exercise response?

5. What has the individual been able to achieve (in the way of muscular strength/flexibility) through physical therapy?

6. Can my client perform high-intensity strengthening exercises?

7. Should they use free weights or machines?

8. Which exercises should they avoid?

9. Should I be ultra-conservative with women who are at risk for osteoporosis?

10. Are weight-bearing exercises feasible for those with arthritis?

11. How important is cardiovascular exercise for the person with osteoporosis?

12. My client prefers water exercise. Isn't this the safest environment for a woman with osteoporosis?

by keeping them mobile, it likely will not promote gains in muscle strength, muscle power or bone mass, which are important factors in preventing the onset of osteoporosis.

Research suggests that athletes involved in activities requiring high-power output and high-impact loads, such as gymnastics (Robinson et al., 1995), high-impact aerobics (Heinonen et al., 1995; Heinonen et al., 1996), wrestling (Bone Research Laboratory, Oregon State University) and jumping (Bassey & Ramsdale, 1994), have higher bone mass than those involved in endurance activities such as walking (Cavanaugh & Cann, 1988) and cycling. In addition, sports with substantial muscular involvement without impact forces (e.g., swimming) are associated with lower bone mass than those with a weight-bearing component (Taaffe et al., 1995). Certainly, water-based training and other forms of non-weight-bearing exercise are beneficial to the cardiovascular system, but weight-bearing activities are essential to provide the optimal stimulus for skeletal development.

There also appears to be an association between lean muscle mass and bone mass, whereby individuals with the highest amount of muscle also tend to have the highest bone density (Khosla et al., 1996). Forceful muscular contractions impose significant bending forces on bone (Granhad, Jonson & Hansson, 1987). Athletes who participate in activities with a high muscular-load component, such as weightlifting (Conroy et al., 1993), display higher bone mass than athletes who train in non-weight-bearing activities (Taaffe et al., 1995). These high-load activities also contain a high muscular-power component, which may suggest a role for forceful muscular contractions in promoting the highest bone mass (Witzke & Snow, 1997; Witzke & Snow, in press), although this has yet to be shown in prospective studies.

Other lifestyle factors such as smoking and alcohol consumption may adversely affect bone. Smoking seems to increase bone resorption, while alcohol decreases bone formation (Seeman, 1996). Excessive caffeine intake may reduce calcium absorption by causing a general **diuresis**, but its effects are minimal compared to smoking and alcohol usage. Prolonged

corticosteroid use and thyroid medications also have been implicated in an increased risk for osteoporosis.

Pre-exercise Screening and Assessment

Bone Density Measurement Techniques

Prior to 1980, traditional X-rays were a physician's only means of diagnosing osteoporosis. Standard radiographs, however, can only detect advanced bone loss and do not include a quantitative measure of bone mineral density. During the past 10 years, an assessment technique called dual-energy x-ray absorptiometry (DXA) has revolutionized this imprecise science. The DXA instrument delivers very low-dose radiation (equal to about 1/20th of a standard two-position chest X-ray), to quantify mineral content per unit area of bone (g/cm^2) at important fracture sites including the wrist (distal radius), hip (proximal femur) and lumbar spine. Although DXA is said to evaluate bone density, the information obtained is area density rather than a true volumetric density. Recently, physicians have utilized computerized tomography (CT) to obtain measures of volumetric (3-dimensional) bone density (g/cm^3). This method allows the physician to more accurately assess the trabecular content of bone, which is more important than cortical bone when assessing fracture risk. Computerized tomography, however, delivers substantially higher amounts of radiation to the patient, so its use is evaluated on the basis of the additional benefit that CT may provide.

The best time for a woman to have her first bone-density assessment is prior to menopause, usually in her late 40s or early 50s. This is especially important for women who are at high risk for the disease. Either technique will allow the physician to determine a patient's risk for osteoporosis and related fractures. If **osteopenia** (low bone mass) or osteoporosis (very low bone mass) is confirmed from the first bone scan, many physicians will perform annual scans to monitor changes in bone density. This information not only is valuable in helping a woman decide if estrogen replacement is advisable, but also assists a physical therapist (if prescribed by the physician) in planning an appropriate exercise regimen, which will prove valuable to you as an ACE-certified Clinical Exercise Specialist. Although results from a bone-density assessment are not required before an individual with osteopenia, osteoporosis or **established osteoporosis** (which describes someone who already has sustained a fracture) becomes a client, a physician referral is required.

While there are no physical assessments that you can perform to determine the presence of osteoporosis, you may want to administer the simple Osteoporosis Risk Questionnaire (see page 372) to all female clients as part of the initial client screening. This is especially true for women approaching menopausal age or who have had a hysterectomy. Women with several risk factors should consult their physician to determine their need for a bone-density assessment.

Exercise Testing for the Osteoporotic Client

Most osteoporotic individuals have relatively poor levels of aerobic fitness and muscular strength, which may be perpetuated by their anxiety about falling. Individuals with a history of falls share certain physical characteristics. They generally have weak hip adductors, quadriceps, hamstrings and ankle dorsiflexors. Fallers also tend to use more antidepressants and other medications, and have poor balance and impaired gait (Spirduso, 1995). These are important considerations for you

when choosing exercises for the older client and in setting up the exercise environment. Improvement in aerobic fitness, muscle mass, strength, flexibility and balance should form the basis of the exercise program for this population.

Traditional exercise-testing protocols may be utilized for osteoporotic clients depending on the degree of limitation imposed by existing fractures and fracture risk. Due to relatively low fitness levels among osteoporotic individuals, ECG and blood pressure monitoring during aerobic fitness testing is indicated. For inactive, frail clients a treadmill protocol with very small increments (1-2 METS per stage) is recommended (Table 23.2).

Exercise heart rates are measured during the last 15 seconds of each stage, and the test is terminated when the client reaches 65 percent to 70 percent of their age-adjusted maximal heart rate (230-age). VO$_2$max can be estimated using the following equation (use the information for the last stage completed):

$VO_2max \ (ml \bullet kg^{-1} \bullet min^{-1}) = [meters \bullet min^{-1} \ x \ 0.1] + [grade \ (as \ a \ decimal) \ x \ meters \bullet min^{-1} \ x \ 1.8] + 3.5$

To convert to absolute values:

$VO_2max \ (ml \bullet min^{-1}) = VO_2max \ (ml \bullet kg^{-1} \bullet min^{-1}) \ x \ body \ weight \ (kg)$ (ACSM, 1991, p. 296)

Forward vision and ventilatory function may be compromised in osteoporotic clients with severe kyphosis. Treadmill testing may impose an increased risk of falling; therefore, aerobic fitness may be more effectively assessed using a bicycle ergometer with 10 to 25 watt (60 to 150 kgm/min) increases every three minutes

Table 23.2
Modified Balke Protocol for Treadmill Testing

MPH	METERS/MIN	% GRADE	MIN/STAGE	METS
2.0	53.6	0	3	2.5
2.0	53.6	3.5	3	3.5
2.0	53.6	7.0	3	4.5
2.0	53.6	10.5	3	5.4
2.0	53.6	14.0	3	6.4
2.0	53.6	17.5	3	7.4
3.0	80.4	12.5	3	8.5
3.0	80.4	15.0	3	9.5
3.0	80.4	17.5	3	10.5
3.0	80.4	20.0	3	11.6
3.0	80.4	22.5	3	12.6

(Bloomfield, 1997). Estrogen replacement therapy may elevate resting blood pressure values, but does not appear to affect exercise values.

Postural stability and gait efficiency in the osteoporotic client also should be assessed be-cause these factors help determine fall risk (Spirduso, 1995). They also determine the client's ability to get around the home and com-munity, thus playing a major role in maintaining the individual's independence. Functional fitness assessments that include walking and balance skills are appropriate since they reflect the health and function of the neuromuscular system. The following are examples of appropriate functional tests; additional information can be found in Chapter 18. Each test is timed, so clients' scores (time) can be compared from baseline to subsequent tests.

General Mobility and Lower-body Strength

- *Time to rise from a chair:* The client is timed from the command "go" until an upright position with hands on hips is reached. Hands may be used for leverage if necessary.
- *Stepping onto and off objects:* Place stable objects of three different heights side-by-side. Starting with feet together, the client steps up with both feet, then down, and repeats on next two objects. Time to complete all three tasks is recorded.

Balance

- *Static balance with visual control:* Stationary balance on two feet (or pre-

ferred foot) with either wide or narrow base of support, and with eyes open. Time maintaining balance is recorded.
- *Static balance without visual control:* Stationary balance on two feet (or preferred foot) with either wide or narrow base of support, and with eyes closed. Time maintaining balance is recorded.

Gait and Mobility Functions

- *Walking a straight, wide path:* Client walks using a natural gait through a pathway 10 feet long and 1 foot wide (use tape or place jump ropes 1 foot apart to denote path; client's feet must stay outside the path). Time, cadence, number of steps and errors are recorded.
- *Maximum gait speed:* Same as above, except client is asked to walk as fast as possible.

Body Agility

- *Walking a wide, curved or circular path at maximum speed:* Client walks through a wide, curved pathway 10 feet long and 1 foot wide as fast as possible, with one curve left and one curve right. (Can be modified to use two right-angle changes of direction.)
- *Moving around obstacles at maximum speed:* Client walks as fast as possible through cones placed at equal distances throughout a 10-foot pathway.

Table 23.3

Typical Activity Guidelines

Young adults

■ High-intensity strength training using free weights and/or high and abnormal impact loads (jumping, etc.). If high-impact activities are contraindicated, weight-bearing activities with the highest impact the individual can tolerate are recommended.

Healthy, nonosteoporotic postmenopausal women

■ High-intensity strength training using free weights and/or dynamic resistance exercises with weighted

vests (as outlined in this chapter) and jumping in place.

Osteoporotic women

■ This population typically is monitored by a physical therapist. However, activities that improve mobility and dynamic balance (lower-body strength and endurance), and promote flexibility and strength of the trunk are recommended. Exercises should be performed slowly and with control as sudden twisting movements and/or large compressive loads may precipitate vertebral fractures.

Muscular strength evaluation for individuals with osteoporosis is critical. Strength testing can be performed using a standard 1-RM test for the quadriceps, hamstrings, hip abductors, biceps and shoulders in individuals without fractures, but a modified strength assessment using a 3 RM or 6 RM is recommended. Strength evaluation using weight machines or dumbbells with close supervision is appropriate, as is an isokinetic dynamometer (e.g., Cybex, KinCom) with a moderate-to-fast speed. Slow settings using an isokinetic machine, and slow, forceful or isometric muscle contractions should be avoided with osteoporotic clients.

Exercise Programming

Published Standards

Only recently have professionals begun to develop specific exercise recommendations for the prevention of osteoporosis, and very little information is available regarding appropriate exercise programs for individuals with established osteoporosis. This is largely due to the lack of conclusive evidence among prospective training studies (Snow, Shaw & Matkin, 1996). In 1995, the American College of Sports Medicine published a Position Stand on Osteoporosis and Exercise. Based on current research, it is the position of the ACSM that:

- Weight-bearing physical activity is essential for the normal development and maintenance of a healthy skeleton. Activities that focus on increasing muscle strength also may be beneficial, particularly for non-weight-bearing bones.
- Sedentary women may increase bone mass slightly by becoming more active, but the primary benefit of the increased activity may be in avoiding the further loss of bone that occurs with inactivity.
- Exercise cannot be recommended as a substitute for hormone-replacement therapy at the time of menopause.
- The optimal program for older women includes activities that improve strength, flexibility and coordination that may indirectly, but effectively, decrease the incidence of osteoporotic fractures by lessening the likelihood of falling (ACSM, 1995).

Published in 1998, the third edition of *ACSM's Resource Manual for Guidelines for Exercise Testing and Prescription* contains a new chapter, titled "Exercise for Skeletal Health and Osteoporosis Prevention." This chapter summarizes pertinent research in the field of exercise and osteoporosis, and includes specific recommendations for weight-training activities for osteoporosis prevention for middle-aged and older adults without documented osteoporosis (Shaw & Witzke, 1998). These guidelines are also included in the Exercise Programming section of this chapter.

Exercise Programming for Osteoporotic Adults

The recommendations for aerobic exercise are similar to those for sedentary individuals, or those at high risk for coronary artery disease. Intensity should be kept low (40 percent to 70 percent peak HR), a minimum of three days per week, for 20 to 30 minutes per session (Bloomfield, 1997). For clients using medications that affect heart rate response to exercise (e.g., blood pressure medications), utilize the RPE scale to monitor intensity, with a recommended range between 10 and 15. General flexibility exercises to improve range of motion should follow all forms of exercise, and place special emphasis on the pectoral muscles, as they often experience shortening in clients with **kyphosis.**

As demonstrated in the literature, and recommended by the ACSM, weight-training activities should be a very important component of the training program (ACSM, 1995). Resistance exercises for the legs, abdomen and back are the most critical since they focus on improving lower-body strength and postural control and may help prevent falls. Adequate lower-body strength helps the individual recover from a stumble. Since the most common and debilitating hip fractures occur from falls to the side, improvements in side-to-side balance may play a critical role in reducing these types of falls (Grisso, Capezuti & Schwartz, 1996; Shaw & Snow, 1998). Therefore, strengthening exercises for the hip abductors and adductors should also be included in the client's program.

Osteoporotic individuals should avoid excessive spinal flexion (e.g., curl-ups, sit-and-reach), because this movement may compromise fragile vertebral bodies. Teach each client proper body mechanics and postural alignment before implementing a weight-training program. Extended periods of standing on one leg also should be avoided as this may lead to a fall due to muscular fatigue. Include flexibility and abdominal exercises (e.g., pelvic tilt) in the warm-up, and emphasize them in the cool-down. Stretching during the warm-up should always follow a general warm-up or range-of-motion exercises. Warm-ups and cool-downs for older individuals should be extended to 10 to 20 minutes since it may take older adults longer to warm the muscles and adjust to circulatory requirements and changes in movement (Spirduso, 1995).

The Resistance Program

An effective resistance-training program for bone must contain weight-bearing exercises. Lower-body exercises on traditional weight machines are usually performed while seated, which reduces forces at the hip. For most individuals, using dumbbells while standing, or a weighted vest or weight belt for resistance, are viable options. A weighted vest provides the opportunity to regulate added resistance and to distribute the load around the torso, thus loading the spine and hips. For those with severe kyphosis, a weight belt worn around the waist will minimize any additional forward shift of the center of gravity, yet still load the hips during exercise. Functional resistance exercises are more likely to improve balance (Shaw & Snow, 1998) and ankle strength and flexibility, which may reduce the risk of a stumble from poor gait mechanics.

Many sporting-goods stores sell quality weight vests specifically designed for resistance work. The vest should fit snugly and not hang below the hips. It should come with many small weights (0.5 to 1 pound each), which allows for small incremental increases. An inexpensive weight vest also can be made using a fishing vest with pockets around the torso. Weight packets made from sand, small stones or pennies in plastic bags can be added to the pockets to provide additional resistance.

Select exercises that emphasize upper- and lower-body development, focusing on the legs, abdominals and back extensors. The client's

health status determines the intensity of the exercises, but the best results occur with intensities greater than 75 percent of 1 RM. If traditional weight machines or free weights are used, begin the program with one to three sets at 10 to 15 RM using five to eight different exercises. Gradually progress to three to four sets at 6 to 10 RM, adding additional exercises as tolerated. Clients should train a minimum of two to three days per week. The following suggested exercises may be easily performed using a weighted vest or hand-held dumbbells for added resistance. Increase the weight in the vest using small increments based on a percentage of the client's body weight (or lean mass if a very overweight client) (Table 23.4). The intensity recommendations previously have been used in adolescents and older adults alike (Fiatarone et al., 1990; Nelson et al., 1994; Shaw & Snow, 1998; Witzke & Snow, 1997), but should be adjusted based on the client's response. Frail elderly clients should begin using a weighted vest only after considerable preconditioning using the same exercises recommended in this section, with body weight alone as the resistance. They should progress more gradually up to 5 percent to 6 percent of body weight for 1-3 sets, 6-12 repetitions.

The periodic inclusion of "recovery days," in which intensity is decreased and repetitions increased, may be helpful to the client, especially when intensity is high. It should also be noted that the intensity recommendations may need to be modified for obese individuals who may have difficulty attaining 15 percent to 20 percent of body weight in their vests or hand-held weights.

Squats or Chair Squats. These exercises strengthen the quadriceps, hamstrings, back extensors and ankles. Standing with feet shoulder width apart, distribute the weight evenly along the soles of the feet. With hands on waist or outstretched directly in front, squat until thighs are parallel with the floor. If necessary, a chair may be placed 6 to 12 inches behind the participant. If the weight shifts to the toes while performing the squat, the buttocks are not reaching back far enough for the chair. *Modification:* Older individuals may opt for a half squat, as symptoms permit. Clients may use the hands to help push off into the standing phase, although hands-free squats should be encouraged.

Front Lunges. This exercise strengthens the quadriceps, hamstrings, hip adductors and hip flexors, and also may improve balance. Starting with feet shoulder width apart and hands on hips, take a large step forward with one leg, drop the hips toward the floor until the knee almost touches the floor, then push back to the starting position. Alternate legs, making sure that the knee of the outstretched leg stays in line over the ankle. *Modification:* Step onto a stair or aerobic bench, and reduce the depth of the lunge. Hands may be outstretched, or the back or seat of a chair used for balance control. To add variety, traveling or walking lunges may be performed.

Side Lunges. This exercise strengthens the quadriceps, hamstrings, hip abductors, hip adductors and ankles, and also may improve balance. Starting with the feet shoulder width apart, take a large step sideways, allowing the knee on the stepping leg to move over the ankle. Push off to return to the starting position. *Modification:* Step onto a stair or aerobic bench, and reduce the depth of the lunge. Hands may be outstretched for balance control. To add variety, perform traveling or walking lunges.

Toe Raises/Heel Drops. This exercise strengthens the ankles and calves, and adds an impact component. Standing on a solid surface, raise up onto the toes, "drop" back down onto the heels with minimal knee flexion and then rock back on the heels. *Modification:* Use the back of a chair for balance control. A small hop may be added to the exercise after the heel rock.

Step-Ups. This exercise strengthens the quadriceps. Using an "up-up, down-down" cadence, step up onto a stair or aerobic bench and return to the floor. Alternate starting leg and increase the height of the bench from 4 to 12 inches. *Modification:* Use the back of a chair for balance control and use a 4-inch step height.

Pelvic Tilt. This exercise strengthens the abdominals without causing excessive spinal flexion. Lie supine on a mat on the floor with the knees bent at 90 degrees, feet flat on the floor. Rotate the pelvis posteriorly and press the lower back into the mat. This position should be held for five to 15 seconds and repeated eight to 10 times.

Press-and-Reach Exercise. This exercise trains the abdominals to stabilize the pelvis against changing resistance. Lie supine on a mat with the knees bent at 90 degrees, positioned over the hips. Focus on keeping the pelvis posteriorly tilted during the exercise. Simultaneously raise the arms overhead and straighten one leg toward the floor until the back begins to pull off the floor. *Modification:* Bend the knee of the leg being lowered to reduce tension on the back.

Upper-body Exercises. A variety of upper-body dumbbell exercises are appropriate for osteoporotic clients, depending on individual limitations. Avoid overhead presses and upright rows, which may aggravate the shoulder joint in older adults. Exercises such as biceps curls, triceps kickbacks, lateral raises, bench press and lat pull-downs are safe and effective exercises for most individuals. If possible, these exercises should be performed while standing to promote the activation of stabilizing muscles and to increase skeletal loads.

Special Considerations

Special attention should be given to the exercise surface. Slick or uneven surfaces, or loose or torn carpet may increase the likelihood of a slip or fall. Be aware of any medications the client is using, and whether or not they may cause dizziness or a loss of balance. If the client wears corrective lenses, ensure that they also are used during exercise. Lastly, advise the client to refrain from wearing excessively baggy clothing that may catch or snag on gym equipment.

Osteoporosis Prevention for Healthy, Non-osteoporotic Adults

As mentioned earlier, prevention of osteoporosis during young adulthood is the key to a

Table 23.4
Weighted-vest Resistance-training Protocol

MONTH	SETS	REPETITIONS	INTENSITY
1-3	1-2	10-15	5-10% of body weight
3-5	2	8-10	10-15% of body weight
5-7	3-4	6-10	15-20% of body weight

stronger skeleton later in life. In addition to resistance exercises, a prevention program for younger and middle-aged healthy adults also should include impact activities to stimulate new bone formation. The use of jumping and plyometric activities, however, is fairly progressive. Individuals with orthopedic limitations, including lower-body joint pain, injuries, arthritis and certainly osteoporosis, should NOT engage in these activities.

Jumping. Simple jumping seems to provide an adequate stimulus for bone, and is a safe and appropriate loading modality for younger and older nonosteoporotic women (Bassey & Ramsdale, 1994; Shaw & Snow, 1998; Shaw & Witzke, 1998). Increases in hip bone density have been observed in premenopausal women who performed 50 two-footed jumps three days per week for six months (Bassey & Ramsdale, 1994). Nonosteoporotic clients seeking to reduce their risk for the disease should perform jumps in stockinged feet on a hard surface, which maximizes ground reaction forces and transmits more load to the hips than if wearing athletic shoes. Stand with feet no more than shoulder width apart, and use the arms while jumping straight up as high as possible. Bend the knees while landing.

Plyometrics. Plyometrics are specialized jumping exercises associated with high-impact loads and forceful muscular take-offs, and include a wide variety of exercises specifically designed to increase muscular strength and power. They are based on the premise that increasing eccentric preload on a muscle will induce the myotatic stretch reflex, thereby causing a more forceful concentric contraction. Plyometrics range in difficulty and intensity level from simple stationary jumping to traveling drills, such as hopping and bounding, to high-intensity box jumps (Chu, 1995; Radcliffe & Farentinos, 1985). The benefit of plyometric exercise on bone only recently has been investigated, but the results appear positive (Witzke & Snow, 1997; Bone Research Laboratory, Oregon State University). An inherent benefit of utilizing these types of activities is that they require little equipment, small blocks of time, and are safe for adolescents and healthy adults to perform (Chu, 1995).

A proper progression of plyometric exercises is important to ensure adequate muscular strength to maintain proper body mechanics during execution and landing. A plyometric program should begin with one to two sets of 10 repetitions of five to seven different exercises and progress slowly to the more strenuous activities, adding sets and repetitions as tolerated. All exercises should be performed on a medium-hard surface such as grass (preferred), aerobic floor or carpet. Plyometrics should not be performed by osteoporotic individuals or older adults with joint concerns. A sample of simple plyometric activities are presented here, but if you are interested in a more comprehen-

---

Figure 23.4

Osteoporosis Risk Questionnaire

RATE YOUR RISK

Check all factors that apply to YOU

Risk factors that CANNOT be controlled

☐ YES	☐ NO	Do you have a family history of osteoporosis?
☐ YES	☐ NO	Are you white, Northern European or Asian?
☐ YES	☐ NO	Do you have a fair complexion?
☐ YES	☐ NO	Do you have a small, thin frame?
☐ YES	☐ NO	Are you postmenopausal?
☐ YES	☐ NO	Have you had an early or surgically induced menopause?

Risk factors that CAN be controlled

☐ YES	☐ NO	Are you physically inactive?
☐ YES	☐ NO	Is your diet low in dairy products and other sources of calcium?
☐ YES	☐ NO	Do you smoke cigarettes or drink alcohol in excess?
☐ YES	☐ NO	Have you ever not menstruated when exercising heavily?

sive program refer to the suggested reading list at the end of the chapter.

Perform all of the following exercises in succession, minimizing time spent on the floor. This maximizes muscle preload and ensures optimal gains in power.

Squat jump. Jump as high as possible, using the arms for propulsion, then land in a squat position.

Box jump progression. Using several 4- to 8-inch steps (aerobic benches work well), spaced two to three feet apart, jump onto and off the succession of steps, spending as little time on the floor as possible. Pauses, if any, should be made on top of the bench rather than on the floor.

Stride jump. Starting from a front lunge position, drive the hips upward and land with the opposite leg forward, again in a lunge position.

Split jump. Starting from a standing straddle position, jump up, quickly bring the legs together and land in the same standing straddle position.

Stair exercises. A variety of exercises can be performed on a flight of stairs, ranging from standard running, or "bounding," skipping several stairs at a time, to a sideways approach. Stand sideways on two successive steps with the trailing leg straight and push the lead leg up to the next step. Move the trailing leg up to the next step, push off and so on. This exercise represents a sort of "seesaw" motion and strengthens hip abductors and adductors.

Alternating leg bounds. These are standard bounds, where the knee on the lead leg drives up and forward, lands, then the opposite knee drives up and forward. Emphasize maximum height and distance, and use the bent arms in a backward circular motion for added propulsion. This exercise also can be performed as a same-leg bound, where the lead leg cycles around and is the only leg to touch the ground.

Double leg butt kicks. From a standing position, jump forward with both legs, kick the buttocks and land on both feet, emphasizing maximum distance.

Hop progressions. Perform basic, small, double-leg hops as quickly as possible for a given distance.

Hurdle hops. Perform large, high, two-footed hops over barriers such as cones or hurdles. Minimize time spent on the ground.

Side cone hops. Perform two-footed lateral hops in succession over cones.

Emergency Procedures

In the event that a client with suspected or documented osteoporosis should suffer injury due to a fall while exercising, or experience sudden extreme back pain, seek professional medical assistance (EMS) immediately. If a hip fracture is suspected, it is extremely important not to move the client, as movement may cause perforation of the femoral artery. If a vertebral fracture is suspected, the client should lie down if possible until EMS arrives.

Conclusion

Of the two types of bone in the human body, trabecular bone is more susceptible to the deleterious effects of osteoporosis. Because of its high trabecular content, the neck of the femur is a common osteoporotic fracture site; hip fractures often cause a loss of independence and death in many cases. Osteoporosis prevention and treatment strategies include estrogen replacement therapy or other pharmacological agents, increased calcium intake and exercise.

The types of exercise that are most beneficial to bone are those that sufficiently overload bone using high-force magnitude rather than a high number of low-force repetitions. High-force magnitude can be produced through direct impact loading of the bone, as with jumping, or through strong muscular contractions that bend bone, as with weight lifting. Non-weight-bearing, non-impact exercise such as swimming does not sufficiently overload bone to increase bone formation or to slow bone loss. Similarly, weight-bearing exercises that are not significantly different from daily loading patterns (in normally ambulating individuals), such as walking, also do not provide a stimulus for new formation.

Osteoporotic clients, especially those prone to falling, may require modifications in exercise-testing protocols. Fitness assessments should include functional tests that mimic activities of daily living and represent skills necessary for the maintenance of independence and effective locomotion. Graded exercise testing may be performed on a treadmill, but clients with extreme kyphosis may have impaired forward vision and should be tested using a bicycle ergometer. Strength assessments using the 3 or 6 RM are preferred over the traditional 1 RM for safety reasons. Osteoporotic clients should avoid exercises that involve forceful and abrupt trunk rotation and large compressive forces on the spine, since these activities may increase the likelihood of a fracture.

An effective exercise program for clients with osteoporosis contains upper- and lower-body resistance training at least two days per week. For clients without osteoporosis, 50 two-footed jumps three times per week may provide an osteogenic stimulus for bone, and may increase bone mass in premenopausal women. General aerobic exercise to improve cardiovascular

health should be performed at least three days per week for 20 minutes or more at low-to-moderate intensities. Postmenopausal women not on estrogen-replacement therapy or anti-resorptive drugs probably will not gain bone mass through exercise, but may effectively slow the natural rate of bone loss.

Case Study 1

Rhonda is a thin, fair-skinned, 35-year-old marathon runner, who has come to you for a strength-training program after finding out that her 50-year-old mother has osteoporosis. She currently runs about 75 miles per week, but would like to add a weight-lifting regimen if it will help reduce her risk for osteoporosis. In the pre-screening assessment, you ask Rhonda to complete an Osteoporosis Risk Questionnaire, which shows that she is at high risk. You also discover that she has-

Table 23.5

Calcium Content of Common Foods

MILK-YOGURT-CHEESE	Serving size	Calcium (mg)
cheese	1 oz or 6 Tbsp	200
cottage cheese	1/2 cup	50
custard, pudding or cream pie	1/2 cup	150
ice cream, frozen yogurt or milk shake	1 cup	200
milk	1 cup	300
soy milk	1 cup	10
yogurt	1 cup	350
macaroni & cheese	1 cup	250
pizza	1/8 of 15"	250
FRUITS & VEGETABLES		
broccoli or cooked greens		
(beet/turnip greens, kale, collards, spinach)	1/2 cup	100
other fruits and vegetables	1/2 cup	30
BREADS-CEREALS-RICE-PASTA		
bread	1 slice	20
rice, noodles or pasta	1 cup	20
pancake, waffle or french toast	1 piece	100
MEAT-FISH-POULTRY-BEANS		
dried beans, cooked	1 cup	50
meat, fish, poultry	3 oz	10
peanuts	1/2 cup	30
egg	1	30
sardines with bones	3 oz	400
shrimp	3 oz	100
tofu	2 1/2" x 2 1/2" x 1"	100

n't had a menstrual period for two years (since she increased her training volume to compete in marathons) and only had a period every other month for three years prior to that. She has had two stress fractures in the past 12 months, but managed to continue her physical activity with non-weight-bearing exercise while they healed. She is very concerned about her dietary fat intake, and claims she consumes about 1,000 calories per day. She is very eager to begin her strength-training program.

Rhonda is probably a classic amenorrheic athlete. You immediately should be concerned that she hasn't menstruated in two years, and has had irregular periods for some time before that. Her high training volume and low caloric intake probably have contributed to her amenorrhea, but a visit to her physician is definitely in order before you begin working with her. Talk to Rhonda about concern over her training volume and associated stress fractures, and discuss amenorrhea, but do not diagnose the problem. You also should educate Rhonda on the usefulness of a bone-density assessment so that she may talk with her physician about getting one. You also may want to question Rhonda about her dietary intake, and recommend a qualified nutritionist.

Once she returns with her physician release and results from her bone-density assessment, you are ready to begin training Rhonda. If her bone mass is below normal (osteopenic), you should implement a conservative program of strength training and stationary jumping. Additional plyometric exercises should not be added for at least three months to ensure that Rhonda tolerates the jumping without injury. Begin with upper- and lower-body resistance exercises for the quads, hamstrings, ankle and hip adductors and abductors, chest, and back using a weighted vest or dumbbells for resistance. Since she is in fairly good shape, she can begin with two sets of 10 repetitions, using 8 percent of her body weight in the vest, or 75 percent of her 1 RM. Every two to three weeks, Rhonda can increase her resistance. Recommend that Rhonda weight train two days per week, substituting one of her running days for a weight day.

Case Study 2

Fiona is a 70-year-old, postmenopausal woman of small build, who has just been told by her physician that she has osteoporosis. She has lost an inch-and-a-half in height, and has upper-back pain, but has been cleared by her physician to begin an exercise program. She performed some upper-body Theraband® exercises with a physical therapist, but is more concerned about a hip fracture. She is otherwise sedentary and has chosen not to use estrogen replacement therapy, although she has heard positive things about these new "bone drugs" from her friends. She wants you to tell her which bone drug she should begin taking, and to start her on a strength-training program to help slow her bone loss. She is on an antidepressant drug that sometimes makes her dizzy, especially when she forgets to wear her glasses. She took a bad fall in her home last month when the kitchen rug caught on her house slippers, and is concerned that she is having trouble climbing the stairs in her home.

Since Fiona has a physician's release to begin working with you, she is ready for screening and program development. Although you can educate Fiona about the new anti-resorptive drugs, all questions about whether or not they are right for her should be directed to Fiona's physician. She should continue performing the regimen her physical therapist prescribed for her to help maintain upper-back flexibility and strength. Since she has a recent history of falling, and experiences episodes of dizziness, you should assess her functional mobility using the mobility, gait, balance and agility tests from this chapter. You also should help Fiona assess safety in her home, and suggest that she wear stable shoes while inside to prevent another house-slipper incident. She also should secure all area rugs in her house and might consider installing handrails in the bathroom. Fiona definitely needs lower-body strength training, especially if she is to continue to climb the stairs in her home. Implement the weighted-vest activities presented in this chapter, but do not include any jumping activities since Fiona's osteoporosis already is established. Make sure that Fiona has her eyeglasses on while training to maximize her safety and minimize her risk of falling.

References

American College of Sports Medicine. (1991). *Guidelines for Exercise Testing and Prescription.* (4th ed.) Philadelphia, Pa.: Lea & Febiger.

American College of Sports Medicine. (1995). ACSM position stand on osteoporosis and exercise. *Medicine and Science in Sports and Exercise*, 27, 4, i-vii.

Bassey, E.J. & Ramsdale, S.J. (1994). Increase in femoral bone density in young women following high-impact exercise. *Osteoporosis International*, 4, 72-75.

Bloomfield, S.A. (1997). Osteoporosis. In *ACSM's Exercise Management for Persons with Chronic Diseases and Disabilities*. Champagne, Ill.: Human Kinetics.

Cavanaugh, D.J. & Cann, C.E. (1988). Brisk walking does not stop bone loss in postmenopausal women. *Bone*, 9, 201-204.

Chrischilles, C., Sherman, T. & Wallace, R. (1994). Cost and health effects of osteoporotic fractures. *Bone*, 15, 377-386.

Chu, D. (1995). *Jumping into Plyometrics*. Champagne, Ill.: Human Kinetics.

Conroy, B.P., Kraemer, W.J., Maresh, C.M., Fleck, S.J., Stone, M.H., Fry, A.C., Miller, P.D. & Dalsky, G.P. (1993). Bone mineral density in elite junior Olympic weight lifters. *Medicine and Science in Sports and Exercise*, 25, 1103-1109.

Cooper, C., Campion, G. & Melton, L.J. III. (1992). Hip fractures in the elderly: A worldwide projection. *Osteoporosis International*, 2, 285-289.

Dawson-Hughes, B. (1996). The role of calcium in the treatment of osteoporosis. In Marcus, Feldman & Kelsey (Eds.) *Osteoporosis*. San Diego, Calif.: Academic Press.

Drinkwater, B.L., Nilson, K. & Chestnut, C.H., III (1994). Bone mineral content of amenorrheic and eumenorrheic athletes. *New England Journal of Medicine*, 311, 277-281.

Drinkwater, B.L. (1994). C.H. McCloy research lecture: Does physical activity play a role in preventing osteoporosis? *Research Quarterly for Exercise and Sport*, 65, 197-206.

Fiatarone, M. S., Marks, D. C., Ryan, N. D., Meredith, C. N., Lipsitz, L. A. & Evans, J. W. (1990). High-intensity strength training in nonagenarians. *Journal of the American Medical Association*, 263, 3029-3034.

Granhad, H., Jonson, R. & Hansson, T. (1987). The loads on the lumbar spine during extreme weight lifting. *Spine*, 12, 146-149.

Grisso, J.A., Capezuti, E. & Schwartz, A. (1996). Falls as risk factors for fractures. In Marcus, Feldman & Kelsey (Eds.) *Osteoporosis*. San Diego, Calif.: Academic Press.

Harman, E., Rosenstein, M., Frykman, P., Rosenstein, R. & Kraemer, W. (1989). Evaluation of the Lewis power output test. *Medicine and Science in Sports and Exercise*, 21, 2, (Supplement), S51.

Hayes, W.C. et al. (1993). Impact near the hip dominates fracture risk in elderly nursing home residents who fall. *Calcified Tissue International*, 52, 192-198.

Heinonen, A., Kannus, P., Sievanen, H., Oja, P., Pasanen, M., Rinne, M., Uusi-Rasi, K. & Vuori, I. (1996). Randomized controlled trial of effect of high-impact exercise on selected risk factors for osteoporotic fractures. *Lancet*, 348, 1343-1347.

Heinonen, A., Oja, P., Kannus, P., Sievanen, H., Haapasalo, H., Manttari, A. & Vuori, I. (1995). Bone mineral density in female athletes representing sports with different loading characteristics of the skeleton. *Bone*, 17, 3, 197-203.

Issekutz, B. Jr., Blizzard, J.J., Birkhead, N.C. & Rodahl, K. (1966). Effect of prolonged bed rest on urinary calcium output. *Journal of Applied Physiology*, 21, 1013-1020.

Kanis, J.A., Delmas, P., Burckhardt, P., Cooper, C. & Torgerson, D. (1997). Position paper: Guidelines for diagnosis and management of osteoporosis. *Osteoporosis International*, 7, 390-406.

Khosla, S., Atkinson, E.J., Riggs, B.L. & Melton, L.J. III. (1996). Relationship between body composition and bone mass in women. *Journal of Bone and Mineral Research*, 11, 6, 857-863.

Lanyon, L.E. (1987). Functional strain in bone tissue as the objective and controlling stimulus for adaptive bone remodeling. *Journal of Biomechanics*, 20, 1083-1095.

Marcus, R. (1987). Normal and abnormal bone remodeling in man. *Annual Review of Medicine*, 38, 129-141.

Montoye, H. J., Christian, J. L., Nagle, F. J. & Levin, S. M. (1988). *Living Fit*. Menlo Park, Calif.: The Benjamin/Cummings Publishing Co.

Nelson, M. E., Fiatarone, M. A., Morganti, C. M., Trice, I., Greenberg, R. A. & Evans, W. J. (1994). Effects of high-intensity strength training on multiple risk factors for osteoporotic fractures. *Journal of the American Medical Association*, 272, 1909-1914.

Radcliffe, J. & Farentinos, R. C. (1985). *Plyometrics: Explosive Power Training*. Champaign, Ill.: Human Kinetics.

Recker, R.R. et al. (1992). Bone gain in young adult women. *Journal of the American Medical Association*, 268, 2403-2408.

Robinson, T.L., Snow-Harter, C., Taaffe, D.R., Gillis, D., Shaw, J. & Marcus, R. (1995). Gymnasts exhibit higher bone mass than runners despite similar prevalence of amenorrhea and oligomenorrhea. *Journal of Bone and Mineral Research*, 10, 26-35.

Sambrook, P.N., Kelly, P.J., White, C.P., Morrison, N.A. & Eisman, J.A. (1996). In Marcus, Feldman & Kelsey (Eds.) *Osteoporosis*. San Diego, Calif.: Academic Press.

Seeman, E. (1996). The effects of tobacco and alcohol use on bone. In Marcus, Feldman, & Kelsey (Eds.) *Osteoporosis*. San Diego, Calif.: Academic Press.

Shaw, J.M., & Snow, C.M. (1998). Weighted vest exercise improves indices of fall risk in older women. *Journal of Gerontology: Medical Sciences*, 53A, M53-M58.

Shaw, J.M. & Witzke, K.A. (1988). Exercise for skeletal health and osteoporosis prevention. In J. Roitman (Ed.) (3rd ed.) *Resource Manual for Guidelines for Exercise Testing and Prescription*.

Snow, C.M., Shaw, J.M. & Matkin, C.C. (1996). Physical activity and risk for osteoporosis. In Marcus, Feldman & Kelsey (Eds.)*Osteoporosis*. San Diego, Calif.: Academic Press.

Snow-Harter, C. & Marcus, R. (1991). Exercise, bone mineral density and osteoporosis. *Exercise and Sport Science Reviews*, 19, 351-388.

Spirduso, W.W. (1995). *Physical Dimensions of Aging*. Champaign, Ill.: Human Kinetics.

Taaffe, D.R., Snow-Harter, C., Connolly, D.A., Robinson, T.L., Brown, M.D. & Marcus, R. (1995). Differential effects of swimming versus weight-bearing activity on bone mineral status of eumenorrheic athletes. *Journal of Bone and Mineral Research*, 10, 586-593.

Whalen, R.T. & Carter, D. R. (1988). Influence of physical activity on the regulation of bone density. *Journal of Biomechanics*, 21, 825-837.

Witzke, K.A. & Snow, C.M. (1997). Effects of high-impact exercise on bone mass in adolescent girls. *Journal of Bone and Mineral Research*, 12, (Supplement 1), T568.

Witzke, K.A. & Snow, C.M. (in press). Lean mass and leg power best predict bone mineral density in adolescent girls. *Medicine and Science in Sports and Exercise*.

Suggested Reading

American College of Sports Medicine. (1995). ACSM position stand on osteoporosis and exercise. *Medicine and Science in Sports and Exercise,* 27, 4, i-vii.

American Council on Exercise. (1998). *Exercise for Older Adults: ACE's Guide for Fitness Professionals.* San Diego, Calif.: American Council on Exercise.

Chu, D. (1995). *Jumping into Plyometrics.* Champagne, Ill.: Human Kinetics.

Drinkwater, B.L. (1994). C.H. McCloy research lecture: Does physical activity play a role in preventing osteoporosis? *Research Quarterly for Exercise and Sport,* 65, 197-206.

Marcus, R., Feldman, D. & Kelsey, J. (Eds.) (1996). *Osteoporosis.* San Diego, Calif.: Academic Press.

Snow-Harter, C. & Marcus, R. (1991). Exercise, bone mineral density and osteoporosis. *Exercise and Sport Science Reviews,* 19, 351-388.

Section Eight

Special Cases

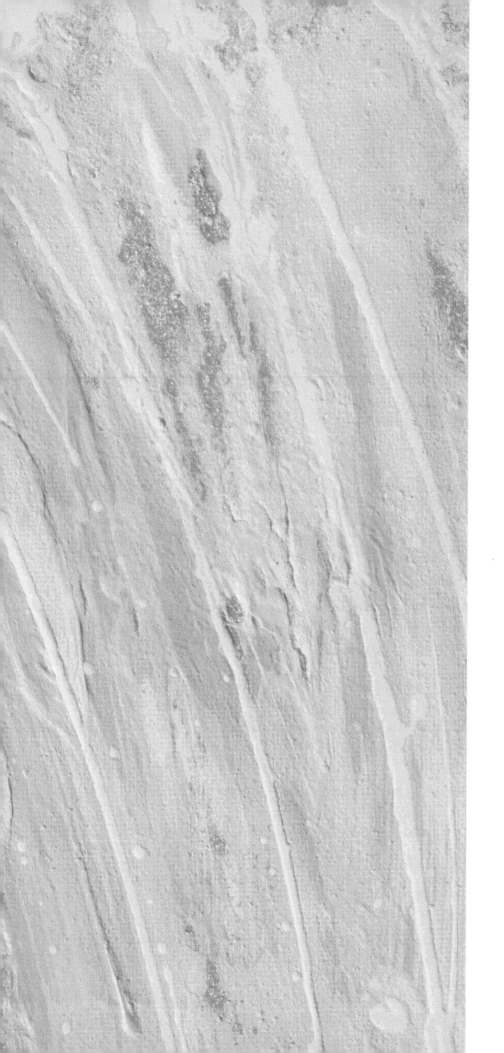

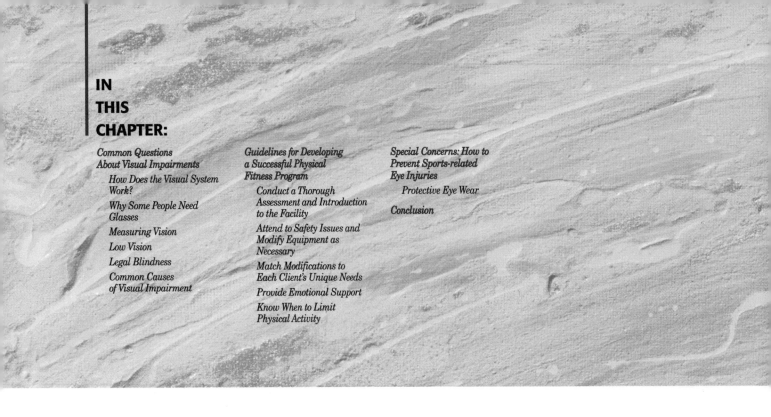

CHAPTER 24

Visual Impairments

LESLEY M. TEITELBAUM
MARY M. JACKOWSKI
CHARLES S. TEITELBAUM

Lesley M. Teitelbaum, Ph.D., is a research assistant professor in the Department of Psychology at Syracuse University. Dr. Teitelbaum is formerly an ophthalmic photographer/technician who has a continued interest in research with persons with visual disabilities.

Mary M. Jackowski, Ph.D, O.D., serves as the coordinator of low vision services at the VA Medical Center in Syracuse. She is also a clinical assistant professor of the Departments of Physical Medicine and Rehabilitation and Ophthalmology, State University of New York, Health Science Center (SUNY, HSC) in Syracuse and is also affiliated with Department of Psychology at Syracuse University. Dr. Jackowski also maintains a private practice specializing in the assessment and treatment of persons with low vision.

Charles Teitelbaum, M.D., is chief of Ophthalmology at the Syracuse VA Medical Center where he oversees medical residency training and education. Dr. Teitelbaum is also a clinical associate professor of ophthalmology at SUNY HSC at Syracuse and maintains a private practice specializing in the treatment of glaucoma and inflammatory eye diseases at the Eye Consultants of Syracuse.

Common Causes
Safety
Issues
Special Concerns

The implementation of the Americans with Disabilities Act has made it possible for more visually-impaired and legally-blind individuals to find their way to your establishment seeking guidance on developing an exercise program that addresses their specific, personal goals. As when training other, healthy clients, some may be referred by their family physician for help coping with health-related problems (e.g., cardiovascular disease, hypertension, obesity or osteoporosis); others may seek the physical and psychological well-being associated with regular exercise. Still others may seek guidance in the initiation or continuation of their athletic training for competitive sports activities. Within the last 20 years, sociopolitical, technological and economic changes have made it possible for physically challenged players to participate in personal recreation, institutional athletic programs and even major athletic competitions. However, those with poor vision have special needs that must be anticipated, understood and addressed. It is necessary to develop a fundamental working knowledge of: 1) the visual system; 2) injuries and diseases that affect the visual system; 3) compensatory strategies for coping with specific types of visual impairment; and 4) devices that prevent eye injury. This chapter is divided into two sections. The first answers some common questions about visual impairment. The second section provides guidelines for the development of a successful physical-training program for visually-impaired persons.

Common Questions About Visual Impairment

How Does the Visual System Work?

The eye works much like a simple camera. The lens in the front of the camera focuses light onto the film located at the back of the camera. Light imprints an image on the film and the picture is "taken." Each structure of the eye has a specific function. The clear cornea and lens at the front of the eye bend and focus light rays, which then pass through the pupil, or adjustable aperture or opening in the iris (the colored part of the eye) and become focused. This narrow beam of light then penetrates the vitreous, a large space in the center of the eye filled with a clear, jelly-like substance. Finally, the light makes its way to the retina, a thin layer of tissue that lines the back of the eye and acts much like the film in a camera. The light focused on the retina initiates a complex visual message sent through the optic nerve to the brain. The brain, acting similar to a computer, organizes and integrates the image. It extracts the different types of visual information (e.g., shapes, sizes, textures, colors), compares it to input from other senses and creates an internal interpretation of the world for the viewer. Thus, both the eye and the brain must be functioning optimally for an individual to see.

Why Do Some People Need Glasses?

Sometimes the size, shape or structure of the eye contribute to a refractive disorder that prevents light from being clearly focused on the retina. For example, the length of the eye may be too short or too long, or the cornea may be shaped like a football instead of a basketball. Corrective therapies (i.e., spectacles, contact lenses or refractive surgery) adjust the visual system and accurately focus the image on the retina. Vision also may be affected by advancing age, which diminishes the elasticity of the lens and reduces the ability to focus at a distance and close up. Corrective lenses compensate for this, especially during reading.

Table 24.1

Client Information to Obtain from Medical Professionals

1) What is the degree of visual impairment that this client experiences (legally blind, low vision, vision in only one eye)? How do they function in their activities of daily living?

2) What is the nature of the impairment (central visual loss, peripheral field loss, glare problems etc.)? (Modifications to routine and equipment should not only be based upon degree of visual loss but also upon type of visual loss.)

3) What is the duration of this impairment (recent or long-standing)? (Adjustment to visual loss takes time.)

4) Has the client has recently undergone an operation or ever experienced and episodes of intraocular bleeding? If so, what specific activity guidelines do you recommend?

5) What are the client's day-to-day changes in visual status? Does the client's vision fluctuate due to systemic diseases (e.g., diabetes, hypertension) or medications (e.g., pilocarpine)? (activities may need to be scheduled accordingly)

6) Is the client's visual loss is secondary to traumatic head injury? Does the client experience any other associated symptoms such as attentional deficits, mood swing, impulsivity, etc.?

Note: For additional information pertaining to these assessment questions, it may be helpful and necessary to consult with other health care specialists working with the client including low visiospecialists and the client's treating opthalmologist.

It is important to differentiate between refractive disorders and eye diseases, which are problems in the visual system that cannot be corrected with glasses.

How is Vision Measured?

Visual function is measured by testing both distance and near vision (known as visual acuity). At times, due to particular disease processes, peripheral vision may be measured, and depth perception, color vision and sensitivity to contrasting tones may be investigated (Rosenberg, 1984). Each type of vision is measured differently, providing vital information about a person's ability to perform in the world around them. Because the brain makes a single image from what both eyes see, all measurements of visual functioning are performed by covering one eye and testing only that eye. Visual acuity and visual field are the two types of measurements most often documented for visually-impaired persons.

Visual Acuity

Visual acuity measures the central portion of visual functioning by testing the ability to recognize and identify objects of varying size at different distances. It is important to note that this measurement is used to indicate "best corrected" vision (which means with corrective lenses if any are needed) and, consequently, visual acuity test results represent the maximum level of visual functioning for distance and near for that person at that time. The test uses different-sized letters viewed at the standard distance-vision and near-vision lengths. Measurements are based upon a ratio: the participant's actual visual performance fixed at 20 feet in the numerator, and the corresponding distance at which a visually non-impaired person could see the same size image (usually ranging from 20 to 400 feet) placed in the denominator. For example, the fully functioning, healthy eye is said to have 20/20 vision because it can resolve standardized small objects (letters, numbers, pictures, etc.) at a viewing distance of 20 feet. In contrast, a visual acuity measured at 20/200 means the participant can see at 20 feet what a fully sighted person can see at 200 feet. Beyond the distance indicator of 400 feet, measurements are taken on the perception of objects: counting fingers (recorded as CF); then hand motion (recorded as HM); then light (re-corded as LP); and finally, the absence of perception of light (recorded as NLP).

Visual Field

Visual-acuity testing measures the function of the central 5 degrees of the retina, even though visual functioning also involves the remaining portion of the retina, which processes images of objects viewed in our peripheral vision. A fully functioning visual field helps us detect the presence and motion of large objects moving toward or away from our central vision. The peripheral visual field of each eye is made up of a three-dimensional area of vision extending approximately 90 degrees to the side, 65 degrees toward the nose, 40 to 45 degrees above, and 50 to 60 degrees below the central visual axis of the eye. Visual-field testing is not always conducted routinely; however, when employed, such testing uses a small pinpoint of light to separately map the visual field in each eye. Impairments discovered by visual-field testing can include a small spot in the peripheral retina of one eye, a missing quarter or half of visual field in one or both eyes, or the entire absence of peripheral vision, which leaves only central vision in tact (often referred to as "tunnel" vision). Damage can occur from neurologic disturbance (e.g., tumor, stroke) or eye disease (e.g., glaucoma, retinal disease).

Low Vision

Low vision is any type or amount of visual loss that reduces a person's optimal visual functioning. For example, with respect to obtaining driving licenses, many states allow for a documented "best corrected" visual acuity of 20/40 (objects at 20 feet are twice as large as those at the 20/20 level). Visual acuity less than 20/40 in the better eye results in the loss of unrestricted driving privileges. People with documented visual acuity of 20/60 or less in their better eye, or those who have substantial visual-field loss, often are labeled as "visually impaired" for legal and compensatory purposes.

There is a large variance in visual functioning in a strange environment for someone with moderate visual impairment compared to the person with legal blindness or no vision. An individual with 20/40 to 20/70 vision still should be able to drive a car during the day if their field of vision is good. They may not, however, be able to read the gauges on the treadmill or the pulse monitor that reveals their progress. Those with vision poorer than 20/70 may not be able to function well in new surroundings, especially those that restrict the field of vision. Magnifying glasses and talking watches are devices commonly used by persons with impaired vision.

Legal Blindness

Government agencies classify legal blindness based on measurements of both visual-acuity and visual-field testing. Measurements are taken using best-corrected vision (i.e., using glasses or other corrective devices). Legal blindness is established when the visual acuity in the better-seeing eye is 20/200 or less, or when the visual field in the better-seeing eye is less than 20-degrees wide. Remember that each eye is tested separately using corrective lenses if necessary. Consequently, a person who may be completely blind in one eye is not considered legally blind if the other eye still sees well.

A visual-impairment classification system has been established by the International Blind Sports Association (IBSA) for competition (Skaggs & Hopper, 1996). The first classification of legally blind athletes (B-1) includes those persons whose visual impairment renders them unable to perceive the contours of any object at any distance or direction, but who may or may not be able to perceive light. The second class (B-2) includes individuals whose visual acuity is documented at 20/600 or less with a visual field not greater than zero to 5 degrees. These people may be capable of perceiving hand movements. The third and final classification (B-3) includes people whose visual acuity ranges from 20/599 to 20/200 with a visual field of 5 to 20 degrees.

What are Common Causes of Visual Impairment?

Population studies in the United States show that about five percent of people are visually impaired, and 0.5 percent are legally blind. That is, their visual loss cannot be corrected with glasses, contact lenses or surgery. The incidence of both visual impairment and blindness is more than 20 times greater for people over age 75 vs. those in their 40s and 50s (Klein, Klein, Linton & DeMets, 1991; see also Tielsch, Sommer, Witt, Kat & Royall, 1990).

A variety of situations can alter the structures of a person's eye, interfere with their ability to see and result in visual impairment or blindness. Cataracts, glaucoma, age-related macular degeneration, diabetes mellitus, disturbances of the light pathway and injury (either to the eye or brain) are common causes of the degradation of visual functioning.

Cataracts

A cataract is a clouding over or darkening of the natural lens of the eye that causes a diffuse decrease in both central and peripheral visual clarity. Cataracts can result from advancing age, injury to the eye or head, severe inflammation of the eye and metabolic problems such as diabetes. This decrease in vision usually progresses over several years. Persons with various stages of cataract development may complain of blurred vision, poor contrast, altered color perception and sensitivity to glare. Though cataracts are usually correctable with surgery, many people put off surgery until their level of functional impairment is severe enough to warrant the risks associated with it.

Glaucoma

Glaucoma is a condition in which the pressure inside the eye increases, damaging the visual system. Glaucoma can result from the inability of the eye's fluid to enter and exit the eye in a balanced fashion. Everyone's eye makes aqueous humor, a clear nutritional fluid that bathes the front chamber of the eye. When this fluid cannot exit the eye through the natural fluid drain, the pressure within the eye rises. A sustained increase in ocular pressure causes damage to the optic nerve fibers (which send visual signals to the brain) and eventually leads to loss of vision. However, visual symptoms related to glaucoma can, at first, go undetected. Pressure increases slowly and resulting visual field losses are imperceptible to the person suffering from glaucoma. Initially there may be some small areas of loss of peripheral vision. If left untreated, or if unresponsive to treatment, glaucoma damage can progress, usually painlessly, until the entire field of vision in one or both eyes is lost. People with glaucoma may have difficulty

Common Questions
About Visual
Impairments

with glare, decreased contrast sensitivity, poor depth perception and, sometimes, dim vision as some eye-drop treatments constrict the pupil and reduce the amount of light entering the eye. Individuals with glaucoma usually are treated with a combination of pharmacotherapy (eye drops and pills), laser treatment or surgery.

Age-related Macular Degeneration (AMD)

The eye's ability to distinguish fine detail is confined to a very small (i.e., one-half millimeter) portion of the central retina in the back of the eye called the macula. This tiny area is responsible for the sharpness and clarity of distance, near and color vision in the central 10 degrees of the visual field. Unfortunately, this area also is vulnerable to systemic and ocular disease processes that can profoundly affect visual functioning (e.g., age-related macular degeneration). There are two classic forms of AMD: 1) atrophic (often referred to as dry) in which there is a gradual loss of the central retinal tissue, and 2) hemorrhagic (often referred to as wet), which involves the growth of abnormal blood vessels within the deeper layers of the retina that can bleed within the retina causing a fibrotic scarred membrane. This problem most often occurs in older persons, and contributing factors include heredity, smoking, hardening of the arteries with poor circulation to the retina, ultraviolet light toxicity, and possible nutritional deficits such as low levels of zinc and vitamins A, C and E . Persons coping with AMD may experience decreased distance, reading and color vision, and glare problems. Treatment is limited. Laser treatment can be used to cauterize abnormal blood vessels if they are growing at a significant distance from the macula. Radiation, surgery and pharmacotheraphy are being studied as methods to reduce vascular membrane growth.

Diabetes Mellitus

Diabetes mellitus is a multi-systemic disease process that may affect the heart, kidneys, eyes, peripheral nerves and extremities. The two primary types of eye disease associated with diabetes, background and proliferative retinopathy, can damage the retina and lead to subsequent visual loss. Problems with insulin metabolism lead to abnormalities of the blood vessel walls and the growth of abnormal blood vessels, which can lead to bleeding and scarring in the retina. Background retinopathy is more common than proliferative retinopathy. It is a condition in which the retinal blood vessels develop microaneurysms and leaky vessel walls that may result in bleeding and the release of fluid and fat within the central retina. Proliferative retinopathy is characterized by abnormal blood vessel growth that fills the vitreous cavity with blood or produces focal areas of poor circulation within the retina. Fibrous scar tissue can also appear and produce a wrinkling or a detachment of the retina. Such alterations of the retina inevitably result in varying degrees (partial to total) of vision loss.

Disturbances of the Light Pathway

Clouding of the normally transparent structures of the eye or disturbance of the retina retards and distorts the passage of light through the eye and reduces image quality and clarity of vision. Examples of light-blocking elements are corneal scars, cataracts, blood or inflammatory cells in the vitreous and irregularities (wrinkling or tears) of the retina. Placing these obstacles in the light's path creates images of objects that appear blurry, hazy, distorted or even doubled. Affected individuals may complain of an increased sensitivity to light, similar to that experienced when looking through a dirty windshield at headlights of oncoming cars at night.

Injury

Any injury to the eye poses the threat of permanent vision loss. Objects such as tree branches can scratch the cornea and leave a permanent scar. Welding sparks and metals, BB bullets, fishing hooks, and other such accidents also can cause permanent damage to eye structures and result in visual impairment or blindness. Individuals also may experience visual dysfunction as a result of brain injury, such as that caused by a stroke (diagnosed or undiagnosed), brain surgery, or any type of head trauma including car accidents, athletic accidents (football or skiing injuries), and the effects of trauma associated with competitive boxing. Brain-injured persons can often suffer from a variety of visual discomforts. At times, after a brain injury, there can be a loss of central or peripheral vision, depending upon the nature and extent of the injury. Other times, visual acuity is measured at a fully functioning 20/20 level but the brain-injured person reports experiencing new, and often intense, sensitivity to light, difficulty focusing the eyes, "ghost-images" or "haloes" around objects, and difficulty (or inability) shifting their focus from images in the distance to those nearby. Symptoms may persist for months or years after even low-impact injury (e.g., whiplash) and may, at times, increase in intensity. It is critical to be aware of the fact that disease processes or injuries affecting brain function can also significantly impact the visual system and, therefore, a person's ability to safely engage in physical activity.

Guidelines for Developing a Successful Physical Fitness Program

Making an exercise program available to visually impaired persons has well-documented and important benefits: improved physical health (e.g., cardiovascular functioning, cholesterol level, bone strength, body fat composition and weight management), improved ocular health (e.g., moderation of intraocular pressure), and improved mental health (mental clarity and alertness, improved sleep patterns, stress management, self-esteem, mood management). Such benefits are recognized by the United States government and increasing levels of physical activity have been included as an objective in the Healthy People 2000 goals set forth by the U.S. Department of Health and Human Services (Skaggs & Hopper, 1996). However, such advantages may never become reality if a visually impaired person does not receive the emotional or functional support they require as they negotiate the many obstacles that cross their path when pursuing physical activity goals. It is critical that you be exceptionally well equipped with the knowledge and skills necessary to modify existing programs and build newly structured programs specific to the needs of your visually impaired clients. This attention and knowledge should also extend to your client's emotional well-being. A dual emphasis on functional and emotional support maximizes the ability of visually impaired clients to achieve their physical fitness goals. Following are guidelines for providing functional and emotional support to your visually impaired clients.

Conduct a Thorough Assessment and Introduction to the Facility

Assessment

Conduct a thorough assessment of your client's unique abilities, limitations and goals for physical activity, and inquire about their particular visual disability (see Table 24.1).

Answers to questions regarding your client's prior experiences with physical activity can be used to help your client overcome past difficulties, and anticipate and cope with future challenges. It is also helpful to elicit information about the effects of your client's visual disability on daily living; ask them to provide examples of activities they can easily engage in as well as those that pose more of a challenge. Assess strengths and weaknesses in their visual functioning.

During the initial visit and assessment you may wish to reassure the client that, while you may not be an expert with regard to visual impairment, you will work to provide a safe environment, modify equipment as is necessary and possible, and achieve mutually agreed upon training goals. Use a collaborative approach when designing the goals and objectives of the training program to maximize the client's motivation and sense of control. Furthermore, using a collaborative approach to goal-setting begins the development of a positive and professional relationship.

Facility Orientation

Conducting an initial orientation plays a central role in helping the low-vision client feel safe, secure and in control. A guided tour of the facility (using guided sight techniques if necessary) that includes the changing room and activity areas is essential, as is a thorough introduction to the mechanics of the exercise machines (which should not be positioned too close together). Use of a combination of physical and auditory cues may be necessary. For example, when you want a participant to sit on the seat of a stationary cycle, place the client's hand on the seat, then move their free hand to the handlebars and use verbal cues to let them know if they are on the left or the right. Teach the client to read the machine displays if they have enough visual function. Repeat the tour and equipment layout orientation three-to-five more times to ensure the visually impaired client learns the layout.

Attend to Safety Issues and Modify Equipment as Necessary

Guiding a Visually-impaired Person

When leading a blind client through their orientation or a walk in an unknown area, stand to the client's left, a half step ahead of them. The client should grasp your right forearm, above the elbow, with their left hand. This allows them to hold their cane in their right hand and use it to explore the area straight ahead, and find objects or the wall to their right. Set your pace at a slow walk and use auditory cues to describe the area and to let them know when you are approaching obstacles (e.g., stairs, doorways, a narrow hall or a chair). (Faye 1984)

Routine Facility Modifications

Modify your facility to increase the likelihood of positive experiences. A blind person may turn off to the many joys and benefits of physical activity for fear of, or the actual experience of, injury by a fall or collision. Consistently keep doors completely open or closed, to reduce collision hazards (Arnheim & Sinclair, 1985). Ensure that work areas are well lighted and control glare as much as possible. Keep indoor and outdoor activity areas uncluttered and free of obstacles, and eliminate protruding bars or sharp edges on equipment. It is critical to monitor running tracks to ensure there are no obstacles (e.g., hurdles or running blocks) before allowing a visually impaired person to run.

Buddy System

Recommend that visually impaired clients exercise with a fully sighted buddy when not working with you. The buddy system promotes increased safety to the visually-impaired client by performing various tasks such as reading displays on aerobic machines, placing pins on weight-training machines and selecting appropriate free weights. Buddies also may provide auditory cues and instructions to visually-impaired runners, swimmers, skiers and bikers. Such helpers can prove to be invaluable to the visually impaired exerciser who, as a result, may engage in a wider variety of activities or participate more frequently, confidently and safely in already-familiar activities. If a buddy is unavailable, guide dogs, and for swimmers, lifeguards, may be helpful in establishing a safe environment within which the visually-impaired person can exercise.

Match Modifications to Each Client's Unique Needs

Each disease process or injury affects the visual system in a unique manner and is associated with a particular type of visual impairment. The fundamental types of visual impairment can be categorized as: 1) central vision loss, 2) peripheral vision loss, 3) visual loss in one eye, 4) complete loss of vision, and 5) disturbances of the light pathway. Following is a discussion of these visual system deficits as well as strategies you may use to modify existing activity programs.

Central Vision Losses

Individuals with reduced visual acuity may have difficulty with any activity that requires recognition of fine detail, such as reading gauges, meters or other visual display units with numbers, letters or other graphics that are too small and/or poorly contrasted to identify. Typically, visual acuity of 20/40 or better is necessary to see symbols the size of normal newsprint.

You may need to use one or several strategies to improve the functioning of persons with central visual losses. For example, small graphics can be replaced with enlarged print, and high-contrast fluorescent tape or flashing lights may substitute for symbols. Tactile cues such as Braille or graphics can replace visual information, and auditory cues such as buzzers, bells or metronomes may be used to signal duration or speed.

Remember that though a client may have profound central vision loss, their peripheral vision may be intact and allow them to be independently mobile and participate in solitary sports (e.g., walking, swimming, gymnastics, dance) that don't require precise and rapid localization of moving objects or accurate eye/hand coordination.

Peripheral Vision Losses

Losses in peripheral vision that cannot be compensated for optically, are often more restrictive for athletes than are central vision losses. Participation in sports that require judgment of body position and motion relative to the environment rely on gross visual cues in the peripheral field. Players who lose large portions of their visual field may have considerable trouble engaging in a variety of activities or participating in sports that incorporate airborne objects (baseball, basketball, kickball, etc.). A hockey or lacrosse stick can appear out of nowhere and be particularly dangerous to persons with constricted visual field function. Inferior visual field losses may make walking or running, especially over curbs, down flights of stairs or around obstacles below the line-of-sight, hazardous. Loss of the entire left or right portions of the visual field may change the perception of midline, which can result in individuals drifting toward unseen walls or objects.

Carefully supervise and continually provide cues to individuals who wish to engage in interactive activities. Eye glasses with prism lenses move the remaining visual field into the missing area and may be used to compensate for some problems with visual field loss. Otherwise, encourage compensatory head turning in the direction of the missing field to "center" the remaining visual field area.

Visual Loss in One Eye

A special subset of clients with vision loss are those who have useful vision in only one eye. If vision loss is recent, monocular vision can create profound spatial disorientation with loss of depth perception and associated problems with balance, judgment of speed and distance, and hand/eye coordination. Long-standing monocular vision may allow for the sensory adaptations that allow players to use other visual/perceptual cues (relative size of objects, placement of shadows, etc.) to compensate for the loss of binocular vision. These individuals have far less trouble with coordinated movements and visually based activities; consider several factors when working with them. First, the nature of the physical activity in which they are participating (e.g., non-interactive vs. interactive competitive activity) and the length of time they have had to adjust to their monocular visual status. During many activities, these persons can be

treated like fully sighted individuals, however, it is important to encourage wearing protective eye wear.

Complete Loss of Vision

Individuals with complete loss of vision in both eyes often demonstrate heightened response levels in their remaining senses, and auditory, proprioceptive or kinesthetic information is used more effectively. To best help blind persons engage in exercise activities, orient the client to space and time using visual memory skills, execution drills and rehearsal of all activities. Break down the rehearsal and drills into simple, repetitive steps. Once the participant is confident of the layout of space and objects and has become physically proficient at the movements of the activity, you may find that their lack of vision is a non-issue in sport or recreation (e.g., weight training, aerobics, wrestling, tandem bicycling and freestyle gymnastics).

Disturbances in the Light Pathway

Glare is the scatter of light as it passes through the eye. It can be caused by aging, injury, surgery, cataract, inflammation that interferes with the direct pathway of light, or the presence of blood, which can scatter light within the eye and reduce vision. Both quality as well as quantity of light is necessary for good vision for all persons, but are especially important considerations in maximizing performance and safety of visually impaired clients.

For problems related to glare, specially-tinted lenses, a hat with a visor, or just controlling illumination sources can be helpful. Visually impaired clients may choose to use dark sunglasses that produce greater visual comfort.

The use of darker tints on glasses may be necessary outdoors, particularly during activities in which glare off snow, sand, water or cement is present. Take care to not over color filter light to affect perception of significant colors such as red and green in traffic lights, or other visual displays. Sometimes the use of light-filtering or polarized lenses, or antireflective lens coatings greatly enhances the sharpness or contrast of the visual image without reducing lighting to unsafe levels. With regard to indoor activities, changing the type (fluorescent or incandescent) or placement of ambient lighting may maximize vision and comfort. Individuals who complain of light sensitivity to fluorescent light may benefit from using yellow lens tints or filters that eliminate short-wavelength (blue) light.

Contrast sensitivity is the ability to notice the difference in brightness between an object and its background. Problems with contrast sensitivity may be caused by aging, disease or dysfunction of the retina. Good sensitivity to contrast allows clients to discern the shape of objects and promotes good depth perception (e.g., noticing the protrusion of a curb or the nature of the incline of stairs). For difficulty related to inadequate contrast, cover shiny, light-reflecting surfaces, such as tile or ceramic floors, or the walls, with dark, non-reflective materials. In addition, lightly colored or transparent objects should be boldly marked or color contrasted to ensure they stand out from the background (Rosenberg, 1984). Problems may arise when exercise areas are painted with similar colors and tones, thereby making it difficult for persons with contrast sensitivity problems to negotiate space (e.g., jog on an indoor track). If possible, paint the walls a contrasting color or pattern, or install a guide rail. Less time-consuming and less costly alternatives include taping paper shapes to the wall to increase visual cues, or suggesting the individual use an extra long cane to help find the wall or edge of a track, or use a sighted buddy or guide dog.

Design a Preliminary Outline for an Exercise Program

After conducting a careful initial assessment, developing an understanding of the nature of the visual impairment and modifying space and equipment as necessary, develop a preliminary outline for an exercise program. Non-interactive physical activities are most appropriate for visually impaired persons just beginning an exercise program. Incorporate a small number of different activities and begin with low degrees of intensity. For visually impaired clients with more experience and skill, consider more sophisticated and challenging routines as well as interactive sports. The four basic components to any exercise program should be addressed: warm up and cool down, aerobic workout, strength training and flexibility training. Every program must be uniquely tailored to each individual's current goals, interests and abilities; over time, suitable modifications to routines will become necessary to best meet your client's evolving goals and abilities.

Provide Emotional Support

The likelihood of achieving success with an exercise program is enhanced when skill and knowledge are combined with emotional support and the development of patience, respect and empathy for each unique human being and their potential. Specifically, promote independence, develop a program that does not induce excessive levels of stress, develop a positive, professional relationship with the client, and utilize available resources when necessary.

Promote Independence

Build an exercise program slowly and break up the routine into easily manageable steps that can be modified as time passes. This approach enhances the client's motivation and self-esteem and helps build upon their successes. Help your client with mobility, routines and equipment only as much as is needed to avoid the pitfalls of being overly protective. Help your client master a level of independence that feels comfortable to improve their sense of control. Anticipate and work to avoid any negative experiences. If a problem emerges, try to determine what went wrong and how the two of you can work together to avoid similar problems in the future.

Attend to Your Client's Level of Stress

Compared to fully sighted individuals, the visually impaired person has additional obstacles to overcome when performing activities of daily living. Furthermore, acquired visual loss in the latter years of life can be especially stressful for persons who must learn to be dependent on someone else for help with driving, shopping, cooking or crossing the street. Therefore, negative experiences related to physical activity (e.g., a serious fall during a hike or while running) may interact with stressful lifestyle experiences and lead to adherence difficulties. Failure to successfully negotiate these difficulties may lead to loss of self-esteem and, eventually, depression.

The perception of stress varies from person to person. What is stressful for one may not be for another. Therefore, it is best to create a dialogue with your clients that allows you to better understand their personal reactions to the program you have developed to meet their exercise needs. A helpful tool for creating such a dialogue is good listening skills. Summarize what your client is telling you and repeat it to them to make sure you understand. Working to reduce stress levels for the visually-impaired client results in a safe and effective program, meets the agreed upon physical activity goals, provides modifications that meet the client's level of physical ability and visual functioning, and is conducted in the context of a positive and interactive relationship.

Build a Positive and Professional Relationship

Incorporate patience, sensitivity and empathy into your interactions. Realize that you may not immediately be successful in your attempts to meet and anticipate your client's needs, and listen to your client's comments. If they do not provide comments, ask. Use the reciprocal feedback process to modify the routine (e.g., type of activity, duration, intensity) as necessary. Remember, working together as a team (trainer and client) is a process. As with any other relationship, the amount of attention the two of you devote to improving the quality and balance of the relationship directly corresponds to the subsequent attainment of joint goals and a sense of personal satisfaction.

Resources

Feel free to consult with other professionals (both in exercise-related as well as health-related areas). Acquiring additional knowledge, from multiple perspectives can prove to be an important tool. Second, become knowledgeable regarding resources for visually impaired clients. Regarding low-vision support, call on The Lighthouse, local public libraries, ophthalmologists and optometrists, and other low-vision experts at hospitals or educational institutions. Build a referral list of agencies and professionals (e.g., psychiatrists, psychologists, social workers and clergy) available in your area.

There are several associations available to facilitate the participation of visually impaired and/or blind persons in various athletic events.

For example, The United States Association for Blind Athletes has national competition events for track and field, gymnastics, wrestling, judo, skiing, tandem cycling, goal ball, power lifting and swimming. (Tseng 1998) Others include the U.S. Blind Golfers Association, the Blind Outdoor Leisure Development, and the American Blind Skiing Foundation (Vinger, 1994). Veterans Administration Rehabilitation Centers across the country provide good examples of training for athletic recreation by blind participants who typically were first introduced to the activity after losing all vision. Visually-impaired persons can participate in activities such as recreational skiing, racing and other timed events with the help of coaches that ski alongside and call out visual details of the slope, instructions and maneuvers.

Know When to Limit Physical Activity

Certain eye diseases and conditions require special attention when training. These include persons who recently have had an eye operation, persons with diabetes and persons with age-related macular degeneration. Below is a brief discussion of each of these conditions and how physical activity may or may not be restricted. Direct consultation with your client's healthcare professionals (in person or in writing) is always recommended.

Post-Surgery

Following any type of eye surgery, contact the client's physician to obtain physical activity guidelines. Below are some general guidelines for glaucoma, cataract and vitreous surgery.

Following surgery for glaucoma (which included cutting a new drain through the wall of the eye), patients typically should refrain from all strenuous physical activity for the first few weeks. Any straining or squeezing could result in damage to the intraocular structures.

Following surgery for retinal detachment, all strenuous physical activity should be avoided for the first month, however, light aerobic activities such as walking may be advised depending upon the status of the patient. For some persons, a fixed head position is required following this type of surgery. After the first month following surgery, activity levels usually, can be incrementally increased back to baseline levels.

The individual who has just had cataract surgery should be limited to walking or easy cycling for the first few weeks. Light weight training using low weights and multiple repetitions helps to reduce the risk of dislocation of the plastic lens implant, bleeding, vitreous separation and retinal detachment.

For the person who has recently had laser treatment, or surgery, to remove blood from inside the eye (vitrectomy), low-impact aerobic exercise such as walking, and light weight training with multiple repetitions and low weights, may be appropriate. See Table 24.2 for general guidelines.

Risk of Intraocular Bleeding

Several disorders are associated with increased risk of intraocular bleeding. They are proliferative diabetic retinopathy, a complication associated with diabetes, and hemorrhagic macular degeneration, a particular form of age-related macular degeneration (AMD). When conducting initial assessment, it is critical to inquire whether or not your client has experienced any episodes of intraocular bleeding. If your client acknowledges a history of such

bleeding or has a diagnosis of either of the conditions described here, special care should be devoted to the modification of their exercise regimen. As mentioned in Table 24.2, when working with clients with these particular disorders it is important to contact their ophthalmologist for specific exercise guidelines. Generally, these restrictions may entail avoiding valsalva activities (e.g., power weight lifting, bench presses, sit-ups on an inclined board); high impact activities such as high impact aerobic dance, jogging, jumping; and other cardiovascular activities that require high levels of perceived exertion. For these clients, as with those post-surgical clients, low-impact aerobic exercise such walking, stationary biking. Flexibility exercises and light weight training with multiple repetitions and low weights may also be appropriate. In all cases, low rates of perceived exertion throughout exercise is required along with regular monitoring of blood pressure throughout the exercise session.

Warning Signs and Symptoms

Exercise should be stopped if the client experiences dimming or loss of vision, new floaters (spots or shapes "floating" through vision) or light flashes in the eye. Note that beta-blocker

Table 24.2

Typical Activity Guidelines

- All clients should use appropriate protective eyewear.
- When the trainer is not physically present during an exercise routine, all visually-impaired persons should be accompanied by a sighted partner to ensure their safety.
- For clients who are new to a particular activity extended introductions and monitoring of the activity is necessary to evaluate client's adaptation to their exercise routine, success of equipment and activity modifications.
- Adjust internal light sources to maximize visual functioning of clients.
- For persons who have undergone recent eye surgery or who are at risk of intraocular bleeding, contact their treating physician for specific activity guidelines. Generally for these patients, it is wise to avoid activities

involving (a) heavy weight lifting (e.g., power lifting, bench press, sit-ups on an inclined board); (b) high levels of impact (e.g., step aerobics, jogging, jumping); and activities which involve high rates of perceived exertion. Instead concentrate on low impact aerobic activities, flexibility training and light weight training with multiple repetitions and low weights. Keep rates of perceived exertion low and monitor blood pressure regularly throughout session.

- Stop exercise if client experiences particular visual symptoms such as dimming of vision, loss of vision, new floaters inside the eye (can look like clouds, strings, spiders, blobs of ink that move), or sees flashes of light. These symptoms require attention from client's treating ophthalmologist.

eye drops used for the treatment of glaucoma can cause bradycardia (slow pulse) and, on rare occasions, blackouts. If any of these situations occur during an exercise training session, the client must receive medical attention and their treating physician should be contacted.

Special Concerns: How to Prevent Sports-related Eye Injuries

The true incidence of eye injuries in sports is unknown because there is no reliable national data collection system for sports or any other type of eye trauma. Though not all serious, eye injuries from sport are extremely common, accounting for 10 percent of all hospital-treated eye injuries; approximately 5.5 percent of all college varsity sports players sustain some form of eye injury each season. In addition, each year, approximately 1.6 to 2.4 million Americans sustain an eye injury, and 40,000 become legally blind. A staggering one-third of these injuries are sports related (Feist and Farber, 1989).

Injury to the eye that results in visual loss can be one of the single most devastating events that occur during a lifetime. Types of injury include punctures or cuts by a sharp or blunt object, blow to the face or head. For example, the eye may be cut by a sharp projectile, frequently a fragment of the athlete's own spectacle lenses, converting blunt trauma into a penetrating injury and permanent impairment. Blows to the eye by small blunt objects, such as BB gun pellets, golf balls or hockey sticks, deliver great forces to the eye itself and expand the eyeball perpendicular to the direction of impact. Such direct impact can have profound and lasting effects upon the external and internal structures of the eye. Energy from blows by blunt objects larger than the eye itself, such as a tennis ball, elbow or fist, are somewhat absorbed by the surrounding bones and tissue, which can fracture easily. Such "blow out" injuries can increase the incidence of internal eye injury. A blow to the skull can create direct or indirect injury to the eye or visual pathways of the brain and create permanent or temporary vision loss. The large forces necessary to create these in-juries are routinely found in many contact/collision sports, as well as skiing, cycling and motorized recreational activities.

Protective Eye Wear

No one is immune to the risk of injury, however, all persons can work to prevent such an unfortunate occurrence. Most sports-related eye injuries or facial bone fractures are preventable with proper protective equipment. Because about half the population wears spectacles, the dispensing of protective impact-resistant lenses can protect a vast number of individuals from permanent visual disability. The use of impact-resistant eyewear (i.e., impact-resistant lenses for glasses, sports goggles, face masks and helmets) cannot be overemphasized.

Impact-resistant Lenses

The impact resistance of a spectacle lens is related to the size of the object hitting the surface. Testing with a variety of objects used in a variety of sports (e.g., golf, lacrosse, tennis) has confirmed the superiority of lenses made with polycarbonate material. That is, polycarbonate glass demonstrated a strength of 10 to 20 times greater than regular spectacle glass and other plastics, which easily shatter upon impact.

Sports Goggles, Face Masks and Helmets

During collision sports in which blows to the skull occur (hockey, football), total head protection is best achieved by a face protector mounted on a well-designed helmet. In sports with far less force transmission potential, only isolated protection is required. A squash ball has little potential for creating brain injury and only eye protection is required. In moderate-impact sports such as tennis, trade-offs between protection, weight, visual field obstruction and even style are important. However, players who have limitations in vision and or reflex time require additional protective wear.

UV Protection

Bright outdoor light can be harmful to visual functioning over time. The ideal sports sunglasses should block ultraviolet light rays, decrease brightness of light and be worn in combination with hats or visors. Such glasses also should be lightweight and form-fitting to the face to prevent loss through rapid head turning. Furthermore, side shields or a rim across the top of the glasses may protect against oblique light rays. Boaters and persons who enjoy fishing often prefer the option of polarization added to lenses to reduce glare produced by sun striking the water. In general, moderate to dark amber polycarbonate lenses in face-fitting, stable frames fill these requirements for protection from outdoor light sources.

Conclusion

This chapter may be used as a beginning guide to advance your knowledge of visual impairment and develop successful programs for visually impaired clients. You should continue to build upon this information base by: 1) asking questions of healthcare professionals (e.g., low-vision experts, ophthalmologists, optometrists, nurses), 2) continued reading on the subject, 3) engaging in the processes of experimentation and elimination to achieve suitable modifications to equipment, facilities, and routines, and, most importantly, 4) continuing a dialogue with your clients and other persons coping with visual impairment so you can learn more and increase the availability of active opportunities that these persons so richly deserve.

References

Arnheim, D.D. & Sinclair, W.A. (1985). *Physical Education for Special Populations*. New Jersey: Prentice-Hall.

Feist, R.M. & Farber, M.D. (1 989). Ocular trauma epidemiology. Archives of Ophthalmology, 107, 503.

Klein, R., Klein, B., Linton, K.L.P. & DeMets, D.L. (1991). *The Beaver Dam eye study: Visual acuity*. Ophthalmology, 98, 1310-1315.

Rosenberg, R. (1984). Light, Glare, and contrast in low vision care. In E.E. Faye (Ed.) *Clinical Low Vision*. Boston: Little Brown & Co. (pp. 197-212).

Skaggs, S. & Hopper, C. (1996). Individuals with visual impairments: A review of psychomotor behavior. *Adapted Physical Activity Quarterly*, 13, 16-26.

Tseng, A.M. (1998). Swimming into the mainstream and other ways the visually-impaired can participate in sports. Journal of Low Vision and Neuro-Optometric Rehabilitation, 11, 6-9.

Tielsch, J.M., Sommer, A., Witt, K., Kat, J., & Royall, R.M. (1990). Blindness and visual impairment in an American urban population: The Baltimore eye survey. *Archives of Ophthalmology*, 108, 286-290.

Vinger, P. (1994). The eye and sports medicine. In Duane, T. & Jaeger, E.A. (Eds.) *Clinical Ophthalmology*. Philadelphia: L.B. Lippincott Company. (pp. 1- 69).

Weitzman, D.M. (1993). Promoting healthful exercise for visually impaired persons with diabetes. *Journal of Visual Impairment & Blindness*, 79, 97-99.

List of Suggested Readings:

Faye, E.E. *Clinical Low Vision* (1984). Little Brown & Company, Inc. New York Second Edition

Tseng, A.M. (1998). Swimming into the mainstream and other ways the visually-impaired can participate in sports. *Journal of Low Vision and Neuro-Optometric Rehabilitation*, 11, 6-9.

Vinger, P.F., Classe, J.G., & Woods, T.A. (1997). *The Eye and Sports Medicine Manual*. International Academy of Sports Vision. Wills Eye Hospital, Philadelphia.

Acknowledgements

We would like to express our gratitude to Charles A. Mango and Mary Lou Mendez for their helpful comments on earlier drafts of this chapter.

CHAPTER 25

Intellectual Disabilities

GREG REID
DAVID L. MONTGOMERY

Greg Reid, Ph.D., is a professor in and chairman of the Department of Physical Education at McGill University in Montreal, Canada. He is a specialist in adapted physical activity and former editor of the Adapted Physical Activity Quarterly. He received his doctorate from Pennsylvania State University and developed a research program on learning and performance of individuals with developmental disabilities, and on fitness for those with intellectual disabilities. The latter research was conducted with Dr. Montgomery.

David L. Montgomery, Ph.D., is a professor in the Department of Physical Education and co-director of the Seagram Sports Science Centre at McGill University. He is an exercise physiologist and fellow of the American College of Sports Medicine. He received his doctorate from Purdue University and pursued a research program focusing on ice hockey and endurance performance. He is currently investigating the use of hyperbaric oxygen therapy in athletic performance and as a treatment for soft tissue injury and cerebral palsy.

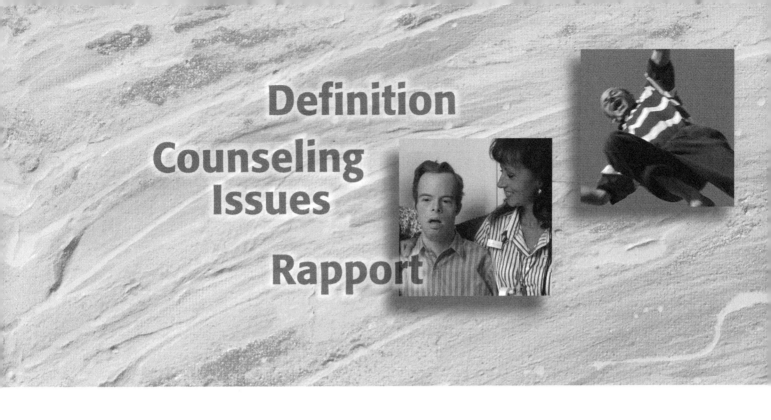

Definition
Counseling
Issues

Rapport

There is a need for fitness professionals who can design exercise programs for people with intellectual disabilities. The latter understand what exercise is, experience motivation to participate in physical activity, and can improve their fitness and health. This chapter discusses the importance of regular physical activity for people with intellectual disabilities as well as assessment and exercise leadership strategies.

Professionals agree that engaging in consistent, moderate-intensity physical activity produces positive health changes (Bouchard, 1997). While exercise programs alone have not been particularly effective in changing the body composition of people with intellectual disabilities, they have had positive effects when combined with other interventions. In addition, research demonstrating positive changes in cardiovascular functioning also has shown rapid reversal once the formal exercise program has ended (Pitetti & Tan, 1991). Thus, physical fitness is only one aspect of needed lifestyle change. Other factors include daily physical activity, nutritional education, personal choice and self-monitoring. All of these aspects must be considered when working with most clients, but especially those with **intellectual disabilities.**

Definition and Etiology

Terminology used in adapted physical activity evolves continuously. While the term "mental retardation" is commonly used in the U.S., it has lost favor in many other countries (Sherrill, 1998). The preferred terms are "intellectually disabled" or "people with intellectual disabilities" — terms that underscore the fact that such individuals are people first. Other terms, such as "developmental disability" and "learning handicap," may be favored depending on the region. Yet the American Association on Mental Retardation (AAMR), in its most recent manual, continued to use "mental retardation" in definition, etiology and classification (Luckasson et al., 1992).

According to the AAMR:

Mental retardation refers to substantial limitations in present functioning. It is characterized by significantly sub-average intellectual functioning, existing concurrently with related limitations in two or more of the following applicable adaptive skill areas: communication, self-care, home living, social skills, community use, self-direction, health and safety, functional academics, leisure and work. Mental retardation manifests before age 18 (Luckasson et al., 1992).

Subaverage intellectual functioning is defined as scoring below 70 to 75 on an IQ test. The adaptive skills include 10 aspects of daily living at which most of us are reasonably adept, independent and flexible. Seidl (1998) suggests that the majority of the 10 adaptive skill areas is directly or indirectly related to motor behavior. In fact, fitness is specifically listed as a component of health and safety in the formal definition (Luckasson et al., 1992). Finally, mental retardation or intellectual disability must be evident prior to age 18. It may surprise you to know that most individuals are not diagnosed until they enter and subsequently fail in school. Only a relatively small number of individuals have clear symptoms from birth or even early childhood.

Prior to the AAMR's 1992 definition, classifications of intellectual disabilities included terms such as mild, moderate, severe and profound. These were based almost solely on IQ and no longer are advocated. Classification now is based on the concept of intensity of support required by the person. Among those with intellectual disabilities, the need for support ranges from almost constant assistance to being nearly self-sufficient. Four levels of support exist: intermittent, limited, extensive and pervasive. Intermittent support is episodic or short term. That is, the individual is largely independent, needing only occasional assistance. Limited support is characterized by consistency over a given time period, although it may be limited in time. Extensive support is regular assistance in at least some environments, such as the workplace. Pervasive support refers to assistance that is constant and crosses several environments. Thus, Luckasson et al. (1992) suggest that individuals should no longer be referred to as having mild mental retardation, but rather as "a person with mental retardation who needs limited support in communication and social skills." A person with intellectual disabilities who requires only limited support may learn academic skills from grades three to six, show no delays in motor skills, be gainfully employed in good economic times, and may marry and have children. Their intellectual disability may lie in problem solving or conceptual thinking, and infrequent support will be required. Those needing limited or extensive support may not enjoy as much academic progress, and may need assistance in learning social and vocational skills, and during employment. Pervasive support is provided to individuals who have significant speech and movement difficulties, who require instruction in basic self-care skills, and who need supervision and support in employment.

The incidence of intellectual disabilities usually is estimated at 3 percent. This translates into 7.5 million U.S. citizens (Sherrill, 1998). The vast majority of these individuals fall within the upper range of functioning (Drew, Logan & Hardman, 1992) and are prime candidates for exercise training with a clinical exercise specialist.

There are hundreds of identified causes of intellectual disability, which often are categorized as prenatal, perinatal and postnatal (Luckasson et al., 1992). Prenatal etiologies include chromosomal disorders, such as **Down's syndrome** and fragile X syndrome; metabolism disorders, such as phenylketonuria, a condition in which an inherited defect affects an individual's ability to metabolize phenylalanine, requiring a diet free of or low in phenylalanine to avoid mental retardation; and environmental problems, such as fetal alcohol syndrome, drug effects and intrauterine malnutrition. Perinatal problems are infections or trauma that occur immediately prior to, during or after birth, such as anoxia (lack of oxygen).

Postnatal causes include head injuries, encephalitis, meningitis, lead and mercury poisoning, malnutrition, and environmental deprivation. Despite the abundance of potential causes, the exact origin of intellectual disabilities in the majority of people is unknown (Drew et al., 1992), and with few exceptions, there is no identified link between etiology and physical activity guidelines. In fact, in the past, researchers usually have ignored etiology in studies of motor behavior.

Thus, whether the etiology of an individual's intellectual disability is known or unknown, as a clinical exercise specialist it is important that you compile a list of medical conditions that may influence the individual's ability to perform physical activity. The only intellectual disability for which guidelines such as these are readily available is Down's syndrome. Though other forms of intellectual disability are associated with medical conditions, the wide variations among this population defy generalizations like those offered for Down's syndrome. While many, if not most, people with an intellectual disability have no additional medical condition that influences participation in physical activity, it is prudent to ascertain if participants experience seizures, emotional problems or other health restrictions, or if they are taking medication that may limit physical activity participation.

Down's Syndrome

Down's syndrome is caused by one of three chromosomal anomalies (Reid & Block, 1996; Sherrill, 1998). People with Down's syndrome may look like members of their family but also have distinctive features, such as short stature, particularly short limbs, slanted eyes, a small mouth (which makes the tongue appear large), and a somewhat flattened face and back of skull. Hypotonic muscle tone in infancy may largely disappear with age and regular exercise. As early as 40 years of age, initial signs of Alzheimer pathology may appear and increase in severity during the decade. There is wide variability in intellectual functioning and adaptive skills. Some individuals with Down's syndrome require only limited support, others pervasive support.

Down's syndrome impacts an individual's physical activity performance; however, they may be quite adept at recognizing music and rhythm (Stratford & Ching, 1988), and may be flexible due to lax ligaments. For these reasons, you may wish to emphasize dance and rhythmic movements. In other measures of fitness or motor performance, these individuals often score below peers with intellectual disabilities but without Down's syndrome (Reid & Block, 1996; Henderson, 1986). Attention to muscular strength and endurance, as well as cardiovascular functioning, appears warranted. Balance is a particular limitation (Jobling, in press), and this disability may cause orthopedic problems (e.g., lordosis), and visual or hearing difficulties. Almost half of all infants with Down's syndrome have a congenital heart defect that usually is corrected by surgery. Hence, you must obtain physician approval prior to cardiovascular assessment. In addition, obesity is prevalent and respiratory infections are common. The prevalence of obesity may be as high as 42 percent in men and 61 percent in women (Rimmer, Braddock & Fujiura, 1992).

Finally, **atlantoaxial instability**, a condition characterized by lax ligaments and muscles around the first two cervical vertebrae, may be present in 17 percent of those with Down's syndrome (Sherrill, 1998). This condition may result in damage to the spinal cord if the neck is forcefully extended or flexed. Atlantoaxial instability can only be confirmed with an X-ray and may restrict certain warm-up activities, gymnastics, soccer, swimming (butterfly stroke and diving start) and high jump. While caution clearly is warranted, remember that most individuals with Down's syndrome will not be affected by atlantoaxial instability, and you may choose from numerous activities that will not pose problems for these participants.

Motor Performance and Fitness

Levels of motor performance and fitness vary widely among those with intellectual disabilities. Some are capable of performance that matches or exceeds those without intellectual disabilities. Watching a Special Olympics event supports this assertion. However, the average performance of individuals with an intellectual disability clearly is inferior to age peers. This has been demonstrated repeatedly in measures of motor performance in children (Francis & Rarick, 1959; Holland, 1987; Ulrich, 1983). Fitness in adults with intellectual disabilities significantly lags behind age peers despite challenges of reliable and valid measurement (Lavay, Reid & Cressler-Chaviz, 1990; Seidl, Reid & Montgomery, 1987; Pitetti, Rimmer & Fernhall, 1993). Following are some of the descriptive adult fitness results that have emerged over the past 15 years.

➤ Reid et al. (1985) reported predicted maximum oxygen uptake scores from a sub-maximal step test protocol with 184 subjects aged 20 to 39 years. The males aged 20 to 29 years achieved the highest mean score, 35.8 ml/kg/min. This corresponded to a second-percentile score for male adults of similar age without a disability. Absolute scores vary with the protocol (Montgomery, Reid & Koziris, 1992), but research consistently demonstrates that individuals with an intellectual disability exhibit low performance levels on cardiovascular tests compared to persons without disability (Beasley, 1982; Fernhall & Tymeson, 1988; Fernhall et al., 1996; Pitetti & Campbell, 1991; Schurrer, Weltman & Brammel, 1985).

➤ Obesity also is a major health risk associated with intellectual disability (Fox & Rotatari, 1982; Kelly, Rimmer & Ness, 1986; Reid et al., 1985; Rimmer, Braddock & Fujiura, 1993). Measurement of skinfold thickness at specific sites is the usual assessment technique; however, the formulas to predict percent fat have varied. It is likely that people with mild disability may be more prone to obesity than those with severe intellectual disability. Also, females are more likely to be obese than males (Fox & Rotatori, 1982; Kelly et al., 1986).

➤ Muscular strength and endurance scores also are low compared to adults without a disability, whether assessed by isometric hand dynamometers, isotonic sit-ups or push-ups (Reid et al., 1985), or isokinetic measures (Horvat, Pitetti & Croce, 1997; Pitetti, Climstein, Mays & Barrett, 1992).

➤ Finally, while flexibility largely has been ignored, both male and female adults with an intellectual disability have demonstrated low performance on the sit-and-reach assessment of trunk flexibility.

Why are fitness scores among people with intellectual disabilities so low? A number of factors have been offered as explanation:

1) A sedentary lifestyle is a major influence (Hoge & Dattilo, 1995), as is the widespread belief that people with intellectual disabilities have fewer opportunities for structured programs.

2) Physical characteristics among people with intellectual disabilities may have a deleterious affect on fitness performance. People with intellectual disabilities are shorter than their nondisabled peers (Reid et al., 1985) and Down's syndrome is associated with unusually stunted limbs. As noted, obesity is common. When body-size differences between children with and without intellectual differences were statistically removed, there were fewer differences in motor performance (Dobbins, Garron & Rarick, 1981).

3) People with intellectual disabilities lack coordination and may perform with less efficiency (Seidl, Montgomery & Reid, 1989), causing predictive measures to underestimate actual performance. For example, the step test is a commonly used cardiovascular test with a skill component that may penalize people with intellectual disabilities.

4) Infrequent opportunities to practice test items may prevent development of optimal strategies and an understanding of test expectations.

5) Authors have noted that individuals with intellectual disabilities are not particularly motivated during tests that demand maximal exertion, and have a tendency to stop

when uncomfortable (Moon & Renzalia, 1982; Reid et al., 1985; Rimmer, 1994).

Exercise Benefits

Though physical fitness may be low, many training studies demonstrate that fitness can be improved. Chanias, Reid and Hoover (1998) recently conducted a meta-analysis to determine the effects of exercise on health-related physical fitness in individuals with intellectual disabilities. A meta-analysis is a quantitative method of synthesizing research studies regardless of the scale of measurement of the dependent variable. Thus, the collective impact of several cardiovascular exercise programs can be quantified from studies using field tests, sub-maximal treadmill protocols or direct measurement of maximum oxygen uptake. A typical study compares an exercising group with a control or nonexercising group. With some relatively simple mathematics, the differences between exercising and nonexercising groups can be standardized regardless of the original measurement. This standardized measure is called an effect size and can be combined across studies.

Chanias et al. (1998) located 21 studies from 1979 to 1996 that yielded 100 effect sizes. Figure 25.1 summarizes five health-related physical fitness components (Chanias et al., 1998). Large effects can be seen for muscular and cardiovascular endurance. That is, across numerous studies, improvement is evident when individuals with intellectual disabilities participate in such programs. The improvement in muscular strength was moderate, and the increase in flexibility was small. No significant effects were found for body composition.

Chanias et al. (1998) limited their review to studies that assessed the sole effect of exercise on body composition. Pitetti et al. (1993) included studies that examined other types of intervention in addition to exercise. There was some support for reduction in body weight when exercise was used with other interventions. However, the researchers pointed out that the studies often included small sample sizes, no control groups and minimal follow-up, and usually assessed only body weight, not body composi-

tion. Clearly more research is needed before definitive conclusions can be offered.

Overall, a relatively optimistic picture evolves. Though fitness levels are low, improvement certainly is possible. People with intellectual disabilities respond to exercise modes, intensity and frequency in the same manner as those without disability. We must continue to investigate the effectiveness of new exercise techniques for all aspects of fitness for those with intellectual disabilities, but should prioritize research that emphasizes increases in strength and flexibility, and body composition modification.

Fitness and physical activity for individuals with intellectual disabilities directly influences vocational pursuits, independent living, leisure activity, health and aging. Coleman, Ayoub and Friedrich (1976) were among the first to recognize that those with intellectual disabilities often are employed in areas that demand at least a minimal level of physical fitness. For example, muscular strength is a prerequisite for a number of industrial vocations (Nordgren & Backstrom, 1971; Croce & Horvat, 1992). In addition, there is evidence that fitness programs may promote work productivity in subjects with intellectual disabilities (Coleman & Whitman, 1984; Beasley, 1982; Croce & Horvat, 1992).

Many facets of community living, such as maintaining a household, cooking, self-care and recreation, require a certain amount of physical stamina, strength and flexibility. Therefore, independent living is more easily maintained with regular physical activity, and minimal levels of fitness enhance the pursuit of a full range of leisure activities.

People with intellectual disabilities are unusually sedentary (Burkhart, Fox & Rotatori, 1985; Hoge & Dattilo, 1995), and because physical inactivity is linked to heart disease, diabetes mellitus, obesity, high blood pressure, osteoporosis, depression and cancer (Shephard, 1995), these individuals will be prone to the health-related difficulties articulated for the nondisabled inactive population. Clearly they need to become more active. While there is a decline in physical fitness with age in the nondisabled population (Blair et al. 1995; Spirduso, 1995), Pitetti and Campbell (1991) speculate this decline may be exacerbated for those with intellectual disabilities. Recently, Graham (1997) provided data to support this speculation. Thirty-two adults with intellectual disabilities, ranging in age from 34 to 57, were reassessed on the Canadian Standardized Test of Fitness after 13 years. The test measures cardiovascular endurance, muscular strength and endurance, flexibility, and body composition. As expected, the fitness levels of the adults were lower than norms for the general population. Perhaps more significantly, the results showed that participants' cardiovascular fitness decreased, and their body fat increased, more

Figure 25.1

Histogram of the differences in effect magnitude on health-related physical fitness components. BC = body composition, CVE = cardiovascular endurance, FLEX = flexibility, ME = muscular endurance, MS = muscular strength, HRPF = health-related physical fitness.

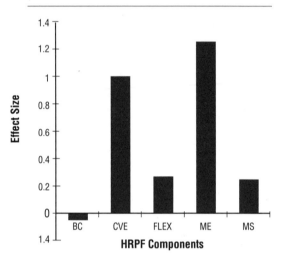

than expected. Overall, their fitness was low and declined at a faster rate than that of their nondisabled peers. Therefore, individuals with intellectual disabilities may have a significant and growing health risk as they age. The sedentary lifestyle and fitness performance of adults with intellectual disabilities must be addressed with all available means.

A Position Statement

In October of 1997, the Board of Directors of the Mental Retardation/Developmental Disabilities Division of the Council for Exceptional Children adopted the following position statement in response to the high prevalence of obesity, below average fitness and greater risk of developing coronary heart disease for those with intellectual disabilities. This position statement underscores the importance of physical activity in the lives of people with intellectual disabilities.

It is the position of the Board that adequate education opportunities and experiences which address health, fitness and wellness concepts must be provided for children and adults with mental retardation and other developmental disabilities. Specifically, all such individuals should be afforded opportunities to participate in educational programs that address: proper nutritional practices, personal hygiene, healthy lifestyle choices, physical fitness and other recreational activities, hazards associated with the use of alcohol, tobacco and illicit substances, stress reduction, sexual responsibility and safety.

Individuals with mental retardation and other developmental disabilities are often not afforded opportunities that promote positive health-related decisions. Educators, counselors and others must provide instruction and assist in development of the necessary decision-making skills that will enable these individuals to change undesirable behaviors and make favorable lifestyle choices.

Education for healthy lifestyle choices should begin during childhood and continue across the life span. As a consequence of such training, many individuals with mental retardation and other developmental disabilities will have enhanced personal health and reduced risk of life-threatening, preventable diseases. As a result, these same individuals will be better able to be active, contributing members of their communities.

Client Assessment

Fitness professionals who lack training in adapted physical activity must increase their theoretical and practical exposure to people with disabilities. Fitness facilities may provide training that enhances the comfort level of clinical exercise specialists who provide services for people with disabilities; if not, the specialist should seek training elsewhere. Sessions should examine your fears and attitudes about working with people with intellectual disabilities, provide opportunities for interaction and enable you to experience a disability. The need for sensitivity and nonpatronizing attitudes should be emphasized, and prevalent myths and misconceptions about disabilities should be addressed (Recommendations for the Fitness Assessment, Programming, and Counseling of Persons with a Disability, 1998).

The fitness appraisal for individuals with intellectual disabilities includes:
- Medical information
- Pre-test screening
- Lifestyle questionnaire

Assessment of:
- Anthropometry
- Aerobic fitness
- Muscular strength and endurance
- Flexibility
- Generating an appraisal report
- Counseling

Medical Information

A wide range of medications are commonly prescribed for persons with intellectual disabilities, and you must know how these medications affect the responses elicited in both the fitness test and the exercise program. It is recommended that you obtain physician approval before accepting clients with intellectual disabilities who are taking prescription medication (Recommendations for the Fitness Assessment, Programming, and Counseling of Persons with a Disability, 1998).

Prior to the fitness assessment, the same standard fitness screening procedures used for the general population should guide the screening process for individuals with intellectual disabilities. If there is a positive response (e.g., heart condition) to any item in the Physical Activity Readiness Questionnaire (**PAR-Q**), the client's physician should complete a form similar to the Physical Activity Readiness Medical Examination (PARmed-X) (See Chapter 2). This form is used to convey clearance for participa-

tion in physical activity or to make a referral to a medically supervised exercise program. The PARmed-X should outline any limitations for participation and provide details on side effects of medications. The PAR-Q and PARmed-X were revised in 1994 and 1995 respectively, and are published in Recommendations for the Fitness Assessment, Programming, and Counseling of Persons with a Disability (1998).

Pre-test Screening

The screening process consists of administration of the PAR-Q (or its equivalent) and consent and release forms, observations of the client, and measurement of resting heart rate and blood pressure. Consent and guidance from the primary caregiver also may be necessary when designing programs for people with intellectual disabilities. When the client is unable to provide sufficient background information, consult the guardian or physician.

Communication is critical in this stage of the assessment process. Clearly explain all procedures and pay attention to the cognizance of the person with the intellectual disability; ensure that your explanation is appropriate for the client's level of disability. It is essential that individuals with intellectual disabilities be allowed equal opportunity to become properly oriented with testing and exercise facilities, as knowledge and understanding are the basis for informed consent. It often is necessary for the client to observe the test before comprehension and confidence can be gained.

To ensure comprehension of test procedure prior to the signing of the informed consent document, Rintala, Dunn, McCubbin and Quinn (1992) suggest a three-stage familiarization period:

Table 25.1

Client Information to Obtain from Medical Professionals

1) Does the client have any condition(s) limiting their participation in a physical activity program (i.e., cardiovascular, musculoskeletal, respiratory, abdominal, other)?

2) Does the client have any sensory or behavioral conditions that would limit their participation in a physical activity program?

3) Is the client taking any medications that may limit their participation in a physical activity program?

4) Does the client have your approval for participation in a physical activity program?

5) Has the PAR-Q or PARmed-X form (or equivalent) been signed?

1. Individually meet with clients in their home environment and review a video tape of the testing environment, equipment and simulated test.
2. Have clients visit the testing laboratory to meet staff and become acquainted with the test equipment.
3. Simulate the formal test in the laboratory without collection of any data.

Therefore, "informed consent should be obtained after familiarizing clients with the test setting, staff, procedures and expectations" (Recommendations for the Fitness Assessment, Programming, and Counselling of Persons with a Disability, 1998).

Resting heart rate and blood pressure often are used as screening tools. Abnormally high or low values that persist upon duplicate measurements separated by a 10-minute period require referral to a physician for a medical examination. Under these circumstances, the physician's permission is necessary prior to completion of the fitness test and exercise prescription.

Contraindications to Exercise Testing

Contraindications to testing include a resting heart rate > 100 bpm or a blood pressure reading > 150/100 mmHg (Canadian Society for Exercise Physiology, 1997). Hypertension (blood pressure reading > 150/100 mmHg (Canadian Society for Exercise Physiology, 1997). Hypotension (blood pressure < 80/50 mmHg) also is considered a contraindication to testing.

There are no special contraindications to exercise for persons with intellectual disabilities. However, cognitive impairments may contribute to a sedentary lifestyle since persons with intellectual difficulties often are unaware of the health benefits of exercise. Limited experience in physical activity may result in low scores on the physical fitness test and influence the intensity and duration of the activities selected for the exercise prescription.

Lifestyle Questionnaire

It is important to gather information on the client's lifestyle and activity level. Questionnaires and checklists are appropriate instruments to establish exercise and leisure habits. Many forms are designed for use with

all clients during the appraisal/consultation process; however, a caregiver or family member may need to assist the person with intellectual disability in completing these forms. Depending upon the situation, the questionnaires can be administered in oral or written form, on-site or at home. Specific, rather than open-ended, questions are recommended for information gathering (Seidl, 1998). For example: "What kind of activities do you participate in?" may be too vague. Labeling the activity may provide more appropriate information. For example, "How many times per week do you go for a walk?"

Health-related Fitness Assessment

Quantitative fitness assessments are necessary to provide appropriate exercise programming and to monitor individual progress during training. In general, fitness test procedures usually do not require modifications for persons with intellectual disabilities, but additional practice may be needed to perform test protocols effectively. It may be necessary to adapt testing procedures for some individuals. The protocol for assessment and counseling should be standardized with respect to both technique and instrumentation. Record any modifications to the initial tests so follow-up procedures can be replicated and accurate comparisons can be made to prior assessments.

The scientific literature stresses the importance of a familiarization period for obtaining reliable and valid results (Rintala, McCubbin & Dunn, 1995; Reid, Dunn & McClements, 1993; Reid, Seidl & Montgomery, 1989). In relation to cardiovascular testing, it is recommended that two practice trials be permitted prior to collection of oxygen consumption data in the laboratory and one practice trial for field tests. Be prepared to spend extra time assessing clients with intellectual disabilities and to communicate with their caregivers.

The health-related fitness appraisal typically contains tests for body composition, musculoskeletal fitness and aerobic endurance. Excess body fat and/or obesity is common among people with intellectual disabilities. Most studies have used skinfold and/or girth measurements with percent fat estimated from regression equations that were developed for nondisabled persons. Using the generalized regression equations of

Jackson and Pollock (1978) for men, and Jackson, Pollock and Ward (1980) for women, it is reported that 45.2 percent of men and 50.5 percent of women with intellectual disabilities were classified as obese (Kelly, Rimmer & Ness, 1986). In many experts' opinion, generalized equations to predict percent fat are appropriate for use with this population, particularly when there is a large data base that has established norms for similar age and gender. Rimmer, Kelly and Rosentsweig (1987) have developed specific equations to predict percent fat for persons with intellectual disabilities, including Down's syndrome. Hydrostatic weighing is seldom used to measure percent fat in persons with intellectual disabilities since they often are uncomfortable and unwilling to remain passive with their heads submerged underwater.

Direct measurement of oxygen consumption is the gold standard for assessment of aerobic fitness; however, Shephard (1990) and Montgomery et al. (1992) have questioned the validity of the peak values obtained when assessing persons with intellectual difficulties. VO_2max values tend to be low when compared to age-matched control subjects. It has been suggested that the concept of competing against time may be too abstract for these persons to comprehend, thus eliciting less than a maximal performance (Fernhall et al., 1988).

We have directly assessed VO_2max using a treadmill test and indirectly using a maximal shuttle-run test, submaximal cycle ergometer test and submaximal step test. (The maximal shuttle-run test is an incremental running test in which speed is increased every minute. In this test, which is similar to a maximal treadmill test, the subject runs back and forth across a 20-meter distance at a controlled velocity. Pace is set by an audiotape that begins at a slow speed and increases until the subject reaches volitional exhaustion.) Five trials were administered on each of the four exercise protocols (Montgomery et al., 1992). Mean values for VO_2max ranged from 19.7 to 36.4 ml/kg/min with moderately functioning adults with intellectual disabilities (n = 18), compared to a much narrower and higher range in VO_2max values (42.1 to 45.5 ml/kg/min) for a control group. For the treadmill test, the range in VO_2max across the five trials was 7.5 ml/kg/min for the experimental group and 4.4 ml/kg/min for the control group. Standard criteria to ascertain that VO_2max has been reached seldom were achieved by participants with intellectual disabilities. The four modes of assessment had similar VO_2max values across trials with intra-class correlations ranging from r = .90 to .97.

Persons with intellectual disabilities may be apprehensive about running on a treadmill. To reduce anxiety, the initial speed of the treadmill should be slower than that used for nondisabled persons. An initial speed of 3 to 4 km/h, with gradual increments (0.3 to 0.5 km/h), is recommended. Discomfort may be exhibited by:

1) constantly holding on to the railings;

Table 25.2

Typical Activity Guidelines

- Use physical and visual prompts to assist in teaching specific movements. A physical prompt is manual guidance; a visual prompt is a demonstration or a cue attached to an exercise machine.

- Give clear, succinct verbal directions, and ensure your message was understood.

- Respect your client's age. Do not treat adults as if they are children.

- When incorporating a series of exercises into a training program for clients with intellectually disabilities, start by linking two of the activities. Add on after the client is able to perform the two, and be prepared to cue the next activity.

- Though some clients enjoy frequent repetition and routine, others are bored by it. Modify the program when appropriate.

- Adapt an exercise or activity to promote success and fun.

- Provide ample praise and encouragement.

- Provide precise performance feedback and chart progress.

- Use reinforcement as necessary, particularly verbal.

- Empower intellectually disabled clients by encouraging them to make choices and participate in setting goals and monitoring progress.

2) reaching out for your assistance as you stand near the treadmill; or

3) verbalizing anxiety (Pitetti et al., 1993).

Preparing people with intellectual disabilities for treadmill testing can be a lengthy procedure, and familiarizing the client with the test environment and equipment is an important part of the process. Practice with a nose clip, mouthpiece and/or heart-rate monitor is necessary. It also is recommended that you teach the client how to walk/run comfortably on the treadmill before using any measurement equipment. The test should not proceed until the client has demonstrated the ability to walk/run comfortably at initial treadmill speeds without physical assistance. Provide verbal and visual feedback throughout the test.

A critique of cardiovascular fitness testing for persons with intellectual disabilities points out some of the confounding variables when interpreting results (Seidl et al., 1987). Motivation, learning, adherence to a specific cadence, pacing, unwillingness to experience uncomfortable symptoms while exercising and physiological efficiency are major concerns. Endurance running performance of intellectually disabled youths is improved when testers use motivational strategies and provide extensive guidance on pacing (Watkinson & Koh, 1988).

At least five field tests to predict cardiovascular fitness have been validated for individuals with intellectual disabilities. These include a stepping test (Montgomery et al., 1992), the Leger and Lambert (1982) shuttle run (Montgomery et al., 1992), cycle ergometry using the Schwinn Air-Dyne (Pitetti et al., 1988), the 1.5-mile walk/run (Fernhall & Tymeson, 1988) and the Rockport 1.0-mile walk/run (Rintala et al., 1992; 1997).

Indirect tests that predict VO_2max from work performance (e.g., shuttle-run test) or heart rate (e.g., cycle ergometer and step tests) assume a constant efficiency. Lower efficiency could be attributed to such factors as poor coordination or lack of experience with the test mode. If adults with intellectual disabilities exhibit less efficient standards than the general population, comparisons using identical prediction equations are inappropriate.

When we assessed 184 adults with intellectual difficulties in a three-stage step test, only 53 percent of the adults stopped the test because their heart rates reached target values (Reid et al., 1985). Lack of motivation was attributed as a cause in the low estimate of aerobic fitness.

Table 25.3 provides a review of some cardiovascular fitness tests that you may use with people with intellectual disabilities. Physical appraisers with experience testing persons with intellectual disabilities have collected the data for these research articles. The treadmill studies are valuable in determining VO_2max, since the researchers have established the validity of these tests for persons with intellectual disabilities and offer suggestions to enhance reliability.

Cardiovascular test results must be interpreted with caution as participants may have low mechanical efficiency, be unable to comprehend the concept of a maximal effort or lack motivation. Be aware of motivational tactics (rewards, incentives and praise) that can be used to help these clients attain valid and reliable results during fitness testing. Since treadmill tests require extensive familiarization, they may not be as feasible as some field tests. For persons with intellectual disabilities, pacers and nondisabled partners can be used during tests such as the Rockport Fitness Walking Test and the Canadian Step Test in which pacing may be problematic.

Few fitness norms are available for persons with intellectual disabilities. The national norms for the general population and the references in Table 25.3 should serve as a guide for interpretation of the results. If a modified protocol is used for individual clients, test and retest results instead of national norms will provide the basis for comparison.

The muscular strength and endurance of persons with intellectual disabilities commonly have been measured using the test battery outlined in the Canadian Standardized Test of Fitness (1987). Grip strength, push-ups and sit-ups are measured. The grip test requires only a single maximal effort and has good reliability (Horvat, Aufsesser, Croce & Roswal, 1994; Montgomery et al., 1988; Pitetti et al., 1988). Using verbal prompts, such as "squeeze hard" may be useful, along with hand-over-hand physical assistance during familiarization. The tester may have to assess whether the client is

Table 25.3
Cardiovascular Fitness Tests for Persons with Intellectual Disabilities

Mode of Exercise	N	Test	Comment	Reference
Treadmill	10	Maximal, direct	5 trials to examine reliability	Montgomery et al., 1992
Treadmill	21	Maximal, direct	Specific physiological criteria for test termination	Fernhall & Tymeson, 1987
Treadmill	38	Maximal, direct	Specific physiological criteria for test termination	Fernhall et al., 1989
Treadmill	12	Maximal, direct	Specific physiological criteria for test termination	Pitetti & Tan, 1991
Treadmill	19	Maximal, direct	Some subjects did not meet criteria for VO_2max	Rintala et al., 1997
Treadmill	6	Maximal, direct	No criteria mentioned	Anchuthengil et al., 1992
Cycle ergometer	10	Submaximal, indirect	5 trials to examine reliability	Montgomery et al., 1992
Cycle ergometer	63	Submaximal, indirect	Problems of cadence and completion of high workloads	Nordgren, 1970
Cycle ergometer	37	Submaximal, indirect	Power output compared at a HR of 170 bpm	Coleman et al., 1976
Cycle ergometer	20	Submaximal, indirect	Power output compared at a HR of 170 bpm	Andrew et al., 1979
Air-Dyne ergometer	16	Submaximal, indirect	Prediction equation for VO_2 max	Pitetti et al., 1988
Step test	10	Maximal, direct	5 trials to examine reliability	Montgomery et al., 1992
Step test	15	Submaximal, direct	Examined stepping efficiency following repeated trials	Seidl et al., 1989
Step test	24	Submaximal, indirect	Peak VO_2 predicted from recovery heart rate	Pitetti et al., 1997
Step test	184	Submaximal, indirect	Battery of physical fitness tests	Reid et al., 1985
Shuttle run	10	Maximal, indirect	5 trials to examine reliability	Montgomery et al., 1992
Shuttle run	10	Maximal	Monitored heart rate	Varela & Pitetti, 1995
Walk-run field test	19	Rockport walking test	Validation study using peak VO_2	Rintala et al., 1997
Walk-run field test	19	Rockport walking test	Test-retest reliability = 0.97	Rintala et al., 1992
Walk-run field test	16	1200 & 2000 m runs	Monitored heart rate	Watkinson & Koh, 1988
Walk-run field test	20	1.5-mile run	Prediction equation for VO_2 max	Fernhall & Tymeson, 1988

really squeezing (grimacing sometimes is a false sign).

Test-retest reliability coefficients were only 0.63 for sit-ups and 0.62 for push-ups, and may require duplicate measurements, as suggested by Reid et al. (1985). Because technique often is poor, push-ups and curl-ups may require a teaching phase prior to testing, and multilevel modifications for these tests frequently are necessary. Measurement criteria for curl-ups and push-ups may require qualitative, as well as quantitative, scoring (Seidl, 1998). Again, test-retest in these circumstances is more appropriate than comparison to national norms.

The Nicholas Manual Muscle Tester also has been used to measure isometric strength in this population. Croce and Hovat (1992) measured elbow flexion (biceps), elbow extension (triceps), shoulder abduction (deltoids), shoulder transverse adduction and thoracic flexion (abdominal) strength with this instrument. Horvat et al. (1995) suggest increasing motivation with verbal cues, giving adequate rest between trials and including contraction times of 2 to 5 seconds. They recommend using the mean of three trials for subjects with intellectual disabilities because replicating a maximal score is difficult.

Nautilus strength machines have been used to establish the 1-repetition maximum (1-RM) prior to initiating weight-training programs (Rimmer & Kelly, 1991). If the 1-RM was not established within three trials, the participant proceeded to the next machine to test another muscle (also helping to prevent fatigue). Retest reliability for the strength measures ranged from 0.95 to 0.99.

Strength testing with a Cybex isokinetic dynamometer has been reported for persons with mild to moderate intellectual disabilities (Pitetti, 1990) and individuals with Down's syndrome (Pitetti et al., 1992). At least two trials were needed to ensure that the individual performed their best effort. When tested on two separate days, the difference between the efforts ranged from 10 percent to 19 percent, suggesting once again the importance of motivation when evaluating this population.

The most common flexibility test for assessment has been the sit-and-reach test to measure trunk flexion. The test is reliable (r = 0.94) for persons with intellectual disabilities (Reid et al., 1985). The AAHPERD Physical Test Battery incorporates the sit-and-reach test in its health-related fitness test (AAHPERD, 1988).

Counseling Issues

The goals of the counseling phase of assessment for the person with a disability follow.

➤ When appropriate, review test results with the client in terms of normative standards.
➤ Define the client's needs and activity preferences within a health context.
➤ Examine past and current patterns of physical activity.
➤ Explore possibilities for future activities.
➤ Discuss realistic fitness goals with the client and help set them.
➤ Discuss and evaluate the means to achieve the goals.
➤ Prescribe an activity program that is agreeable to the client.
➤ Use worksheets and charts that can be understood by the client.
➤ Use the same training principles that apply to the general population.
➤ Agree to a follow-up mechanism to examine fitness and adherence. Persons with intellectual disabilities require a greater number of follow-up sessions than the general population (Recommendations for the Fitness Assessment, Programming, and Counseling of Persons with a Disability, 1998; Seidl, 1998).

Reid, Montgomery and Seidl (1990) developed a model for fitness counseling and exercise prescription for persons with intellectual disabilities. The model, which combines fitness training principles with an objective-based approach to teaching motor skills, includes goal sheets, progress charts, intermittent reinforcement and regular follow-up. The counseling process includes strategies to facilitate adherence to the exercise program, and considers the client's living situation, existing and potential support networks, and location of community facilities.

A seven-step approach for counseling is outlined by the Canadian Physical Activity, Fitness & Lifestyle Appraisal (1997). This approach is based on a simple problem-solving model. It integrates physical activity participation, health-related fitness and healthy lifestyle components. The seven-step approach is:

➤ Establish rapport and structure.
➤ Gather information.
➤ Conduct the Health-related Fitness Appraisal.
➤ Interpret the Health-related Fitness Appraisal Results.
➤ Generate and evaluate alternatives for change.
➤ Develop an action plan.
➤ Follow-up.

The following case study incorporates the seven-step model.

Case Study 1

Setting the Scene

Robert is a 30-year-old male, employed in a supported work environment requiring moderate physical exertion. He enjoys sports and watching games on television while snacking on chips and beer. Robert participates in a 10-week physical activity program once a week during the winter months in which he works out with a university student as part of an internship program. He lives independently with a co-worker, and both receive periodic assistance from social services. He looks forward to the university exercise program each year, but does not actively participate in any sport or activity during the remainder of the year. He recognizes the importance of physical fitness, but does not have the motivation to begin. Robert's parents have guided him to you.

Initial Observations

Robert is a bit nervous and shy, as he has never had a formal fitness appraisal. He avoids eye contact. Robert is unsure of what is required and is afraid you will expect more than he is capable of.

Step 1: Rapport and Structuring

You suggest going for a walk and touring the facilities. During the tour you mention you enjoy baseball. Robert indicates that basketball is his favorite sport and the Bulls are his team. This is the opening that helps to establish rapport and confidence for Robert. You remind him that even Michael Jordan must stay fit to play effectively, and this leads to a discussion of Robert's level of fitness. You invite Robert to view a video that explains the fitness evaluation. Since Robert is eager to continue, the decision is made to continue the appraisal process.

Step 2: Gathering Information Using the PAR-Q & PARMED-X

Robert's parents assist him in completing the PAR-Q and a questionnaire that examines physical activity involvement and preferences. It is agreed that the optimal time to exercise is after work, but Robert is concerned about how to get to the facility from his job. His parents offer to assist in teaching him the bus route. Looking at the PAR-Q, you know that Robert is able to perform the fitness test if he desires. "Robert, we can find out a bit about your fitness by trying some of the tests that you are comfortable performing. It helps to know your initial levels so that we can help you improve your fitness, and I suggest that we try some of the tests. We can discuss ways of exercising and eating that may help you. How does that sound?" Robert agrees to give it a try.

Step 3: Conduct the Health-related Fitness Appraisal

You permit Robert to practice each item in the fitness-test battery normally used at his facility. Each test is verbally explained and demonstrated. Robert is then guided to the appropriate position. Robert does not like the pinch of the skinfold caliper on each site, and Robert's father volunteers to have his skinfolds measured to assure Robert that the procedure is safe. Modify the cardiovascular treadmill test by starting with a low speed and adding gradual increments for each workload. Only the treadmill test required more than one practice trial. Additional familiarization was needed before Robert was able to walk on the treadmill without holding on to the side railings. A note was added to the result sheet to describe the modified procedure. It was agreed that

Robert would return in two days to repeat the test battery. On his second visit, Robert's parents again accompany him and show him where to meet bus 12. You measure Robert's body composition, muscular strength and endurance, flexibility, and cardiovascular endurance.

Step 4: Interpret the Health-related Fitness Results

After the appraisal is completed, the results are compared to norms for males aged 30 to 39 years. The appraiser asks Robert if he is ready to change his scores by following a physical activity program. Robert is told that his results are:

Fitness Component	Rating compared to adults (30 – 39 years)
Body Composition	Overfat – 27 percent fat, 15th percentile
Musculoskeletal Fitness	Good – 70th percentile
Flexibility	Good – 75th percentile
Aerobic Endurance	Fair – 20th percentile

The meaning of the ratings is explained to Robert, with the initial comments directed at the positive aspects of the appraisal (musculoskeletal fitness and flexibility). To help Robert understand percentile scores, a bar graph with scores from zero to 100 is used as a visual aid.

Step 5: Generate and Evaluate Alternatives for Change

Next, relate Robert's passion for television and sport to sedentary living so that Robert understands he must become more active in his leisure time to improve his body composition and cardiovascular fitness. The relationship between lifestyle habits and the risks of an inactive lifestyle are discussed. "After looking at your results, it seems like you need to do some aerobic exercise. Here is a list of activities that could improve your aerobic fitness." If Robert does not read, provide pictures. "Which activities would be most enjoyable for you? Would you like to sign up for basketball and some aerobics classes? Prior to each session, I will meet with you for 20 minutes of training. I'll meet you immediately after work at the fitness center." During the initial weeks of the program, you may need to train with Robert for the entire exercise session, and then decrease your involvement during the basketball or aerobics classes.

Step 6: Developing an Action Plan

When you ask Robert how he feels about traveling to the fitness center, joining a class and working out one-on-one, you find he is excited about the chance to play basketball and to practice with you. Suggest alternative activities that Robert can participate in on the days he does not come to the fitness center. It is decided that Robert will walk for 20 minutes each evening prior to watching any television, and record the time on a chart that you provide. You and Robert agree that he gradually will increase his walking time so he reaches a goal of 40 minutes after two months. This period seems like a long time for Robert, so, as an incentive, the personal trainer offers to take Robert to an NBA game when this goal is reached.

Step 7: Follow-up

You outline the process of tracking/recording Robert's physical activity and plan to begin the exercise program the following day. Remind Robert to bring his basketball shoes and gym attire and of the 5 p.m. start time. Tell Robert that you will participate with him during the first week of classes to assist him with the movements. You agree to repeat the fitness test in two months to check Robert's progress and establish new goals. Although Robert could use some counseling on nutrition, you decide to wait until the exercise routine is well established. Introducing too many lifestyle changes at once could be overwhelming for Robert.

Exercise Programming and Leadership

Mode of Exercise

The emphasis of exercise programming is placed on the mode of exercise. The guidelines on duration and frequency of exercise are the same as those used for the non-disabled population. It is well documented that persons with intellectual disabilities have low cardiovascular fitness. Therefore, when designing an exercise program, the intensity must begin at the low end of the aerobic training zone.

Because intellectual disability is a disability of cognition rather than a medical condition or physical limitation, the activities you select with nondisabled clients are appropriate for individuals with an intellectual disability. There is no mode of exercise that "works" in

the sense that it is used with 99 percent of the people to the exclusion of other activities. There are no magical activities. The corollary also is true; there is no mode that "doesn't work." However, there are some considerations that will influence the mode of exercise for a specific person.

Ascertain the person's interest. Just as there are dedicated runners who trek outside in all kinds of weather, and others who won't budge from the confines of the gym and treadmill, everyone has personal preferences. For example, if an individual likes to dance, use music to your advantage. Speak to the person to determine what is meaningful and fun for them, and remember that the individual may be able to articulate personal fitness and activity goals.

Another consideration is necessary skill. Remember that many individuals have problems with coordination, so it may be necessary to refrain from activities with high skill demands. On the other hand, evaluate the real need for skill. If individuals are engaged in aerobic dance, even missing a step now and again, they may be quite active and enjoying themselves immensely. Other activities may require concomitant life skills. For example, outdoor cycling requires adherence to the rules of the road.

There are advantages in selecting activities that can be used with other members of the community. Can the participant use your resistance-training program at the local gym on days they are not working with you? Select activities and individual exercises that are adaptable for interaction with others. Continuity is important. If you select resistance exercises requiring specialized equipment that is only available at your exercise facility, the opportunity for continuity at another facility is limited.

Age is an important factor that should be respected. Remember that if your clients are adults, they likely are sensitive to being treated as children. Show dignity and respect commensurate with age. The prescribed program for persons with intellectual disabilities should be based on chronological, not mental, age. Age-appropriate programming minimizes stereotyping and maximizes community acceptance and socialization with nondisabled persons.

Specific Guidelines for Health-related Fitness

Cardiovascular fitness. Cardiovascular programming has been quite successful for persons with intellectual disabilities (Chanias et al., 1998). Walking, dance, water activities and circuit training are recommended (Rimmer, 1992, 1994; Sherrill, 1998). For example, walking can be done almost everywhere, requires minimal skill and can be engaged in for longer periods of time than other forms of exercise. Lavay and McKenzie (1991) showed that five men with intellectual disabilities were able to elevate and maintain their heart rates in the training zone with walking and running. Millar, Fernhall and Burkett (1993) used 30 minutes of brisk walking and running to test young adults and adolescents with Down's syndrome. The researchers noted, however, that participants required much encouragement. Koh and Watkinson (1988) also have indicated that verbal encouragement and prompting were necessary for children with an intellectual disability to sustain vigorous activity with heart rates above 150 for a period of 15 minutes. Low-impact aerobic dance may be effective for those who enjoy music. Start with basic movements and build.

Circuits with clearly marked stations also can be effective. Two minutes of exercise at six stations and 30 to 60 seconds between each station is sufficiently taxing for most beginners. To ensure independence, teach by demonstrating the exercise. If you are leading a group, you also may want to place arrows on the floor or wall to indicate the direction of the next station. Reid et al. (1990) used aerobic dance, circuits, ropes, hoops and walking/running to promote cardiovascular fitness. Many individuals with intellectual disabilities learned to swim as youngsters and, therefore, swimming laps or water exercise may be attractive.

Cardiovascular fitness also has been improved with training on stationary cycle ergometers. For example, Pitetti and Tan (1991) taught seven men and five women with intellectual disabilities to exercise at an intensity that improves cardiovascular functioning on a Schwinn Air-Dyne ergometer. Target heart rates during exercise were monitored via telemetry by both the participants and staff. The 16-week program was effective in promoting cardiovascular improvement, but there was regression to original baseline levels after six months. Subjects had stopped using the ergometers in their workplace, leaving the researchers to speculate that an "escort" might be needed to take participants to the ergometers and maintain their exercise regimes. You may find that cycling produces local muscular fatigue in those with particularly low fitness. Thus, cycling may need to be combined with other cardiovascular exercise such as walking or exercising on a stair climber (Rimmer, 1994).

Muscular strength and endurance. Muscular strength and endurance programs also have been successfully implemented (Chanias et al., 1998). Calisthenics (Reid et al., 1990), surgical tubing (Croce & Horvat, 1992) and progressive resistance training on Nautilus machines (Rimmer & Kelly, 1991) have been reported. Rimmer (1994) has offered guidelines for developing resistance-training programs for adults with intellectual disabilities. He recommends that participants practice using the equipment for a minimum of two sessions before baseline data are collected.

Some practical tips include:
➤ Teach the client to identify fitness supervisors and to ask for help when assistance is needed.
➤ Teach the client to move from station to station and, if one station is crowded, move to a different station and return later.
➤ Provide adequate rest between machines and much verbal encouragement.
➤ If possible, teach clients to record their own scores using pictograms for each exercise. Match pictures with a number on the apparatus.
➤ Label the machines by name of movement, for example the "Pec Deck" can be called the "bring the arms together" machine. Finally, Rimmer (1994) reminds us that the first six to eight sessions require much supervision, with participants needing appropriate feedback on movement speed, body position and breathing.

Body composition. Recall that the meta-analysis of Chanias et al. (1998) demonstrated that exercise training did not alter the body composition of individuals with an intellectual disability when exercise was the only intervention variable. A more optimistic picture emerges when exercise is combined with verbal reinforcement and/or a token economy (Croce, 1990).

Without question, regular exercise is part of a multiple-component strategy for alteration of body composition and weight reduction. Weight reduction for those with intellectual disabilities has been a concern for many years. Successful weight-loss programs often have included various techniques of behavior therapy and support, including self-monitoring of food intake and external reinforcement in terms of money (Foreyt & Parks,1975), self-monitoring of weight (Joachim & Korboot, 1975), manipulation of emotional responses to food, food-cue elimination, alternative activities to eating and modeling of new behaviors (Rotatori Fox & Switzky, 1980), buddy reinforcement (Fox, Haniotes, Rotatori, 1984), and parental involvement (Fox, Rosenberg & Rotatori, 1985). Weight reduction is clearly an area that requires the holistic approach outlined in the introduction of this chapter. You are encouraged to promote weight control among your clients with intellectual disabilities, but success will be enhanced if it occurs with self-monitoring, nutrition education, appropriate reinforcement and the assistance of important people in clients' lives. Again, establish the exercise regimen, then take steps to make changes in nutritional lifestyle.

General Guidelines to Promote Physical Activity

Interacting with people with an intellectual disability may be more productive and positive if you use the following suggestions that have been generated by several authors (Houston-Wilson, 1995; Reid et al., 1990; Reid & Hermo, in press; Sherrill, 1998; Watkinson, 1990).

Physical and visual prompts assist in teaching specific movements. A physical prompt is manual guidance, either complete or partial, that places the individual's limb or body in the correct position. A visual prompt is a demonstration or other helpful visual cue. If you demonstrate a movement, do it slowly and point to the most important aspect. For example, if you are emphasizing "bent knees," point to your knees during the demonstration. A visual cue also may be a strip of tape on an apparatus that reminds the client where to place their hands. Only use prompts that are necessary and remove them as independence is gained.

Verbal directions should be clear and succinct. Avoid idioms or "play on words" that may be misunderstood or taken literally. Watch for comprehension cues from the individual, and ask the client what they expect to ensure your message was understood. As you get to know the person, you will learn which level of verbal interaction is correct.

Do not speak to adults as if they are children. If a parent or guardian is present, never talk about the individual as if they are not present.

People with intellectual disabilities have short-term memory problems (though once something is learned, it is well retained). Thus, asking them to perform a series of five activities will prove difficult. Start by linking two of the activities before adding others, and be prepared to prompt the next activity, perhaps by a partial demonstration.

Some individuals enjoy the security of frequent repetition and routine, but watch your clients carefully — they are just as susceptible to boredom as nondisabled participants.

Be prepared to modify an activity to promote success and fun. If push-ups are too difficult, let the client do them on their knees or on a wall. If a flexibility exercise seems boring, have them reach for colorful scarves. If you are playing one-on-one basketball, lower the rim to promote success.

Provide ample praise and encouragement to help combat lack of motivation. An enthusiastic instructor will produce surprising results.

In addition to general encouragement, provide precise performance feedback. "Last week you walked three-quarters of a mile, today you reached a mile." Charting progress often is motivational as well.

Use reinforcement as necessary. Many types of reinforcement have been used in fitness and physical activity programs, including token economies, music, visual stimulation, trinkets, stars and certificates (Caouette & Reid, 1985, 1991; Croce, 1990; Deener & Horvat, 1992; Sechrest, 1968). Such reinforcements usually are provided for specific accomplishments in terms of duration or intensity of exercise and, if possible, should gradually be discontinued. Try to use verbal reinforcement as much as possible and typical motivational means such as, "After we walk those two miles continuously, we can treat ourselves to a movie."

Self-determination is an important factor in motivation and empowerment (Wehmeyer, 1996). Too frequently, parents, teachers or employers control individuals with intellectual disabilities. They are given little opportunity to make decisions that influence their lives. The result is an individual who shows little initiative and has minimal confidence. We can begin to reverse this cycle in physical activity programs by allowing individuals with intellectual disabilities to make more choices (which is why it is crucial to ascertain individual likes and dislikes in physical activity). In addition, involve clients in goal setting and monitoring their own progress. Coleman and Whitman (1984) taught adults with intellectual disabilities to count the number of repetitions in calisthenics, to record the number on charts and to self-reinforce. Ellis, Cress and Spellman (1992) encouraged self-management of exercise by having adolescents use a digital kitchen timer to prompt treadmill walking and a lap counter for walking in school halls. Deener and Horvat (1995) used self-recording to note improvement in walking/running.

Attribute successes to the individual's effort and skill, not your great leadership. As they gain control, motivation should increase and they will interact in society with greater confidence.

Conclusion

There is enormous variability among people who have intellectual disabilities. We have emphasized assessment and training, as well as practical tips to use with relatively high-functioning adults. Those who require pervasive support may need assistance from instructors with thorough knowledge and expertise in behavior therapy.

There is growing literature supporting the idea that individuals with profound disabilities benefit from physical activity. Though exercise alone has not been shown to improve body composition, when combined with other interventions such as nutrition education and self-reinforcement, people with intellectual disabilities receive many health-related exercise benefits. These include small reductions in body weight, and improved muscular and cardiovascular endurance, work productivity, and independent living skills. Bouchard (1998) has completed extensive research showing that increased physical activity can result in health benefits for individuals without an increase in physical fitness. The key is physical activity. Young adults with an intellectual disability lead sedentary lifestyles (Hoge & Dattilo, 1995), and their fitness levels decline at a much faster rate throughout middle age than those of their nondisabled peers (Graham, 1997). It is apparent that parents and health professionals must encourage physical activity in individuals with intellectual disabilities.

One of the major goals of clinical exercise specialists working with people with intellectual disabilities is motivation. Like most adults, they need encouragement to participate and to take personal responsibility for their activities and health by making choices and selecting goals. Assuming more personal responsibility and working with a fitness professional are not incongruent. With support from family, friends and you, important lifestyle changes are possible, resulting in more active and healthier individuals.

References

American Alliance for Health, Physical Education, Recreation and Dance. (1988). *Physical Best*. Reston, Va.: AAHPERD.

Anchuthengil, J.D., Nielson, D.H., Schulenburg, J., Hurst, R. & Davis, M.J. (1992). Effects of an individualized treadmill exercise training program on cardiovascular fitness of adults with mental retardation. *Journal of Orthopaedic and Sports Physical Therapy*, 16, 220-228.

Andrew, G.M., Reid, J.G., Beck, S. & McDonald, W. (1979). Training of the developmentally handicapped young adult. *Canadian Journal of Applied Sport Sciences*, 4, 289-293.

Beasley, C.R. (1982). Effects of a jogging program on cardiovascular fitness and work performance of mentally retarded adults. *American Journal of Mental Deficiency*, 86 (6), 609-613.

Blair, S.N., Kohl, H.W. III, Barlow, C.E., Paffenbarger, R.S. Jr., Gibbons, L.W. & Macera, C.A. (1995). Changes in physical fitness and all-cause mortality. A prospective study of healthy and unhealthy men. *Journal of the American Medical Association*, 273 (14), 1093-8.

Bouchard, C. (1997). Biological aspects of the active living concept. In J.E.Curtis & S.J.Russell (Eds.) *Physical Activity in Human Experience*, pp. 11-58, Champaign, Ill.: Human Kinetics.

Bouchard, C. (1998). Individual differences in the response to regular physical activity: Implications for research and practice. Paper presented at the AAHPERD National Convention, Reno, Nevada.

Burkhart, J.E., Fox, R.A. & Rotatori, A.F. (1985). Obesity of mentally retarded individuals: Prevalence, characteristics and intervention. *American Journal of Mental Deficiency*, 90, 303-312.

Canadian Standardized Test of Fitness — Operations Manual, (1987), Fitness Canada, Ottawa, Fitness and Amateur Sport.

Canadian Society of Exercise Physiology. (1997). *The Canadian Physical Activity, Fitness & Lifestyle Appraisal Manual*. Ottawa, Canada.

Caouette, M. & Reid, G. (1985). Increasing the work output of severely retarded adults on a bicycle ergometer. *Education and Training of the Mentally Retarded*, 20, 296-304.

Caouette, M. & Reid, G. (1991). Influence of auditory stimulation on the physical work output of adults who are severely retarded. *Education and Training in Mental Retardation*, 26, 43-52.

Chanias, A.K., Reid, G. & Hoover, M.L. (1998). Exercise effects on health-related physical fitness of individuals with an intellectual disability: A meta-analysis. *Adapted Physical Activity Quarterly*, 15, 119-140.

Coleman, R.S., Ayoub, M.M. & Friedrich, D.W. (1976). Assessment of physical work capacity in institutionalized mentally retarded males. *American Journal of Mental Deficiency*, 80, 629-635.

Coleman, R.S. & Whitman, T.L. (1984). Developing, generalizing and maintaining physical fitness in mentally retarded adults: Toward a self-directed program. *Analysis and Intervention in Developmental Disabilities*, 4, 109-27.

Croce, R.V. (1990). Effects of exercise and diet on body composition and cardiovascular fitness in adults with severe mental retardation. *Education and Training in Mental Retardation*, 25, 176-187.

Croce, R.V. & Horvat, M. (1992). Effects of reinforcement-based exercise on fitness and work capacity in adults with mental retardation. *Adapted Physical Activity Quarterly*, 9, 148-178.

Deener, T.M. & Horvat, M.H. (1995). Effects of social reinforcement and self-recording on exercise duration in middle school students with moderate mental retardation. *Clinical Kinesiology*, 49 (1), 28-33.

Dobbins, D.A., Garron, R. & Rarick, G.L. (1981). The motor performance of educable mentally retarded and intellectually normal boys after covariate control for differences in body size. *Research Quarterly for Exercise and Sport*, 52, 1-8.

Drew, C.J., Logan, D.R. & Hardman, M.L. (1992). Mental Retardation: A Life Cycle Approach. (5th ed). New York: Macmillan Publishing.

Ellis, D.N., Cress, P.J. & Spellman, C.R. (1992). Using timers and lap counters to promote self-management of independent exercise in adolescents with mental retardation. *Education and Training in Mental Retardation*, 27, 51-59.

Fernhall, B., Pitetti, K.H., Rimmer, J.H., McCubbin, J.A., Rintala, P., Millar, A.L., Kittredge, J. & Burkett, L.N. (1996). Cardiorespiratory capacity of individuals with mental retardation including Down's syndrome. *Medicine and Science in Sport and Exercise*, 28 (3), 366-371.

Fernhall, B. & Tymeson, G.T. (1987). Graded exercise testing of mentally retarded adults: A study of feasibility. *Archives of Physical Medical Rehabilitation*, 68, 363-365.

Fernhall, B. & Tymeson, G.T. (1988). Validation of cardiovascular fitness field test for adults with mental retardation. *Adapted Physical Activity Quarterly*, 5, 49-59.

Fernhall, B., Tymeson, G.T. & Webster, G.E. (1988). Cardiovascular fitness of mentally retarded individuals. *Adapted Physical Activity Quarterly*, 5, 12-28.

Fernhall, B., Tymeson, G., Millar, L. & Burkett, L. (1989). Cardiovascular fitness testing and fitness levels of adolescents and adults with mental retardation including Down's syndrome. *Education and Training of the Mentally Retarded*, 24, 133-138.

Foreyt, J.P. & Parks, J.T. (1975). Behavioral controls for achieving weight loss in the severely retarded. *Journal of Behavior Therapy and Experimental Psychiatry*, 6, 27-29.

Fox, R.A., Haniotes, H. & Rotatori, A.F. (1984). A streamlined weight loss program for moderately retarded adults in a sheltered workshop setting. *Applied Research in Mental Retardation*, 5, 69-79.

Fox, R.A., Rosenberg, R. & Rotatori, A.F. (1985). Parent involvement in a treatment program for obese retarded adults. *Journal of Behavior Therapy and Experimental Psychiatry*, 16, 45-48.

Fox, R. & Rotatori, A.F. (1982). Prevalence of obesity among mentally retarded adults. *American Journal of Mental Deficiency*, 87, 228-230.

Francis, R.J. & Rarick, G.L. (1959). Motor characteristics of mentally retarded. *American Journal of Mental Deficiency*, 63, 792-811.

Graham, A. (1997). Physical fitness of persons with an intellectual disability: A 13-year follow-up study. Unpublished Master's Thesis, McGill University, Montreal, Quebec.

Henderson, S.E. (1986). Some aspects of the development of motor control in Down's syndrome. In: H.T. Whiting & M.G. Wade (Eds.) *Themes in Motor Development*. Boston, Mass.: Martinus Nijhoff.

Hoge, G. & Dattilo, J. (1995). Recreation participation of adults with and without mental retardation. *Education and Training in Mentally Retardation and Developmental Disabilities*, 30, 283-298.

Holland, B.V. (1987). Fundamental motor skill performance of non-handicapped and educable mentally impaired students. *Education and Training in Mental Retardation*, 22, 197-203.

Horvat, M, Aufsesser, P, Croce, R. & Roswal, G. (1994). Utilization of a single trial versus maximal or mean values for evaluating muscular strength in atypical populations. *Research Quarterly for Exercise and Sport*, 65, (Supp. A-101).

Horvat, M., Croce, R., Roswal, G. & Seagraves, F. (1995). Utilization of a single trial versus maximal or mean values for evaluating upper-body strength in individuals with mental retardation. *Adapted Physical Activity Quarterly*, 12, 52-59.

Horvat, M., Pitetti, K.H. & Croce, R. (1997). Isokinetic torque, average power and flexion/extension ratios in non-disabled adults and adults with mental retardation. *Journal of Orthopaedic Sports and Physical Therapy*, 25 (6), 395-399.

Houston-Wilson, K. (1995). Program Development.

In: A.J. Seaman (Ed.) *Physical Best and Individuals with Disabilities: A handbook for inclusion in fitness programs,* pp. 125-137. AAHPERD.

Jackson, A.S. & Pollock, M.L. (1978). Generalized equations for predicting body density of men. *British Journal of Nutrition,* 40, 497-504.

Jackson, A.S., Pollock, M.L. & Ward, A. (1980). Generalized equations for predicting body density of women. *Medicine and Science in Sports and Exercise,* 12, 175-182.

Joachim, R. & Karboot, P. (1975). Experimenter contact and self-monitoring of weight with the mentally retarded. *Australian Journal of Mental Retardation,* 3, 222-225.

Jobling, A. (In press). The attainment of motor proficiency in school aged children with Down's syndrome. *Adapted Physical Activity Quarterly.*

Kelly, L.E., Rimmer, J.H. & Ness, R.A. (1986). Obesity levels in institutionalized mentally retarded adults. *Adapted Physical Activity Quarterly,* 3, 167-176.

Koh, S.M. & Watkinson, E.J. (1988). Endurance run pacing of moderately mentally handicapped children. *CAHPER Journal* (Nov/Dec), 12-15.

Lavay, B. & McKenzie, T.L. (1991). Development and evaluation of systemic run/walk program for men with mental retardation. *Education and Training in Mental Retardation,* 26, 333-341.

Lavay, B., Reid, G. & Cressler-Chaviz, M. (1990). Measuring the cardiovascular endurance of persons with mental retardation: A critical review. In K. Pandolf (Ed.) *Exercise and Sport Sciences Reviews,* pp. 263-290. Baltimore, Md.: Williams & Wilkins.

Leger, L.A. & Lambert, J.A. (1982). A maximal multistage 20 m shuttle run test to predict VO_2max. *European Journal of Applied Physiology,* 49, 1-12.

Luckasson, R., Coulter, D., Polloway, E., Deiss, S., Schalock, R., Snell, M., Spetalnik, D. & Stark, J. (1992). Mental Retardation: Definition, Classification and Systems of Support, (9th ed.) Washington, DC: *American Association of Mental Retardation.*

Millar, A.L., Fernhall, B. & Burkett, L.N. (1993). Effects of aerobic training in adults with Down's syndrome. *Medicine and Science in Sport and Exercise,* 25, 270-274.

Montgomery, D.L., Reid, G. & Koziris, L.P. (1992). Reliability and validity of three fitness tests for adults with mental handicaps. *Canadian Journal of Sport Sciences,* 17 (4), 309-315.

Montgomery, D.L. Reid, G. & Seidl, C. (1988). The effects of two physical fitness programs designed for mentally retarded adults. *Canadian Journal of Sport Sciences,* 13 (1), 73-78.

Moon, M.S. & Renzalia, A. (1982). Physical fitness and the mentally retarded: A critical review of literature. *Journal of Special Education,* 16, 269-287.

Nordgren, G. & Backstrom, L. (1971). Correlations between strength and industrial work performance in mentally retarded persons. *Acta Paediatrica Scandinavica,* (supp. 217), 122-126.

Pitetti, K.H. & Campbell, K.D. (1991). Mentally retarded individuals — A population at risk? *Medicine and Science in Sport and Exercise,* 23, 586-593.

Pitetti, K.H., Climstein, M., Mays, M.J. & Barrett, P.J. (1992). Isokinetic arm and leg strength of adults with

Down's syndrome: A comparative study. *Archives of Physical Medicine and Rehabilitation,* 73, 847-850.

Pitetti, K.H., Fernandez, J.E., Pizarro, D.C. & Stubbs, N.B. (1988). Field testing: Assessing the physical fitness of mildly mentally retarded individuals. *Adapted Physical Activity Quarterly,* 5, 318-331.

Pitetti, K.H., Fernhall, B., Stubbs, K. & Stadler, L.V. Jr. (1997). A step test for evaluating the aerobic fitness of children and adolescents with mental retardation. *Pediatric Exercise Science,* 9, 127-135.

Pitetti, K.H., Rimmer, J.H. & Fernhall, B. (1993). Physical fitness and adults with mental retardation: An overview of current research and future directions. *Sports Medicine,* 16 (1), 23-56.

Pitetti, K.H. & Tan, D.M. (1990). Cardiorespiratory responses of mentally retarded adults to air-brake ergometry and treadmill exercise. *Archives of Physical Medicine and Rehabilitation,* 71, 318-321.

Pitetti, K.H. & Tan, D.M. (1991). Effects of minimally supervised exercise program for mentally retarded adults. *Medicine and Science in Sports and Exercise,* 23, 594-601.

Rarick, G.L., Dobbins, D.A. & Broadhead, G.D. (1976). The motor domain and its correlates in educationally handicapped children. Englewood Cliffs, NJ: Prentice-Hall.

Recommendations for the Fitness Assessment, Programming, and Counseling of Persons with a Disability. (1998). *Canadian Journal of Applied Physiology,* 23 (2), 119-130.

Reid, G. & Block, M.E. (1996). Motor development and physical education. In B. Stratford & P. Gunn, (Eds.) *New Approaches to Down's Syndrome.* (pp. 309-341). London, GB: Cassell.

Reid, G., Dunn, J.M. & McClements, J. (1993). People with disabilities as subjects in research. *Adapted Physical Activity Quarterly,* 10, 346-358.

Reid, G. & Hermo, J. (In Press). Beyond skill development. *Journal of Practical Approaches to Developmental Handicap.*

Reid, G., Montgomery, D.L. & Seidl, C. (1985). Performance of mentally retarded adults on the Canadian standardized test of fitness. *Canadian Journal of Public Health,* 76, 187-190.

Reid, G., Seidl, C. & Montgomery, D.L. (1989). Fitness tests for retarded adults: Tips for test selection, subject familiarization and interpretation. *Journal of Physical Education, Recreation and Dance* 60 (6), 76-78.

Reid, G., Montgomery, D.L. & Seidl, C. (1990). *Stepping Out for Fitness: A Program for Adults Who are Mentally Handicapped.* Ottawa: Canadian Association for Health, Physical Education and Recreation.

Rimmer, J.H. (1992). Cardiovascular fitness programming for adults with mental retardation: Transplanting research into practice. *Adapted Physical Activity Quarterly,* 9, 237-248.

Rimmer, J.H. (1994). *Fitness and Rehabilitation Programs for Special Populations.* Dubuque, Iowa: William C. Brown.

Rimmer, J.H., Braddock, D. & Fujiura, C. (1992). Blood lipid and percent body fat levels in Down's syndrome versus non-DS persons with mental retardation. *Adapted Physical Activity Quarterly,* 9, 123-129.

Rimmer, J.H., Braddock, D. & Fujiura, C. (1993). Prevalence of obesity in adults with mental retardation: Implications for health promotion and disease prevention. *Mental Retardation,* 31,105-110.

Rimmer, J.H. & Kelly, L.E. (1991). Effects of a resistance-training program on adults with mental retardation. *Adapted Physical Activity Quarterly,* 8, 146-153.

Rimmer, J.H., Kelly, L.B. & Rosentsweig, J. (1987). Accuracy of anthropometric equations for estimating body composition of mentally retarded adults. *American Journal of Mental Deficiency,* 91, 626-632.

Rintala, P., Dunn, J.M., McCubbin, J.A. & Quinn, C. (1992). Validity of a cardiovascular fitness test for men with mental retardation. *Medicine and Science in Sport and Exercise,* 24 (8), 941-945.

Rintala, P., McCubbin, J.A. & Dunn, J.M. (1995). Familiarization process in cardiorespiratory fitness testing for persons with mental retardation. *Sports Medicine, Training and Rehabilitation,* 6, 15-27.

Rintala, P., McCubbin, J.A., Downs, S.B. & Fox, S.D. (1997). Cross validation of the 1-mile walking test for men with mental retardation. *Medicine and Science in Sport and Exercise,* 29 (1),133-137.

Rotatori, A.F., Fox, R. & Switzky, H. (1980). A multicomponent behavioral program for achieving weight loss in the adult mentally retarded person. *Mental Retardation,* 18, 31-33.

Schurrer, R., Weltman, A. & Brammel, H. (1985). Effects of physical training on cardiovascular fitness and behavior patterns of mentally retarded adults. *American Journal of Mental Deficiency,* 90, 167-169.

Sechrest, L. (1968). Exercise as an operant response for retarded children. *Journal of Special Education,* 2, 311-317.

Seidl, C. (1998). Considerations for fitness appraisal, programming and counseling of people with intellectual disabilities. *Canadian Journal of Applied Physiology,* 23, 185-211.

Seidl, C., Montgomery, D. & Reid, G. (1989). Stair stepping efficiency of mentally handicapped and non-mentally handicapped adult females. *Ergonomics,* 32(5), 519-526.

Seidl, C., Reid, G. & Montgomery, D.L. (1987). A critique of cardiovascular fitness testing with mentally retarded persons. *Adapted Physical Activity Quarterly,* 4, 106-116.

Shephard, R.J. (1990). *Fitness in Special Populations.* Champaign, Ill.: Human Kinetics.

Shephard, R.J. (1995). Physical activity, fitness and health: The current consensus. *Quest,* 47 (3), 288-303.

Sherrill, C. (1998). *Adapted Physical Activity, Recreation and Sport: Cross Disciplinary and Lifespan.* (5th ed). Dubuque, Iowa.: Brown and Benchmark.

Spirduso, W.W. (1995). *Physical Dimensions of Aging.* Champaign, Ill.: Human Kinetics.

Stratford B. & Ching, E.Y. (1989). Responses to music and movement in the development of children with Down's syndrome. *Journal of Mental Deficiency Research,* 33, 13-24.

Ulrich, D.A. (1983). A comparison of qualitative motor performance of normal, educable and trainable mentally retarded students. In: R.L. Eason, T.L. Smith & F. Caron (Eds.) *Adapted Physical Activity: From Theory to Application.* (pp.219-226). Champaign, Ill.: Human Kinetics.

Varela, A.M. & Pitetti, K.H. (1995). Heart-rate responses to two field exercise tests by adolescents and young adults with Down's syndrome. *Adapted Physical Activity Quarterly,* 12 (1), 43-51.

Watkinson, E.J. (1990). Preparing children with mental disabilities for active living. In H.A. Quinney, L. Gauvin & A.E.T. Wall (Eds.) *Toward Active Living: Proceedings from the International Conference on Physical Activity, Fitness and Health,* pp.164-171.

Watkinson, E.J. & Koh, S.M. (1988). Heart-rate response of moderately mentally handicapped children and youth on the Canada fitness award adapted endurance run. *Adapted Physical Activity Quarterly,* 5, 203-211.

Wehmeyer, M.L. (1996). Self-determination as an educational outcome: Why is it important to children, youth and adults with disabilities? In D.J. Sands & M.L. Wehmeyer (Eds.) Self-determination across the lifespan (pp.17-36). Baltimore: Paul H. Brooks.

Suggested Reading

Recommendations for the Fitness Assessment, Programming, and Counseling of Persons with a Disability (1998). *Canadian Journal of Applied Physiology,* 23 (2), 119-130.

Rimmer, J.H. (1994). *Fitness and Rehabilitation Programs for Special Populations.* Dubuque, Iowa: William C. Brown.

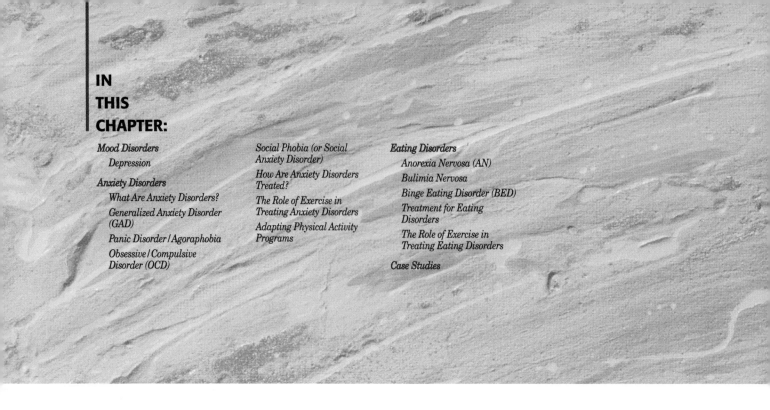

CHAPTER 26

The Role of Exercise in Recovering from Psychological Disorders

SUSAN BARTLETT

Susan J. Bartlett, Ph.D., is a clinical psychologist and instructor of medicine at the Johns Hopkins School of Medicine in Baltimore, Md. Dr. Bartlett's research and clinical interests focus on weight and eating disorders as well as the development of effective strategies healthcare providers can use to motivate lifestyle changes in their patients.

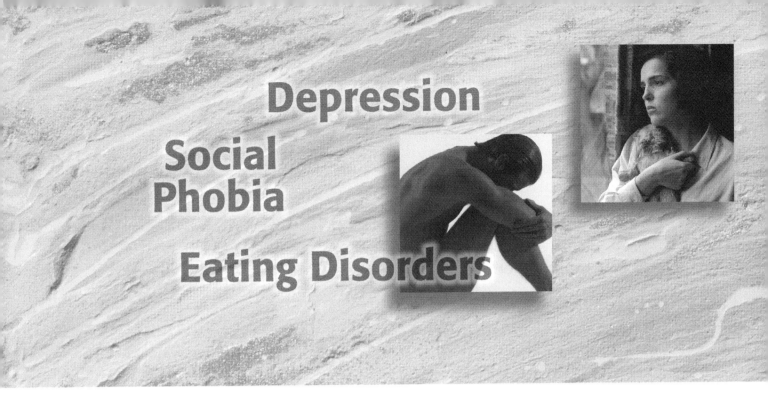

Depression
Social
Phobia

Eating Disorders

Regular physical activity plays an important role in overall psychological health. For nearly two decades, thousands of American businesses have developed employee fitness centers and programs and incentives to improve work-related behaviors. Decreased absenteeism, increased job satisfaction, employee retention, decreased stress and reduced healthcare costs all have been associated with employee physical activity programs. Across a wide variety of medical populations, from cardiac patients to new moms, exercise has been shown to improve mood, self-esteem and general well-being. Similarly, exercise often is considered an effective component of comprehensive treatment of several psychological disorders.

This chapter reviews several psychological disorders for which exercise can act as a clinical intervention to facilitate recovery, and also discusses psychological disorders manifested through the compulsive need to exercise. Recommendations are offered on how to adapt physical activity programs to meet the needs of individuals suffering from selected psychological disorders. Because of the widespread prevalence of conditions such as depression, anxiety and eating disorders, this chapter will focus on activity programs designed specifically for people suffering from such conditions. Descriptions of the selected psychological disorders are drawn from the Diagnostics and Statistical Manual (DSM IV) of the American Psychiatric Association.

Mood Disorders

Depression

Depression is the most common of mood disorders. It is estimated that 10 percent to 25 percent of women and 5 percent to 12 percent of men suffer from depression at some time during their lives (DSM IV). Clinical depression is characterized by a period (at least two weeks) of depressed mood or loss of interest in most activities that the person formerly enjoyed (DSM-IV). All areas of an individual's life are affected, including their performance at work and interaction in social settings and with family. People experiencing clinical depression feel sad, hopeless, discouraged or "down in the dumps." Often, they report that they "just don't care about anything anymore." In some cases, individuals who are clinically depressed report feeling more irritable than sad.

Depression involves changes in neurotransmitter levels and, hence, affects many systems of the body. Several medical conditions also may result in depressed mood or symptoms of anxiety. For example, up to 40 percent of individuals with neurological disorders (e.g., Parkinson's, Alzheimer's and Huntington's disease, stroke and multiple sclerosis) experience a mood disorder. Other medical conditions associated with depression include endocrine disorders (e.g., hyperthyroidism or hypothyroidism), autoimmune disorders (e.g., lupus), infections (e.g., hepatitis, mononucleosis, HIV) and certain cancers. Medications (antihypertensives, cardiac agents, hormone therapy and oral contraceptives, among others) also can induce depression.

Depression is associated with changes in the way an individual functions, thinks and feels about himself. Functional changes include increases or decreases in appetite (with resultant change in weight), sleep disturbance (trouble falling asleep, remaining asleep and/or waking too early), lack of energy, and psychomotor activity (agitation such as pacing, hand-wringing and difficulty sitting still, or retardation such as slowed speech, thinking and/or body movements). Cognitive changes include trouble concentrating and difficulty making decisions, as well as feeling hopeless about the future. Depressed persons report feeling worthless and guilty, and often have recurrent thoughts of death or suicide. They are frequently tearful, especially when discussing how they feel.

Depression ranges from mild (significant distress and some impairment in functioning) to severe (inability to function at work or with others). Symptoms of depression often develop slowly over a period of weeks to months. When left untreated, most major depression can last six months or more, and some symptoms linger for longer periods. It is likely that the majority of sufferers do not seek help, which is especially worrisome since up to 15 percent of all depressed persons will eventually attempt suicide. Any client whom you suspect may be clinically de-

Table 26.1

Client Information to Obtain from Medical Professionals

1) What are the primary psychological symptoms and how are they expressed?

2) Do you anticipate that the client will have any difficulties with adopting an exercise program?

3) If motivation to exercise becomes a problem, do you have suggestions on how to address this with this client?

4) Have you (or anyone else) prescribed any medications that may potentially influence exercise tolerance (i.e., beta blockers for anxiety)?

pressed should be referred for evaluation. Clinicians who are qualified to assess and treat depression include psychiatrists and other physicians, psychologists and clinical social workers. A summary of depression characteristics is outlined in Table 26.2.

How Is Depression Treated?

Treatment for depression typically involves psychotherapy, which may be combined with antidepressant medication. Common medications are listed in Table 26.3. Older antidepressants were accompanied by various unwelcome side effects, including dry mouth, constipation and weight gain. In some cases, the medications required significant dietary restrictions. Second- and third-generation antidepressants, such as Prozac and Zoloft, are much more specific in their action on brain receptors and, therefore, are associated with fewer side effects. Common side effects of these newer antidepressants may include insomnia and sexual difficulties. In some cases (e.g., venlafaxine), blood pressure (BP) can be elevated through regular use of the medication. Thus, ongoing monitoring of BP by a healthcare provider may be necessary. Severe cases of depression may be alleviated with electroconvulsive therapy (ECT). This therapy may result in temporary or permanent short-term memory loss of events occurring during the period in which the patient receives treatment, but otherwise does not appear to cause adverse long-term effects.

The Role of Exercise in Treating Depression

Exercise has been shown to be effective in treating depression when combined with psychotherapy and medication. In the short term (i.e., immediately after exercising), exercise improves mood and well-being. A growing body of empirical research also suggests that exercise has long-term effects. Improvements in mood and well being have been reported by regular exercisers in both clinical and nonclinical populations and with most types of exercise. In at least one major clinical trial sponsored by the National Institutes of Health, exercise and group counseling are being tested by clinicians (who are qualified to assess and monitor the disorder) as a primary treatment for mild depression. Though more research is warranted to confirm these findings,

preliminary studies suggest that moderate-intensity lifestyle exercise, such as walking, is as effective as traditional vigorous aerobic exercise in improving mood.

Adapting Physical Activity Programs

Many clinicians who treat depression recommend their patients begin exercising if they are sedentary, or continue to exercise if they are active. If the client's heart rate is greater than 100 bpm at rest, the client should be evaluated and cleared for exercise by a primary care provider (PCP). Similarly, clients who report feeling faint during exercise should be referred to their PCP. It is rare that limitations (other than those that preceded the depression) are placed on the type or intensity of physical activity performed by depressed individuals. The gradual increases in intensity and duration of exercise associated with any sound training program are optimal.

Depression may influence one's ability to exercise in several important ways. Most importantly, depression depletes motivation. A depressed individual has little to no desire to exercise, and regular physical activity is not likely to occur without structure, encouragement and support.

Another common barrier depressed individuals face is a feeling of chronic exhaustion — even upon awakening in the morning. Physical

---

Table 26.2
Characteristics of a Major Depressive Episode

Five or more of the following symptoms have been present during the same two-week period and represent a change from previous functioning. At least one of the symptoms is either depressed mood or a loss of interest or pleasure.

1. Depressed mood most of the day, nearly every day (e.g., feels sad or empty, is tearful). Note: In children and adolescents, this can be an irritable mood
2. Markedly diminished interest or pleasure in all or almost all activities most of the day, nearly every day
3. Significant weight loss when not dieting, significant weight gain or changes in appetite
4. Insomnia or hypersomnia nearly every day
5. Psychomotor agitation or retardation nearly every day
6. Fatigue or loss of energy nearly every day
7. Feelings of worthlessness, or excessive or inappropriate guilt nearly every day
8. Diminished ability to think or concentrate, or indecisiveness nearly every day
9. Recurrent thoughts of death or suicide

Summarized from DSM-IV criteria

Clinical Exercise Specialist Manual

419

activity may be viewed as yet another drain on a client's already limited mental and physical energy. Encouragement and support are necessary to help depressed clients become active enough to experience the energy boost that accompanies regular physical activity.

Since persons who are suffering from depression already feel overwhelmed, it is important that their work with you not be perceived as an additional burden or something at which they can fail. Set simple, easily attainable goals that may be reached gradually to increase feelings of achievement. Remember that exercise facilitates recovery from depression by improving mood. In that respect, any type of exercise (i.e., aerobic, strength or lifestyle) that the person is able to perform consistently is likely to be beneficial in improving mood and self-esteem.

Strive for the mental and physical health benefits offered by physical activity rather than improvements in fitness. Since sunshine also has been associated with improvements in mood in some depressed persons (e.g., those with seasonal affective disorder), it may be helpful to encourage clients to exercise outdoors whenever possible. As the depression lifts, more rigorous training programs that focus on enhanced cardiovascular conditioning and overall physical fitness may be developed.

Your client's exercise program adherence is greatly influenced by their level of depression. Lack of adherence between training sessions most likely reflects the psychological and motivational effects of this disorder. This is your cue to increase the frequency of your contact, if possible, and provide more specific (and perhaps more limited) short-term goals between training appointments. As the depression improves, so will your client's ability to follow through with less supervision and support. The link between exercise and mood makes documenting adherence and reporting it to the primary clinician on a regular basis (i.e., every two months) an important marker of recovery from depression.

Table 26.3
Common Antidepressant Medications

Drug Classification	Brand name
Tricyclic Antidepressants (TCAs)	
imipramine*	Tofranil
amitryptyline*	Elavil
desipramine*	Norpramin
nortriptyline*	Pamelor
Monoamine Oxidase Inhibitors (MAOIs)	
tranylcypromine*	Parnate
phenelzine*	Nardil
Selective Serotonin Reuptake Inhibitors (SSRIs)	
fluoxetine*	Prozac
sertraline*	Zoloft
paroxetine*	Paxil
Other Antidepressants (Atypical)	
fluvoxamine*	Luvox
venlafaxine	Effexor
bupropion	Wellbutrin
nefazodone	Serzone

*May also be used to treat symptoms of anxiety or anxiety disorders

Table 26.4

Typical Activity Guidelines — Depression

- Moderate-intensity lifestyle activity which is done consistently is as effective as vigorous aerobic activity in elevating mood and feelings of well-being.

- The best exercise for client with depression is the one they are most comfortable with. For many individuals, a structured walking program is the optimal way to begin. Even small amounts of activity (i.e., a 10-minute walk) can improve mood.

- Feeling unmotivated, tired, and having little energy are common symptoms of depression. Develop a plan with your clients who are depressed to deal with days when they don't feel like exercising. Help clients remember they rarely regret having exercised, once they got started.

- Identify short-term (i.e., daily and weekly) goals and be liberal with praise when they are achieved. Stay in close contact. Between workout sessions, have clients call or e-mail you with updates on adhering to their exercise program.

- Encourage clients to exercise outdoors in the sunshine whenever possible.

Anxiety Disorders

What Are Anxiety Disorders?

Anxiety disorders are prevalent among both adults and children. While mild to modest anxiety enhances performance (for example, during athletic competition), higher levels of anxiety can detract from performance and become problematic. Chronic anxiety that is severe enough to interfere significantly with a person's ability to function is termed an anxiety disorder. The four types of anxiety disorders that will be reviewed in this chapter are: Generalized Anxiety Disorder, Panic Disorder/ Agoraphobia, Obsessive/Compulsive Disorder and Social Phobia.

Generalized Anxiety Disorder (GAD)

Approximately 3 percent to 8 percent of the population experiences GAD (DSM-IV). GAD is characterized by excessive anxiety and worry about a number of events or situations on most days, for at least six months. (Relax, the anxiety you feel about taking the upcoming ACE Clinical Exercise Specialist exam is not indicative of GAD.) Individuals with GAD feel unable to control a tendency to worry and experience other symptoms such as restlessness, lack of energy, muscle soreness (from tension), irritability and insomnia. Worries often focus on life circumstances such as job, children, finances, health, or even minor matters such as being late for appointments. Likewise, the intensity of the worrying is disproportional to the actual likelihood or the consequences of the feared event. As with

Table 26.5
Characteristics of Generalized Anxiety Disorder

- Excessive anxiety and worry (apprehensive expectation) about a number of events or activities (such as work or school performance), occurring most days, then ceasing, for at least six months
- Difficulty in controlling the worry
- The anxiety and worry are associated with three (or more) of the following:
  - restlessness or feeling keyed-up or on edge
  - being easily fatigued
  - difficulty concentrating or mind going blank
  - irritability
  - muscle tension
  - difficulty falling asleep or staying asleep, or restless, unsatisfying sleep

Summarized from DSM-IV diagnostic criteria

depression, all areas of an individual's life are affected, including work performance and interaction in social settings and with family. Table 26.5 lists the symptoms of GAD.

People who are experiencing GAD may not always identify their worrying as excessive (many individuals say they have felt this way as long as they can remember). However, they may speak of other common anxiety symptoms, such as having a lump in their throat, sweating, having cold and/or clammy hands, feeling nauseated, and having a dry mouth or pounding heart. These individuals often jump excessively when startled. Symptoms of depression also may be present. Persons with GAD are likely to appear very anxious, pacing nervously while talking with you or sitting on the edge of the chair, unable to relax. Their expectations of themselves (and others) often are unrealistically high, and they may describe themselves as perfectionists.

Anxiety disorders are thought to result from a sensitive nervous system combined with a cognitive style (i.e., thinking too much), as well as potential alternations in neurotransmitter levels. Women are affected more often than men. Medications such as nonsedating antihistamines, thyroid replacement therapy and even antidepressants can make people feel very anxious. As with depression, you should refer for evaluation any client whom you suspect may be clinically anxious. Clinicians who are qualified to assess and treat anxiety include psychiatrists and other physicians, psychologists, and clinical social workers.

Panic Disorder/Agoraphobia

Panic disorder is characterized by recurrent panic attacks — an acute episode of intense anxiety and apprehension, accompanied by feelings of doom and overwhelming terror. During a panic attack, many individuals feel unable to breathe or as if they are being smothered, and experience heart palpitations and/or chest pain. When people first experience panic attacks, they may feel as though they are having a heart attack or are going crazy, and may lose control.

When some individuals experience panic attacks in public places (especially when alone), they begin to fear being in situations or places they cannot readily escape from if an attack occurs. Agoraphobia is the widespread avoidance of places or situations in which panic attacks have previously occurred, or may potentially occur. A primary characteristic of agoraphobia is a fear of having panic symptoms, and agoraphobics often avoid restaurants, theaters, stores or traveling far from home.

Individuals who suffer from panic disorder and/or agoraphobia often are highly attuned to sensations in their body, and they label these sensations in negative ways. For example, any increase in heart rate (even when exercise-induced) may be perceived as the onset of a panic attack.

Obsessive/Compulsive Disorder (OCD)

OCD is characterized by recurrent intrusive obsessions (i.e., thoughts, ideas or images) and/or compulsions (i.e., irresistible urges to behave in a certain manner) that significantly interfere with a person's life. Often, the individual is aware that the obsessions and/or compulsions are unreasonable and may perceive them as silly or irrational. Regardless, they are unable to control them. The most common obsessions include fear of contamination, such as exposure to germs by shaking hands or touching doorknobs; having relentless doubts (e.g., wondering whether one has completed a task properly, such as turning off the stove or unplugging an iron); and the need to have things in a particular order (e.g., everything in the cupboard arranged in alphabetical order). Often, the individual feels compelled to neutralize the obsessions with ritualistic or repetitive behaviors. Examples of compulsions include hand washing

(to undo contamination), continual checking to verify task completion, or mental tasks such as repeating a phrase or counting. While individuals derive little pleasure from such compulsive activities and may wish to resist them, they generally feel unable to stop.

Obsessions also may revolve around perfectionist impulses to obtain an ideal body shape or level of fitness. Compulsion may include the irresistible impulse to exercise excessively to attain these goals. (Obsession and compulsion to eat in prescribed manners to achieve similar results are discussed later in the chapter.) Thus, persons with OCD may seek out a clinical exercise specialist to help them optimize their programs. Their preoccupation with rigid exercise schedules, muscle definition or weight loss will appear excessive and all-consuming.

Social Phobia (or Social Anxiety Disorder)

Phobias result when individuals feel clinically anxious in response to certain objects or situations they fear. Phobias most often are handled by avoiding the feared object or situation. Social phobia is characterized by anxiety to social situations, especially those involving some type of performance in front of others. Many individuals avoid health clubs altogether or attend only when they are confident few will be present to view them exercising. Another common manifestation of social phobia is overwhelming embarrassment when disrobing in locker rooms. Persons with social phobia will be particularly sensitive to any feedback you may provide.

Table 26.6

Typical Activity Guidelines — Anxiety Disorders

- Before beginning any exercise program, be certain clients understand the normal body sensations associated with exertion (i.e., increasing heart rate, mild shortness of breath, sweating).
- Work very closely in the beginning to ensure that heart rate is elevated slowly. The primary goal initially is to increase comfort with exercise and help clients recognize that they can both increase and decrease exercise-related sensations.

- Vigorous aerobic exercise produces optimal decreases in anxiety in both the short- and long-term. Moderate intensity lifestyle activity also appears to decrease high anxiety levels over time.
- Keep the program and exercise sessions predictable and structured. Provide as much advance notice as possible of changes in the program, training schedule, or substitute trainers.
- Schedule indoor training sessions during off-peak hours.

How Are Anxiety Disorders Treated?

Treatment for anxiety disorders typically involves cognitive-behavioral therapy, which has proven to be highly effective. The individual in cognitive-behavioral therapy learns two primary techniques: 1) To decrease their level of physiological arousal through techniques such as relaxation or breathing exercises, and 2) To talk to themselves in supportive, comforting ways rather than continuing an internal conversation that makes them more anxious. (An example of supportive self-talk is having people remind themselves that it is only a panic attack, that they are not really having a heart attack and that they will be fine as soon as they calm down.)

When individuals are so anxious that they are unable to utilize these techniques effectively, medication also may be used in combination with therapy. Of these medications, the benzodiazepines should be utilized only for relatively brief periods, as they carry the risk of dependence over time. Examples of common anti-anxiety medications are shown in Table 26.7. Several antidepressant medications also have mild anti-anxiety properties. Side effects related to anti-anxiety medications usually are mild and usually disappear over time. However, when the medications are discontinued, particularly if withdrawal is abrupt, symptoms such as anxiety, nausea, insomnia and sadness may appear. Beta blockers occasionally are used to treat anxiety disorders as well. These drugs suppress heart rate and must be considered when designing an exercise program.

The Role of Exercise in Treating Anxiety Disorders

As with depression, exercise, in addition to therapy and/or medication, may play a central

Table 26.7
Common Anti-anxiety Medications

Drug Classification	Brand name
Benzodiazepines	
diazepam	Valium
alprazolam	Xanax
lorazepam	Ativan
clonazepam	Klonopin
buspirone	Buspar
Beta Blockers	
atenolol	Tenormin
propranolol	Inderal

For antidepressants that may be used to treat anxiety, see Table 26.3.

role in treating anxiety disorders. In the short term (i.e., immediately after exercising), exercise decreases anxiety and induces a more relaxed state. Aerobic exercise may be particularly effective. Several studies show that baseline levels of anxiety are lower in individuals who exercise regularly compared to sedentary adults. Thus, exercise appears to be a potent stress reducer, further enhancing its benefits in anxious persons.

Adapting Physical Activity Programs

Many clinicians who treat anxiety also recommend their patients begin exercising if they are sedentary, or continue to exercise if they are active. Specific adaptations to exercise may be helpful for highly anxious clients. For example, carefully choose the type of exercise and calculate the rate of progression, which is likely to be much slower than the progression you use with other clients. Individuals with panic disorder who usually interpret physiological arousal as a danger signal (e.g., an impending heart attack) may experience a great deal of psychological discomfort in purposefully bringing on these sensations. Thus, a primary initial goal may be to help your client learn to tolerate low levels of arousal and to recognize that arousal can be decreased and increased voluntarily.

It is important to follow some basic principles that minimize the onset of anxiety as a result of exercise.

- Ensure clients know what to expect regarding physiological arousal that occurs with exercise (e.g., increased heart rate, some shortness of breath, etc.).
- Keep exercise sessions highly structured and predictable.
- Inform clients in advance of any planned changes, including vacations and/or when a substitute may train for you. (Try to allow a minimum of three weeks' notice.)

Carefully monitor your client's anxiety levels when changing their exercise program. Develop an ongoing dialogue that encourages clients to talk about any exercise-related concerns, such as fears about achieving an elevated heart rate. Never ridicule or diminish concerns; instead, discuss factual knowledge about the issue in a supportive and positive fashion. Acknowledge that some apprehension about physical activity is normal for many people when they begin to exercise.

Because high levels of anxiety are physically exhausting, individuals with anxiety disorders often feel very tired, especially toward the end of the day. Therefore, morning may be the most productive time for exercise sessions. Anxious clients need encouragement and support to stick with an exercise program long enough to experience the stress reduction and energy boost that accompany regular physical activity.

If you suspect a client is socially anxious, take their fears seriously. If exercising in a facility, try to schedule sessions during off-peak times. Socially anxious persons are keenly sensitive about being watched and often fear that every observation is coupled with a resultant criticism.

Initially, be liberal with praise and careful with corrections. A good rule is to sandwich any corrective comment inside at least two positive ones.

Eating Disorders

Eating disorders are characterized by severe disturbances in eating and related behaviors. Three types of eating disorders have been identified: anorexia nervosa, bulimia nervosa and binge eating. An individual with anorexia nervosa reduces eating to the point that they refuse to maintain a minimally normal body weight. With bulimia nervosa, recurrent episodes of binge eating are accompanied by desperate and unhealthy attempts to compensate for the calories that were consumed. Binge eating is similar to bulimia nervosa in that large amounts of food are eaten; however, no compensatory behaviors are used and the individual typically becomes, or remains, overweight. Exercise may play a central role in both anorexia and bulimia, as the fear of fatness that is typical of anorexia or bulimia may drive individuals to exercise excessively in an attempt to burn calories and lose weight.

Anorexia Nervosa (AN)

Anorexia nervosa, present in about 1 percent of the population, is most prevalent in cultures in which food is abundant and thinness is highly valued. More than 90 percent of anorexic individuals in the U.S. are female and Caucasian (although these statistics are beginning to change). Anorexia is prevalent among female athletes, especially gymnasts, dancers and runners. Onset typically begins in adolescence and early adulthood. Table 26.8 summarizes the characteristics of anorexia nervosa.

The threshold of weight for anorexia nervosa is approximately 85 percent or below what is considered normal for a person's height (see Table 26.9). This is approximately equal to a body mass index of 17.5 kg/m2. Low body weight is accompanied by an intense fear of becoming fat; paradoxically, as the individual loses weight, the fear of fat seems to increase. Individuals suffering from AN are dissatisfied with the size and shape of their body, and may frequently comment that they feel fat or ask others whether they look fat. Women stop menstruating when their body fat falls below the critical weight threshold.

Anorexics generally lose weight by reducing total caloric intake, frequently excluding any food from their diet that they perceive as being "bad," or fattening. It is not uncommon for elaborate rituals to be developed around eating or the avoidance of food. While relentlessly avoiding eating, the anorexic appears preoccupied with thoughts of food and eating, often collecting recipes or reciting the nutritional content of most foods. Excessive exercise also may be used to reduce body weight. A common marker may be taking back-to-back group classes at a health club. Because family and friends are concerned with the individual's weight, anorexics often exercise in secret and are dishonest about the amount of physical activity they perform each day. Inability to exercise often results in feelings

---

Table 26.8
Characteristics of Anorexia Nervosa

1. Refusal to maintain body weight at or above a minimally normal weight for age and height (e.g., weight loss leading to maintenance of weight less than 85 percent of that expected, or failure to make expected weight gain during period of growth, leading to body weight less than 85 percent of that expected)
2. Intense fear of gaining weight or becoming fat, even though individual is underweight
3. Disturbance in the way in which one's body weight or shape is experienced, undue influence of body weight or shape on self-evaluation, or denial of the seriousness of the current low body weight
4. In post-puberty females, amenorrhea (i.e., the absence of at least three consecutive menstrual cycles)
5. Types:
    a. Restricting (person does not binge eat or purge)
    b. Binge-eating/purging

Source: Summarized from DSM-IV criteria

Table 26.9
Metropolitan Height and Weight Tables

MEN					WOMEN				
Height		Frame			Height		Frame		
Feet	Inches	Small	Medium	Large	Feet	Inches	Small	Medium	Large
5	2	128-134	131-141	138-150	4	10	102-111	109-121	118-131
5	3	130-136	133-143	140-153	4	11	103-113	111-123	120-134
5	4	132-138	135-145	142-156	5	0	104-115	113-126	122-137
5	5	134-140	137-146	144-160	5	1	106-118	115-129	123-140
5	6	136-142	139-151	140-164	5	2	108-121	118-132	128-143
5	7	138-145	142-154	149-168	5	3	111-124	121-135	131-147
5	8	140-148	145-157	152-172	5	4	114-127	124-138	134-151
5	9	142-151	148-160	155-176	5	5	117-130	127-141	137-155
5	10	144-154	151-163	156-180	5	6	120-133	130-144	140-159
5	11	146-157	154-166	161-184	5	7	123-136	133-147	143-163
6	0	149-160	157-170	164-188	5	8	126-139	136-150	146-167
6	1	152-164	160-174	168-192	5	9	129-142	139-153	149-170
6	2	155-168	164-178	172-197	5	10	132-145	142-156	152-173
6	3	158-172	167-182	176-202	5	11	132-148	145-159	155-176
6	4	162-176	171-187	181-207	6	0	138-151	148-162	158-179

Weight according to frame (ages 25 to 59) for men wearing indoor clothing weighing 5 lbs.; for women wearing indoor clothing weighing 3 lbs. Source: Reprinted with permission from the Metropolitan Life Insurance Company, New York.

of terror, anxiety and stress, as the individual fears rapid weight gain will occur. The most common long-term physical complication of anorexia nervosa is osteoporosis, which can lead to stress fractures caused by exercise. And while anorexic individuals often believe exercise will strengthen their bones, it is important to realize that the risk of exercise to the underweight individual far exceeds any possible benefits to bone density. Indeed, attaining a normal body weight is the only definitive way to halt progressive osteoporosis in anorexia nervosa.

Most individuals with AN do not voluntarily seek help, and in many cases family or friends refer anorexics for treatment. Coaches and trainers often are instrumental in helping individuals who exercise intensely to seek treatment. Clinical signs of the disorder include bradycardia, constipation, cold intolerance, hypotension, hypothermia, and either lethargy or excessive energy. About 10 percent of anorexics who receive inpatient hospitalization eventually die from starvation, suicide or electrolyte imbalance.

Bulimia Nervosa

Bulimia nervosa is thought to be, in part, culturally related and exacerbated by Western soci-

ety's preoccupation with thinness. Bulimia is characterized by binging on large amounts of food, followed by unhealthy behaviors to avoid weight gain and heightened attempts to further restrict food intake. (These behaviors generally must occur at least twice a week for three months before diagnosis.) The prevalence of BN ranges from 1 percent to 3 percent of adolescents and adults. About 90 percent of individuals with this disorder are females who

Figure 26.1
Binge Triggers

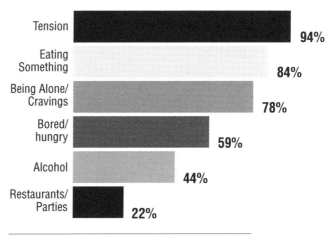

Tension — 94%
Eating Something — 84%
Being Alone/ Cravings — 78%
Bored/ hungry — 59%
Alcohol — 44%
Restaurants/ Parties — 22%

Source: Abraham & Beaumont, 1982

are of average weight or are slightly over-weight. Bulimia nervosa is characterized by an intensive fear of gaining weight, a strong desire to lose weight, high levels of dissatisfaction with one's body, and excessive emphasis on the importance of weight and shape as determinants of one's self-worth. A summary of characteristics of bulimia nervosa is outlined in Table 26.10.

A binge is defined as eating an unusually large amount of food in a short period (e.g., less than two hours), accompanied by a feeling of loss of control. Binge foods often are sweet, high-calorie foods such as ice cream or cake, and typically are considered forbidden at any other time. Binges often are planned in advance, occur in secrecy and continue well beyond the point when the person feels full. Binging can be triggered by feeling bad, boredom, feeling overwhelmed or unable to cope, or high levels of hunger after eating very little (see Figure 26.1).

Binges are followed by inappropriate compensatory behaviors. Individuals force themselves to vomit to rid themselves of the food approximately 80 percent to 90 percent of the time. Other purging-type behaviors include the abuse of diuretics (over-the-counter as well as prescription) and/or laxatives. Excessive exercise also may be used to "purge" the body of the excess calories in an attempt to prevent weight gain. According to the DSM-IV:

> Exercise may be considered to be excessive when it significantly inter-feres with important activities, when it occurs at inappropriate times or in inappropriate settings, or when the individual continues to exercise despite injury or other medical complications. (p. 546)

Psychological symptoms of depression, anxiety and substance abuse are common among individuals who suffer from bulimia. Often, more serious personality disorders also are present, making this type of eating disorder a challenge to treat. Other clinical signs include dental erosion (from recurrent vomiting), enlargement of the salivary glands, menstrual difficulties, cardiac arrhythmia, and potentially life-threatening fluid and electrolyte imbalances.

Binge Eating Disorder (BED)

Of the three eating disorders, binge eating is by far the most common, though it only recently has been studied and treated in clinical settings. Both men and women suffer from binge eating disorder, and in clinical weight-management programs, about 25 percent to 30 percent of participants are thought to suffer from BED. As with bulimics, individuals with BED also consume unusually large amounts of food in a short period, and feel a loss of control over their eating habits. However, with BED, there is little or no compensatory behavior. As a result, individuals with BED almost always are overweight. Binges often are triggered by negative moods, stressful situations or even eating small amounts of "forbidden" foods. As with other eating disorders, BED involves an intense fear of gaining weight, a strong desire to lose weight, high levels of body dissatisfaction, and an excessive emphasis on the importance of weight and shape. Individuals with BED also feel ashamed of their disorder and believe their eating is "out of control." Frequently, binge eating also is referred to as compulsive overeating. Characteristics of BED are shown in Table 26.11.

Treatment for Eating Disorders

Eating disorders are psychological disorders manifested through food and eating. Treatment always involves psychotherapy by qualified eating disorders specialists (i.e., psychiatrists, psychologists, family therapists and social workers) who most often work within a multi-discipli-

---

**Table 26.10
Characteristics of Bulimia Nervosa**

1. Recurrent episodes of binge eating. An episode of binge eating is characterized by the following:
    a. Eating, in a discrete period of time (e.g., usually within a two-hour period), an amount of food that is definitely larger than most people would eat during a similar period and under similar circumstances
    b. A sense of lack of control over eating during the episode (i.e., a feeling that one cannot stop eating or control what or how much one is eating)
    c. Recurrent inappropriate compensatory behavior to prevent weight gain, such as self-induced vomiting; misuse of laxatives, diuretics, enemas or other medications; fasting; or excessive exercise
    d. Binge eating and inappropriate compensatory behaviors occur, on average, at least twice a week for three months
    e. Self-evaluation is heavily influenced by body shape and weight.
2. Types: Purging or nonpurging (i.e., use of inappropriate compensatory behaviors such as fasting or excessive exercise, but does not vomit, misuse laxatives or enemas)

Source: Summary of DSM-IV diagnostic criteria

---

nary team that may include nutritionists and occupational therapists, among others. In severe cases, individuals are hospitalized and stabilized until they are able to continue with outpatient treatment. Since depression may accompany the eating disorder, antidepressant medications often are used as part of treatment. Medical nutrition therapy is provided to teach individuals the principles of healthy eating and normal portion sizes.

The Role of Exercise in Treating Eating Disorders

Exercise plays a complex and varied role in treating eating disorders. When excessive exercise is part of the disorder, exercise intensity and duration should be diminished during treatment. Likewise, anorexic individuals who need to gain weight should not exercise until they have achieved a healthy weight and BMI of at least 20.

If you suspect a client has an eating disorder, it is critical that you refer them to a qualified specialist for evaluation. No amount of exercise or nutritional therapy alone will sufficiently address the eating disorder. Many times, individuals with eating disorders seek out the assistance of allied health and fitness professionals to reassure themselves that they are getting "professional help" for their problem. However, such alliances prevent people with eating disorders from dealing with the issue directly and getting the help they need. Therefore, it is not wise to work with these individuals unless a therapist clears them for participation in an exercise program.

How do you approach the topic of an eating disorder with a client? This is never easy, as individuals often feel ashamed of their behaviors and typically go many years before seeking assistance. Nonetheless, it is important that you provide a clear, personal and compassionate message of concern. For example:

"I'm Mary, and as a clinical exercise specialist my role is to provide you with feedback about your current nutrition and exercise practices. I have to be honest with you, I'm concerned about... [state concerns, using the client's words whenever possible]. It's important to have someone with more expertise in this area evaluate you, and I'd like to refer you to Dr. X. (And if this is the case you might add...) I've worked with Dr. X in the past and other clients have found her to be helpful."

Table 26.11
Characteristics of Binge Eating Disorder

1. Recurrent episodes of binge eating. An episode of binge eating is characterized by the following:
   a. Eating, in a discrete period of time (e.g., usually within any two-hour period), an amount of food that is larger than most people would eat during a similar period and under similar circumstances
   b. A sense of lack of control over eating during the episode (i.e., a feeling that one cannot stop eating or control what or how much one is eating)
   c. Binge episodes are associated with three (or more) of the following:
      - Eating much more rapidly than normal
      - Eating until feeling uncomfortably full
      - Eating large amounts of food when not feeling physically hungry
      - Eating alone to avoid embarrassment over how much one is eating
      - Feeling disgusted with oneself, depressed or very guilty after overeating
   d. Marked distress regarding binge eating
   e. Binges occur at least two days a week for six months, on average
   f. There is no use of inappropriate compensatory behaviors

Source: Summary of DSM-IV diagnostic criteria

Table 26.12

Typical Activity Guidelines — Eating Disorders

- Because excessive exercise is often a major symptom of eating disorders, exercise must be carefully regulated by the health care provider who is coordinating treatment. For individuals with anorexia nervosa, exercise must often be avoided until a minimally safe body weight is achieved and maintained.

- The health care provider should determine the minimally safe body weight.

- When clients with eating disorders have a history of exercising excessively, the goal is to teach how to exercise in moderation (i.e., appropriate levels of duration, frequency, and intensity).

Locate the eating disorders programs offered in your area and provide your client with phone numbers and addresses whenever possible. A good place to look for eating disorders programs is the psychiatry departments at medical schools and/or large hospitals.

Case Study I

Clarence is a 45-year-old African-American stockbroker who is 6 feet tall and weighs 290 pounds. He suffers from severe sleep apnea (episodes of complete, brief cessation of breathing during sleep) and was referred to you by a sleep disorders center. He tells you that a sleep study revealed he experiences more than 60 episodes of apnea an hour each night. Though his physicians have recommended the use of a CPAP (continuous positive air pressure) machine, he also has been told that losing weight will reduce or eliminate his problems entirely. He wants to begin exercising, as part of an overall lifestyle change.

Together, you develop an appropriate exercise program using the American College of Sports Medicine guidelines for sedentary overweight adults. The plan is to have Clarence work with you twice a week, and exercise on his own two additional times during the week. He tells you he knows what to do in terms of eating to lose weight. During the first week, Clarence misses his second session with you. When you call, he tells you that he simply forgot about the appointment. In the second week, he cancels the second appointment because he feels too tired. When you meet the next time, he confides that he hasn't been doing any exercise outside of your work together.

Clarence tells you that he is always tired, from the time he awakens in the morning until he falls asleep at night, and asks you not to take it personally when he misses appointments. On most days, he falls asleep in the recliner before dinner, and often takes brief naps during the work day when he can get away. He states that he feels unmotivated because of his overwhelming fatigue. In fact, he's even stopped going to NFL games, even though he holds Redskins season tickets. Clarence reaffirms his commitment to change his lifestyle, and pleads for another chance to prove he can begin exercising. He is convinced his lack of motivation is completely related to the sleep apnea.

During week four, Clarence does not attend either appointment. He leaves a message for you saying he will be in next week, and you decide to hold your next meeting in your office rather than in the weight room. When you meet, you tell him you are concerned that his lack of motivation may reflect more than just fatigue and recommend that he talk with his doctor about the matter. With his permission, you contact his physician and outline your concerns about his mood and consistent inability to follow through with plans.

It takes Clarence four weeks (and several prompts from you) to see his doctor. Once he does, he is placed on antidepressant medication and begins weekly sessions with a therapist. He tells you that he still thinks his problems are related to his sleep apnea, but he's willing to take medication and attend some counseling sessions. Together, you begin developing new exercise goals. You agree that you will train together at a moderate intensity for 30 minutes, two times a week, and that he will go for a 20-minute walk with his wife one night each week. (He consents to call you and leave word on your voice mail once he has completed the walk.) You agree that in one month, if he has been unable to lose weight, you will refer him to a dietitian for assistance in developing a meal plan that promotes weight loss.

Simpler goals, more frequent contact and having his depression evaluated all appear to improve Clarence's adherence to his exercise program. The real changes in mood, motivation and energy become apparent as Clarence loses weight and reduces both the severity and frequency of his sleep apnea episodes. Treatment of the depression proved essential in making these gains.

Case Study 2

Karen is a 36-year-old physical education instructor who is 5 feet 5 inches and weighs 115 pounds. Her BMI is 19. She comes to you for post-rehabilitative supervision following a rotator cuff repair. An avid swimmer, she wants assistance developing a cross-training program that will be intensive, but not place too much demand on her shoulder musculature. She tells you that not being able to swim was unbearable and she is very anxious to increase her physical activity.

During your interview, Karen confides that she is looking for an intensive aerobic program to help her lose the 5 pounds she has gained since her shoulder surgery. When you suggest a running and step-climbing routine, she tells you about repetitive injuries to her right knee that now preclude her from running or doing weight-bearing exercise. She seems anxious, worried and preoccupied with beginning a new exercise routine. She asks you to estimate her body fat on a regular basis. She also asks your opinions regarding the optimal protein content of her diet.

As you discuss her diet, you become increasingly uncomfortable with Karen's decisions about what she will eat. She wants to avoid all red meat and chicken, and occasionally allows herself to have some fish or egg whites as protein sources. She has eliminated any sources of added fat from her diet. However, she tells you that she's not overly rigid about this; on occasion, she will allow herself to splurge on fat calories and enjoy either ice cream or a large value meal at the local fast food restaurant.

You begin to suspect that Karen's interest in food, her intense desire to be thinner and her preoccupation with exercise may reflect a pattern of disordered eating. When you begin to broach your concerns with her, she immediately makes it clear that this is not open to discussion. Though unwilling to talk initially, after several openings to discuss the subject during subsequent meetings, Karen tells you that she used have an eating disorder (bulimia nervosa), but hasn't had problems with it for a long time.

It is important for Karen to be evaluated for the recurrence of the eating disorder by a qualified mental health specialist. Though she may initially balk at the suggestion, over time she will hopefully take your concerns seriously and seek necessary help. In the interim, it is important to not fuel her eating disorder by condoning inappropriate exercise levels or offering nutritional advice.

References

American Psychiatric Association. (1994). *Diagnostic and Statistical Manual of Mental Disorders.* (4th ed.) Washington, DC: American Psychiatric Association.

Bartlett, S.J. (1996). Counseling, communication, and group dynamics. In R. T Cotton (Ed) *Lifestyle and Weight Management Consultant Manual.* (pp. 1-21) San Diego, Calif.: American Council on Exercise.

Beck, A., Emery, G. & Greenberg, R. (1985). *Anxiety Disorders and Phobias: A Cognitive Perspective.* New York: Basic Books.

Beck, A., Rush, A., Shaw, B. & Emery, G. (1979). *Cognitive Therapy of Depression.* New York: Guilford Press.

Brownell, K.D. & Fairburn, C.G. (Eds.) (1995). *Eating Disorders and Obesity.* New York: Guilford.

Burns, D.D. (1989). *The Feeling Good Handbook: Using the New Mood Therapy in Everyday Life.* New York: William Morrow.

Fairburn, C. & Wilson, G. (1993). *Binge Eating: Nature, Assessment and Treatment.* New York: Guilford Press.

Grilo, C., Brownell, K.D. & Stunkard, A.J. (1993). The metabolic and psychological importance of exercise in weight control. In A.J. Stunkard & T.A. Wadden (Eds.) *Obesity: Theory and Therapy.* (pp. 253-273) New York: Raven Press.

Kaplan, H.I. & Saddock, B.J. (1996). *Comprehensive Textbook of Psychiatry VI.* (6th ed.) Baltimore, Md.: Williams & Wilkins.

Rodin, J. & Plante, T. (1989). The psychological effects of exercise. In R. Sanders, W. Wallace & A. Wallace (Eds.) *Biological Effects of Physical Activity.* (pp. 127-137) Champaign, Ill.: Human Kinetics.

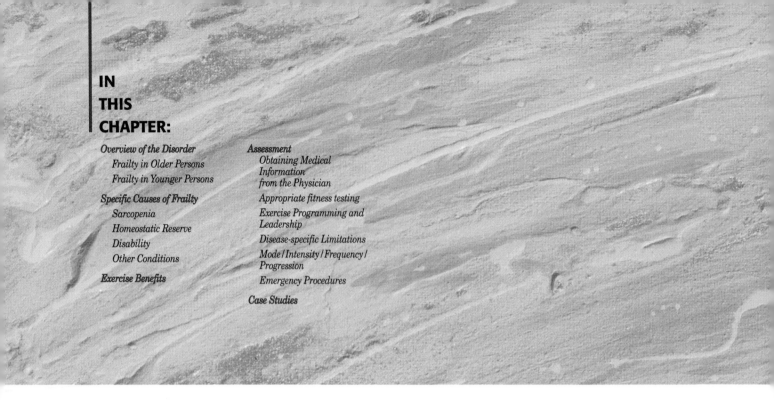

CHAPTER 27

Frailty

BROCK BEAMER

Brock Beamer, M.D., received his graduate medical and geriatric fellowship training at the Johns Hopkins University School of Medicine and completed an internal medicine residency and chief-residency at the UCLA-San Fernando Valley Program. His interest in the clinical exercise specialist's role in the care of frail elderly persons stems from his belief that better health, improved functional status and greater independence are realistic goals for most, if not all, older adults. Successfully reaching these goals not only adds years to one's life, but life to one's years.

Overview
Specific
Causes

Disease-Specific Limitations

When many people think of frailty, the image of older adults comes to mind. While frailty is a common condition among the elderly, it also occurs in younger persons. Imagine that frailty represents the next-to-last portion of a continuum be-

tween maximal health and death or severe disability. Now recognize that the goal of healthcare professionals is to push everyone up the continuum, away from frailty and toward maximal health. This chapter not only helps in working with those who are already frail, but in recog-

nizing the importance of preventing frailty.

To guard against frailty we must first define "frail." Unfortunately, this isn't an easy term to define as the definition continually changes. Currently, frailty is being redefined as a medical term with specific implications that do not necessarily match its former meaning of "easily damaged, delicate or fragile." The medical community, particularly those caring for older adults, began using the word (both accurately and innocently) to describe those whose health or functional status appeared fragile or delicate. Frail individuals are those who are at high risk for illness, disability, nursing-home placement or death.

"Frail" is now used to describe people who are fragile in different ways (Rockwood 1994), and definitions of the word are now given most every time it is used. Often "frail" is used to describe institutionalized elders, mostly in nursing homes. Some healthcare professionals use frail to describe anyone who requires assistance with activities of daily living (ADL), regardless of place of residency. Some look at underlying traits and define **frailty** as a single parameter — typically loss of strength or muscle mass. Some retrospectively define frailty as a constellation of traits shared by people who have already experienced a negative outcome (e.g., nursing home placement). Others refer to it as a loss of physiologic reserve or an increase in social dependency.

Because of its various meanings, use of the work frailty sometimes causes controversy in geriatric healthcare. When a social worker, geriatrician, physical therapist and nutritionist all use the same term, but mean something slightly different, a great deal of confusion ensues. For our purposes, "frail/frailty" represents very nonspecific, general descriptors much like the original or lay definition. In addition to giving readers a working definition, this chapter also covers the complexity and importance of the concept of frailty. We will focus on one important cause of frailty of special interest to clinical exercise specialists: **sarcopenia**.

When working with a frail individual, you must be aware of their apparent feeling of being prone to a bad outcome, or being at the "point just before something bad happens." Certainly many people who are frail do suffer from an illness or several illnesses. Frailty may not be an integral part of the illness itself but a result of the illness, or perhaps the predisposing state that allowed the illness to occur. In many cases, treatment of the illness will not decrease the frailty. And it is frailty that causes the person to be more prone to further negative outcomes (e.g., disease, disability or death).

Those at the highest end of the frailty continuum are almost completely healthy and may not be typically recognized as "frail." Those at the lowest end represent the most extreme cases, clients for whom being frail is like being a camel with the next-to-last straw placed on your back. It does not matter if you were once a strong camel who had many heavy straws loaded on over years and years, or if you were always a weak camel who just had a few straws loaded on. It does not matter if the load is all straws, or if it is mostly bricks. All that matters is that one more straw cannot be accommodated.

Technically, precisely or conceptually, the definition of frailty should be as outlined above — someone is frail when there is no more reserve capacity to withstand even minor insults; however, given our current ability to measure physiologic parameters and predict which insults will happen and how they will be withstood, this definition doesn't work. We don't want to wait until someone has had a bad outcome to be able to say they were at risk for a bad outcome. We want the ability to predict who will not be able to withstand reasonably expected insults, so that they may be prevented or their impact lessened.

Why do we want to prevent or treat frailty? To avoid the prolonged suffering inherently associated with frailty and, ultimately, to reduce the cost of healthcare. Current investments in increased muscle strength and bone density, decreased drug interactions and improved control of diabetes/hypertension/arthritis yield big savings in hip replacement, hospitalization and other costs.

Overview of the Disorder

Similar to defining frailty, diagnosing the disorder also is controversial. For our purposes, frailty is not diagnosed, it's recognized; neither a disease nor a syndrome, it is a state of being. Controversy arises because the medical community likes to "diagnose" things. There are some who believe we need to agree upon diagnostic criteria for frailty, and others who feel that this is inappropriate, if not impossible. Some have published proposed guidelines for diagnosing frailty that are useful in designing research studies to ensure we compare data from similar subjects. However, caution must be used when incorporating these guidelines into the clinical setting (Rockwood, 1994; Jarrett, 1995; Northridge, 1995; Gealey, 1997; Strawbridge, 1998) as they group together frailties from different etiologies and can be too restrictive to include all frail persons. While they are useful under some circumstances, do not let these guidelines heavily influence your judgment. Following are specific characteristics sometimes experienced by frail people as well as common illnesses often associated with frailty. Remember that not all frail people necessarily have these traits, and not all people with these illnesses are necessarily frail.

Frailty in Older Persons

Many, if not most, people over age 85 are frail. In fact, some people think we should assume that all very old people are frail based on the fact that as people age they lose physiologic reserve in numerous parameters. Not all people lose function in all areas, but few are completely unscathed. An exhaustive list is not needed here, but an example may be helpful. Beginning around age 30, people experience gradual reductions in their pulmonary-function gait (Hazzard, 1994) from loss of the cells that exchange gases between blood and air, as well as a loss of elasticity of lung tissue, and loss of elasticity and strength in the thorax. The rate of decline of each specific component may vary, but decline appears inevitable. Under ordinary circumstances, for many people this is not a problem as organs have great reserve capacity from which this loss is absorbed. However, when the rate of decline is more rapid due to genetic differences in the lungs' protective mechanisms or to external insults such as smoking, the reserve capacity may be depleted. This leads to diseases, such as emphysema, that interfere with normal life. People with less reserve capacity are more susceptible to negative outcomes from the same degree of illness experienced by those without diminished reserve capacity. They get sicker, require longer and more aggressive hospital treatment, and recover less quickly and less often.

Similar age-related declines in reserve capacity in the kidneys, brain, heart, and immune and endocrine systems (Hazzard, 1994) are well documented. Declines also occur in muscle tis-

sue, bone density and the nervous system. As with the lungs, the decline in any given system may include several different aspects, each of which may have several different etiologic paths that lead to the decline. Of particular research interest is the relationship of these various paths in various systems. Is there one underlying "aging" mechanism that accounts for all of the changes? Do several different hormonal or enzymatic changes affect multiple systems? Is "aging" the result of myriad changes in separate systems that happen to coincide? Some links have been made. For example, it is very clear that menopause results from the depletion of ovarian follicles, leading to dramatic changes in hormone levels. Subsequently, these hormonal shifts cause dramatic changes in bone, connective tissue, fat and muscle composition, as well as neuropsychiatric and cardiovascular changes. However, even this relatively straightforward example is not entirely straightforward. First, estrogen is not the only hormone altered by menopause, though replacement of it improves most or all of the particular changes mentioned. Second, most of the systems that rapidly decline after menopause began declining (albeit at a slower rate) before menopause. After a peak in early adulthood, women as well as men steadily lose bone density, regardless of estrogen levels. Third, we do not know that treating all of the many conditions of menopause with the single therapy of estrogen replacement is necessarily better than treating each condition with separate, specific therapies. (Currently there are few effective "separate, specific therapies," but conceptually it is important to assume there may be some.) There is evidence that many aspects of "the normal decline of aging" may have similar endocrine bases. However, there also is evidence that many cell types are programmed with finite lifespans and division capacities. Furthermore, some evidence suggests that years of cumulative exposure to the environment – even from glucose and oxygen – is detrimental. Though there are other plausible theories about the etiology of the aging process in general, in particular the frailty associated with aging, none fully explain the phenomenon we see every day. Suffice it to say that older people are more prone to a wide variety of diseases, that their physiologic reserve is diminished, and that they are generally at increased risk from even relatively minor insults.

Frailty in Younger Persons

Young people most often experience frailty as a result of malnutrition. Lack of adequate protein intake leads to catabolism of muscle to supply amino acids for vital functions such as immunity, digestion and hematopoeisis. Lack of adequate caloric intake has the same effect because after fat stores are gone, muscle protein is used for energy. Lack of both adequate caloric and protein intake (**protein-energy malnutrition**) is perhaps the most common cause of frailty in young people worldwide. As the body's protein-energy reserves (largely muscle) are depleted, vital functions are affected, including increased susceptibility to infection, decreased ability to digest food, anemia and decreased function of most organ systems. The effect of starvation on growth and development may be permanent but, if it ends before vital functions are seriously compromised, frailty is reversible (i.e., muscle mass, immunity, digestion, etc., return to full function).

Closely related causes of frailty in younger persons include digestive disorders (malnutrition in spite of adequate intake), and eating disorders such as anorexia and bulimia. This latter group may be of particular importance to you as a clinical exercise specialist as it is common for young people with eating disorders to exercise excessively.

Another source of frailty in younger persons results not from inadequate nutritional intake but excessive nutritional needs. Catabolic states such as chronic infections also can deplete the body's protein reserves and lead to increased frailty. Malignancies often result from both decreased intake as well as excess catabolism, and chemotherapy frequently makes persons frail, if only temporarily. Not all frail young people have a problem with protein-energy malnutrition. Persons with AIDS are often at risk for adverse outcomes, as are those with other diseases that affect multiple organ systems, such as cystic fibrosis. Virtually any serious chronic disease (e.g., renal, cardiac, neurologic) can cause frailty in some or most of its victims. In general, any catabolic state, any combination of multiple-organ-system impairments, and any severe impairment in even one organ system is likely to result in some degree of frailty. This is true in young or old individuals, but younger persons generally have greater reserve capacity and a greater ability to recuperate if the offending condition can be reversed.

Specific Causes of Frailty

Sarcopenia

The single trait most commonly associated with frailty is decreased muscle mass or sarcopenia. In fact, in some cases, sarcopenia is a necessary precondition for frailty. It often is used specifically to indicate an age-related decrease in muscle mass. Closely related terms include loss of lean body tissue, decreased lean-tissue-to-fat ratio, loss of power and others. These terms may be used somewhat interchangeably in describing the same phenomenon, and are conceptually distinct from terms such as weakness, deconditioned, paralysis or disability (though terms from either group may be applied to the same individual). Sarcopenia is reliably part of inflammatory diseases or malignancies, and present in the end stages of heart failure and emphysema. Because some experts consider sarcopenia the sine qua non of frailty, and because you may be able to provide the best defense against it, it is important to spend time exploring sarcopenia.

Decreased muscle mass is a common condition in older people. In fact, there is reason to believe that it is closely related to the aging process itself. Many studies have demonstrated that people with sarcopenia are at increased risk of disease, disability, dependence and death. Perhaps most studied is the effect of sarcopenia on the risk of falling (see Chapter 19). Sarcopenia leads to weakness, in terms of loss of both muscle strength and power. Therefore, sarcopenia increases the risk of falls by: 1) causing a person to depend upon momentum (or even reckless speed), 2) causing them to "right" themselves when balance is lost after tripping and 3) causing the person to become less able to resist a forcible blow to the chest. Sarcopenia also increases the risk of injury from a fall because: 1) a weak, powerless person is less able to turn or twist to facilitate landing on their cushioned backside; 2) that backside is less cushioned with a withered gluteus maximus; 3) it is harder to get one's hands in front of one's face quickly; 4) it is even harder to use one's hands to prevent the face from contacting the pavement without upper-body strength/power.

Not only does sarcopenia and its resulting weakness lead to increased injury from falls, it also leads to decreased function of other systems. For instance, inactivity is a major risk factor for atherosclerosis and diabetes. Weakness and decreased ambulation frequently result in lack of proper personal hygiene, decreased access to medical care and social isolation. In extreme cases, these conditions result in persons becoming homebound or even bedbound, which may contribute to psychological problems such as extreme fear of falls, paranoia and depression.

Men and women develop sarcopenia with different patterns. Men begin to lose muscle mass and increase fat mass around age 30, with a more rapid decline beginning around age 50. By age 70, most men have lost an average of about 30 percent of their muscle strength, and a comparable amount of skeletal muscle tissue. These changes are more dramatic after age 80 and still more so after age 90. In women, the decline in muscle mass is most rapid after menopause. In most individuals, the degree of muscle loss is "hidden" by increased fat deposits within the remaining muscle. Even people who maintain vigorous exercise have been found to lose some muscle mass and strength (as well as aerobic power) between the ages of 60 and 80 (Hazzard, 1994; Pollock, 1997; Metter, 1997; Kehayias, 1997). Why does this occur? The fact that it is so common suggests that loss of strength may be related to aging itself, rather than the result of a particular illness. This does not mean that it absolutely cannot be avoided, but it does mean we do not yet understand how to do so. Hormonal influences may play a role, and there is evidence that the gradual decrease in levels of sex steroids, particularly androgens, may contribute to sarcopenia. Similarly, decreased levels of growth hormone are a near universal accompaniment of aging, and may contribute to the loss. As people become very old, they often lose appetite and experience decreased taste, a combination that leads to protein/energy mal-

nutrition. As previously mentioned, this leads to loss of muscle mass and, eventually, impairment of many vital functions. Also, many elders have increased catabolism from what appears to be an immune disregulation or a nonspecific chronic inflammatory state. Such individuals have elevated markers of inflammation in ESR and TNF levels and, similar to having cancer or an infection, increased protein loss and decreased lean body mass (Hazzard, 1994).

Regardless of what initial events lead to sarcopenia, as one ages it often appears a vicious cycle is created. As people become weaker, they exercise less frequently and develop disuse atrophy or deconditioning. Decreased activity further decreases appetite, so that the body must use its "stored" energy and protein to continue normal maintenance of vital functions. Quite simply, the weaker you get, the weaker you get.

How Sarcopenia is Diagnosed

Too often, it is determined a person has sarcopenia after they have experienced a negative outcome, such as a hip fracture. When the reason for the fracture is examined, it becomes obvious that the person is thin and weak, with loose skin hanging on their gaunt. Because these cases are not easily treated, it is necessary to identify at-risk persons earlier to prevent frailty and the injuries that accompany it.

Given the statistics mentioned above, it is reasonable to assume that everyone experiences some sarcopenia after a certain age, and that it eventually worsens. Those in more advanced stages of sarcopenia demonstrate weakness and loss of power on any number of tests of strength. Similarly, anyone who reports a decrease in activity should be suspected of having begun the vicious cycle of protein-energy loss. Commonly used measures of protein-energy malnutrition, such as serum albumen levels, are abnormal only at the end stage, when there is too little "expendable" muscle mass left to be scavenged. These measures are not useful in determining who is at risk of becoming weak from sarcopenia, but rather in determining which of those weak persons is at risk of dying from the malnutrition itself. In short, everyone should be suspected of becoming weak as they age, and those with demonstrable weakness should be assumed to be on their way to becoming frail.

Homeostatic Reserve

A less easily understood component of frailty is a loss of homeostatic reserve. People normally are able to compensate for a variety of insults; for example, most of us can eat a bag of potato chips and excrete the added salt load with no trouble, contract a cold and quickly recover, or break an arm but still function with the pain. In fact, most of us could break an arm, eat a bag of potato chips on the way to the ER then catch a cold in the waiting room, and still do pretty well. When we are no longer able to do so, we are frail. Losing any one of our compensatory mechanisms may not be so bad; however, the cumulative loss of multiple compensatory mechanisms leads to frailty. This is a rather common companion of aging and, like sarcopenia, is not fully understood. People lose renal, pulmonary and immune function with age. The rate of loss varies from person to person, and if influenced by other factors, such as disease or smoking, the rate can increase rather quickly. The addition of sarcopenia makes one even more likely to be frail in such a state.

Disability

Frailty often leads to disability and disability may contribute to frailty, but disability and frailty are not synonymous. Certainly, there are many persons who experience difficulties in mobility or in carrying out ADLs who otherwise remain strong, healthy and at relatively low risk of further disability or death. Nonetheless, frailty and disability are closely linked for many persons. Often an underlying condition, such as rheumatoid arthritis (RA), leads to both frailty and disability. Recognize that RA predisposes people to particular disabilities and frailty and work toward preventing them. When disability and frailty are so closely tied to the same underlying condition, presume that both will occur without intervention, and that each will make the other more likely to occur.

Sometimes it is clear that frailty results from disability (a person with a stroke moves less and develops weakness on their unaffected side), and often it is frailty that leads to a disability (which can lead to greater degrees of frailty). Frail people can fall and break their hip, and develop a complication from the fracture. such as pneumonia or pulmonary embolism. The end result is not only a sore and stiff hip, but decreased muscle strength and endurance. Recognizing the aspects of a particular disability that lead to increased frailty allows healthcare professionals to target preventive interventions. In this case, resistance training and range-of-motion exercises, even in bed, may prevent deconditioning and resultant frailty.

Other Conditions

Many medical conditions lead to some degree of frailty by causing specific disabilities or by having disease- (or therapy-) specific effects on homeostatic reserve. Several diseases covered in previous chapters are common contributors to frailty. We will briefly look at one as an example, though others are equally important. Remembering our working definition of frailty as being prone to a bad outcome, it is easy to see that many diseases lead to frailty when they are severe.

For example, a relatively young individual with well-preserved muscle mass may have severe cardiovascular disease with a very high likelihood of death from myocardial infarction (MI) or disability from heart failure. The individual may not represent the picture of frailty that we have in mind, but may be prone to a negative outcome. Are they as likely to survive a bout of pneumonia as a similar person without heart disease? No. Are they as likely to survive an auto accident? No. Technically, one might call this person frail. Practically, many would not. Regardless, treatment is required for cardiovascular disease. If surgical or medical management leads to decreased risk of MI or heart failure, then the person may no longer be frail. If there are complications from therapy, or persistent angina that leads to inactivity and deconditioning, then the person is becoming more frail. This is an example of potentially reversible, or at least postponed, frailty.

Some of the conditions mentioned in other chapters are less amenable to dramatic improvement from medical or surgical therapy than heart disease and therefore are more likely to lead to persistent frailty. Some are especially troublesome when combined with sarcopenia and decreased strength. Increased risk of falling as a result of sarcopenia makes many elders more susceptible to osteoporosis. Add neurologic impairment, particularly balance or gait difficulties, and the reason so many frail elders break their hips becomes clear. Not only are the disabilities and frailty related to these conditions confounded by sarcopenia, but many conditions also contribute to the development of sarcopenia. As mentioned, inflammatory disorders such as cancer, rheumatoid arthritis and AIDS are highly catabolic states that lead to loss of muscle mass. Emphysema and end-stage heart failure also are highly catabolic states that lead to wasting syndromes. Neuromuscular disorders such as stroke and Parkinson's disease, as well as joint or orthopedic problems, lead to inactivity, which can propel someone into the vicious cycle of muscle loss.

Exercise Benefits

Other chapters have discussed various pulmonary, cardiac, rheumatologic, orthopedic and neurologic conditions for which exercise produces benefits. Many, if not all, of these conditions can contribute to an individual's frailty. Fortunately, the positive effects of exercise on these conditions carry over to affect an individual's frailty. Little has been done to examine the effects of exercise on immunity or homeostatic reserve, but a great deal of research has been done on sarcopenia. As mentioned, sarcopenia may have many underlying mechanisms that result in a negative protein-energy balance. Treatment with hormonal manipulation using androgens or growth hormone has not yet been found effective. Similarly, nutrient supplementation with calories, protein, micronutrients and/or specific amino acids has not shown benefit. Exercise, however, has repeatedly produced benefits in a number of measures. Maximal oxygen consumption (VO_2 max) and other markers of improved cardiovascular fitness increase with aerobic training in sarcopenic individuals. Balance and flexibility training (including t'ai chi and yoga) improve balance and gait (Province, 1995). However, the effects of aerobic training have little effect on functional measures, and most improvements in balance, mobility, gait, func-

tion, levels of physical activity and risk of injury from falls result from strength training (Fiatarone, 1994, Chandler 1998).

It is clear that resistance training increases strength and muscle mass in elderly sarcopenic individuals, though perhaps less effectively than in younger individuals (Welle, 1996). It is not clear if resistance training improves the altered physiology of aged muscle or simply compensates with increased amounts of disordered muscle. Intensive resistance training in elderly persons has been shown to induce type-I fiber hypertrophy, while the fiber number ratio remains unchanged (Sipila, 1997). Strength training also increases energy requirements and appetite, improves protein retention, increases bone mass, and restores the relationship of whole-body potassium and muscle strength, which tends to decline with sarcopenia (Evans, 1997).

Perhaps the best-publicized evidence supporting the use of physical training in frail elders came from the FICSIT (Frailty and Injuries: Cooperative Studies of Intervention Techniques) trials, sponsored by the National Institute on Aging and the National Institute on Nursing Research. Seven of these independent clinical trials included a physical training component, though each study had a different patient-recruitment scheme and interventions. Some exercise interventions were aimed at improving flexibility or balance and produced a reduction in falls (Province, 1995). Particularly relevant to the problem of sarcopenia, the FICSIT trial site in Boston studied resistance training in 100 nursing-home residents over the age of 70. The intervention group underwent resistance training of the hip and knee for 10 weeks, using the program described below. Subjects showed significant improvement in muscle strength (>100 percent) and in cross-sectional muscle area as measured by CT scans of the mid thigh. Exercising subjects also showed improvement in several measures of mobility, including gait velocity, stair-climbing power and level of spontaneous activity (Fiatarone, 1994). Other studies involving high-intensity, dynamic resistance training have shown impressive improvements in upper-body strength (about 50 percent in elbow flexion), and increases in lower-extremity strength in community-dwelling elders (Evans, 1997; Chandler, 1998). While less intense resistance training results in lower strength improvements, it has been shown to improve mobility and/or decrease falls (Province, 1995).

Assessment

Obtaining Medical Information from the Physician

Training a frail person is greatly facilitated by communication with their primary-care physician. The physician may address every question or concern listed below, either immediately or after consultation with other healthcare providers. If the primary physician is not fully aware of the opinions and treatment plans of other physicians caring for the client, it is necessary to communicate with each physician. It may be as simple as asking if they have concerns about the client participating in strenuous exercise, particularly intense resistance training. Specialists or subspecialists such as neurologists, endocrinologists, urologists and opthalmologists usually do not indicate contraindications. However, a cardiologist, rheumatologist, orthopedist or physical therapist may have input.

Address the cardiac status of your elderly clients. Coronary artery disease is common in the elderly, and often goes undiagnosed due to a lack of typical symptoms or sufficient exercise that elicits symptoms. Whether or not a client has a known history of CAD, a current stress test may be indicated. A prior history of CAD or a positive stress test is likely not a contraindication to exercise regimens, unless it is suggestive of severe disease. People who experienced an early onset of symptoms, or who showed ECG changes after relatively little exertion, may be at high risk of heart attack with exercise. Those who have had a stable pattern of angina with moderate-to-heavy exertion are likely to experience greater benefits than risks with exercise.

There are contraindications to exercise for some co-morbid conditions of frailty. Please review chapters 5, 6, 7, 14 and 18-24 for further information. With regard to resistance training, note the following relative/absolute contraindications: diabetic retinopathy; significant valvular heart disease; poorly controlled angina or hypertension; some cardiac arrhythmias; advanced heart block; aortic aneurysm; recent heart attack; stroke; abdominal surgery; active rheumatoid arthritis; history of joint surgery; nerve impingement from spinal disease (e.g., cervical or lumbar radiculopathy, spinal stenosis); and anticoagulant therapy. Ask the client's physician for intensity limitations and specific precautions.

Because most exercise programs for the elderly are low intensity (e.g., walking and stretching), explicitly query the physician about intense resistance training. Because many physicians may be unaware of the physiology of weight training, it may be wise to "remind" them that this may result in significant, though transient, blood pressure elevation. If the physician has general vague concerns about the safety of such a program, it may be helpful to provide a copy of a published review on the subject (Fiatarone, 1994).

A discussion of treatment goals is reasonable. The more strength training a frail person performs, the stronger they become, though it is unlikely they will ever return to their previous maximal functional capacity. The amount of strength a person wants to regain may depend upon multiple medical and social factors, such as life expectancy, living arrangements and personal preferences. Remember (and remind the physician if necessary) that a dramatic improvement in one's life may arise from even a partial return of function (such as being able to walk to the bathroom unassisted).

Appropriate fitness testing

Fitness testing during the initial consultation must be specific to the individual. Some clients may be too weak to perform even the simplest of measures, and others may not have walked in years, regardless of their ability to do so. Expect improvements in strength within weeks. No long-term data are available to estimate what the maximal effects may be, so use intermittent re-testing to revise program goals.

Exercise Programming and Leadership

Disease-specific Limitations

Limitations for frail clients include those outlined in other chapters for co-morbid conditions, and those provided by the client's physician. Remember that much of the current American elderly population may be unfamiliar with scheduled exercise of any type – resistance training in particular. Take special care to avoid injury from improper use of equipment.

Mode/Intensity/Frequency/Progression

When designing a resistance-training program remember that each client requires individual assessment and program design. As a starting point, consider adapting the guidelines below, based upon those used by Fiatarone et al. in their FICSIT trial (Fiatarone, 1994). See Chapter 19 for instructions on balance exercises.

Mode: High-intensity progressive dynamic resistance training.

Intensity/Progression: 80 percent of the one-repetition maximum, increased as tolerated, with retest adjustment of baseline maximum at least bimonthly.

Frequency: Eight reps per set, three sets per session. Each rep should last six to nine seconds with a one- to two-second rest in-between, and a two-minute rest between sets. Schedule sessions three times a week for a minimum of 10 to 12 weeks with at least one day of rest between sessions. Follow with at least one session per week of training; three sessions per week when a loss of strength is evident.

Blood pressure: Monitor blood pressure before, during and after exercise in the first several sessions. Do not proceed with a session if the starting diastolic blood pressure is > 100 or the systolic blood pressure is > 180. Expect a rise during and after the session; be concerned by a drop, which may represent only a vagal response to increased abdominal pressure, but may also suggest significant cardiac disease. If a drop in blood pressure occurs, refer the client to their physician before resuming the program.

Biceps tendon: Rupture in the form of a lump in the upper arm may be more common in this age group than in younger adults. This may occur with or without pain. Do not unduly alarm the individual, but recommend they see their physician. It is not likely that surgical repair is warranted unless significant strength loss results.

Muscle soreness: Initial soreness is to be expected.

Focal pain or joint tenderness: This should raise concerns about tendinitis or bursitis, and the affected area should be promptly evaluated and treated to prevent limited exercise participation. If exercise is interrupted due to injury involving one muscle group, continue training other muscle groups during regular sessions to keep the individual accustomed to the exercise routine.

Cardiac disease: Cardiac disease in the elderly may manifest in unusual ways. Be mindful of typical symptoms, such as left chest/arm/neck/jaw pain or pressure, dyspnea, diaphoresis, nausea, and palpitations. The disease also

---

Table 27.1

Client Information to Obtain from Medical Professionals

1) What are the goals of treatment?

2) Are there resources for maintenance and/or further strengthening if those goals are met?

3) What advance directives have been discussed?

4) Who is the client's power of attorney for health (healthcare agent)?

5) Does the client have any specific contraindications for strenuous exercise, specifically intense resistance training?

6) For example, does this person have critical or unstable coronary artery disease, uncontrolled hypertension, specific rheumatologic or orthopedic concerns or contraindications for Valsalva (e.g., recent CVA, diabetic retinopathy, significant aortic stenosis, known aortic aneurysm)?

7) What precautions should be used to counter those specific conditions or concerns?

8) What medications is the client taking? Do any of these require special precautions (e.g., Coumadin)?

9) Are there other healthcare providers that you feel I should contact? (e.g., cardiologist, surgeon, rheumatologist)

may present itself as mid-epigastric or upper-back pain.

Emergency Procedures

There are no emergency procedures specific to frail individuals; in fact, this group may be more likely not to want CPR. If this is the case, the individual's preferences should be well documented (and observed). If the physician does not provide this information, insist that it be done before beginning training. As mentioned, it is wise to have names and telephone numbers of the primary care physician, family and/or power of attorney at hand, as well as a list of medications and medical problems.

Case Studies

Case Study 1

Mr. Smith recently celebrated his 92nd birthday in the hospital sick with pneumonia. He has mild emphysema and "prostate trouble," and prior to being hospitalized, was feeling well. For most of his adult life, Mr. Smith has weighed about 180 pounds. Over the past few years, however, his weight dropped to 150 pounds.

His pneumonia was rather serious and required an eight-day hospital stay, all of which was spent in bed. He now is feeling unsteady on his feet, and has difficulty walking to the bathroom even with assistance. In fact, he now prefers a wheelchair, which he is able to self-propel with less effort than it takes to walk. Unfortunately, he lives in a two-story house and believes there is no way he can climb the stairs.

Comments: Mr. Smith is a typical 92-year-old. Though he lost muscle mass in recent years, he maintained just enough strength to "get by" until forced bed rest led to further decline. He is a very good candidate for resistance training that will help him regain leg strength, increase safety in his ambulation and improve his ability to independently climb stairs. After a couple of months, it is likely that he will be stronger than before his hospitalization. However, without strength exercise, he is likely to remain confined to bed and chair.

Case Study 2

Mrs. Jones has lived in the same house since returning from her honeymoon 62 years ago. Lately, her neighbors have been concerned because she no longer sits out on the porch or works in her garden. In fact, since she experienced a fall a year ago, they rarely see her out of the house. Her groceries and meals are delivered, and a nurse visits once a month to give her a vitamin B12 shot. She has not seen a doctor since she left the hospital following her fall, though she is mindful of his advice to avoid another fall so she does not break a hip.

Comments: It seems Mrs. Jones heeds her doctor's advice too well. Because her mother and sister both broke their hips and never walked again, Mrs. Jones no longer leaves her home for fear of falling, rearranged her furniture so she can navigate throughout her home without ever being more than a step from a handhold, and carefully plans her activities to avoid extra steps. Upon questioning, Mrs. Jones reports that she does not trust her balance. Upon examination, it appears that she has very little trouble with her balance or her sensation in her legs. She does, however, have significant weakness in both legs, making it difficult for her to rise from a chair or walk more than 20 feet without rest. It's possible that Mrs. Jones may have been frail before her fall, but she definitely is now. She is an excellent candi-

Table 27.2

Typical Activity Guidelines

- Exercise whenever possible, including normal daily activities such as walking, cooking, shopping, housework or gardening.
- Encourage clients to do things for themselves, relying on others as little as possible.
- Remember, clients are more likely to fall and hurt themselves if they are weak and out of shape.
- Clients can keep weights (even a can of vegetables, which weighs about a pound) by their favorite chair and periodically lift them over their head.
- Clients should use their legs only, not their arms, for support when rising from a chair (only use the arm rest for balance).
- Once clients become stronger they should keep working and exercising to prevent loss of strength.

date for resistance training for her leg strength, as well as for balance training and t'ai chi to improve her self-confidence. Mrs. Jones may resist exercise due to her fear of injury, and may require significant coaxing and coaching. Remind her that she is more likely to fall and to be injured if she does not exercise.

Conclusion

Frailty occurs both in young and old individuals, though more frequently in older adults. Many parameters influence frailty, and many conditions predispose one to it. This chapter focused primarily on sarcopenia, or loss of muscle mass, in the elderly. The only therapy that consistently demonstrates improvements in sarcopenia is high-intensity resistance training. Several other exercise interventions may improve other parameters of frailty, such as risk of falls and poor mobility and balance. Though a combination of these exercises may be of value, the cornerstone of therapy for frailty should be a focus on increased strength.

References

Please note that most geriatric-medicine textbooks include excellent chapters on frailty. Of those below, the Rockwood, Province, Fiatarone and Evans articles are highly recommended.

Chandler, J.M., Duncan, P.W., Kochersberger, G. & Studenski S. (1998). Is lower extremity strength gain associated with improvement in physical performance and disability in frail, community-dwelling elders? *Archives of Physical Medicine and Rehabilitation,* 79, 24-30.

Evans, W. (1997). Functional and metabolic consequences of sarcopenia. *Journal of Nutrition,* 127, 998s-1003s.

Fiatarone, M.A., O'Neill, E.F., Ryan, N., Clements, D.M., Solares, G.R., Nelson, M.E., Roberts, S.B., Kehayias, J.J., Lipsitz, L.A. & Evans, W.J. (1994). Exercise Training and Nutritional Supplementation for Physical Frailty in Very Elderly People. *New England Journal of Medicine,* 330, 1769-1775.

Gealey, S.G. (1997). Quantification of the elderly as applied to the elderly client. *Journal of the American Academy of Nurse Practitioners,* 9 (11), 505-510.

Hazzard, W.R., Bierman, E.L., Blass, J.P., Ettinger, W.H., Halter, J.B. & Andres, R., (Eds.) (1994). *Principles of Geriatric Medicine and Gerontology,* (3rd ed.) McGraw-Hill, Inc.

Jarrett, P.G., Rockwood, K., Carver, D., Stolee, P. & Cosway, S. (1995). Illness presentation in elderly patients. *Archives of Internal Medicine,* 155 (10), 1060-1064.

Keyayias, J.J., Fiatarone, M.A., Zhuang, H. & Roubenoff, R. (1997). Total body potassium and fat: Relevance to aging. *American Journal of Clinical Nutrition,* 66 (4), 904-910.

Metter, E.J., Conwit, R., Tobin, J. & Fozard, J.L. (1997). Age-associated loss of power and strength in the upper extremities in women and men. *Journals of Gerontology,* 52 (5), B267-276.

Northridge, M.E., Nevitt, M.C., Kelsey, J.L. & Link, B. (1995). Home hazards and falls in the elderly: the role of health and functional status. *American Journal of Public Health,* 85(4), 509-515.

Pollock, M.L., Mengelkoch, L.J,. Graves, J.E., Lowenthal, D.T., Limacher, M.C., Foster, C. & Wilmore, J.H. (1997). Twenty-year follow-up of aerobic power and body composition of older track athletes. *Journal of Applied Physiology,* 82 (5), 1508-1516.

Province, M.A., Hadley, E.C., Hornbrook, M.C., Lipitz, L.A, Miller, J.P., Mulrow, C.D., Ory, M.G., Sattin, R.W., Tenetti, M.E. & Wolf, S.L. (1995). The Effects of Exercise on Falls in Elderly Patients: A Preplanned Meta-Analysis of the FICSIT Trials. *Journal of the American Medical Association,* 273, 1341-1347.

Rockwood, K., Fox, R.A., Stolee, P., Robertson, D. & Beattie, B.L. (1994). Frailty in Elderly People: An Evolving Concept. *Canadian Medical Association Journal,* 150, 489-495.

Sipila, S., Elorinne, M., Alen, M., Suominen, H., & Kovanen, V. (1997). Effects of strength and endurance training on muscle fibre characteristics in elderly women. *Clinical Physiology,* 17, 459-474.

Strawbridge, W.J., Shema, S.J., Balfour, J.L., Higby, H.R. & Kaplan, G.A. (1998). Antecedents of frailty over three decades in an older cohort. *Journals of Gerontology,* 53 (1), s9-16.

Welle, S., Totterman, S. & Thornton, C. (1996). Effect of age on muscle hypertrophy induced by resistance training. *Journals of Gerontology,* 51, M270-275.

Appendix A

10-Step Decision-making Approach

I. Introduction
A. Purpose of this module
1. To familiarize CESs with a step-wise approach based on the principles of exercise science and clinical medicine, to the management of clients with chronic diseases, disabilities, and special health conditions.
2. To provide CESs with a model for reasoning/thinking through (vice memorizing) the critical steps of exercise programming for clients with any of a variety of health conditions.

B. Model premise
1. For a client with any particular disease or disability, the clinical exercise specialist must understand the effects of each of the following on all of the body's major organ systems:
   a. exercise, both acute and long-term
   b. disease/disability pathophysiology
   c. medications
2. With knowledge of the above information, the clinical exercise specialist will be able to determine:
   a. Mechanisms by which the disease/disability alters the exercise response,
   b. Benefits of exercise (usually related to long-term exercise adaptations),
   c. Risks of exercise (usually related to acute exercise response).
3. Knowledge of the exercise benefits and risks for each organ system will then direct all subsequent steps in the management of clients with chronic diseases, disabilities, or special health conditions.

C. Module outline
1. Review of normal exercise physiology
2. General guidelines for modifying exercise programs when the exercise response is altered by disease or disability
3. The 10-Step Decision-Making Approach

II. Review of Normal Exercise Physiology
A. Normal acute physiological responses to aerobic exercise
1. Cardiovascular responses to exercise.
   Primary purpose-to transport nutrients, remove waste products, and help maintain homeostasis at rest and during exercise.
   a. Increased heart rate.
   b. Increased stroke volume (volume of blood ejected per heart beat).
   c. Increased cardiac output (stroke volume x heart rate)
   d. Increased systolic blood pressure (force generated during ventricular contraction).
   e. Increased diastolic blood pressure with static exercise.
   f. Decreased peripheral resistance (dilation of arteries in active muscle).
2. Respiratory responses to exercise
   Primary purpose — to exchange carbon dioxide and oxygen.
   a. Increased VO_2 (volume of oxygen consumed).
   b. Increased respiratory rate (frequency of breathing).
   c. Increased ventilation (volume of air passing through pulmonary system).
   d. Increased tidal volume (volume of air expired per breath).
3. Metabolic responses to exercise
   Primary purpose — to provide energy source to exercising tissues.
   a. Increased glucose utilization.
   b. Increased insulin sensitivity.
   c. Increased fats utilization.
   d. Increased lactic acid production (by-product of anaerobic ATP production).
4. Neuromuscular responses to exercise
   Primary purpose — to produce bodily movement.
   a. Increased blood flow to working muscles.
   b. Increased motor unit recruitment.
   c. Increased mechanical force production.
5. Thermoregulatory responses to exercise.
   Primary purpose — to maintain the body's temperature within a safe zone.
   a. Increased heat production.
   b. Increased core temperature.
   c. Increased skin temperature.
   d. Increased sweating.

B. Long-term physiological adaptations to aerobic exercise training (benefits)
1. Cardiovascular adaptations to aerobic exercise training
   a. Decreased resting heart rate.

b. Decreased submaximal exercise heart rate.

c. Increased stroke volume (resting & exercise).

d. Increased cardiac output.

2. Respiratory adaptations to aerobic exercise training
   a. Increased VO$_2$ max.
   b. Increased aerobic endurance.

3. Metabolic adaptations to aerobic exercise training
   a. Increased glycogen stores.
   b. Increased ability to mobilize fat from tissues.
   c. Decreased insulin resistance.

4. Neuromuscular adaptations to aerobic exercise training
   a. Dependent upon the complexity of the aerobic modality

5. Thermoregulatory adaptations to aerobic exercise training
   a. Sweating begins at a lower body temperature.
   b. Larger volumes of more dilute sweat is produced during exercise.
   c. Acclimatization to heat after approximately 10-14 days of exposure.

C. Normal physiological responses to strength training

1. Cardiovascular responses to strength training
   a. Increased heart rate.
   b. Increased stroke volume (eccentric phase).
   c. Increased cardiac output.
   d. Increased systolic blood pressure.
   e. Increased diastolic blood pressure during isometric contraction.

2. Respiratory responses to strength training
   a. Increased oxygen consumption.
   b. Increased respiratory rate.
   c. Increased ventilation.
   d. Increased tidal volume.

3. Neuromuscular responses to strength training
   a. Increased blood flow to working muscles.
   b. Increased motor unit recruitment.
   c. Increased mechanical force production.

4. Metabolic responses to strength training
   a. Increased resting metabolic rate

5. Thermoregulatory responses to strength training
   a. Increased heat production.
   b. Increased core temperature.
   c. Increased skin temperature.
   d. Increased sweating.

D. Physiological adaptations to strength training

1. Cardiovascular adaptations to strength training
   a. Increased heart size.

2. Respiratory adaptations to strength training
   a. Generally no significant changes in respiratory system.

3. Neuromuscular adaptations to strength training
   a. Increased muscle strength and endurance.
   b. Increased anaerobic power.
   c. Increased muscle fiber size.
   d. Increased neuromuscular activation

4. Metabolic adaptations to strength training
   a. Increased energy stores (ATP, CP, glycogen).
   b. Decreased percentage body fat.

I. Guidelines for Modifying Exercise Programs When the Exercise Response is Altered by Disease or Disability

A. How to use these guidelines

1. The following guidelines are provided to assist CESs in developing a clinically based organ-systems approach to managing clients with any of a number of diseases and disabilities.

2. Each set of guidelines pertains to an altered exercise response in one distinct organ system. Many chronic diseases coexist. Some diseases affect multiple organ systems. For the client with multiple organ system involvement, the CES should refer to all applicable sets of organ-system guidelines.

3. Exercise-related risks are identified for each organ system. The lists are not intended to be all-inclusive. Only the risks of greatest medical consequence are identified.

4. The guidelines are general recommendations. Not all recommendations will apply to all clients, in all cases. CESs should manage each client as an individual case with unique characteristics and exercise needs and limitations.

5. The guidelines should be used only in conjunction with consultation from the client's physician and other appropriate health team members.

6. Guidelines are based on currently available scientific and clinical information. Because exercise medicine is a new and rapidly advancing field, CESCs are advised of the critical necessity of staying current with the latest research in this area and of updating their program guidelines accordingly.

B. Altered central cardiovascular response

1. Examples: coronary artery disease, cardiomyopathies

2. Effect on exercise response: reduced capacity to deliver oxygen and blood to the myocardium and exercising muscles

3. Risks: myocardial ischemia, adverse cardiac event

4. Exercise Modifications

   a. Reduce intensity (all modes of exercise). Exercise at levels below "symptom threshold."

   b. Prolong warm-up and cool-down periods.

   c. Avoid exercise to fatigue.

   d. Avoid exercise in extremes of temperature (hot or cold).

   e. Avoid isometric strength exercises.

   f. Progress exercise very gradually.

   g. Avoid Valsalva maneuvers.

C. Altered peripheral cardiovascular response

1. Examples: peripheral artery disease (due to arteriosclerosis)

2. Effect on exercise response: reduced capacity to deliver oxygen and blood to the exercising muscles

3. Risks: muscle ischemia and associated pain (intermittent claudication)

4. Exercise modifications

   a. Reduce intensity.

   b. Use intermittent exercise (repetitive exercise-rest periods: exercise to onset of moderate claudication pain, stop until pain resolves, and restart exercise).

   c. Prolong warm-up and cool-down periods.

5. Special considerations: Central cardiovascular disease frequently coexists in clients with peripheral artery disease.

D. Altered respiratory response

1. Examples: asthma, chronic obstructive pulmonary disease

2. Effect on exercise response:

   a. reduced oxygen supply to myocardium, exercising muscles, brain

   b. reduced capacity to eliminate excess carbon dioxide

3. Risks

   a. hypoxemia (decreased oxygenation of arterial blood) with resultant potential hypoxic effect on myocardium and central nervous system (CNS)

   b. hypercapnia (excess carbon dioxide) with potential toxic effect on CNS

4. Exercise modifications

   a. Reduce intensity. Use client's rating of perceived dyspnea (breathlessness) to monitor exercise intensity.

   b. Prolong warm-up and cool-down periods. (Prolonged cool-downs will help prevent post-exercise bronchospasm.)

   c. Use very gradual exercise progression, with emphasis on progressing duration over intensity.

   d. Use repetitive exercise-rest periods for the more dyspneic clients, especially during initial exercise sessions.

   e. Avoid exercise during periods of acute exacerbation of symptoms (e.g. increased coughing, wheezing, dyspnea).

   f. Avoid exercise in environments with poor air quality (e.g. high air pollution, automobile exhaust)

   g. Avoid exercise in climates with extremes of temperature or humidity. Especially for asthmatics, avoid exercise in cold, dry climates.

   h. Avoid exercise in the early morning hours, when pulmonary symptoms frequently are worse.

5. For advanced disease:

   a. Include exercises that improve breathing efficiency.

b. Use pursed lip breathing technique.

c. Use supplemental oxygen during exercise.

6. Special considerations: COPD frequently coexists with cardiovascular disease such as coronary artery disease, hypertension, and peripheral artery disease.

E. Altered metabolic response

1. Examples: diabetes mellitus

2. Effect on exercise response: varies with the specific disease pathophysiology

3. Risks: specific to the disease pathophysiology

4. Exercise modifications

a. Dependent on the disease pathophysiology and resultant effect on the exercise response.

b. Refer to the individual disorder guidelines.

F. Altered Neuromuscular response - joint disorders

1. Examples: arthritis, acute or overuse injuries (e.g. sprains, strains, meniscal tears)

2. Effect on exercise response

a. reduced capacity of affected joint(s) to sustain increased or repetitive mechanical loads

b. possible limited range of motion

3. Risks:

a. further joint damage

b. delayed healing of injuries

c. increased pain and decreased function of affected joint

d. for unstable joints, subluxations and dislocations

4. Exercise Modifications

a. Avoid exercises that place excessive or repetitive loads on affected joint (e.g. 1-RM knee extension or running for client with chronic patellofemoral syndrome).

b. Avoid exercising affected joints during acute exacerbations of symptoms (e.g. red, hot, swollen, painful joint in client with rheumatoid arthritis).

c. Use intermittent exercise-rest periods if exercise endurance is limited by joint pain.

d. Include flexibility and joint range of motion exercises as key exercise compo-

nents, but avoid over-stretching and hypermobility.

e. Use caution (controlled movements, careful spotting) when exercising affected joints at extremes of motion.

f. Avoid poorly controlled movements of the affected joints.

g. Condition supporting muscles prior to exposing affected joints to more vigorous activity.

h. Alternate exercise modalities to avoid overuse of affected joints.

i. For unilateral joint involvement, use independent vice dependent exercise modalities (e.g. use unilateral heel raises and not bilateral heel raises in client with resolving ankle sprain) to provide targeted exercise effect and to prevent compensation by the unaffected side.

j. Avoid exercise modalities that result in altered biomechanics due to the limited capacity of the affected joint (e.g. running with a limp in a client with a resolving ankle sprain). Altered biomechanics frequently lead to secondary injuries.

k. For unstable joints, avoid exercises that place joint in vulnerable positions (e.g. shoulder abduction plus external rotation, such as in behind-the-neck lat pulldowns, in client with anterior shoulder subluxation)

G. Altered neuromuscular response - muscle, tendon, and associated soft tissue injuries

1. Examples: strains, tears, tendinitis, fasciitis

2. Effect on exercise response

a. reduced capacity of affected tissues to sustain increased or repetitive mechanical loads

b. reduced capacity of affected muscles to generate increased or repetitive mechanical forces

3. Risks:

a. further tissue damage

b. delayed healing

c. increased pain and decreased function of affected tissue

4. Exercise Modifications

a. Avoid exercises that place excessive or repetitive loads on affected tissues (e.g. breaststroke swimming for client with hip adductor muscle strain).

b. Use carefully controlled stretching techniques to avoid over-stretching and re-injury of the affected tissues.

c. Use caution (controlled movements, careful spotting) when exercising affected tissues at extremes of motion.

d. Alternate exercise modalities to avoid overuse of affected tissues.

e. For unilateral injuries, use independent vice dependent exercise modalities (e.g. use unilateral heel raises and not bilateral heel raises in client with right gastrocnemius strain) to provide targeted exercise effect and to prevent compensation by the unaffected side.

f. Avoid exercise modalities that result in altered biomechanics secondary to the limited capacity of the affected tissue (e.g. running with a limp in a client with a quadriceps strain).

H. Altered neuromuscular response - systemic disease

1. Examples: multiple sclerosis, muscular dystrophy, poliomyelitis, amyotrophic lateral sclerosis

2. Note: These diseases have complex pathophysiologies. They can present with a variety of clinical manifestations, a range of degrees of disease severity, and with multiple organ-system involvement. Exercise research in these populations is very limited. For all these reasons, it is not possible to provide general guidelines for exercise management. CESs who manage clients with these conditions should work very closely with other members of the client's healthcare team.

I. Altered thermoregulatory response

1. Examples: obesity; diseases that can affect the autonomic nervous system (e.g. diabetes mellitus, multiple sclerosis, Parkinson's Disease)

2. Effect on exercise response: reduced capacity to regulate body temperature during exercise.

3. Risks: heat and cold stress injuries

4. Exercise Modifications
   a. Avoid exercise in extremes of temperature.
   b. Insure adequate hydration before, during, and after exercise.
   c. Dress appropriately for climate.
   d. For warmer environments, utilize air-conditioners and fans, when possible.

The 10-Step Approach

A. The 10 steps

Step 1. Perform pre-exercise health risk assessment

Step 2. Obtain physician clearance

Step 3. Identify exercise benefits and goals

Step 4. Determine acute exercise risks

Step 5. Prepare for medical emergencies

Step 6. Obtain informed consent

Step 7. Plan baseline "fitness" testing

Step 8. Design exercise program

Step 9. Plan exercise program implementation

Step 10. Double check established guidelines

Critical components of each step are presented below.

B. Step 1: Perform pre-exercise health risk assessment

1. Purpose
   a. To maximize client safety by assisting in the detection of known and unknown conditions that may increase exercise-related risks
   b. To assist in individualizing client's exercise program
   c. To provide CESs with some level of protection from potential liabilities.

2. This is probably the most important step of all because it "defines the problems". All other decisions are made based upon the results of step 1.

3. The procedures and tools used for the pre-exercise health risk assessment are covered in more detail in the Screening, Evaluation, and Programming Module.

C. Step 2: Obtain physician clearance

1. Determining requirement for a physician clearance
   a. ACSM guidelines
   b. Other established exercise guidelines from professional medical groups (e.g. American Heart Association, American College of Obstetricians and Gynecologists).
   c. As a general rule, it is probably prudent, from both a medical and legal perspective, to obtain a physician clearance for all clients with an identified chronic disease, disability, or injury, even if a clearance is not explicitly recommended in any of the established guidelines. When in doubt, CESs should be conservative with these higher risk clients.

2. Essential elements of the physician clearance
   a. Diagnosis(es)
   b. Associated conditions and disease complications
   c. Disease status (stable vs. progressing)
   d. Medications and doses
   e. MD's goals for exercise
   f. Limitations/contraindications for exercise
   g. Results of any clinical exercise screening tests
   h. Other members of the health care team

D. Step 3: Identify exercise benefits & goals

1. Questions to answer
   a. What are the client's goals?
   b. What are the health team's goals?
   c. What role does exercise play in the management of the disease/disability?
   d. Is there documented evidence of the benefits of exercise?

2. Recommended strategies to answer questions
   a. Client's goals
   - Use interviews, surveys, informal discussions.
   b. Health team's goals
   - Include question as part of the medical clearance form.
   - Interview health team members (phone, personal visits, if possible).

- Note: The medical team's goals will most likely relate to the health benefits gained through exercise.
   c. Role of exercise/benefits
   - Apply organ-systems model. (Based on what you know about the normal long-term effects of exercise on each organ system, and on what you know about how the disease affects each organ system, how do you think exercise may affect disease progression and/or the general health of the client?)
   - Perform medical/scientific literature reviews.
   - Refer to exercise medicine texts and journals.
   - Review any established guidelines.

E. Step 4: Determine acute exercise risks

1. Questions to answer
   a. What are the risks of exercise?
   b. Are there any absolute and/or relative contraindications to exercise?
   c. Has the physician identified any special limitations/contraindications?

2. Recommended strategies to answer questions
   a. Apply organ-systems model. (Based on what you know about each organ system's normal acute response to exercise, and on what you know about how the disease affects each organ system, what risks do you think may be associated with exercise?)
   - primary disease
   - associated conditions
   - medications
   b. Consult with health care team.
   c. Review established guidelines.

F. Step 5: Prepare for medical emergencies

1. Questions to answer
   a. What are the potential exercise-related medical emergencies?
   b. How will I recognize a medical emergency?
   c. How should I respond?

2. Recommended strategies to answer questions
   a. Proper completion of Step 4 will identify the most common potential emergencies.

b. Learn the signs and symptoms of the events identified in Step 4.
  - Refer to first aid, medical, and/or sports medicine texts and manuals.
  - Take a basic first aid course.
c. Develop an emergency plan based on your qualifications. CESs should know, at a minimum, standard CPR and basic first aid.(ACE requires CPR certification and highly recommends basic first aid certification.)
d. Practice the emergency plan.

G. Step 6: Obtain informed consent.

1. The purpose and procedure for obtaining informed consent are the same as for apparently healthy clients.
2. Clients should be informed of the potential risks, identified in Step 4, associated with exercise. These risks should be clearly documented on the informed consent.
3. Informed consent should be obtained prior to performance of any fitness screening tests.

H. Step 7: Plan baseline "fitness" screening tests

1. Questions to be answered
  a. Is fitness testing safe?
  b. Is it necessary?
  c. What should I measure?
  - Fitness variables?
  - Health variables?
  - Ability to perform activities of daily living(ADLs)?
2. Strategies to answer questions
  a. Refer to Steps 3 and 4 and to the appropriate "altered-organ-system exercise guidelines" (section III above) for guidance.
  b. Safety: Remember that fitness testing is exercise! The answers derived in Step 4 will provide guidance.
  c. Include measurements that will allow tracking of goals and expected benefits.
  d. Refer to any established guidelines.

I. Step 8: Plan exercise program design.

1. Questions to be answered
  a. What exercise program will most effectively maximize the benefits and minimize the risks?
2. Strategies to answer questions

a. Refer to steps 3 and 4 and to the appropriate "altered-organ-system exercise guidelines" (section III above) for guidance.
b. Consider all components of a balanced exercise program (aerobic, muscle conditioning, flexibility, balance and gait, warm-up and cool-down). Determine frequency, intensity, mode, and duration.
c. For clients with advanced diseases and/or disabilities, focus on improving ability to perform activities of daily living.
d. Remember that many individuals with chronic diseases and disabilities lead sedentary lifestyles. In many cases, exercise capacity frequently will be more limited by poor general conditioning than the disease/disability.
e. Refer to established guidelines.

J. Step 9: Plan exercise program implementation

1. Questions to be answered
  a. What should I include in the pre-exercise session (prior to every exercise session) screen?
  b. What should I monitor during each exercise session?
  c. What program variables should I monitor over time?
  - Fitness variables?
  - Health variables?
  - Ability to perform ADLs?
  d. How quickly should I progress the client's program?
  e. What are indications for
  - program modification?
  - referral to a physician?
  f. What type of follow-up should I provide my client's physician?
2. Strategies for answering questions
  a. For all questions
  - Refer to Steps 3 and 4 and to the appropriate "altered-organ-system exercise guidelines" (section III above) for guidance.
  - Consult members of health care team, as needed.
  - Review established guidelines.

b. Pre-exercise session screen:
- Primarily a safety screen
c. Monitoring during exercise session
- Signs and symptoms of medical problems (e.g. ratings of perceived dyspnea in client with COPD; pre- and post-exercise session blood pressure in client with hypertension).
- Exercise variables central to program design (e.g. RPE for client with coronary artery disease on program limited to moderate intensity).
d. Monitoring long-term program variables
- Measurements, preferably objective, that will track goals and expected benefits.
- Signs and symptoms of evolving medical problems (e.g. increased severity or frequency of disease symptoms; increased medication requirements).
e. Physician follow-up
- This topic is covered in the Effective Communication with Healthcare Professionals lecture.

J. Step 10: Double check established guidelines
1. Importance
   a. client safety
   b. liability
2. Resources
   a. *ACE Clinical Exercise Specialist Manual*
   b. ACSM guidelines
   c. Medical specialty colleges
   Examples:
   - American College of Obstetricians and Gynecologists
   - American College of Cardiology
   a. Other medical and public education groups
   Examples:
   - American Heart Association
   - American Cancer Society
   - American Diabetes Association
3. Staying current in the field
   a. Most exercise research to date addresses the prevention of chronic diseases.
   b. The role of exercise in the management of most chronic diseases has not been well-studied.

c. For most chronic diseases, there is insufficient scientific data for the development of specific exercise guidelines.
d. Clinical exercise specialists must continually review the exercise medicine literature to stay informed of new research findings and practice guidelines.

References

American College of Sports Medicine. (1998). *ACSM's resource manual for guidelines for exercise testing and prescription* (3rd ed.). Baltimore, Md.: Williams & Wilkins.

American College of Sports Medicine. (1997). *ACSM's exercise management for persons with chronic diseases and disabilities*. Champaign, Ill.: Human Kinetics.

American College of Sports Medicine. (1995). *ACSM's guidelines for exercise testing and prescription* (5th ed.). Baltimore, Md.: Williams & Wilkins.

American Council on Exercise. (in press). *Clinical Exercise Specialist Manual*.

American Red Cross. (1993). *Standard first aid*. St. Louis, Mo.: Mosby Lifeline.

American Red Cross & Handal, K. A. (1992). *The American Red Cross first aid and safety handbook*. Boston, Ma.: Little, Brown, & Co.

Goroll, A. H., May, L. A. & Mulley, A. G. (1995) *Primary care medicine: Office evaluation and management of the adult patient* (3rd ed.). Philadelphia, Pa.: J. B. Lippincott & Co.

Guyton, A. C., & Hall, J. E. (1998). *Pocket companion to textbook of medical physiology*. Philadelphia, Pa.: W. B. Saunders Co.

Jenkins, J. L., Loscalzo, J. & Braen, G. R. (1995). *Manual of emergency medicine* (3rd ed.). Boston, Ma.: Little, Brown, & Co.

Lamb, D. R. (1984). *Physiology of exercise: Responses and adaptations*. New York:McMillan Pub.

McArdle W. D., Katch F. I. & Katch V. L. (1994). *Essentials of exercise physiology*. Philadelphia, Pa.:Lea & Febiger.

Sallis, S. & Massimino, F. (eds.). (1997). *ACSM's Essentials of Sports Medicine*. St. Louis, Mo.: Mosby.

Appendix B

GENERIC NAME	BRAND NAME	EXERCISE PRECAUTIONS
Antarrhthmic		
Quinidine	Quinidex, Quinaglute Cardioquin	May increase HR and decrease BP.
Disopyramide	Norpace	
Procainamide	Pronestyl, Procan SR	Little or no effect
Moricizine	Ethmozine	Little or no effect
Mexiletine	Mexitil	Little or no effect
Phenytoin	Dilantin	Little or no effect
Tocainide	Tonocard	Little or no effect
Flecainide	Tambocor	Little or no effect
Propafenone	Rhymol	May decrease HR
Amiodarone	Cordarone	May decrease HR
Beta-blockers		
Acebutolol	Sectral	Decrease Resting and Exercise Heart Rate, consider using RPE to monitor exercise intensity
Atenolol	Tenormin	
Betaxol	Kerlone	
Bisoprolol	Zebeta	
Carteolol	Cartrol	Decrease Resting and Exercise BP
Metoprolol	Lopressor, Toprol	
Nadolol	Corgard	Decrease Myocardial Contractility
Penbutolol	Levatol	
Pindolol	Visken	Decrease Maximum Oxygen Uptake
Propranolol	Inderal	
Timolol	Blocadren	
Sotalol	Betapace	May cause fatigue and limit exercise capacity in non-ischemic, hypertensive individuals.
		May exacerbate asthma in individuals with hyperactive airways.
		May worsen claudication in individuals with PVD
Alpha & Beta-blocker		
Carvedilol	Coreg	Same as beta-blocker
Labetalol	Trandate	
Alph-Adrenergic blocker		
Doxazosin Mesylate		
Prazosin	Cardura	
Terazosin	Minipres	No effect on HR
	Hytrin	
Digitalis	Lanoxin	May decrease HR in patients with Atrial Fib., No effect on BP, May result in Non-specific ST-T wave changes at Rest and ST depression with exercise.
Digoxin		
Diuretics		
Thiazides		No influence on HR
		May decrease BP
Chlorothiazide	Diuril	Can cause hypovolemia (dehydration), reduced CO and PVC's due to hypokalemia and/or hypomagnesemia.
Hydorchlorathiazide (HTCZ	Esidrex, Hyodrodiuril, Microzide	
	Zaroxolyn. Mykrox	
Metolazone		
"Loop"	Lasix	
Furosemide	Edecrin	
Ethacrynic Acid	Demadex	
Torsemide		

GENERIC NAME	BRAND NAME	EXERCISE PRECAUTIONS
Potassium Sparing Spironolactone Triamterene Amiloride *Combination* Triamterene & HTCZ Amiloride & HTCZ	Aldactone Dyrenism Midamor Dyazide, Maxide Moduretic	
Calcium Channel Blockers Amlodipine Bepridil Diltiazem Felodipine Isradipine Mibefradil Nicardipine Nifedipine Nisoldipine Reserpine Verapamil Nimodipine	 Norvasc Vascor Cardizem, Dilacor, Tiazac Plendil DynaCirc Posicor Cardene Procardia, Adalat Sular Serpasil, Sandril Calan, Isoptin, Verelan, Covera Nimotop	Variable effects on HR, Diltiazem, Verapamil and Bepridil may decrease resting and exercise HR, Nifedipine may increase HR. Consider using RPE to monitor exercise intensity. Decrease resting and exercise BP.
Hyperlipedemic Cholestyramine Colestipol Clofibrate Dextrothyroxine Gemfibrozil Lovastatin Nicotinic Acid Pravastatin Probucol Simvastatin	Questran, LoCholest Colestid Atromids Choloxin Lopid Mevacor Nicobid Pravachol Lorelo Zocor	Dextrothyroxine may increase HR and BP and along with Clofibrate can provoke arrhythmias. Nicotinic Acid may decrease resting and exercise BP, be careful of hypotension following exercise.
Nitrates Isorbide Nitroglycerin Nitroglycerin Patch	Isordil, Sorbitrate, Monoket, Ismo, Dilatrate Nitrostat, Nitro-bid Transderm Nitro, Nitrodisc, Nitro-Dur, Minitran, Deponit	May increase resting and exercise HR, decrease resting and exercise BP and improve exercise capacity in individuals with angina.
Vasodilators Hydralazine Minoxidil	Apresoline Loniten	May cause reflex tachycardia. Decrease resting and exercise BP. May accentuate post exercise hypotension.
Other Dipyridamole Warfarin Pentoxifylline	Persantine Coumadin Trental	Generally no effect on exercise except Pentoxifylline which may increase exercise capacity in patients with peripheral vascular disease.

GENERIC NAME	BRAND NAME	EXERCISE PRECAUTIONS
Angiotensin-Converting Enzyme (ACE) Inhibitors.		
Benazepril	Lotensin	Little or no effect on HR or BP.
Captopril	Capoten	
Enalapril	Vasotec	
Fosinopril	Monopril	
Lisinopril	Prinivil, Zestril	
Perindopril	Aceon	
Quinapril	Accupril	
Rampril	Altace	
Trandolopril	Mavik	

Appendix C

CLINICAL EXERCISE SPECIALIST

Purpose

In September 1997, the American Council on Exercise (ACE) and Columbia Assessment Services, Inc., conducted a role delineation study to identify primary tasks performed by Clinical Exercise Specialists. The purpose of this study was to establish and validate appropriate content areas for the ACE Clinical Exercise Specialist Certification Exam. The results of this process include this exam content outline, which sets forth the tasks, knowledge and skills necessary for a Clinical Exercise Specialist to perform job responsibilities at a minimum professional level. It is the position of ACE that these recommendations are not exhaustive to the qualifications, but represent a minimum level of proficiency and theoretical knowledge.

Please note that not all knowledge and skill statements listed in the exam content outline will be addressed on each exam administration.

Description

In conjunction with other healthcare professionals, ACE-certified Clinical Exercise Specialists design, implement and manage exercise and physical-activity programs for individuals who want to return to physical activity following treatment for clinically documented chronic disease and disabilities.

The ACE Clinical Exercise Specialist Certification Exam is available to those who meet the following prerequisites:

(1) current adult CPR certification.

(2) Three hundred hours of work experience specifically in designing and implementing exercise programs for apparently healthy individuals and/or those with health challenges who have been cleared by their physician.

(3a) a Bachelor of Science/Arts in physical education, exercise science, kinesiology, exercise physiology, adapted physical education, athletic training, physical therapy OR

(3b) current certification from the American Council on Exercise, American College of Sports Medicine (clinical track or higher) or the National Strength and Conditioning Association (CSCS only). The certification will be valid for a two-year period at which time it may be renewed. Requirement for renewal will be 4.0 continuing education credits (CECs) and applicable fee.

These recommendations apply specifically to those individuals working with apparently healthy individuals and/or those with chronic disease and disabilities who have been cleared by their physician for participation in exercise and physical-activity programs. It is not the intent of ACE to provide recommendations for ACE-certified Clinical Exercise Specialists to deliver specialized programs outside of their scope of practice, such as those requiring a registered or licensed healthcare professional such as physical therapist, occupational therapist, dietitian, clinical psychologists, nurse, etc.

CONTENTS

Percentages indicate how much of the exam is devoted to each area.

I. Screening and Assessment (35%)

A. Obtain health/medical information to determine appropriateness for physical activity.

B. Obtain lifestyle information to aid program design and optimize program adherence.

C. Identify the client's readiness, expectations and personal preferences.

D. Perform baseline and follow-up evaluations of physical-activity levels and physical limitations.

E. Maintain detailed records of all screening and assessment data using accepted documentation procedures.

II. Program Design (20%)

A. Establish realistic, measurable short- and long-term goals.

B. Apply the principles of exercise science in designing and modifying an individualized program.

III. Program Implementation and Management (45%)

A. Orient the client to an individualized program using various instructional techniques.

B. Enhance compliance using appropriate motivation and adherence strategies.

C. Modify the program and/or session using health, clinical and performance measures.

D. Attend to the client's changing needs by referring to, or consulting with, other healthcare providers.

E. Instruct the client in correct technique and self-monitoring skills.

F. Document program activity and the client's health status using accepted record-keeping systems.

Performance Domain I. Screening and Assessment

Task 1. Obtain health/medical information to determine appropriateness for physical activity, aid program design and identify the need for referral by establishing rapport with the client and using questionnaires, interviews and consultation with physicians and other healthcare providers, as indicated.

Knowledge of:

Domain-specific Content

1. Physical and psychological conditions that may require referral to appropriate allied health professional.
2. Various disease risk factors and their implication on health and physical activity participation.
3. Appropriate content for health history and risk-assessment forms.
4. Clinically significant information regarding the chronic disease or disability.
5. Disorders associated with a specific chronic disease or disability.
6. Contraindications for participation in physical activity or exercise.
7. The typical prognosis for an individual challenged with a specific chronic disease or disability.

Clinical Exercise Sciences

8. Risks and benefits of physical activity on chronic disease and disabilities.
9. Exercise science as it relates to the rehabilitation of chronic disease and disability.
10. The effects of aging on performance.
11. The effects of chronic disease and disability on performance.
12. The benefits of exercise directly related to the treatment or rehabilitation of the chronic disease or disability.
13. The benefits of exercise directly related to the maintenance of function given the reconditioning or other effects of the chronic disease or disability.

Education, Behavior Change and Counseling

14. Communication techniques (e.g., active listening, appropriate eye contact, reflecting, body language, non-verbal behavior, other attending behaviors).
15. Techniques that build and enhance rapport.
16. Individual differences that may influence behavior (e.g., gender, age, culture, ethnicity).
17. Psychological implications of various chronic diseases and/or disabilities (e.g., motivation, mood).

Pathophysiology and Pharmacology of Clinical Conditions and Related Disease-specific Guidelines

18. How to obtain disease-specific guidelines.
19. Pathophysiology of chronic diseases and disabilities.
20. Signs and/or symptoms of chronic diseases and disabilities.
21. Pharmacology of various medical conditions.
22. Established physical guidelines or standards for individuals with specific chronic disease and disabilities.

Professional and Administrative Responsibility

23. Scope of practice and personal bounds of competence of a certified clinical exercise specialist.
24. Roles of a diversified treatment team (e.g., physicians or other healthcare providers).
25. How to obtain necessary and appropriate medical records.
26. The responsibilities and scope of practice for all members of the treatment team.
27. The implications and responsibilities of procuring and maintaining medical and other information provided by physicians or other healthcare professionals.
28. Appropriateness of physician referral in order to participate in community-based training.

Skill in:

Domain-specific Content

1. Choosing general and specialized evaluation tools.
2. Recognizing indications for referral.
3. Making appropriate referrals.

Clinical Exercise Sciences

4. Evaluating health conditions in terms of exercise and physical-activity participation.

Education, Behavior Change and Counseling

5. Effective interviewing and communicating.
6. Interpreting body language and recognizing incongruities between verbal and non-verbal behaviors.
7. Building rapport.
8. Modifying interaction style and content appropriate to client's personal characteristics (e.g., gender, age, culture, ethnicity), chronic disease and/or disabilities and individual behavioral style.
9. Exercising professional tact in all communications (e.g., explaining services, avoiding prejudicial statements, exhibiting appropriate body language).
10. Recognizing client learning style preferences.

Pathophysiology and Pharmacology of Clinical Conditions and Related Disease-specific Guidelines

11. The implications of disease and disabilities on health conditions (e.g., endocrine disorders, cardiovascular disorders, musculoskeletal disorders) on the selection of evaluation tools.
12. Obtaining and applying disease-specific guidelines.
13. Applying medical and other information to screening and assessment.
14. Applying pharmacological information in collecting assessment data.

Professional and Administrative Responsibility

15. Recognizing the responsibilities and scope of practice for all members of the treatment team.
16. Soliciting information from, interacting with, and interpreting information from healthcare providers (e.g., insurance, physicians).

Task 2. Obtain lifestyle information as needed in order to aid program design and optimize program adherence using interviews and questionnaires.

Knowledge of:
Domain-specific Content

1. Implications of lifestyle as it relates to the health of the client.
2. Knowledge of appropriate content of lifestyle forms.

3. The profile of a typical client that has been cleared to participate in a community-based exercise program.

Skill in:
Domain-specific Content

1. Administering and analyzing assessment data.

Task 3. Identify the client's readiness, expectations and personal preferences to aid in program design using interviews and questionnaires.

Knowledge of:
Education, Behavior Change and Counseling

1. Theories of behavior change (e.g., stages of change, health belief model) and the implications for tailoring treatment.
2. Mental and physical barriers associated with various conditions.
3. Methods used to identify and address unrealistic expectations as they relate to underlying medical conditions.

Pathophysiology and Pharmacology of Clinical Conditions and Related Disease-specific Guidelines

4. Mental and physical barriers associated with various medical conditions.
5. Procedures typically followed to communicate with healthcare providers to safely screen a client with a chronic disease or disability.

Skill in:
Education, Behavior Change and Counseling

1. Utilizing appropriate methods to assess client's readiness, expectations and preferences.
2. Assessing client's readiness, expectations and preferences.
3. Applying behavior-change assessment methods.
4. Identifying barriers associated with various medical conditions that may affect assessment.
5. Adapting the assessment in accordance with the identified barriers.
6. Contraindications to exercise and physical activity given the chronic disease or disability.

Pathophysiology and Pharmacology of Clinical Conditions and Related Disease-specific Guidelines

7. Identifying and/or addressing unrealistic expectations as they relate to underlying medical conditions.

Task 4. Perform baseline and follow-up evaluations of physical-activity levels and physical limitations using recommended guidelines and established protocols to aid program design, ensure safety and monitor effectiveness.

Knowledge of:

Domain-specific Content

1. Appropriate assessments and modifications.
2. Appropriate types of assessments (e.g., strength, cardiovascular, flexibility, functionality, body composition).
3. Applying disease-specific guidelines during assessment.
4. The proper use and application of testing equipment.
5. Appropriateness of non-clinical fitness testing.

Clinical Exercise Sciences

6. Administering assessments at appropriate intervals.
7. Variables that affect interpretation of test results.
8. Appropriate intervals for re-evaluation for various medical conditions.
9. The proper use and application of equipment during assessment.
10. Appropriate types of assessments (e.g., strength, cardiovascular, flexibility, functionality, body composition).
11. Standard therapeutic modalities and treatments that precede involvement in community-based exercise programs (e.g., cardiac rehabilitation, diabetes education, physical therapy).

Pathophysiology and Pharmacology of Clinical Conditions and Related Disease-specific Guidelines

12. Variables that affect interpretation of test results.
13. Physiological effects of medications and appropriate precautions for a client taking medications and/or other substances during physical-activity evaluation (e.g., antihypertensives, NSAIDs, insulin, antihistamines, antidepressants, alcohol, cold medications, caffeine, nicotine, illicit drugs).
14. Typical medications prescribed for a given chronic disease or disability.
15. Influence or other relevant responses of medications on exercise responses.
16. Side effects or other relevant responses to medications.

Skill in:

Domain-specific Content

1. The selection of appropriate assessments.
2. Administering assessments at appropriate intervals.
3. Individualizing the assessment.
4. Analyzing physical-activity assessment data.

Pathophysiology and Pharmacology of Clinical Conditions and Related Disease-specific Guidelines

5. Identifying and recognizing symptoms of various diseases and disabilities before, during and after physical-activity evaluation.
6. Applying disease-specific guidelines during physical-activity assessment.

Task 5. Maintain detailed records of all screening and assessment data using accepted documentation procedures to aid in program development.

Knowledge of:

Professional and Administrative Responsibility

1. Adequate baseline documentation and associated liabilities.
2. Components of an adequate client record (e.g., progress notes, SOAP notes, etc.).
3. Confidentiality guidelines.
4. The appropriate information to be documented.
5. Appropriate information to be reported to a physician/healthcare provider.

Skill in:

Domain-specific Content

1. Summarizing data objectively.
2. Making appropriate recommendations

based on assessment data.

3. Maintaining the privacy and security of records.

Performance Domain II. Program Design

Task 1. Establish realistic, measurable short- and long-term goals by acknowledging the client's expectations and interpreting assessment and reassessment data to design and/or modify a safe and effective program for individuals with existing special health needs.

Knowledge of:

Domain-specific Content

1. Principles of goal setting as it relates to individuals with chronic disease and/or disabilities.
2. Expected progression given the individual's limitation to physical function (mild, moderate, severe).

Clinical Exercise Sciences

3. Safe and effective rates of change (e.g., physical, psychological).
4. Goal setting based on fitness, health and lifestyle assessments and utilization of this data in goal setting.
5. Appropriate guidelines to follow to progress an exercise program.

Education, Behavior Change and Counseling

6. Obstacles that may interfere with the attainment of goals (e.g., time restraints, weather changes, family obligations, financial issues).
7. Motivation, exercise adherence and behavior modification and their relationship to goal setting.
8. Principles of adult learning (e.g., readiness, success, practice).
9. Appropriate educational materials based on cognitive, affective and psychomotor factors and learning.

Pathophysiology and Pharmacology of Clinical Conditions and Related Disease-specific Guidelines

10. Genetic psychological and physiological factors that influence goal setting.

Professional and Administrative Responsibility

11. Appropriate design and use of record-keeping materials.
12. Ethics and scope of practice in relation to coordinating programs for individuals with chronic disease and/or disabilities.
13. Methods used to facilitate the client's acceptance, responsibility and accountability for program goals.

Skill in:

Domain-specific Content

1. Establishing a well-stated goal (e.g., specific, measurable, action-oriented, realistic, timed).
2. Identifying barriers and developing options.

Pathophysiology and Pharmacology of Clinical Conditions and Related Disease-specific Guidelines

3. Researching new information to assist in determining appropriate goals (e.g., libraries, databases, Internet, research journals).
4. Interpreting and understanding research.

Task 2. Apply the principles of exercise science in designing and modifying an individualized program by integrating the specific, measurable goals and interpreting assessment and re-assessment data to develop safe and effective programs for individuals with chronic disease and/or disabilities.

Knowledge of:

Domain-specific Content

1. Designing a safe, well-balanced and comprehensive physical-activity program specific to the client's health status, special needs, desires and goals.
2. Applicable standards, guidelines and position statements published by accepted organizations (e.g., ACSM, ACOG, ADA, AHA, IOM, NCEP, USAA, YMCA) for use in program design.

3. Strategies for interpreting the client profile as it relates to established guidelines.
4. Current nutrition guidelines and concepts (e.g., macronutrient, micronutrient, ergogenic aids) as they relate to chronic disease and/or disabilities.
5. Appropriate guidelines for designing an exercise program (mode, intensity, frequency, duration, progression) for a given chronic disease or disability.
6. Exercises specific to the continued rehabilitation of the chronic disease or disability.

Clinical Exercise Sciences

7. Methods to determine appropriate loads, resistance or intensity for program design.
8. Concepts, principles and techniques related to program design utilizing the health components of fitness (e.g., muscular strength and endurance, cardiorespiratory endurance, flexibility, body composition) and skill-related components of fitness (e.g., agility, balance, reaction time, coordination, power).
9. Concepts, principles and techniques related to overload, specificity, periodization, reversibility and training effects.
10. Environmental conditions (e.g., heat, cold, humidity, altitude, smog) and their impact on physical activity.
11. Identified dose-response relationship for a given exercise(s).

Education, Behavior Change and Counseling

12. Test results and their implications for motivational strategies and techniques.

Pathophysiology and Pharmacology of Clinical Conditions and Related Disease-specific Guidelines

13. Designing a safe, well-balanced and comprehensive physical-activity program specific to the client's health status, special needs, desires and goals.
14. Educational resources (e.g., Arthritis Foundation, American Diabetes Association, American Heart Association).
15. Environmental conditions (e.g., heat, cold, humidity, altitude, smog) and their impact on physical activity.
16. Contraindications and side effects of prescription and nonprescription medications.

17. Interaction between medications, exercise and diet.
18. Resources for obtaining information on pathological conditions and drug effects.
19. Signs and symptoms that should be monitored before, during and after exercise.
20. Absolute or relative contraindications for performing specific exercises.

Professional and Administrative Responsibility

21. Copyright laws as they apply to music, video, written text and trademark usage.
22. Currently accepted standards of care.
23. Contributions of other allied health/fitness professions (e.g., athletic training, physical therapy, chiropractic) to the client.

Skill in:
Clinical Exercise Science

1. Designing safe exercises for all major muscle groups.
2. Identifying joint type, action and the normal degree of range of motion and/or movements.

Education, Behavior Change and Counseling

3. Selecting and integrating appropriate educational materials for use in client instruction.
4. Facilitating the client's acceptance, responsibility and accountability for program goals.

Pathophysiology and Pharmacology of Clinical Conditions and Related Disease-specific Guidelines

5. Interpreting test results and their implications for program design.
6. Designing a safe, well-balanced and comprehensive physical-activity program specific to the client's health status, special needs, desires and goals.

Professional and Administrative Responsibility

7. Documenting pertinent, day-to-day information (e.g., subjective, objective, assessment and planning data).
8. Researching new information to assist in determining safe, well-balanced and comprehensive physical-activity program

goals (e.g., libraries, databases, Internet, research journals).

9. Interpreting information from healthcare providers (e.g., insurance, physicians).

10. Recognizing scope of practice and ethical standards in relation to chronic disease and/or disabilities.

11. Recognizing scope of practice of certified clinical exercise specialists and personal bounds of competence.

Performance Domain III. Program Implementation and Management

Task 1. Orient the client to an individualized program using various instructional techniques to set the foundation for program implementation.

Knowledge of:
Clinical Exercise Sciences

1. Application of advanced exercise physiology principles as they relate to cardiovascular, metabolic and musculoskeletal conditions relative to individuals with chronic disease and/or disabilities.

2. The rationale for appropriate programming factors (e.g., frequency, intensity, duration, mode, progression) as they apply to individuals with chronic disease and/or disabilities.

3. Benefits of physical activity as they affect the function and performance of the individual with chronic disease and/or disabilities.

Pathophysiology and Pharmacology of Clinical Conditions and Related Disease-specific Guidelines

4. Pathophysiology of cardiovascular, metabolic and musculoskeletal conditions.

5. Selection of appropriate exercises at varying program phases.

6. The proper use and application of equipment and/or modalities in program implementation.

Skill in:
Education, Behavioral Change and Counseling

1. Instructing, cueing and/or supervising the client in the safe and proper execution of exercise.

2. Communicating effectively with the client and/or healthcare team.

3. Recognizing life-threatening situations and implementing appropriate emergency procedures.

Task 2. Enhance compliance using appropriate motivation and adherence strategies to maximize the effectiveness of the program.

Knowledge of:
Education, Behavioral Change and Counseling

1. Appropriate motivation and adherence strategies to meet individual needs (e.g., rewards, contracts).

2. Appropriate strategies to facilitate behavior change.

3. Factors related to chronic disease and disabilities that affect compliance.

4. Different communication styles required to interact effectively with individuals with chronic disease and disabilities, as well as older adults and individuals from different social/cultural backgrounds.

Pathophysiology and Pharmacology of Clinical Conditions and Related Disease-specific Guidelines

5. Disease-specific factors that influence compliance and adherence.

Professional and Administrative Responsibility

6. Ethical strategies to augment client compliance and adherence.

Skill in:
Education, Behavior Change and Counseling

1. Using interpersonal communication for enhanced motivation and adherence relative to individual needs and responses.

2. Interpreting and applying clinical and exercise data as a basis for client motivation.

3. Communicating effectively with the client and healthcare team.

4. Applying motivational techniques to enhance and assist training.

Task 3. Modify the program and/or session as indicated using health, clinical and performance measures to aid program progression and ensure safety and effectiveness.

Knowledge of:
Clinical Exercise Sciences
1. Appropriate programmatic changes based on current health status and/or response to physical activity.
2. Modifying program design based upon assessment and/or reassessment.

Pathophysiology and Pharmacology of Clinical Conditions and Related Disease-specific Guidelines
3. The need to consult with the physician based on the physiological effects and interaction between medication and physical activity.

Skill in:
Clinical Exercise Sciences
1. Identifying adverse signs and symptoms that may require modifications to exercise.
2. Recognizing and adjusting the program to the needs of individuals with chronic disease and/or disabilities (e.g., dose response).

Education, Behavior Change and Counseling
3. Modifying motivational strategies based upon assessment and/or reassessment.

Task 4. Attend to the client's changing needs by referring to, or consulting with, other healthcare providers, as necessary, to facilitate a safe and effective program.

Knowledge of:
Domain-specific Content
1. Physiological and/or psychological changes and responses to the program that may indicate referral.

Professional and Administrative Responsibility
2. Qualified local health/medical health professionals to use as referrals.
3. Recognized scope of practice and personal bounds of competence.

Skill in:
Clinical Exercise Sciences
1. Assessing the client's changing health needs.
2. Recognizing factors and conditions that necessitate referral.

Professional Responsibility
3. Communicating effectively with other healthcare providers.

Task 5. Instruct the client in correct technique and self-monitoring skills by evaluating the client's objective and subjective responses to the program to achieve program objectives safely and effectively.

Knowledge of:
Domain-specific Content
1. Appropriate objective monitoring techniques required for individuals with chronic disease and/or disabilities (e.g., heart rate, blood pressure, glucose, body weight).
2. Appropriate subjective monitoring techniques required for individuals with chronic disease and/or disabilities (e.g., RPE, observation, talk test).
3. Safe and effective spotting procedures.
4. Safe and effective exercise techniques.

Clinical Exercise Sciences
5. Adverse signs and symptoms that indicate exercise intolerance and overwork and necessitate modification.
6. Correct biomechanical technique.

Pathophysiology and Pharmacology of Clinical Conditions and Related Disease-specific Guidelines
7. Criteria indicating when to defer, delay or terminate physical activity.
8. Contraindicated activities specific to the chronic disease or disability.

Professional and Administrative Responsibility
9. Appropriate emergency procedures relative to chronic disease/disability and the program environment.
10. Safety guidelines as they relate to program implementation (e.g., facilities, equipment, location).
11. Environmental conditions that may affect

exercise performance and tolerance (e.g., floor surface, temperature, access to equipment or facilities).

12. Current understanding of the principles of CPR.

13. Current understanding of the principles of first aid.

Skill in:

Clinical Exercise Sciences

1. Obtaining and interpreting subjective-monitoring techniques.

2. Obtaining and interpreting objective-monitoring techniques.

3. Demonstrating and instructing the client in self-monitoring techniques.

4. Instructing the client in the importance of self-reporting signs and symptoms that may be present before, during or after exercise.

5. Recognizing signs and symptoms of exercise intolerance or overwork.

6. Using appropriate spotting techniques specific to individual needs and conditions.

7. Demonstrating and instructing correct biomechanical exercise technique.

Task 6. Document program activity and the client's health status and response to the program using accepted record keeping systems to maintain appropriate records and communicate with other members of the treatment team.

Knowledge of:

Clinical Exercise Science

1. The use of appropriate documentation procedures (e.g., progress recording, Subjective, Objective, Assessment and Plan [SOAP] notes).

2. Physiological variables of importance (e.g., blood pressure, heart rate, workload, intensity, weight, body composition).

Pathophysiology and Pharmacology of Clinical Conditions and Related Disease-specific Guidelines

3. The documentation of disease status, progression and medication response.

4. How to convey information to the client in a meaningful manner.

Skill in:

Domain-specific Content

1. Integrating and communicating information to the client and the healthcare team.

ACE Clinical Exercise Specialist

Role Delineation Panel

Susan Bartlett, Ph.D.
Clinical Psychologist
Johns Hopkins Weight Management Center
Baltimore, Md.

Stephen A. Black, P.T., A.T.C.
Physical Therapist
Sports Performance, LTD
Boulder, Colo.

Jack L. Boyer, M.D.
Cardiologist
Alpine, Calif.

Richard Cotton, M.A.
Chief Exercise Physiologist
American Council on Exercise
San Diego, Calif.

Ted E. Dreisinger, Ph.D., F.A.C.S.M.
Vice-President for Cumulative Trauma Prevention
Prevention First, Inc.
Minneapolis, Minn.

Dolores Eckert-Cook, M.A., R.D.
Registered Dietitian
Northwest Covenant Medical Center
Dover, N.J.

Denise Fandel, M.S., A.T.C.
Chief Administrative Officer
NATABOC
Omaha, Neb.

Kathleen Hargarten, M.D., F.A.C.E.P.
Emergency Medicine Physician
Oconomowoc, Wis.

Dale Huff, R.D., C.S.C.S.
Registered Dietitian/Personal Trainer
Nutriformance, Inc.
Creve Coeur, Mo.

Gwen Hyatt, M.S.
Desert Southwest Fitness, Inc.
Tucson, Ariz.

Ralph LaForge, M.S.
Clinical Exercise Physiologist
Durham, N.C.

Steven Loy, Ph.D., F.A.C.S.M.
Professor of Kinesiology
California State University, Northridge
Northridge, Calif.

Tim Moore, Ph.D., C.H.E.S., C.S.C.S.
Fitness Editor
Shape Magazine
Woodland Hills, Calif.

Tony Ordas, M.A.
Director of Certification
American Council on Exercise
San Diego, Calif.

Brad Roy, Ph.D.
Director, The Summit
Kalispell, Mont.

Rich Seibert, M.S.
American Council on Exercise
San Diego, Calif.

Kevin C. Stevens, M.A., M.P.H.
New York, N.Y.

Janice Slater, M.S., M.B.A.
Director of Fitness
East Bank Club
Chicago, Ill.

Dan Trone, M.A.
Exercise Epidemiologist
Naval Health Research Center
San Diego, Calif.

David Upton, Ph.D.
The David Upton Company , Inc.
Fort Worth, Texas

Larry Verity, Ph.D., F.A.C.S.M.
Professor of Kinesiology
San Diego State University
San Diego, Calif.

Greg Welch, M.S.
Exercise Physiologist/President
SpeciFit
Seal Beach, Calif.

Appendix D

ACE-certified Professional
Code Of Ethics

As an ACE-certified Professional, I am guided by the American Council on Exercise's principles of professional conduct whether I am working with clients, the public or other health and fitness professionals. I promise to:

- Provide safe and effective instruction.
- Provide equal and fair treatment to all clients.
- Stay up-to-date on the latest health and physical activity research and understand its practical application.
- Maintain current CPR certification and knowledge of first-aid services.
- Comply with all applicable business, employment and copyright laws.
- Protect and enhance the public's image of the health and fitness industry.
- Maintain the confidentiality of all client information.
- Refer clients to more qualified fitness, medical or health professionals when appropriate.

Glossary

Acquired immune deficiency syndrome (AIDS) A syndrome of the immune system caused by the human immunodeficiency virus (type HIV-1 or HIV-2) and characterized by opportunistic infection and disease.

Activities of daily living (ADL) Activities normally performed for hygiene, bathing, household chores, walking, shopping and similar activities.

Acute Describing a disease of rapid onset, severe symptoms and brief duration, or any intense symptom, such as severe pain.

Adherence The degree to which an individual follows a recommended health- or illness-related recommendation.

Adiadochokinesia Inability to perform rapidly alternating movements, such as forearm supination and pronation.

Afterload The pressure in the aorta and pulmonary trunk respectively that the left and right ventricles of the heart must overcome to eject blood.

AIDS-dementia complex The effect of HIV-related encephalitis or inflammation of the brain, the most common neurological complication in the later stages of HIV infection; characterized by memory loss and progressive dementia, accompanied by motor abnormalities

AIDS-related complex (ARC) Common pattern of nonspecific symptoms occurring in the symptomatic stage of HIV infection, characterized by fever, lymphadenopathy, diarrhea, weight loss and moderate reduction in CD4+ cell count.

Akinesia An inability to initiate movement.

Alveolar ventilation The volume of fresh air that reaches the area of gaseous exchange (respiratory zone) of the lungs.

Ambulatory The ability to walk and move from one place to another.

Amenorrhea Cessation of menstrual periods due to a lack of estrogen, high intensity/volume of physical training, poor nutrition, low body weight or a combination of these factors.

Analgesia A complete loss of pain sensibility.

Anatomical dead space Represents the conduction zone (tubes) of the lungs.

Aneurysm A localized abnormal dilation of a blood vessel; associated with a stroke when the aneurysm bursts.

Angina pectoris Pain associated with insufficient blood flow to the heart muscle. Usually described as chest, neck or jaw pressure/pain, arm/elbow pain (usually left) or back pain.

Unstable angina Sudden increase in intensity/duration (severity) of symptoms, occurring at lower levels of exertion and even at rest; often a precursor to acute myocardial infarction (heart attack).

Ankylosing spondylitis Inflammatory arthritis of the spine, resembling rheumatoid arthritis, that may progress to bony ankylosis with lipping of vertebral margins; the disease is more common in the male.

Ankylosis Stiffening or fixation of a joint as the result of arthritis, with fibrous or bony union across the joint.

Antibody An immunoglobulin molecule produced by lymphocytes in response to an antigen and characterized by reacting specifically with the antigen.

Antigen Any substance that induces a state of sensitivity and/or immune responsiveness and which evokes lymphocyte production of antibodies that react specifically with the antigen.

Antigen-presenting cell A cell of the immune system that breaks down antigen into peptide fragments and presents them on the cell surface in a context where they can interact with T-cell receptors.

Antinuclear antibody Autoantibody that reacts with nuclear material.

Apraxia A disorder of voluntary learned movement that is characterized by an inability to perform purposeful movements and that cannot be accounted for by inadequate strength, loss of coordination, impaired sensation, attention deficits or lack of comprehension.

Arteriosclerosis Pathological thickening, hardening and loss of elasticity of the walls of blood vessels, especially pertaining to arteries.

Arteriovenous O$_2$ difference The difference between oxygen saturation in arterial and venous blood.

Arthralgia Joint pain.

Arthritis Inflammation of a joint or a state characterized by inflammation of joints.

Asthenia A generalized muscle weakness associated with cerebellar lesions.

Ataxia A general term used to describe uncoordinated movement.

Atherosclerosis A form of arteriosclerosis. The inner layers of artery walls are made thick and irregular by deposits of a fatty substance.

Athetosis Slow, involuntary, writhing, twisting, worm-like movements.

Atlantotaxial instability Congenital condition involving a misalignment or displacement of the C1 to C2 vertebrae. Enlargement of the space between these vertebrae allows excessive movement during flexion or hyperextension of the neck, exposing the spinal cord to potential danger.

Autoimmune disease A process in which the body's immune system causes illness by attacking body cells that are normal and essential for health.

Autonomic dysreflexia A pathological autonomic reflex seen in patients with high-level spinal cord injuries. It is precipitated by a noxious stimulus below the level of the lesion, and produces an acute onset of autonomic activity.

Basal ganglia Masses of gray matter located beneath the cerebral cortex and just lateral to the dorsal thalamus; included are the caudate nucleus, putamen, globus pallidus, substantia nigra and subthalamus.

Bisphosphonates A class of synthetic pharmaceutical agents that act to slow bone loss by inhibiting the process of bone resorption.

Body composition The makeup of the body in terms of the relative percentage of fat mass and fat-free mass.

Body mass index (BMI) The measure of an individual's body weight to body height used for determining obesity; expressed as kg/m2.

Bradykinesia Extreme slowness of movement.

Bruit An abnormal sound heard on auscultation.

Cachexia General malnutrition, weight loss and wasting occurring in the course of a chronic disease

Calcitonin: A naturally occurring hormone that acts to slow bone loss by inhibiting the process of bone resorption.

Cancer An abnormal tissue that grows by cellular proliferation more rapidly than normal, and continues to grow after the stimuli that initiated the new growth cease. Also called tumor or neoplasm. The growth may be benign or malignant, i.e., capable of invading surrounding tissues and producing metastases (the spread of cancer cells from one part of the body to another).

Candidiasis Infection caused by the fungus Candida (usually C. albicans), characterized by itching, burning sensation and white discharge.

Capsid The protein shell that surrounds and protects the viral RNA.

Carcinoma Any of the various types of malignant cancers derived from epithelial tissue (the lining or covering cells of tissues).

Cardiac output The amount of blood pumped from the ventricle per unit of time, usually expressed as L/min.

Cardiac rehabilitation The process by which the person with cardiovascular disease is restored to, and maintained at, optimal physiological, psychological, social, vocational and emotional status.

Cardiomyopathy Disease of the myocardium.

Catabolic state A state of increased energy demand, which results in skeletal muscle catabolism; often the result of infection or malignancy.

Cauda equina Peripheral nerve roots below the first lumbar vertebra.

Causalgia Painful, burning sensation, usually along the distribution of a nerve.

CD4 Abbreviation for cluster-of-differentiation 4, an antigen marker found on various immune cells (including the T helper lymphocyte); CD markers are used to identify leukocytes and categorize their function.

Cerebellum Part of the brain located in the posterior fossa of the skull.

Cerebral vascular accident (CVA) (stroke) Loss of blood supply to the brain.

Chemotherapy Treatment of cancer by means of chemical substances or drugs.

CHF Congestive heart failure Inability of the heart to pump blood forward at a sufficient rate to meet the metabolic demand or the ability to do so only when the cardiac filling pressures are abnormally high, frequently resulting in lung congestion.

Chorea Involuntary, rapid, irregular, jerky movements.

Chronic Describing a disease of long duration and often of gradual onset, involving very slow changes; does not indicate the severity of the disease.

Clonus Cyclic hyperactivity of antagonistic muscles occurring at a regular frequency.

Cognition The process by which an organism becomes knowledgeable and includes such functions as thoughts, emotion, memory, judgment and learning.

Computed tomography (CT) A development of X-ray technology to examine the soft tissues of the body. Involves recording "slices" of the body with a CT scanner. A cross-sectional image is then formed by computer integration.

G

M

O

P

stenosis, 58
   aortic, 87, 89
   mitral, 87-90
stenotic valves, 86
stent, 58, 67
step, 293
step climbing, 126, 217, 371, 404
   for clients with multiple sclerosis, 322
   on and off, 299
step length, 293, 297
step test, 404
step width, 297
steroids
   anabolic, 106
   epidural, 341
   inhaled, 101-102
sex, 435
sterotaxic surgery, 324
strength training. *See* resistance exercise
stress, 57
   and clients with visual impairment, 389-390
   and fibromyalgia syndrome, 274
   management, 190
stress fractures, 424
stress incontinence, 314
stress test, 50-51
   for clients with diabetes, 145-146, 148, 154-155
stretching. *See* flexibility exercises
stretch response, 309
stride, 290, 293, 297
stride jump, 373
stride length, 290, 293, 296
stride velocity, 296
Stringer, W. W., 233
stroke. See cerebral vascular accident (CVA)
stroke volume, 59, 60, 62, 88, 112, 120
strongyloidiasis, 230
ST segment depression, 62, 64, 66, 89, 97
ST-T wave changes, 89
Studenski, S., 293
subluxation, 218, 316, 327, 353
submaximal fitness testing, 13, 14, 90
   and cardiac risk factors, 61, 62
   for clients with stable disease, 14, 64
substance abuse, 425
substantia nigra, 323
suicide, 418, 424
sulfanomides, 262
sulfasalazine, 215
sulfones, 262

supplemental oxygen, 118, 125
support reactions, 317
support systems, 145
supraspinatus, 352
supraventricular arrhythmias, 89
supraventricular tachycardia, 90, 95
sway, area of, 291
swing, 292, 293
symptomatic HIV infection, 229, 234
syncope, 87, 89
synergistic patterns, 309, 311
synovial membrane, 214
syphilis, 328
syphilitic aortitis, 87
systemic lupus erythematosus (SLE), 214, 218, 243
   cardiovascular manifestations, 252
   case studies, 255-256
   classification and diagnosis, 250-251
   common treatments, 253
   constitutional features, 251-252
   cutaneous (dermatologic) features, 252
   defined, 250
   epidemiology, 250
   etiology, 251
   exercise programming for clients with, 254-255
   hematological features, 252
   musculoskeletal features, 252
   neuropsychiatric features, 253
   pathophysiology of, 251-253
   physiological responses to exercise in clients with, 253-254
   pre-exercise screening and assessment for clients with, 254
   renal features, 253
   respiratory manifestations, 252
   and serositis, 252
systolic blood pressure, 45, 48, 62, 75

T

tachypnea, 114
tai chi, 235, 276, 437
talofibular ligament, 350
Tan, D. M., 409
target-heart-rate range, 164
Teitelbaum, Charles S., 380
Teitelbaum, Lesley M., 380
television watching, 160
temporomandibular joint syndrome, 274
tender points, 274, 275-276